Atherosclerosis XIII

Atherosclerosis XIII

Proceedings of the 13th International Atherosclerosis Symposium, held in Kyoto, Japan, between 28 September and 2 October 2003

Editors:

Yuji Matsuzawa
Sumitomo Hospital
Osaka
JAPAN

Toru Kita
Graduate School of Medicine
Kyoto University
Kyoto
JAPAN

Ryozo Nagai
Graduate School of Medicine
The University of Tokyo
Tokyo
JAPAN

Tamio Teramoto
Teikyo University School of Medicine
Tokyo
JAPAN

ELSEVIER

2004

ELSEVIER B.V.
Sara Burgerhartstraat 25
P.O. Box 211, 1000 AE
Amsterdam
The Netherlands

ELSEVIER Inc.
525 B Street, Suite 1900
San Diego, CA 92101-4495
USA

ELSEVIER Ltd
The Boulevard, Langford Lane
Kidlington, Oxford OX5 1GB
UK

ELSEVIER Ltd
84 Theobalds Road
London WC1X 8RR
UK

First edition 2004

Library of Congress Cataloging in Publication Data
A catalog record from the Library of Congress has been applied for.

British Library Cataloguing in Publication Data
International Atherosclerosis Symposium (13th : 2003 : Kyoto, Japan)
Atherosclerosis XIII : proceedings of the 13th International Atherosclerosis Symposium, held in Kyoto, Japan, between 28 September and 2 October 2003. - (International congress series ; 1262)
1. Atherosclerosis - Congresses
I. Title II. Matsuzawa, Yuji 616.1'36

ISBN 0444514481

International Congress Series No. 1262
ISBN: 0-444-51448-1
ISSN: 0531-5131

∞ The paper used in this publication meets the requirements of ANSI/NISO Z39.48-1992 (Permanence of Paper).
Printed in The Netherlands.

International Congress Series 1262 (2004) v–vi

ELSEVIER

www.ics-elsevier.com

Preface

On behalf of the XIIIth International Symposium on Atherosclerosis (ISA) organizing committee, the International Atherosclerosis Society (IAS) and the Japan Atherosclerosis Society (JAS), we are pleased to publish this book, the Proceedings of the XIIIth ISA. We would like to thank all participants, speakers and presenters who attended the XIIIth ISA in Kyoto from September 28 to October 2, 2003. In spite of the sudden epidemic of SARS in the world, approximately 3000 researchers from more than 60 countries attended this symposium. We also appreciate the great support of many sponsors. As a representative of the Asia/Pacific region, we were very proud to be hosting the first ISA symposium of the 21st century. We hoped to summarize the scientific and technological achievements in the field of atherosclerosis during the 20th century and to look ahead to our potential for future progress and development in this new millennium. Our research topics encompassed all aspects of atherosclerosis, including epidemiology, pathogenesis, diagnosis and prevention as well as its treatment. We are convinced that all participants to this triennial conference were satisfied and encouraged by its contents.

This symposium highlighted the recent advances in the research of vascular biology, angiogenesis and atherogenesis, the importance of multiple risk factor clustering and the mechanism of metabolic syndrome. The mechanism of plaque rupture as a cause of acute coronary syndrome and the recent development of methods for non-invasive and invasive diagnosis of atherosclerosis were extensively discussed. Furthermore, we held sessions about how translational research can contribute to the field of atherosclerosis; how lifestyle is correlated to the incidence of atherosclerotic cardiovascular diseases; and how newly discovered drugs such as statins can be used for clinical applications in addition to their effectiveness. We also shed light into the features of atherosclerosis in the Asia/Pacific region in comparison to those of other populations and discussed, along global standards and guidelines, the prevention of atherosclerosis with consideration to regional and ethnic backgrounds.

Moreover, we took this opportunity to support the many talented young scientists from the Asia/Pacific region with an educational grant from JAS. The Executive Committee is indebted to the Young Investigator Award Committee, led by Dr. John Chapman, for its hard and skillful work in selecting 11 awardees out of 399 applicants. The Young Investigator Award was granted to the 11 scientists for their outstanding research achievement and scientific merit in the poster presentation.

We hope you found some time to enjoy the city of Kyoto. This international city was once the ancient capital of Japan for over 1000 years. Today, its past is represented by temples, shrines and a UNESCO World Heritage Site. Along with the wonderful ancient

0531-5131/
doi:10.1016/j.ics.2004.01.002

architecture you may have experienced Japanese arts, music and cultural activities in various locations throughout the city.

The International Satellite Symposia in Hong Kong, Taipei, Okinawa, Fukuoka, Kobe, Kanazawa and Tokyo were held in connection with the main symposium. We hope you may have visited and enjoyed them. Each Satellite Symposia focused on seven different specified topics with further interest and insight and undoubtedly produced a more concentrated dialogue. If you chose to attend one of the International Satellite Symposia, you definitely had the prospect of further expanding your experience in Oriental culture.

It is our sincere wish that this volume would convince you that the XIIIth ISA really brought new knowledge to the scientific community of atherosclerosis research.

Yuji Matsuzawa
Chairman
Toru Kita
Chairman
Ryozo Nagai
Chairperson of Scientific Program Committee
Tamio Teramoto
Chairperson of Scientific Program Committee

International Congress Series 1262 (2004) vii

www.ics-elsevier.com

Young Investigator Award

The Young Investigator Award was bestowed to the 11 young scientists listed alphabetically by name:

Christoph Binder, University of California San Diego, USA
L-5 links adaptive and innate atheroprotective immunity specific for OxLDL

Radjesh Bisoendial, AMC University Hospital, Netherlands
Restoration of endothelial function by increasing HDL in subjects with isolated low-HDL

Tsuyoshi Chiba, Tokyo Medical and Dental University, Japan
Leptin-deficiency suppressed progression of atherosclerosis

Naoki Ishimori, The Jackson Laboratory Bar Harbor, USA
Quantitative trait locus analysis for atherosclerosis susceptibility between inbred mouse strains C57BL/6J and 129S1/SvImJ; implications for evaluating gene function in knockout mice

David Lamb, University of Surrey, United Kingdom
Ligation of ErbB1 induces monocyte chemotaxis and macrophage mitogenesis

Martin Merkel, University Hospital, Hamburg-Eppendorf, Germany
Apo AV accelerates chylomicron catabolism and augments chylomicron uptake into liver and adipose tissue in vivo

Stephen Nicholls, The Heart Research Institute, Australia
Periarterial collar induced pro-oxidant and proinflammatory changes are inhibited by reconstituted high-density lipoprotein

Nobutaka Ohgami, Dartmouth Medical School, USA
Identification of NPC1 protein as a cholesterol binding protein by photoaffinity labeling

Roshni Singaraja, University of British Columbia, Canada
Biochemical characterization of mutations in ABCA1 correlate with disease severity

Morgan Treguier, INSERM, France
Transcriptional regulation of the expression of scavenger receptor Cla-1 by sterol regulatory element binding protein (SREBP)-2

Miranda Van Eck, LACDR, Netherlands
Macrophage ABCA1 overexpression inhibits atherosclerotic lesion progression

doi:10.1016/S0531-5131(04)00413-3

International Congress Series 1262 (2004) viii–ix

www.ics-elsevier.com

International Atherosclerosis Society

Member Societies (September 2003)

Argentine Chapter of the Latin American Atherosclerosis Society (SOLAT)
Asian Pacific Society of Atherosclerosis and Vascular Diseases
Atherosclerosis, Thrombosis, and Vascular Biology Council / American Heart Association
Australian Atherosclerosis Society
Austrian Society of Atherosclerosis
Belgian Atherosclerosis Society
British Atherosclerosis Society
CIS Atherosclerosis Society
Canadian Society of Atherosclerosis, Thrombosis and Vascular Biology
Chinese Atherosclerosis Society
Croatian Atherosclerosis Society
Cuban Atherosclerosis Society
Czech Atherosclerosis Group
Czech Atherosclerosis Society
Department of Atherosclerosis, Brazilian Cardiology Society
Dutch Atherosclerosis Society
Egyptian Society of Atherosclerosis
European Atherosclerosis Society (EAS)
French Atherosclerosis Society (FAS)
Georgian Atherosclerosis Association
German Atherosclerosis Society
Hellenic Society of Lipidology and Atherosclerosis

doi:10.1016/S0531-5131(04)00419-4

Hungarian Atherosclerosis Society
Indian Society for Atherosclerosis Research
Indonesian Cardiovascular Society (ICS), Council on Atherosclerosis
Iranian Heart Foundation - Council on Atherosclerosis, Nutrition & Lipid Research
Israel Medical Association - Society for Research, Prevention and Treatment of Atherosclerosis
Italian Society for the Study of Arteriosclerosis (SISA)
Italian Working Groups for the Study of Metabolic Diseases and Atherosclerosis
Japan Atherosclerosis Society
Korean Society of Lipidology and Atherosclerosis
Latin American Atherosclerosis Society (SOLAT)
Lipid Working Group of the Turkish Cardiology Association
Lipid and Atherosclerosis Society of Southern Africa (LASSA)
Mediterranean Society of Atherosclerosis
Mexican Society of Atherosclerosis
Moroccan Society of Atherosclerosis (SMA)
New Zealand Atherosclerosis Society
Philippine Lipid Society
Polish Society for Atherosclerosis Research
Portuguese Atherosclerosis Society
Romanian Association for Atherosclerosis and Lipidology (RAAL)
Scandinavian Society for Atherosclerosis Research (SSAR)
Serbian Association for Arteriosclerosis, Thrombosis and Vascular Biology
Slovak Atherosclerosis Section of Slovak Medical Association
Sociedad Iberolatinoamericana de Aterosclerosis (SILAT)
Spanish Society of Arteriosclerosis
Swiss Working Group on Lipids and Atherosclerosis
Taiwan Society of Atherosclerosis & Vascular Diseases
Taiwan Society of Lipids & Atherosclerosis
Venezuelan Atherosclerosis Association (AVA)
Yugoslav Atherosclerosis Society

International Congress Series 1262 (2004) x–xiii

www.ics-elsevier.com

XIIIth International Symposium on Atherosclerosis

Hajime Orimo, Honorary Chairman
Yuji Matsuzawa, Chairman
Toru Kita, Chairman

Executive Committee
Secretary-General: Yasuyoshi Ouchi
Members: Yasuo Ikeda
Masunori Matsuzaki
Ryozo Nagai
Yasushi Saito
Katsuo Sueishi
Akira Takeshita
Mitsuhiro Yokoyama
Shinji Yokoyama

Supervising Committee
Chairpersons: Yuichiro Goto† and Akira Yamamoto
Members: Takao Fujinami
Hisashi Fukuzaki
Yoshiya Hata
Masakuni Kameyama
Akira Kumagai
Hiroshi Mabuchi
Seiitsu Murota
Chikayuki Naito
Haruo Nakamura
Motoomi Nakamura
Fujio Numano
Kenzo Oshima
Akinobu Sumiyoshi
Shigeo Takebayashi
Kenzo Tanaka
Seiichiro Tarui

† Deceased

doi:10.1016/S0531-5131(04)00414-5

Yoshio Yazaki
Yoji Yoshida
Teruo Watanabe

Scientific Program Committee
Chairpersons: Ryozo Nagai and Tamio Teramoto
Members: Atsunori Kashiwagi
Makoto Kinoshita
Koichi Kozaki
Ikuro Maruyama
Masunori Matsuzaki
Akira Miyazaki
Ryuichi Morishita
Kazuwa Nakao
Toshio Ogihara
Yasufumi Sato
Koji Suzuki
Makiko Ueda
Hirotsugu Ueshima
Kazuo Yamada
Shizuya Yamashita
Masayuki Yokode
Kotaro Yokote

Fund Raising Committee
Chairperson: Yasushi Saito
Vice-Chairperson: Tamio Teramoto
Members: Hiroshi Mabuchi
Yuji Matsuzawa
Fujio Numano
Katsuo Sueishi
Kotaro Yokote
Mitsuhiro Yokoyama
Shinji Yokoyama

Organizing Committee
General Affairs
Chairperson: Yasuyoshi Ouchi
Vice-Chairperson: Nobuhiro Yamada
Members: Keisuke Fukuo
Koichi Kozaki
Masataka Sata
Hitoshi Shimano

Public Relations
Chairperson: Shinji Yokoyama
Vice-Chairperson: Kentaro Shimokado
Members: Mariko Shiba
Masayuki Yoshida

Finance
Chairperson: Katsuo Sueishi
Vice-Chairperson: Shinichi Oikawa
Members: Sadatoshi Biro
Yuichi Ishikawa
Junji Koizumi
Yasushi Saito
Norio Tada
Kotaro Yokote

Social Events
Chairperson: Yasuo Ikeda
Vice-Chairperson: Makiko Ueda
Member: Minoru Yoshiyama

Site Operation
Chairperson: Mitsuhiro Yokoyama
Vice-Chairperson: Jun Sasaki
Members: Noriaki Kume
Takahiro Taniguchi
Shizuya Yamashita
Masayuki Yokode

Health Affairs
Chairperson: Mitsuhiro Yokoyama
Vice-Chairpersons: Masayuki Yokode and Shizuya Yamashita
Members: Hidenori Arai
Kenichi Hirata
Koichi Kozaki
Naohiko Sakai

Exhibition
Chairperson: Masunori Matsuzaki
Vice-Chairperson: Ikuro Maruyama
Members: Takeshi Kimura
Mitsuhiro Yokoyama

Program Preparation
Chairperson: Tamio Teramoto
Members: Makoto Kinoshita
Koichi Kozaki
Akira Miyazaki
Shizuya Yamashita
Masayuki Yokode
Kotaro Yokote

International Congress Series 1262 (2004) xiv–xv

ELSEVIER

www.ics-elsevier.com

International Advisory Board

doi:10.1016/S0531-5131(04)00416-9

International Congress Series 1262 (2004) xvi

ELSEVIER

www.ics-elsevier.com

Young Investigator Award Committee

Chairman: John M. Chapman, France
Co-chairman: Shinji Yokoyama, Japan
Members: Ulrike Beisiegel, Germany
Gordon R. Campbell, Australia
Alberico L. Catapano, Italy
Steve E. Humphries, UK
Robert W. Mahley, USA
Ernst J. Schaefer, USA
Wolfgang J. Schneider, Austria
Bart Staels, France
Seppo Ylä-Herttuala, Finland

doi:10.1016/S0531-5131(04)00802-7

International Congress Series 1262 (2004) xvii–xx

www.ics-elsevier.com

Acknowledgements

The organizing committee of the XIIIth International Symposium on Atherosclerosis gratefully acknowledges the generous financial support of the following:

Platinum Sponsors
AstraZeneca
Fournier Pharma
Pfizer

Silver Sponsors
GlaxoSmithKline
MSD
MSD Schering-Plough
Novartis Pharma AG

Bronze Sponsors
Roche
Bayer

Foundations
Japan Arteriosclerosis Prevention Fund
Kowa Life Science Foundation
Manpei Suzuki Diabetes Foundation
Sankyo Foundation of Life Science
Setsuro Fujii Memorial The Osaka Foundation For Promotion of Fundamental Medical Research
Takeda Medical Research Foundation
The Kao Foundation for Arts and Sciences
The Naito Foundation
Uehara Memorial Foundation

Sponsors
The Pharmaceutical Manufacturers' Association of Tokyo
Osaka Pharmaceutical Manufacturers Association

Abbott Japan Co., Ltd.
Amgen Ltd.

doi:10.1016/S0531-5131(04)00417-0

Asahi Kasei Corporation
AstraZeneca K.K.
Aventis Pharma Ltd.
Azwell Inc.
Banyu Pharmaceutical Co., Ltd.
Bayer Yakuhin, Ltd.
Bristol Pharmaceuticals K.K.
Chugai Pharmaceutical Co., Ltd.
Daiichi Pharmaceutical Co., Ltd.
Dainippon Pharmaceutical Co., Ltd.
Eiken Chemical Co., Ltd.
Eisai Co., Ltd.
Elmed Eisai Co., Ltd.
Fujisawa Pharmaceutical Co., Ltd.
Fuso Pharmaceutical Industries, Ltd.
GlaxoSmithKline K.K.
Grelan Pharmaceutical Co., Ltd.
Japan Tobacco Inc.
Kaken Pharmaceutical Co., Ltd.
Kaken Shoyaku Co., Ltd.
Kanebo, Ltd.
Kirin Brewery Co., Ltd.
Kissei Pharmaceutical Co., Ltd.
Kowa Shinyaku Co., Ltd.
Kyorin Pharmaceutical Co., Ltd.
Kyowa Hakko Kogyo Co., Ltd.
Maruho Co., Ltd.
Maruishi Pharmaceutical Co., Ltd.
Meiji Dairies Corporation
Meiji Seika Kaisha, Ltd.
Merck Hoei Ltd.
Mikasa Seiyaku Co., Ltd.
Minophagen Pharmaceutical Co., Ltd.
Mitsubishi Pharma Corporation
Mochida Pharmaceutical Co., Ltd.
Morinaga Milk Industry Co., Ltd.
Nihon Pharmaceutical Co., Ltd.
Nihon Schering K.K.
Nikken Chemicals Co., Ltd.
Nippon Boehringer Ingelheim Co., Ltd.
Nippon Chemiphar Co., Ltd.
Nippon Kayaku Co., Ltd.
Nippon Shinyaku Co., Ltd.
Nippon Zoki Pharmaceutical Co., Ltd.
Nipro Pharma Corporation

Novartis Pharma K.K.
Ono Pharmaceutical Co., Ltd.
Otsuka Pharmaceutical Co., Ltd.
Otsuka Pharmaceutical Factory, Inc.
Pfizer Pharmaceuticals Inc.
Rohto Pharmaceutical Co. Ltd.
Sankyo Co., Ltd.
Santen Pharmaceutical Co., Ltd.
Sanwa Kagaku Kenkyusho Co., Ltd.
Sato Pharmaceutical Co., Ltd.
Sawai Pharmaceutical Co., Ltd.
Schering-Plough K.K.
Shinnihon Seiyaku Co., Ltd.
Shionogi & Co., Ltd.
Snow Brand Milk Products Co., Ltd.
SSP Co., Ltd.
Sumitomo Pharmaceuticals Co., Ltd.
Taiho Pharmaceutical Co., Ltd.
Taisho Pharmaceutical Co., Ltd.
Takeda Chemical Industries, Ltd.
Tanabe Seiyaku Co., Ltd.
Teijin Limited
Teikoku Hormone Mfg. Co., Ltd.
Terumo Corporation
Toa Eiyo Pharmaceutical Company
Torii Pharmaceutical Co., Ltd.
Towa Pharmaceutical Co., Ltd.
Toyama Chemical Co., Ltd.
Tsumura & Co.
Wakamoto Pharmaceutical Co., Ltd.
Wyeth Lederle Japan, Ltd.
Yakult Honsha Co., Ltd.
Yamanouchi Pharmaceutical Co., Ltd.

Other Contributors
Abbott Vascular Devices Japan Co., Ltd.
Boston Scientific Japan K.K.
Colin Corporation
Daiichi Pure Chemicals Co., Ltd.
Eli Lilly Japan K.K.
Fuji Oil Co., Ltd.
Fujimoto Pharmaceutical Corporation
Guidant Japan K.K.
Japan Immunoresearch Laboratories Co., Ltd.
Johnson & Johnson Company Cordis

Kao Corporation
Kowa Company, Ltd.
Kuraray Medical Inc.
Kyowa Medex Co., Ltd.
Medtronic Japan Co., Ltd.
Omron Corporation
Sanki International Congress Information Center
Hatsumi Goto
Masayuki Shinoda
Ryuzo Ueno

Contents

Oxidized lipoprotein and atherosclerosis

Image analysis of atherosclerotic lesions and therapeutic application

Proliferation and differentiation of smooth muscle cells

Vascular tissue engineering and clinical applications

Life style and vascular disease – the West and the East meet together

Scavenger receptors

Asian sessions: Metabolic syndrome in Asian countries

Lp(a) – Still a mystery

Aging and blood vessels

ABC transporters and related disorders

Geographic epidemiology of atherosclerotic diseases in different populations

Plenary lectures

International Congress Series 1262 (2004) 3–8

www.ics-elsevier.com

The origin of the statins

Akira Endo *

Biopharm Research Laboratories, Main Office, 2-1-31, Minamicho, Kokubunji, Tokyo 185-0021, Japan

Abstract. In the early 1970s we isolated the first statin, mevastatin (formerly called compactin or ML-236B), from *Penicillium citrinum*, as a potent inhibitor of 3-hydroxy-3-methylglutaryl coenzyme A (HMG-CoA) reductase, the rate-controlling enzyme in cholesterol synthetic pathway. By the end of the 1970s we had demonstrated that mevastatin was highly effective in lowering serum total and low-density lipoprotein (LDL) cholesterol in both experimental animals and patients with primary hypercholesterolemia. The discovery of mevastatin paved the way for the worldwide development of its analogues (statins), and since then several statins—lovastatin, simvastatin, pravastatin, fluvastatin and atorvastatin—have been approved in many countries and are currently used by millions of patients.

Keywords: Cholesterol; HMG-CoA reductase inhibitors; Statins; Mevastatin; Lovastatin

1. Introduction

Coronary heart disease is the main clinical manifestation of atherosclerosis and is the major cause of death in modern, industrialized countries and increasingly a cause in developing countries; atherosclerosis might also affect the peripheral arteries and the cerebral circulation, leading to other debilitating or life-threatening conditions. One of the major risk factors for atherosclerosis and coronary heart disease is hypercholesterolemia.

2. Background

In the mid-1960s fascinated with several excellent reviews on cholesterol biosynthesis by Konrad Bloch of Harvard University (Boston, MA) [1,2], who received the Nobel Prize in 1964, I became interested in the biochemistry of cholesterol and other lipids. In early December 1965, I wrote to Bloch, inquiring about postdoctoral research in his laboratory.

Unfortunately, the postdoctoral fellowship was no longer available for the year 1966–1967. Soon after, I wrote to P. Roy Vagelos at the National Institute of Health (Bethesda, MD), inquiring about research into fatty acid synthesis in his laboratory. But after a month I still had no answer, so, in late January 1966, I determined to study phospholipids at the

* Tel.: +81-42-329-1070; fax: +81-42-329-8070.
E-mail address: aendo@biopharm.co.jp (A. Endo).

0531-5131/
doi:10.1016/j.ics.2003.12.099

Department of Molecular Biology (Bernard Horecker, chair), at the Albert Einstein College of Medicine (AECM), New York for 2 years (1966–1968) (soon after this appointment had been made, Vagelos answered me that he would grant my request).

In AECM, under the guidance of L. Rothfield, I isolated, purified, and worked out the mechanism of action of a bacterial phospholipid-requiring enzyme involved in the biosynthesis of cell wall lipopolysaccharide [3,4]. Rothfield had worked as a physician for nearly 10 years in the New York University Hospital before he joined AECM. I learnt from him that hypercholesterolemia was a major risk factor for coronary heart disease, the No. 1 killer in Western countries. In addition, my stay in the U.S. gave me the opportunity to learn about the regulation of the cholesterol metabolism. At that time, experiments with animals and humans by other groups had shown that cholesterol could either be absorbed from diet, or if diet was lacking sufficient cholesterol to meet the body's needs, then it could be synthesized mainly in the liver. However, if a diet was rich in cholesterol then synthesis within the body virtually stopped. HMG-CoA reductase, an enzyme that catalyzed conversion of HMG-CoA into mevalonate, was shown to be the rate controlling enzyme in cholesterol synthesis [5]. My experiences from those days aroused my curiosity about developing a cholesterol-lowering agent.

3. Discovery of mevastatin

In 1968, I returned to Sankyo, and in 1970, I hypothesized that levels of plasma cholesterol could be lowered more effectively by inhibiting hepatic HMG-CoA reductase than by decreasing absorption from the diet; and postulated that some microbes would produce secondary metabolites that inhibited HMG-CoA reductase, possibly as a defense mechanism against other microbes that required sterols and/or other mevalonate-derived isoprenoid compounds for their growth.

In April 1971, we created a research unit to isolate such products. We focused on fungi and mushrooms as a source of these metabolites. The search for a suitable compound took 2 years and involved 6000 microbes. As a result, the fungus, *Penicillim citrinum* was shown to inhibit lipid synthesis. The major inhibiting compound from *P. citrinum* broths, ML-236B (now known as mevastatin), was isolated by solvent extraction, silica gel chromatography and crystallization [6].

The lactone ring of the mevastatin molecule was reversibly converted to an open acid that resembled the HMG portion of HMG-CoA, the substrate of the reaction catalyzed by HMG-CoA reductase. In the reaction HMG-CoA is reduced to mevalonate, a key precursor to cholesterol. Mevastatin was shown to be an ideal potent competitive inhibitor to the enzyme reaction [7]. Although some early experiments carried out in rats indicated that mevastatin would only work in the very short term, in 1976–1977, we were able to show that mevastatin dramatically lowered plasma cholesterol levels in hens, dogs and monkeys. In early 1978, Akira Yamamoto (Osaka, Japan) and I showed that mevastatin dramatically lowered plasma cholesterol of patients with serious hypercholesterolemia [8]. In November 1978, based on these results, formal clinical trials of mevastatin were started in Japan. By mid 1980, these trials had shown that mevastatin lowered plasma total and LDL-cholesterol by 20–40% at 15–60 mg/day; no serious side effects were noticed [9].

4. Discovery of lovastatin

At the end of December 1978, I left Sankyo and joined the School of Agriculture at Tokyo Noko University in Tokyo. In February 1979, I isolated three mevastatin analogues—monacolin J, monacolin K, monacolin L—from *Monascus ruber* M1005 (Monacolin K was filed for a patent in February 1979 [10][1]; monacolin J in April 1979 [11]; and monacolin L in October 1979 [12])[1]. Of these three compounds, monacolin K, the major product, was slightly more effective in inhibiting HMG-CoA reductase than mevastatin.

Back in 1966, P. Roy Vagelos and Alfred Alberts from the NIH had moved to Washington University School of Medicine (St. Louis, MO), where they showed that animal cells required cholesterol to maintain their normal membrane structure. In 1975, taking Alberts with him, Vagelos joined Merck as senior vice-president in charge of research (President of the Merck Sharp and Dohme Research Laboratories-MSDRL-Division) [13]. In April 1976, H. Boyd Woodruff (Executive Administrator of MSDRL) who had noted the Sankyo patent application covering mevastatin, inquired of Sankyo about the possibility to obtain a sample of mevastatin for evaluation at MSDRL under a confidentiality agreement. Sankyo accepted Merck's request[2] and in July 1976, it provided MSDRL with samples (crystals) of mevastatin and confidential data of our biochemical, pharmacological and toxicological studies of mevastatin[2].

During the next two or so years, researchers at MSDRL studied mevastatin in cultured mammalian cells, with a cell-free enzyme system; and in vivo in rats and dogs, and by October 1978 had obtained results that corresponded closely to those obtained by my group[3]. On April 6, 1979, I gave a lecture at MSDRL in Rahway, NJ on the development of mevastatin; after which, Vagelos, Alberts and I discussed the experimental results of mevastatin obtained by both Alberts' and my groups. However, the discovery of other statins never came up in our discussion.

At the end of August, 1979, the discovery of monacolin K was published in a scientific journal [14], and soon after Alberts and Woodruff who had noticed the article flew to Tokyo and said: In September 1978, Alberts and his assistant Julie Chen started searching for an HMG-CoA reductase inhibitor, and on 16 November 1978, found that the extract of a soil fungus, *Aspergillus terreus*, strongly inhibited HMG-CoA reductase. In February 1979, Carl Hoffman and his associates at MSDRL isolated the pure inhibitor, called mevinolin (now called lovastatin), from cultured broths of *A. terreus*. In June 1979, Merck filed mevinolin for patent. Merck was anxious to know if it was distinct from monacolin K or not [13,15].

In October 1979, it was accepted that monacolin K and mevinolin were the same compound. Mevinolin had been discovered three months before monacolin K (November

[1] This patent was also applied in the following 30 countries: USA, UK, FRG, France, Italy, Switzerland, Spain, Belgium, The Netherlands, Canada, Sweden, South Korea, USSR, Ireland, Austria, Mexico, Australia, Argentina, The Philippines, South Africa, East Germany, Hungary, Poland, Finland, Norway, India, Pakistan, Formosa, New Zealand and Yugoslavia.

[2] A disclosure agreement on this matter was reached between B. Woodruff (Merck) and H. Okazaki (Sankyo) on July 21, 1976.

[3] A report covering these data was sent by mail from B. Woodruff (Merck) to R. Yamamoto (Sankyo) on October 19, 1978.

1978 vs. February 1979), but its patent application came four months after monacolin K (June 1979 [16] vs. February 1979 [10]). As a result, it became clear that patents were to be approved for mevinolin but not for monacolin K in the U.S. and several countries that gave priority to 'time of invention'. In some other thirty countries[1] that gave priority to 'time of application', patents were to be granted for monacolin K but not for mevinolin.

In November 1979, the patent right of monacolin K was passed to Sankyo; who paid Tokyo Noko University 35 million yen as an equivalent for the patent right[4]. This transfer made Merck unable to commercialize mevinolin (lovastatin) in the above-mentioned thirty countries without getting a license from Sankyo. Although Sankyo neither gave Merck the license nor commercialized monacolin K itself, it would get billions of dollars by blocking Merck's commercialization of mevinolin in the major countries except the U.S. (In 1981, Merck synthesized another statin-simvastatin and commercialized it world-wide in the 1990s [17].)

Meanwhile, rumors appeared from time to time that the work on the discovery of monacolin K from *M. ruber* M1005 had been done at Sankyo when I was there; that is pure invention. It is clear that the work on the isolation of monacolin K, together with its two analogues, monacolin J and monacolin L, from *M. ruber* M1005 was started and completed at Tokyo Noko University [18][4]. That work, then, had no legal connection with Sankyo.

In April 1980, Merck began clinical studies of lovastatin (mevinolin) [13]. Several months later, Sankyo discontinued clinical trials of mevastatin, which had been carried out since 1978, apparently because intestinal tumors were found in dogs. Although there was some question that the company's decision was right, on learning this in September 1980, Merck halted its clinical studies of lovastatin and undertook further pharmacological and toxicological studies.

In 1982, several clinicians, including Roger Illingworth (Portland, OR), David Bilheimer and Scott Grundy (Dallas, TX) began to give lovastatin to patients with serious hypercholesterolemia who were unresponsive to available agents [13]. These trials showed that lovastatin dramatically lowered plasma cholesterol, and very few side effects were noted.

In November 1983, based on these results as well as the recommendation of Daniel Steinberg (San Diego, CA) and Jean Wilson (Dallas, TX), formal clinical trials of lovastatin were started [13]. Large-scale clinical studies began in May 1984. In the 2 years that followed, the clinical trials and long-term safety studies were completed; and in November 1986, Merck submitted a new drug application for lovastatin to the Food and Drug Administration (FDA). The FDA moved rapidly and in late February 1987, an FDA

[4] On November 30, 1979, an agreement confirming the following terms under which Endo shall grant to Sankyo patent right of the Japanese Patent Application No. 54-17, 856, filed by Endo on February 20, 1979, with the title of 'Novel physiologically active substance monacolin K and process for producing the same' was entered into between both parties: ① Endo shall grant to Sankyo the worldwide patent right of this application. ② Sankyo shall pay 35,000,000 yen to the organization designated by Endo (Tokyo Noko University) as an equivalent to the patent right. ③ Sankyo shall file worldwide applications for this patent at its own expense. ④ Sankyo shall grant to Merck a non-exclusive license to develop and commercialize monacolin K worldwide, except for Japan. In case the license is granted to Merck, Sankyo shall pay to Tokyo Noko University a royalty of 0.75% of Merck's net sales of the monacolin K products.

advisory committee reviewed the company's application. The committee recommended approval of the drug for certain patients whose elevated cholesterol levels cannot be lowered through diet or other non-pharmacological methods. On September 1, 1987, the FDA announced that it had approved lovastatin (Mevacor®) [13].

5. Other statins

The following years witnessed the development in many countries of other statins based on mevastatin and lovastatin. Three main approaches have been utilized. First, chemical alteration of fungal products created statin drugs such as simvastatin. Second, microbial alteration of fungal compounds led to drugs such as pravastatin. Finally, synthetic compounds such as fluvastatin and atorovastatin were produced. Research in this area has concentrated on replacing the decaline ring of the fungal compounds with an aromatic ring [17]. These statins have been all well established as effective and safe cholesterol-lowering agents and have been used by tens of millions of patients. Several landmark clinical trials with statins demonstrated that the lipid-lowering therapy reduces cardiovascular morbidity and mortality in both primary and secondary prevention [19].

References

[1] K. Bloch, The biological synthesis of cholesterol, Science 150 (1965) 19–28.

[2] K. Bloch, Biogenesis and transformations of squalene, in: G. Wolftenholme, M. O'Connor (Eds.), Biosynthesis of Terpenes and Sterols, J. and A. Churchill, London, 1959, pp. 4–9.

[3] A. Endo, L. Rothfield, Studies of a phospholipid-requiring bacterial enzyme: 1. Purification and properties of uridine diphosphate galactose: lipopolysaccharide α-3-galactosly transferase, Biochemistry 8 (1969) 3500–3507.

[4] A. Endo, L. Rothfield, Studies of a phopholipid-requiring bacterial enzyme: 2. The role of phosholipid in the uridine diphosphate galactose: lipopolysaccharide α-3-galactosly transferase reaction, Biochemistry 8 (1969) 3508–3515.

[5] J. Dietschy, J. Wilson, Requlation of cholesterol metabolism, N. Engl. J. Med. 282 (1970) 1128–1138; 1179–1183; 1241–1249.

[6] A. Endo, M. Kuroda, Y. Tsujita, ML-236A, ML-236B, and ML-236C, new inhibitors of cholesterogenesis produced by *Penicillium citrinum*, J. Antibiot. 29 (1976) 1346–1348.

[7] A. Endo, K. Tanzawa, M. Kuroda, Competitive inhibition of 3-hydroxy-3-methylglutaryl coenzyme A reductase by ML-236A and ML-236B, fungal metabolites, having hypocholesterolemic activity, FEBS Lett. 72 (1976) 323–326.

[8] A. Yamamoto, H. Sudo, A. Endo, Therapeutic effects of ML-236B in primary hypercholesterolemia, Atherosclerosis 35 (1980) 259–266.

[9] Abstract Book of the 7th International Symposium on Drugs Affecting Lipid Metabolism, The Lorenzini Foundation, Milan, 1980 (May 28–31).

[10] A. Endo, Novel physiologically active substance monacolin K and process for producing the same, Japanese Patent Application 54-17856, filed on February 20, 1979.

[11] A. Endo, Novel physiologically active substance monacolin J and process for producing the same, Japanese Patent Application 54-44249, filed on April 13, 1979.

[12] A. Endo, Novel physiologically active substance monacolin L and process for producing the same, Japanese Patent Application 54-133991, filed on October 17, 1979.

[13] Merck and Co. (Rahway, NJ), The scientific search for an effective weapon against cholesterol, Press Release, November, 1987.

[14] A. Endo, K. Monacolin, A new hypocholesterolemic agent produced by a *Monascus* species, J. Antibiot. 32 (1979) 852–854.

[15] R. Vagelos, Are prescription drug prices high? Science 252 (1991) 1080–1084.

[16] R. Monaghan, A. Alberts, C. Hoffman, G. Albers-Schonberg, Hypocholesterolemic fermentation products and process of preparation, US Patent No. 4, 231, 938, 11/1980(549/292), filed on June 15, 1979.
[17] A. Endo, Discovery and development of the statins, in: A. Gaw, C. Packard, J. Shephered (Eds.), Statins The HMG-CoA Reductase Inhibitors in Perspective, Martin Dunitz, London, 2000, pp. 35–47.
[18] A. Endo, The story of HMG-CoA reductase inhibitor: 1. Details of the discovery of lovastatin (monacolin K), Igaku No Ayumi 172 (1995) 131–133.
[19] D. Steinberg, A. Gotto Jr., Preventing coronary artery disase by lowering cholesterol levels, JAMA 282 (1999) 2043–2050.

International Congress Series 1262 (2004) 9–14

ELSEVIER

www.ics-elsevier.com

New frontiers in atherosclerosis prevention and treatment: HDL as a novel therapeutic target

Cesare R. Sirtori*

University of Milano, Director University Center for Dyslipidemias, Niguarda Hospital, Milan, Italy

Abstract. The high-density lipoprotein (HDL) system offers an attractive target for novel therapeutic approaches to prevent or treat atherosclerosis. Clinical preventative studies with HDL modulators, both increasing HDL levels [peroxisome proliferator activator receptor (PPAR) α agonists] and stimulating turnover [cholesteryl ester transfer protein (CETP) activators] have led to favorable outcomes. Treatment of preexisting atherosclerosis with novel HDL mimetics, i.e., wild-type recombinant apo A-I, reconstituted HDL from human serum, large unilamellar phospholipid vesicles (LUV), and the recombinant apo A-I_{Milano} dimer (AIM) offer exciting opportunities. Recent findings with AIM are consistent with the hypothesis that direct HDL administration can rapidly regress coronary plaques. © 2003 Published by Elsevier B.V.

Keywords: HDL; Apolipoprotein A-I; Apolipoprotein A-I_{Milano}; Atherosclerosis; CETP

1. Introduction

Circulating high-density lipoprotein (HDL) cholesterol levels show an independent, inverse relationship with coronary disease risk [1]. The antiatherogenic effects of HDL are largely due to their major protein component, apolipoprotein (apo) A-I. HDL and apo A-I mediate reverse cholesterol transport, by which free cholesterol is transferred from peripheral tissues, such as the arterial wall, to the liver [2]. They also exert antioxidant effects [3], reduce platelet aggregation [4], stimulate fibrinolysis [5], and modulate endothelial dysfunction induced by dyslipidemia or atherosclerosis [6]. A number of well-controlled studies have clearly indicated a 20–40% reduction of major cardiovascular events after low-density lipoprotein (LDL) lowering therapies. This remarkable effect also underlines, however, the need for additional interventions. Supporting the hypothesis that increasing HDL levels may be beneficial are studies with HDL raising drugs, such as the

Abbreviations: PPAR, peroxisome proliferator activator receptor; CETP, cholesteryl ester transfer protein; ABCA1, ATP binding cassette A1; SRB1, scavenger receptor B1; POPC, polyoleylphosphatidylcholine.

* Department of Pharmacological Sciences, University of Milano, Via Balzaretti 9, 20133 Milan, Italy. Tel.: +39-2-5031-8303, 8311; fax: +39-2-5031-8394.

E-mail address: cesare.sirtori@unimi.it (C.R. Sirtori).

0531-5131/ © 2003 Published by Elsevier B.V.
doi:10.1016/j.ics.2003.12.026

Helsinki Heart Study and the VA-HIT Study with gemfibrozil [7,8]. Similar findings have been provided by other HDL raising agents, e.g., nicotinic acid and fenofibrate [9,10].

The HDL system, due to its complexity, offers a number of other potential intervention strategies, thus proving an enticing therapeutic target for the prevention or direct treatment of atherosclerosis.

2. Therapeutic approaches

Surprisingly, understanding of HDL metabolism remains incomplete owed in part to the fact that HDL generation is not a linear pathway, such as VLDL→LDL, but the end result of extensive recycling–exchange processes. In humans, cholesterol acquired by HDL from the periphery (e.g., the arterial wall) by way of the ATP binding cassette A1/scavenger receptor B1 (ABCA1/SRB1) systems, can be exchanged for triglycerides from VLDL, thus leading to LDL, subsequently taken up by the liver [11]. This exchange system is largely absent in many species, most notably rodents. Therefore, treatments can be aimed at directly influencing metabolic processes to accelerate catabolism of triglyceride (TG)-rich lipoproteins, releasing redundant material, which contributes to HDL maturation and concomitantly reduces catabolism. Conversely, treatment can be aimed at the exchange/transfer system, i.e., cholesteryl ester transfer protein (CETP), an ambiguous target, in view of the inadequate understanding of the consequences of raised HDL levels after CETP antagonism. Other therapeutic strategies build on novel molecular knowledge of HDL formation, affecting in a number of ways ABCA1/SRB1 expression. Finally, the availability of "HDL mimetics" offers an exciting opportunity for direct plaque removal.

3. Small molecule HDL modulators: current and future

Fibrates were the major lipid lowering drugs until the advent of statins. Fibrates, as well as other "fraudulent fatty acids", by activating the peroxisome proliferator activate receptor (PPAR) α-system, influence a range of metabolic activities via PPAR response elements (PPRE) present in target genes [12]. Fibrates, in particular, upregulate lipoprotein lipase and down regulate expression of the apo C-III gene [13], thus accelerating catabolism of TG-rich lipoproteins, and releasing redundant material contributing to HDL maturation. The HDL rise exerted by fibrates results in a significant reduction of coronary risk in primary and particularly secondary prevention [7,8,10].

Activators/antagonists of the CETP system represent an ambiguous topic in atherosclerosis prevention. CETP, when activated, leads to enhanced cholesteryl ester turnover and reduced HDL cholesterolemia [2]. The original findings by our group clearly indicated powerful CETP activating properties of probucol, a major therapeutic mechanism of this agent [14]. The efficacy of probucol in coronary prevention has been recently supported by the Fukuoka Study, indicating both a reduction of carotid intima media thickness and of coronary events in a high-risk elderly population [15]. Studies with a stable analogue of probucol, AGI 1067, have shown both a reduction of HDL cholesterolemia and an improved luminal area after coronary angioplasty [16].

CETP antagonists have also been developed. One of these, JTT-705 was initially proven to reduce plaque area in cholesterol-fed rabbits [17]. More recently, however, another Japanese group failed to see atheroma regression when using rabbits with higher choles-

Table 1
CETP antagonism attenuates atherosclerosis in rabbits?

	T. Chol (mg/dl)	HDL	Lesion area (%)
0.2% cholesterol diet			
Control, 6 months	129	15.2	30.3
JTT-705, 300 mg/kg	98	30.0**	9.2**
Okamoto et al [17], p. 203			
0.25% cholesterol diet			
Control, 3 months	757	27.0	58
JTT-705, 300 mg/kg	601	57.0**	60
Huang et al [18], p. 587			

**Mean $P<0.01$.

terolemia [18] (Table 1). These data have raised skepticism about the possibility that CETP antagonists, significantly increasing HDL in man [19] may, in fact, be clinically useful.

4. Biopharmaceuticals: the HDL mimetics

Apo A-I has become a prime candidate for the development of apolipoprotein-like pharmaceuticals. In early studies wild-type pro-A-I combined with soybean PL, at a dose of 1.6 g iv, raised HDL cholesterol levels markedly for up to 3 days [20]. More recently, reconstituted HDL (rHDL) from serum has been used to evaluate direct vascular effects. In hypercholesterolemic individuals with an impaired vasodilator response, infusion of rHDL (80 mg of protein), remarkably improved endothelial dependent vasodilation [21]. Similar findings were very recently described on carriers of ABCA1 mutations [22].

Apolipoprotein A-I_{Milano} (apo A-I_M) the first described mutant of apo A-I, differs from wild-type apo A-I for an $Arg^{173} \rightarrow Cys$ substitution, leading to the formation of disulfide-linked dimers [23]. Apo A-I_M carriers, all heterozygotes and with low HDL cholesterol, have a reduced cardiovascular risk. Among the circulating forms of apo A-I_M, the homodimer apo A-I_M/A-I_M appears to be the "protective" component [24,25]. Recombinant A-I_M/A-I_M has been expressed in *Escherichia coli* and formulated as synthetic HDL with PL (AIM).

In cholesterol-fed rabbits AIM markedly reduces intimal thickening after balloon injury, as well as after perivascular manipulation [26]. In apo E-deficient mice, 18 injections (40 mg/kg) of AIM prevented progression of lesions; a higher dose (80 mg/kg) induced a clear regression [27].

The hypothesis of inducing significant regression/stabilization of plaques by single administrations of AIM was recently tested. AIM (400 mg/kg of protein) promoted a rapid cholesterol mobilization from atheromas in E-deficient mice [28]. In a new rabbit model allowing direct measurement of carotid plaque areas by intravascular ultrasound (IVUS), a reduction in plaque size of up to 30% was observed after a 90-min. infusion, associated to a striking increase of HDL cholesterolemia [29].

In healthy volunteers, AIM proved safe and well tolerated, with an up to threefold free cholesterol increase in HDL, proportional to the administered dose (Fig. 1). A phase II trial

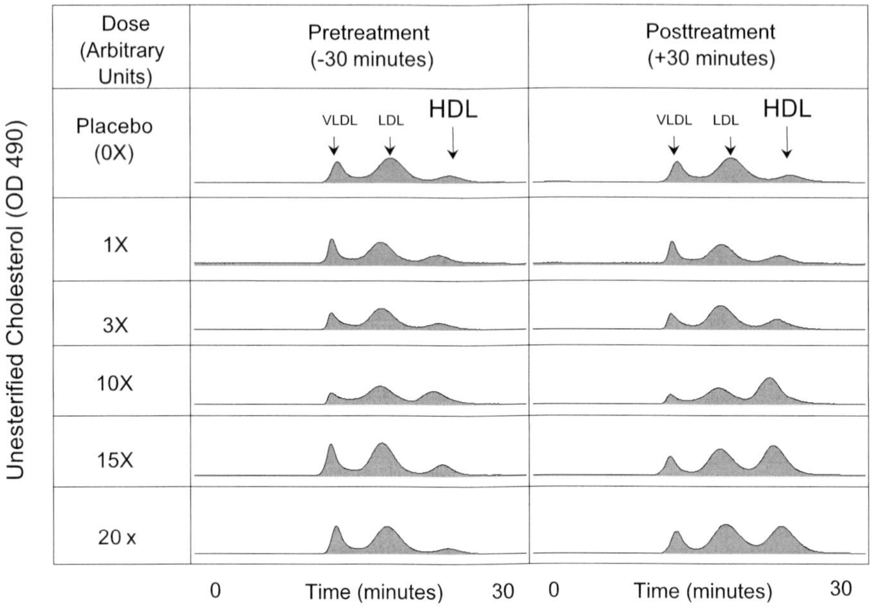

Fig. 1. Acute effect of a single intravenous dose of A-I_{Milano} on serum HDL unesterified cholesterol in normal human male subjects.

on coronary patients has been very recently completed [30]. Patients were randomized into three groups, receiving five weekly infusions of placebo or AIM at 15 or 45 mg/kg. IVUS evaluation was performed at baseline and at the end of the treatments. In the placebo group, percent atheroma volume increased by 0.14%, whereas it was reduced by 14.1 mm^3 or 4.2% in the combined treatment groups ($p<0.001$). These findings provide the first clinical demonstration of the potential of HDL therapy to induce a rapid plaque regression.

5. Other aspects of HDL therapy and future developments

Apo A-I has been known for many years to exert a direct fibrinolytic activity in vitro [6]. In an in vivo model of arterial thrombus in rats, AIM produced both inhibition of platelet aggregation and delayed thrombus formation [31].

Other options may be offered by HDL mimetics such as the large unilamellar vesicles (LUV) of PL, i.e., spherical particles of natural polyoleylphosphatidylcholine (POPC), hydrated and made into 100–200 nm particles by extrusion [32]. Repeated bolus injections (1 g/kg) reduce lesions in E-deficient mice by accelerating reverse cholesterol transport.

Future approaches to vascular disease may involve the use of AIM by direct infiltration into the coronary wall during stent application; recent results indicate a remarkable reduction of intrastent proliferation in pigs [33]. A dramatic reduction of myocardial damage following postischemia revascularization was recently also shown after AIM infusion.

Therapeutic uses of HDL mimetics will depend largely on the availability of novel technologies for direct vascular evaluation. Ongoing studies suggest that novel MRI technologies can offer a very satisfactory resolution of arterial plaques, not significantly different from IVUS. If such techniques prove sufficiently reliable and widely available, these will allow continued evaluation of vascular lesions over time in patients treated by novel HDL-based approaches.

Acknowledgements

Supported in part by the Italian Ministry of University and Scientific Research and by Esperion Therapeutics.

References

[1] D.J. Gordon, B.M. Rifkind, High density lipoprotein: the clinical implications of recent studies, N. Engl. J. Med. 321 (1989) 1311–1316.
[2] G.H. Rothblat, M. de la Llera-Moya, V. Atger, G. Kellner-Weibel, D.L. Williams, M.C. Phillips, Cell cholesterol efflux: integration of old and new observations provides new insight, J. Lipid Res. 40 (1999) 781–796.
[3] M. Navab, J.A. Berliner, A.D. Watson, S.Y. Hama, M.C. Territo, et al, The yin and yang of oxidation in the development of the fatty streak, ATVB 16 (1996) 831–842.
[4] T.Z. Naqvi, P.K. Shah, P.A. Ivey, M.D. Molloy, A.M. Thomas, S. Panicker, et al, Evidence that high-density lipoprotein cholesterol is an independent predictor of acute platelet-dependent thrombus formation, Am. J. Cardiol. 84 (1999) 1011–1017.
[5] K. Saku, M. Ahmad, P. Glas-Greenwalt, M.L. Kashyap, Activation of fibrinolysis by apolipoproteins of high density lipoproteins in man, Thromb. Res. 39 (1985) 1–8.
[6] L. Calabresi, M. Gomaraschi, G. Franceschini, Endothelial protection by high-density lipoproteins. From bench to bedside, ATVB 23 (2003) 1724–1731.
[7] M.H. Frick, O. Elo, K. Haapa, O.P. Heinonen, P. Heinsalmi, et al, Helsinki heart study: primary-prevention trial with gemfibrozil in middle-aged men with dyslipidemia, N. Engl. J. Med. 317 (1987) 1237–1245.
[8] H.B. Rubins, S.J. Robins, D. Collins, C.L. Fye, J.W. Anderson, et al, Gemfibrozil for the secondary prevention of coronary heart disease in men with low levels of high-density lipoprotein cholesterol. Veterans affairs high-density lipoprotein cholesterol intervention trial study group, N. Engl. J. Med. 341 (1999) 410–418.
[9] B.G. Brown, X.-Q. Zhao, A. Chait, L.D. Fisher, M.C. Cheung, et al, Simvastatin and niacin, antioxidant vitamins, or the combination for the prevention of coronary disease, N. Engl. J. Med. 345 (2001) 1583–1592.
[10] Effect of fenofibrate on progression of coronary-artery disease in type 2 diabetes: the diabetes atherosclerosis intervention study, a randomised study, Lancet 357 (2001) 905–910.
[11] A. von Eckardstein, J.R. Nofer, G. Assmann, High density lipoproteins and arteriosclerosis. Role of cholesterol efflux and reverse cholesterol transport, ATVB 21 (2001) 13–27.
[12] H. Vosper, G.A. Khoudoli, T.L. Graham, C.N.A. Palmer, Peroxisome proliferator-activated receptor agonists, hyperlipidaemia, and atherosclerosis, Pharmacol. Ther. 95 (2002) 47–62.
[13] R.W. James, A helping hand for the good guy; novel pharmacological approaches for augmenting the cardiovascular benefits of high density lipoproteins, Curr. Med. Chem. 10 (2003) 955–966.
[14] G. Chiesa, S. Michelagnoli, M. Cassinotti, G. Gianfranceschi, J.P. Werba, et al, Mechanisms of high-density lipoprotein reduction after probucol treatment: changes in plasma cholesterol esterification/transfer and lipase activities, Metabolism 42 (1993) 229–235.
[15] Y. Sawayama, C. Shimizu, N. Maeda, M. Tatsukawa, N. Kinukawa, et al, Effects of probucol and pravastatin on common carotid atherosclerosis in patients with asymptomatic hypercholesterolemia. Fukuoka atherosclerosis trial (FAST), JACC 39 (2002) 610–616.
[16] J.-C. Tardif, J. Grégoire, L. Schwartz, L. Title, L. Laramée, et al, Effects of AGI-1067 and probucol after percutaneous coronary interventions, Circulation 107 (2003) 552–558.

[17] H. Okamoto, F. Yonemori, K. Wakitani, T. Minowa, K. Maeda, H. Shinkai, A cholesteryl ester transfer protein inhibitor attenuates atherosclerosis in rabbits, Nature 406 (2000) 203–206.
[18] Z. Huang, A. Inazu, A. Mohara, T. Higashikata, H. Mabuchi, Cholesteryl ester transfer protein inhibitor (JTT-705) and the development of atherosclerosis in rabbits with severe hypercholesterolaemia, Clin. Sci. 103 (2002) 587–594.
[19] G.J. de Grooth, J.A. Kuivenhoven, A.F.H Stalenhoef, J. de Graaf, A.H. Zwinderman, et al, Efficacy and safety of a novel cholesteryl ester transfer protein inhibitor, JTT-705, in humans, Circulation 105 (2002) 2159–2165.
[20] L.A. Carlson, Effect of a single infusion of recombinant human proapolipoprotein A-I liposomes (synthetic HDL) on plasma lipoproteins in patients with low high density lipoprotein cholesterol, NMCD, Nutr. Metab. Cardiovasc. Dis. 5 (1995) 85–91.
[21] L.E. Spieker, I. Sudano, D. Hurlimann, P.G. Lerch, M.G. Lang, et al, High-density lipoprotein restores endothelial function in hypercholesterolemic men, Circulation 105 (2002) 1399–1402.
[22] R.J. Bisoendial, K. Hovingh, H. Levels, P.G. Lerch, I. Andresen, et al, Restoration of endothelial function by increasing high-density lipoprotein in subjects with isolated low high-density lipoprotein, Circulation 107 (2003) 2944–2948.
[23] K.H. Weisgraber, S.C. Rall Jr., T.P. Bersot, R.W. Mahley, G. Franceschini, C.R. Sirtori, Apolipoprotein AI_{Milano}. Detection of normal AI in affected subjects and evidence for a cysteine for arginine substitution in the variant AI, J. Biol. Chem. 258 (1983) 2508–2513.
[24] P. Roma, R.E. Gregg, M.S. Meng, R. Ronan, L.A. Zech, et al, In vivo metabolism of a mutant form of apolipoprotein A-I, apo A-IMilano, associated with familial hypoalphalipoproteinemia, J. Clin. Invest. 91 (1993) 1445–1452.
[25] G. Franceschini, L. Calabresi, G. Chiesa, C. Parolini, C.R. Sirtori, et al, Increased cholesterol efflux potential of sera from ApoA-IMilano carriers and transgenic mice, ATVB 19 (1999) 1257–1262.
[26] G. Chiesa, C.R. Sirtori, Recombinant apolipoprotein $A\text{-}I_{Milano}$: a novel agent for the induction of regression of atherosclerotic plaques, Ann. Med. 35 (2003) 267–273.
[27] P.K. Shah, J. Nilsson, S. Kaul, M.C. Fishbein, H. Ageland, et al, Effects of recombinant apolipoprotein A-IMilano on aortic atherosclerosis in apolipoportein E-deficient mice, Circulation 97 (1998) 780–785.
[28] P.K. Shah, J. Yano, O. Reyes, K.Y. Chyu, S. Kaul, et al, High-dose recombinant apolipoprotein A-IMilano mobilizes tissue cholesterol and rapidly reduces plaque lipid and macrophage content in apolipoprotein E-deficient mice, Circulation 103 (2001) 3047–3050.
[29] G. Chiesa, E. Monteggia, M. Marchesi, P. Lorenzon, M. Laucello, et al, Recombinant apolipoprotein A-I Milano infusion into rabbit carotid artery rapidly removes lipid from fatty streaks, Circ. Res. 90 (2002) 974–980.
[30] S.E. Nissen, T. Tsumoda, E.M. Tuczu, P. Schoenhagen, C.J. Cooper, et al, Effect of recombinant apo A-I Milano on coronary atherosclerosis in patients with acute coronary syndromes, JAMA 290 (2003) 2292–2300.
[31] D. Li, S. Weng, B. Yang, D.S. Zander, T. Saldeen, et al, Inhibition of arterial thrombus formation by ApoA-I Milano, ATVB 19 (1999) 378–383.
[32] K.J. Williams, R. Scalia, K.D. Mazany, W.V. Rodrigueza, A.M. Lefer, Rapid restoration of normal endothelial functions in genetically hyperlipidemic mice by a synthetic mediator of reverse lipid transport, ATVB 20 (2000) 1033–1039.
[33] S. Kaul, V. Rukshin, R. Santos, B. Azarbal, C.L. Bisgaier, et al, Intramural delivery of recombinant apolipoprotein A-IMilano/phospholipid complex (ETC-216) inhibits In-stent stenosis in porcine coronary arteries, Circulation (2003) 2551–2554.

ELSEVIER

International Congress Series 1262 (2004) 15–18

www.ics-elsevier.com

Therapeutic angiogenesis

Seppo Ylä-Herttuala*

Department of Medicine, A.I. Virtanen Institute, Molecular Medicine, University of Kuopio P.O. Box 1627 FIN-70211 Kuopio, Finland

Abstract. Therapeutic angiogenesis is a new, promising option for the treatment of severe ischaemia in myocardium and peripheral muscles. Both recombinant growth factors and gene therapy have been used in therapeutic angiogenesis trials. Most common growth factors belong to the vascular endothelial growth factor (VEGF) family and fibroblast growth factor (FGF) family. Encouraging results have resulted from several small clinical trials. However, final proof of efficacy as measured by clinically relevant endpoints will only be obtained from large phase II/III trials, which should be finished within 2–3 years. © 2003 Elsevier B.V. All rights reserved.

Keywords: VEGF; FGF; Angiogenesis; Arteriogenesis; Clinical trials

1. Introduction

Myocardial ischaemia and peripheral vascular disease are very significant clinical problems in the elderly population. Long-term improvement in the condition of ischaemic muscles would require improved perfusion of the affected muscles. This can be achieved by several treatment strategies, such as angioplasty and vascular surgery. Many patients are also able to compensate for reduced blood flow by growing new collateral vessels around occluded arteries. Therapeutic angiogenesis tries to mimic this natural process in ischaemic muscles.

2. Therapeutic angiogenesis

The concept of therapeutic angiogenesis involves generation of new capillaries, collateral vessels, or both, in ischaemic muscles, using either recombinant growth factors or their genes [1]. Most commonly used growth factors for therapeutic angiogenesis are vascular endothelial growth factors (VEGF) and fibroblast growth factors (FGF) [1]. Some other cytokines and growth factors may also have angiogenic effects in vivo (Table 1). In addition to growth factors, other mediators, such as nitric oxide, seem to be important for this process.

* Tel.: +358-17-162075; fax: +358-17-163751.
E-mail address: seppo.ylaherttuala@uku.fi (S. Ylä-Herttuala).

doi:10.1016/S0531-5131(03)01735-7

Table 1
Factors that can be used for therapeutic angiogenesis

VEGF-A, -B, -C, -D, PlGF
FGF-1, -2, -4
Hepatocyte growth factor, Del-1
MCP-1, GM-CSF

PlGF: Placental growth factor, MCP-1: monocyte chemotactic protein-1, GM-CSF: granulocyte-macrophage colony-stimulating factor, Del-1: Development early locus-1.

Recombinant growth factors can be injected into the blood stream or directly in the ischaemic muscles. Repeated injections are usually required. Genes encoding growth factors can be delivered via the same routes using either non-viral or viral gene transfer vectors. Most commonly used vectors are naked plasmids, plasmid/liposomes and adenoviruses [1]. Direct delivery of recombinant growth factors allows precise control of the delivered dose, but the short half-life of the growth factors in vivo may limit their efficacy. Gene therapy can lead to a long-lasting therapeutic effect after a single administration of the vector but suffers from a less precise control of the delivered dose and an unknown safety profile [1].

3. Mechanisms of therapeutic angiogenesis

Improved perfusion in the ischaemic muscle can be achieved by angiogenesis and arteriogenesis. Angiogenesis means sprouting of new blood vessels from pre-existing ones as a result of the proliferation and migration of endothelial cells. Arteriogenesis is a process caused by increased sheer stress at the arteriolar level resulting in the formation of large conduit vessels from preexisting small vessels. Optimally, both angiogenesis and arteriogenesis should be achieved in order to improve muscle perfusion [1]. There is increased evidence that therapeutic angiogenesis may be more difficult to achieve in older and in diabetic patients.

4. Clinical trials

Clinical trials of angiogenic therapy with recombinant proteins or genes have been mostly conducted in patients with inoperable chronic critical limb ischaemia or in severe myocardial ischaemia. Early, non-controlled phase I studies have shown promising results, but so far, only a few phase II/III trials have been published (Table 2). According to this information, recombinant VEGF protein delivery for the treatment of coronary heart disease did not meet its primary endpoint based on exercise tolerance test (ETT) 60 days after the VEGF administration (VIVA Trial) [2]. Also, recombinant FGF-2 protein delivery was ineffective in improving ETT in myocardial ischaemia patients 90 days after the FGF delivery (FIRST Trial) [3] but has shown efficacy in peripheral vascular disease (TRAFFIC Trial) [4]. On the other hand, adenovirus-mediated FGF-4 gene delivery into coronary arteries produced some improvement at 4 weeks ETT (AGENT Trial) [5]. Adenovirus- and plasmid-mediated VEGF gene delivery into ischaemic legs during angioplasty operations have been shown to improve vascularity of the treated limbs 3 months after the VEGF gene therapy [6]. Also, adenovirus-mediated VEGF treatment

Table 2
Phase II/III angiogenesis trials

Trial	Therapeutic agent	n	Endpoint	Results	Reference
VIVA Trial	Recombinant VEGF protein	178	ETT[a] at 60 days	Negative	[2]
FIRST Trial	Recombinant FGF-2 protein	337	ETT at 90 days	Negative	[3]
TRAFFIC Trial	Recombinant FGF-2 protein	190	ETT at 90 days	Positive	[4]
AGENT Trial	Adenovirus-FGF-4	79	ETT at 4 weeks	Positive	[5]
VEGF Peripheral Vascular Disease Trial	Adenovirus-VEGF Plasmid-VEGF	54	Increased vascularity in angiography at 3 months	Positive	[6]
KAT Trial	Adenovirus-VEGF Plasmid-VEGF	103	Increased myo-cardial perfusion at 6 months	Positive	[7]

[a] ETT: exercise tolerance test.

improved myocardial perfusion at a 6-month time point in coronary heart disease patients (KAT Trial) [7].

Safety records from published trials seem to indicate that no major problems have been encountered. However, therapeutic angiogenesis can theoretically lead to severe side effects, such as growth stimulation of tumors or tumor blood vessels and worsening of retinopathy. It is obvious that larger phase II/III trials need to be conducted before safety and efficacy of recombinant protein or gene-based treatment strategies can be fully evaluated.

5. Conclusions and future directions

Therapeutic angiogenesis may provide a novel treatment option for patients with myocardial and peripheral ischaemia not amenable to conventional revascularization. However, solid evidence from large phase II/III clinical trials showing efficacy of the primary endpoints needs to be obtained before these new treatments can enter clinical practice. Also, better vectors and more efficient gene delivery tools are needed to further improve the efficacy of angiogenic gene therapy.

References

[1] S. Ylä-Herttuala, K. Alitalo, Gene transfer as a tool to induce therapeutic vascular growth, Nat. Med. 9 (2003) 694–701.

[2] T.D. Henry, B.H. Annex, G.R. McKendall, M.A. Azrin, J.J. Lopez, F.J. Giordano, P.K. Shah, J.T. Willerson, R.L. Benza, D.S. Berman, C.M. Gibson, A. Bajamonde, A.C. Rundle, J. Fine, E.R. McCluskey, The VIVA trial. Vascular endothelial growth factor in ischemia for vascular angiogenesis, Circulation 107 (2003) 1359–1365.

[3] M. Simons, B.H. Annex, R.J. Laham, N. Kleiman, T. Henry, H. Dauerman, J.E. Udelson, E.V. Gervino, M. Pike, M.J. Whitehouse, T. Moon, N.A. Chronos, Pharmacological treatment of coronary artery disease with recombinant fibroblast growth factor-2, Circulation 105 (2002) 788–793.

[4] R.J. Lederman, F.O. Mendelsohn, R.D. Anderson, J.F. Saucedo, A.N. Tenaglia, J.B. Hermiller, W.B. Hillegass, K. Rocha-Singh, T.E. Moon, M.J. Whitehouse, B.H. Annex, Therapeutic angiogenesis with recombinant fibroblast growth factor-2 for intermittent claudication (the TRAFFIC study): a randomised trial, Lancet 359 (2002) 2053–2058.

[5] C.L. Grines, M.W. Watkins, G. Helmer, W. Penny, J. Brinker, J.D. Marmur, A. West, J.J. Rade, P. Marrott, H.K. Hammond, R.L. Engler, Angiogenic Gene Therapy (AGENT) Trial in patients with stable angina pectoris, Circulation 105 (2002) 1291–1297.

[6] K. Mäkinen, H. Manninen, M. Hedman, P. Matsi, H. Mussalo, E. Alhava, S. Ylä-Herttuala, Increased vascularity detected by digital subtraction angiography after VEGF gene transfer to human lower limb artery, Molec. Ther. 6 (2002) 127–133.

[7] M. Hedman, J. Hartikainen, M. Syvänne, J. Stjernvall, A. Hedman, A. Kivelä, E. Vanninen, H. Mussalo, E. Kauppila, S. Simula, O. Närvänen, A. Rantala, K. Peuhkurinen, M.S. Nieminen, M. Laakso, S. Ylä-Herttuala, Safety and feasibility of catheter-based local intracoronary vascular endothelial growth factor gene transfer in the prevention of postangioplasty and in-stent restenosis and in the treatment of chronic myocardial ischemia, Circulation 107 (2003) 2677–2683.

International Congress Series 1262 (2004) 19–24

ELSEVIER

www.ics-elsevier.com

Genetics, obesity, and the metabolic syndrome: The Professor Donald S. Fredrickson Memorial Lecture

Scott M. Grundy*

University of Texas Southwestern Medical Center at Dallas, Center for Human Nutrition, 5323 Harry Hines Boulevard, Y3.206, Dallas, TX 75390-9052, USA

Abstract. The metabolic syndrome consists of a clustering of metabolic risk factors in one individual. These risk factors consist of atherogenic dyslipidemia (high triglycerides, high apolipoprotein B [apo B], small LDL particles, and low HDL), elevated blood pressure, insulin resistance ± elevated plasma glucose, a prothrombotic state, and a proinflammatory state. Although the metabolic syndrome is increasingly common around the world and represents an important cause of cardiovascular disease (CVD), its pathogenesis is not well understood. The two major underlying causes appear to be obesity or other disorders of adipose tissue and insulin resistance. There is little doubt that genetic susceptibility plays an important role in the development of the metabolic syndrome. This paper addresses the question of the interaction between obesity and genetic susceptibility in the etiology of the metabolic syndrome. Genetic susceptibility appears to exist at three levels: within adipose tissue itself, in insulin signaling pathways, and in regulation of individual risk factors. A major research challenge for the future is to unravel the complex genetic architecture that gives rise to the metabolic syndrome once a person becomes obese.

Keywords: Metabolic syndrome; Insulin resistance; Obesity; Genetic susceptibility

The metabolic syndrome is a multiplex risk factor for cardiovascular disease (CVD). It has emerged as one of the most important contributing causes of CVD in the world. Its prevalence is increasing rapidly in many countries. This increased occurrence is due in large part to the "epidemic" of obesity in both developed and developing countries. The metabolic syndrome is characterized by a clustering of metabolic risk factors in one person. The principal CVD risk factors of the metabolic syndrome include:

- atherogenic dyslipidemia
- elevated blood pressure
- insulin resistance ± elevated glucose
- proinflammatory state
- prothrombotic state

* Tel.: +1-214-648-2890; fax: +1-214-648-4837.
E-mail address: scott.grundy@utsouthwestern.edu (S.M. Grundy).

0531-5131/
doi:10.1016/S0531-5131(03)01817-X

Atherogenic dyslipidemia consists of elevations of serum triglycerides, remnant lipoproteins, total apolipoprotein B (apo B), and small LDL particles along with reductions in serum HDL cholesterol. Blood pressure often is increased only moderately. Insulin resistance is present in most persons with the metabolic syndrome, and it predisposes to development of elevated glucose in some persons. When the glucose level reaches a defined threshold, the person is said to have type 2 diabetes. Arterial wall inflammation is secondary to several factors including proinflammatory lipoproteins, elevated blood pressure, possibly insulin resistance, elevated glucose, and inflammatory cytokines. The presence of arterial wall inflammation can be recognized clinically by elevations of C-reactive protein (CRP). Finally, a prothrombotic state is identified by elevations of plasma fibrinogen and PAI-I.

The United States National Cholesterol Education Programs (NCEP) Adult Treatment Panel III (ATP III) [1] recently proposed a simple way to recognize the metabolic syndrome in clinical practice. ATP III proposed that a diagnosis of the metabolic syndrome can be made in any person who has three of five for the following characteristics:

- Abdominal obesity (elevated waist circumference)
- Serum triglycerides ≥ 150 mg/dl
- Serum HDL cholesterol < 40 mg/dl in men and < 50 mg/dl in women
- Blood pressure $\geq 130/85$ mm Hg
- Plasma glucose ≥ 110 mg/dl

For the United States, an elevated waist circumferences was defined as ≥ 102 cm in men and ≥ 88 cm in women. This level of waist circumference usually is associated with a significant degree of insulin resistance. An elevated waist circumference can be taken as a surrogate marker for insulin resistance. ATP III noted that many men have insulin resistance when the waist circumference is in the range of 94–101.9 cm; this range can be used as one of the criteria. In other regions, significant insulin resistance develops at lesser degrees of abdominal obesity; thus, lower waist circumferences will be used to define abdominal obesity in some countries. Elevations of triglyceride and reductions of HDL cholesterol are indicative of atherogenic dyslipidemia. Most patients with higher triglyceride and lower HDL cholesterol with or without elevated fasting glucose will be insulin resistant. According to ATP III, the metabolic syndrome is still present in a person who has glucose levels >126 mg/dl (categorical hyperglycemia) if other defining components are present. The presence of elevations in CRP (≥ 3 mg/l), fibrinogen, and PAI-1 are not required for a clinical diagnosis of metabolic syndrome; however, if such abnormalities are detected, their presence will add confirmation for the existence of the syndrome.

1. Obesity versus insulin resistance as the dominant underlying cause

The metabolic syndrome is a complex disorder that undoubtedly is multifactorial in origin. ATP III identified obesity as the major driving force underlying the increasing prevalence of metabolic syndrome in the United States. Many studies have shown that obesity is associated with the presence of several of the metabolic risk factors. On the other hand, some investigators [2, 3] hold that insulin resistance plays a direct causative role in causation of the other metabolic risk factors. Various mechanisms have been proposed whereby insulin resistance is linked causally with these risk factors. These investigators believe that at the least, insulin resistance is more central in the development of the syndrome than is obesity. This viewpoint is illustrated by the World Health Organization (WHO) criteria [4] for diagnosis of the syndrome. These criteria require more direct evidence for the presence of insulin resistance than the indirect evidence required by ATP III. For example, to qualify for having the metabolic syndrome, WHO require either elevated glucose, hyperinsulinemia, or reduced glucose disposal under glucose-clamp conditions. At present, it is not possible to determine whether obesity or insulin resistance is mechanistically the more closely related to the metabolic syndrome. Both are strongly associated, and the mechanisms underlying the metabolic risk factors are not well understood. Moreover, obesity and insulin resistance are tightly interrelated themselves. Perhaps a more interesting question is how do obesity and insulin resistance interact together to produce the metabolic syndrome.

2. Acquired versus genetic causes

There is growing evidence that both acquired factors and genetic factors contribute to the metabolic syndrome. The major acquired factor is obesity, although others, such as physical inactivity, also appear to be involved as well [1]. A role for obesity is suggested by the correlation between rise in prevalence rates of both metabolic syndrome and obesity in the United States and other populations [5]. On the other hand, only about a third of people who are obese develop the metabolic syndrome. This suggests that other factors, such as genetic, also play an important role. One attractive hypothesis is that the syndrome develops largely through the interaction between obesity and genetics. The current manuscript will explore this hypothesis.

If the metabolic syndrome results largely from the interaction of obesity and genetic factors, the three levels of genetic variation can be visualized. The first is at the level of adipose tissue itself. Various genetic abnormalities in adipose tissue metabolism could be accentuated with weight gain. Second, individuals could have genetic forms of insulin resistance that adversely affect metabolic risk factors. Third, there could be genetic variation at the level of risk factor regulation. At this level, too, obesity could have an adverse influence. Genetic variation at each of these three levels can be considered for the impact of increasing obesity.

3. Adipose tissue variations and disorders

The most recognized variant in adipose tissue distribution associated with the metabolic syndrome is upper body obesity. This pattern is usually called "abdominal obesity" because it is recognized clinically by increased waist circumference. In reality, however, upper body obesity is accompanied by increases in adipose tissue in both truncal subcutaneous and intra-abdominal regions. Persons with this pattern can be contrasted to those with lower body obesity in which most of the excess body fat occurs in the gluteofemoral region. Persons with predominant lower body obesity are less prone to the metabolic syndrome than are those with upper body obesity. The causes of upper body obesity may be multifactorial. Men are especially likely to have this pattern, thus, its alternate name "android obesity;" in contrast, women typically manifest lower body obesity (gluteofemoral or "gynoid" obesity). Hormonal factors thus likely are one factor responsible for the difference. Still, genetic influences may be at play because some women exhibit upper body obesity, whereas men vary in the distribution of fat between upper and lower body. The mechanistic connections between upper body obesity and metabolic syndrome are not well understood. Nonetheless, those with upper body obesity typically have greater insulin resistance and metabolic risk factors are more severe than in persons with lower body obesity [6]. For the general population, the more severe forms of upper body obesity may have a polygenic origin; on the other hand, there are rare monogenic disorders of adipose tissue in which the distribution of body fat is markedly deranged, and the metabolic syndrome is severe.

One of these rare disorders is called familial partial lipodystrophy. This condition is characterized by progressive loss of subcutaneous adipose tissue and overloading of intra-abdominal adipose tissue pools with fat. Patients with familial partial lipodystrophy commonly manifest insulin resistance and atherogenic dyslipidemia. They often develop premature type 2 diabetes. Several monogenic conditions have been identified as being responsible for this condition. They include mutations in the structural protein lamin A/C [7–9], a protein required for the conversion of prelamin to lamin [10], and PPAR gamma [11]. Another monogenic disorder of adipose tissue is congenital partial lipodystrophy. It is characterized by almost total loss of adipose tissue, severe insulin resistance, severe hypertriglyceridemia, and premature diabetes; it further results from a mutation in the enzyme required for the synthesis of triglyceride in adipose tissue [12]. Although these disorders are responsible for severe forms of metabolic syndrome, it is possible that less severe mutations or sets of polymorphisms in adipose tissue function contribute to more common forms of upper body obesity that are associated with this syndrome.

4. Primary insulin resistance

Since insulin resistance is strongly associated with other metabolic risk factors, some investigators [3, 4] hypothesize that genetic forms of insulin resistance are critical for development of the metabolic syndrome in populations. Strong support for this hypothesis is the apparent genetic susceptibility of certain populations for insulin resistance and premature type 2 diabetes. Most notable is the population of South Asia. In this population, insulin resistance is commonly observed with even mild obesity [13]. Furthermore, in the Caucasian population, there is considerable variability in insulin resistance at given levels of body fat content [14]. Rare mutations of the insulin receptor produce severe insulin resistance, but whether they are associated with other metabolic risk factors has not been extensively studied. More likely, common forms of reduced insulin sensitivity have a polygenic basis. A variety of gene polymorphisms have been reported to be associated with reduced insulin sensitivity. However, these associations have not been extensively replicated in various cohorts. One polymorphism of interest occurs in the membrane protein PC-1, which has been reported to be associated with increased insulin resistance [15]. In a recent study, Abate et al. [16] found that this polymorphism is strongly associated with insulin resistance in the South Asian population.

However, it is doubtful that this polymorphism alone can account for all of the insulin resistance that is observed in this population. Nonetheless, variation in PC-1 could be one of several genes responsible for the high prevalence of insulin resistance among South Asians. When primary insulin resistance is associated with obesity, insulin resistance likely will be increased further, as will the frequency of other metabolic risk factors.

5. Genetic regulation of metabolic risk factors

The third level of genetic variation affecting metabolic risk factors exists at the risk factors themselves. In other words, there is genetic control of lipoprotein metabolism, blood pressure, insulin secretion, and inflammatory and thrombotic responses. Variation in the genetics of risk factor regulation is high in the general population. For example, it has been estimated that approximately 40–50% of the variation in serum levels of triglycerides and HDL is genetically determined. The same undoubtedly holds for hypertension. Only a portion of obese and/or insulin-resistant persons will develop type 2 diabetes; this is because of variation in ability to secrete insulin to offset insulin resistance. To date, little is known about the sources of genetic variation in risk-factor control in the population. Indeed, in the fields of lipoproteins and blood pressure, debate continues whether variation in expression of these parameters is determined by a few major genes or many, i.e., whether dyslipidemia and hypertension are largely oligogenic or polygenic in origin. Regardless, this third level of control undoubtedly plays a significant role in the expression of the metabolic risk factors in patients who are obese and/or insulin resistant.

6. Interaction of obesity and genetics in causation of the metabolic syndrome

In summary, the metabolic syndrome appears to represent an important example of the interaction of acquired factors (especially obesity) and genetic factors in the causation of cardiovascular risk. Genetic variation exists at three levels: adipose tissue, insulin responsiveness, and risk factor regulation. The rise in prevalence of the metabolic syndrome worldwide is being fueled largely by increasing obesity. However, the pattern and severity of metabolic risk factors within and between populations varies greatly depending on the genetic substratum. Gradually, more information is accruing on the genetic architecture of the metabolic syndrome. However, much remains to be determined. One important question is whether the interaction of obesity and genetics is additive for risk factors, or whether it is synergistic. The answer to this question awaits further investigation.

References

[1] Third report of the National Cholesterol Education Program (NCEP) expert panel on detection, evaluation, and treatment of high blood cholesterol in adults (Adult Treatment Panel III). Final Report, Circulation 106 (2002) 3143–3421.

[2] G.M. Reaven, Banting lecture 1988. Role of insulin resistance in human disease, Diabetes 37 (1988) 1595–1607.

[3] E. Ferrannini, S.M. Haffner, B.D. Mitchell, M.P. Stern, Hyperinsulinemia: the key feature of a cardiovascular and metabolic syndrome, Diabetologia 34 (1991) 416–422.

[4] K.G. Alberti, P.Z. Zimmet, Definition, diagnosis and classification of diabetes mellitus and its complica-

tions: part 1. Diagnosis and classification of diabetes mellitus provisional report of a WHO consultation, Diabet. Med. 15 (1998) 539–553.
[5] E.S. Ford, W.H. Giles, W.H. Dietz, Prevalence of the metabolic syndrome among US adults. Findings from the Third National Health and Nutrition Survey, JAMA 287 (2002) 356–359.
[6] P. Bjorntorp, Body fat distribution, insulin resistance, and metabolic diseases, Nutrition 13 (9) (1997) 795–803.
[7] J.M. Peters, R. Barnes, L. Bennett, W.M. Gitomer, A.M. Bowcock, A. Garg, Localization of the gene for familial partial lipodystrophy (Dunnigan variety) to chromosome 1q21–22, Nat. Genet. 18 (1998) 292–295.
[8] H. Cao, R.A Hegele, Nuclear lamin A/C R482Q mutation in Canadian kindreds with Dunningan-type familial partial lipodystrophy, Hum. Mol. Genet. 9 (2000) 109–112.
[9] R.A. Speckman, A. Garg, F. Du, et al, Mutational and haplotype analyses of families with familial partial lipodystrophy (Dunnigan variety) reveal recurrent missense mutations in the globular C-terminal domain of lamin A/C, Am. J. Hum. Genet. 66 (2000) 1192–1198.
[10] A.K. Agarwal, J.P. Fryns, R.J. Auchus, A. Garg, Zinc metalloproteinase, ZMPSTE24, is mutated in mandibuloacral dysplasia, Hum. Mol. Genet. 12 (2003) 1995–2001.
[11] A.K. Agarwal, A. Garg, A novel heterozygous mutation in peroxisome proliferator-activated receptor-gamma gene in a patient with familial partial lipodystrophy, J. Clin. Endocrinol. Metab. 87 (2002) 408–411.
[12] A.K. Agarwal, E. Arioglu, S. De Almeida, et al, AGPAT2 is mutated in congenital generalized lipodystrophy linked to chromosome 9q34, Nat. Genet. 31 (2002) 21–23.
[13] M. Chandalia, N. Abate, A. Garg, J. Stray-Gundersen, S.M. Grundy, Relationship between generalized and upper body obesity to insulin resistance in Asian Indian men, J. Clin. Endocrinol. Metab. 84 (1999) 2329–2335.
[14] C.N.O. Jones, F. Abbasi, M. Carantoni, K.S. Polonsky, G.M. Reaven, Roles of insulin resistance and obesity in regulation of plasma insulin concentrations, Am. J. Physiol. Endocrinol. Metab. 278 (2000) E501–E508.
[15] A. Pizzutti, L. Frittitta, A. Argiolas, R. Baratta, I.D. Goldfine, M. Bozzali, T. Ercolino, G. Scarlato, L. Iacoviello, R. Vigneri, V. Tassi, V. Trischitta, A polymorphism (K121Q) of the human glycoprotein PC-1 gene coding region is strongly associated with insulin resistance, Diabetes 48 (1999) 1881–1884.
[16] N. Abate, L. Carull, A. Cabo-Chan, Jr., M. Chandalia, P.G. Snell, S.M. Grundy, Genetic polymorphism PC-1 K121Q and ethnic susceptibility to insulin resistance, J. Clin. Endocrinol. Metab. (in press).

International Congress Series 1262 (2004) 25–29

www.ics-elsevier.com

PPAR-α and atherosclerosis from basic research to clinical applications

Jean-Charles Fruchart*, Patrick Duriez

INSERM U545-Unité de Recherche sur l'Athérosclérose, Institut Pasteur de Lille, 1, rue du Professeur Calmette, BP245, F-59019 Lille Cedex, France

Abstract. Peroxisome proliferator-activated receptors (PPARs) are a subfamily of the nuclear receptors. Three distinct PPARs termed α, δ(β) and γ, each encoded by a separate gene and showing a distinct tissue distribution pattern, have already been described. All PPARs are activated by fatty acids (FAs). In addition, fibrates bind to and activate PPAR-α. Activated PPARs alter the transcription of target genes after binding to specific peroxisome proliferator response elements (PPREs). PPAR-α activation by fibrates leads to: – decreased hypertriglyceridaemia, – increased HDL-cholesterol, apo A-I and apo A-II levels, – reduced LDL-cholesterol in combined hyperlipidemia by decreasing the levels of atherogenic dense LDL, while increasing buoyant LDL which display high affinity to this receptor. © 2004 Published by Elsevier B.V.

Keywords: Peroxisome proliferator-activated receptor-α; Atherosclerosis; Lipoprotein; Inflammation

1. Effect of PPHR-alpha activators (fibrate) on triglycerides

Recent studies have shown that the effects of fibrates on triglyceride-rich lipoprotein are partly due to an increase in cellular fatty acid (FA) catabolism and the resulting inhibition of hepatic VLDL triglyceride secretion. Peroxisome proliferator-activated receptor (PPAR)-α is highly expressed in tissues with elevated rates of FA catabolism, where it regulates genes involved in FA uptake, degradation via the peroxisomal and mitochondrial β-oxidation pathways. Nevertheless, PPAR-α activators decrease plasma triglyceride concentrations by increasing VLDL- and chylomicron-triglyceride hydrolysis. LPL gene expression is induced by PPAR activators. A sequence element was identified as a peroxisome proliferator response element (PPRE) in the human LPL promoter that mediates the functional responsiveness to PPAR-α activators (fibrates) and PPAR-γ activators (glitazones).

Apo C-III acts by delaying the catabolism of triglyceride-rich particles by inhibiting their lipolysis by LPL. PPAR-α activators decrease human and rat liver apo C-III

* Corresponding author. Tel.: +33-3-20-87-77-52; fax: +33-3-20-87-73-60.
E-mail address: Jean-Charles.Fruchart@pasteur-lille.fr (J.-C. Fruchart).

0531-5131/
doi:10.1016/j.ics.2004.01.051

expression. PPAR-α activators may induce the expression of repressor proteins, such as ARP-1, Ear3/COUP-TF or Rev-erb-α.

Comparison of genomic DNA sequences from human and mouse revealed a new apolipoprotein gene (apo A-V) located on human 11q23. Mice expressing a human apo A-V transgene showed a decrease in plasma triglyceride concentrations; conversely, knockout mice lacking apo A-V had four times as much plasma triglycerides as controls. Human primary hepatocytes treated with Wy 14,643 or fenofibrate displayed a strong induction of apo A-V mRNA [1,2]. By deletion, site-directed mutagenesis and binding analysis, a PPRE located 271-bp upstream of the transcription start site was identified.

2. Effect of PPAR-α activators (fibrate) on HDL metabolism and reverse cholesterol transport (RCT)

RCT is a pathway transporting cholesterol from extrahepatic cells and tissues to the liver, and perhaps intestine, for excretion. RCT consists of seven steps.

PPAR-α activators modify the expression and therefore the synthesis and activity of proteins governing HDL metabolism, and so these drugs could significantly modify RCT. The role of PPAR-α and the effects of PPAR-α activators will be present at the different stages of the RCT.

2.1. Acceptors of cellular cholesterol (step 1)

Fenofibrate increased apo A-I by increasing its synthetic rate. The fibrate effect on human apo A-I is mediated by the transcription factor PPAR-α, which interacts with a positive PPAR-response element (PPRE) in its promoter. The weaker effect of gemfibrozil, in comparison to fenofibrate on human apo A-I and HDL-cholesterol levels correlated with a less pronounced impact on ACO mRNA levels suggesting that the level of the induction of human apo A-I gene is related to the PPAR-α activating potency of the fibrate used [3]. Using transfection assays fenofibrate and gemfibrozil were found to activate PPAR-α with a similar affinity. However, maximal activation was significantly lower for gemfibrozil than fenofibrate using a reporter gene driven by the apo A-I DR-2 PPRE, while using an Aco-like Dr-1 PPRE. This differential activity correlated with the ability to promote co-activator recruitment to PPAR-α. Whereas fenofibrate induced co-activator recruitment to a similar extent on both DR-1 and DR-2 sites, recruitment by gemfibrozil was less efficient on the DR-2 site. Therefore, whereas fenofibrate behaves as a full agonist, gemfibrozil appears to act as a partial agonist depending on the nature of the PPAR-α response element, which dictates its ability to recruit co-activators to the promotor [3]. In apoE-deficient mice expressing a human apo A-I transgene, fenofibrate increased human apo A-I plasma and hepatic mRNA levels without affecting plasma lipid levels. This increase in human apo A-I expression was accompanied by a significant reduction in the lesion surface area in the aortic sinus [4].

Apolipoprotein (apo) A-II is a major protein constituent of HDL. Administration of fenofibrate to patients resulted in a marked increase in plasma apo A-II concentrations. This increase in plasma apo A-II was due to a direct effect on hepatic apo A-II production. Transient transfection experiments of a reporter construct driven by the human apo A-II gene promoter indicated that fenofibrate induced apo A-II gene expression at the transcriptional level. A sequence element located in the J-site of the apo A-II promoter mediates the responsiveness to fibrates and fatty acids. This element contains two imperfect half sites similar to a PPRE.

2.2. Lipoprotein receptors (step 2)

The ATP-binding cassette transporter A1 (ABCA1) mediates apolipoprotein A-I-mediated cellular cholesterol efflux. PPAR-α and PPAR-γ activators induce the expression of the gene encoding ABCA1. These effects are probably due to enhanced expression of liver-x-receptor α, an oxysterol-activated nuclear receptor which induces ABCA1-promoter transcription. Moreover, PPAR-α and PPAR-γ activators increase apo A-I-induced cholesterol efflux from normal macrophages. It has recently been shown that PPAR-α activation decreases cholesterol esterification in macrophages, resulting in enhanced availability of free cholesterol for efflux through the ABCA1 pathway. The scavenger receptor SRBI may be involved in cholesterol efflux. Activation of PPAR-α and PPAR-γ resulted in the induction of CLA-1 protein expression in monocytes and in differentiated macrophages. SR-BI expression increased in the atherosclerotic lesions of apoE-deficient mice treated with either PPAR ligands.

2.3. Esterification of cholesterol within HDL by lecithin/cholesterol acyltransferase (LCAT) (step 3)

LCAT activity increased in children and in adults who were treated with fenofibrate.

Rat hepatic LCAT mRNA levels decreased after treatment with the fibric acid derivatives. Fenofibrate lowered liver LCAT mRNA levels in a dose-dependent manner in rat, which was paralleled by a decrease in plasma LCAT activity. The expression of hepatic LCAT in Human Apo A-I transgenic mice was not significantly modified by fenofibrate despite a significant decrease in plasma cholesterol esterification activity.

2.4. Transfer of lipids to apo B-containing lipoproteins (cholesteryl ester transfer) (step 4)

The next RCT step involves the exchange of accumulated cholesteryl esters for triglycerides through the action of the cholesteryl ester transfer protein (CETP) and the transfer of phospholipid through the action of phospholipid transfer protein (PLTP) between atherogenic apo B containing lipoproteins (VLDL, IDL, LDL) and anti-atherogenic apo A-I containing lipoproteins (HDL). In humans, the promoter activity of the PLTP gene is significantly reduced by fenofibrate. The DNA sequence analysis suggests DNA sequences, which are homologous to a PPRE.

2.5. Remodelling of HDL (step 5)

Hepatic lipase (HL) hydrolyses the triglycerides and the phospholipids of the resulting HDL. PPAR-α activators do not appear to significantly modify HL activity in humans as there is no significant increase in the activity of plasma hepatic lipase after treatment of patients with fibric acids.

2.6. Uptake of HDL cholesterol by the liver and possibly also by kidney and small intestine through lipoprotein receptors (cholesterol uptake) (step 6)

The hepatic expression of SR-BI plays a critical role in lipoprotein metabolism, mainly due to its ability to mediate selective cholesterol uptake. This effect is concomitant with the down-regulation of CLAMP, a putative SR-BI stabilizing protein found in the hepatic plasma membrane, which was also not associated with changes in CLAMP mRNA levels.

2.7. Bile secretion (step 7)

Fibrate treatment causes adverse changes in biliary lipid composition and decreases bile acid excretion and increases fecal cholesterol excretion, leading to an increased incidence of cholesterol gallstones. Decreased bile acid production by PPAR-α-mediated down-regulation of cholesterol 7α-hydroxylase and sterol 27-hydroxylase may contribute to the increased risk of gallstone formation after fibrate treatment. PPAR-α activators inhibit biliary acid secretion and increase fecal cholesterol excretion [5].

3. Effect of fibric acids on insulin sensibility and adiposity

Selective PPAR-α activators reduce insulin resistance without any significant effects on body weight and adipose tissue mass in rodent models of insulin resistance.

4. Effect of fibric acids on thrombosis

Fibric acids decrease PAI-1 production in cultured cynomolgus hepatocytes. Fibric acids influence plasma fibrinogen levels. It has been shown that in mice, fibric acids, decreased hepatic fibrinogen α-, β- and γ-chain mRNA levels. It has been reported that PPAR-α activation negatively regulates human fibrinogen gene expression via inhibition of CCAAT box/enhancer-binding protein β. Fibric acids inhibit tissue factor expression in human monocytes and macrophages.

5. Effect of fibric acids on vascular inflammation

Atherosclerosis development is a long-term process which involves the recruitment and the activation of different cells such as macrophages. PPAR-α is expressed in atherosclerotic plaques and in primary cultures of vascular wall cells. Fenofibric acid treatment prevented the formation of 6-keto-PGF_{1a} by preventing COX-2 induction by IL-1 as a result of a negative regulation of COX-2 transcription through a negative regulation of NF-κB transcription activity. The negative interference of PPAR-α with AP-1 signalling explains the repression of thrombin-induced endothelin-1 (ET-1) expression in endothelial cells by PPAR-α ligands. Activation of PPAR-α by fibric acids negatively regulates the vascular inflammatory gene response by negative cross-talk of activated PPAR-α with transcription factors NF-κB and AP-1 (protein–protein interaction with p65 and c-jun).

6. Discussion

PPAR-α regulates lipid metabolism, insulin sensibility and inhibits inflammatory response in the vascular wall. PPAR-α activators such as fibrates inhibit atherosclerosis development through their normolipidaemic activities but it is highly credible that other effects such as inhibition of vascular inflammation and thrombogenesis also participate in this beneficial effect.

References

[1] N. Vu-Dac, et al., Apolipoprotein A5, a crucial determinant of plasma triglyceride levels, is highly responsive to peroxisome proliferator-activated receptor alpha activators, J. Biol. Chem. 278 (2003) 17982–17985.

[2] X. Prieur, et al., The human apolipoprotein AV gene is regulated by PPAR alpha and contains a novel FXR response element, J. Biol. Chem. 278 (2003) 25468–25480.

[3] B. Staels, Modulation of the PPAR-alpha signalling pathway: relevance for the metabolic syndrome and atherosclerosis, 2003. Second International Symposium on PPARS: From Basic Science to Clinical Applications, Florence (Italy).

[4] H. Duez, et al., Reduction of atherosclerosis by the peroxisome proliferator-activated receptor alpha agonist fenofibrate in mice, J. Biol. Chem. 277 (2002) 48051–48057.

[5] T. Kok, et al., Peroxisome proliferator-activated receptor alpha (PPARalpha)-mediated regulation of multi-drug resistance 2 (Mdr2) expression and function in mice, Biochem. J. 369 (2003) 539–547.

International Congress Series 1262 (2004) 30–38

www.ics-elsevier.com

Risk assessment of myocardial infarction and stroke

Gerd Assmann[a,b,*], Paul Cullen[a], Helmut Schulte[a]

[a] *Institute of Arteriosclerosis Research, University of Münster, Domagkstrasse 3, Münster 48149, Germany*
[b] *Institute of Clinical Chemistry and Laboratory Medicine, University of Münster, Münster, Germany*

Keywords: CHD risk; Myocardial infarction; Estimation

1. Introduction

Over the past approximately 10 years, there has been a steady change in emphasis in the assessment of risk of myocardial infarction and stroke, with a movement away from individual risk factors or risk factor quotients towards the concept of overall or "global" risk. The idea of global risk is that it attempts to combine information on as many independent risk factors as possible in order to provide a more accurate risk assessment. The aim of the present short review is to present some of the approaches to global risk assessment that have been published in recent years. This report is divided into three sections. Section 2 deals with methods for scoring risk of myocardial infarction that have been developed in Münster as part of the *Pro*spective *Ca*rdiovascular *M*ünster (PROCAM) study [1]. Section 3 deals with application of risk algorithms developed in PROCAM to the assessment of risk of stroke, while Section 4 compares and contrasts the PROCAM risk algorithms with risk algorithms presented elsewhere, most notably the recommendations of the Adult Treatment Panel III of the National Cholesterol Education Program of the United States of America [2] and the recently published Third Joint European Guidelines [3].

2. Scoring risk of myocardial infarction in PROCAM

2.1. Design of PROCAM

In discussing the risk algorithms derived from PROCAM, it is important to briefly review the design of this study [4].

The PROCAM study data in this report were obtained between 1979 and 1985. During this time, 20,060 employees of 52 companies and government authorities in the region of Münster and the northern Ruhr Valley region of Germany participated in the study. Since only people in employment were included, the results of PROCAM are subject to the

* Corresponding author. Tel.: +49-251-83-47222; fax: +49-251-83-47225.
E-mail address: assmann@uni-muenster.de (G. Assmann).

0531-5131/ © 2004 Published by Elsevier B.V.
doi:10.1016/j.ics.2004.01.100

"healthy worker" effect and possibly underestimate the true extent of morbidity and mortality in the German population.

The examination at study entry included a case history using standardized questionnaires, measurement of blood pressure and anthropometric data, a resting electrocardiogram, and collection of a blood sample after a 12-h fast for the determination of more than 20 laboratory parameters. The examination was carried out during paid working hours. Participation was voluntary, and between 40% and 80% (average 60%) of employees participated. There was no charge to the volunteers or to their employers (apart from time lost from work). All findings were reported to the participant's general practitioner, and the participant was told whether the results of the examination were normal or a check-up by the general practitioner might be advisable. The investigators neither carried out nor arranged for any intervention.

After the initial examination, questionnaires were sent to the participants of PROCAM every 2 years to determine the occurrence of myocardial infarction, stroke, or death. The response rate to these questionnaires was 96% after a maximum of two reminders per participant by mail and telephone, as required. In cases where the participant had died, the death certificate was reviewed. In cases where mortality and morbidity data were obtained from the questionnaire, hospital records, records from the attending physician, and an eyewitness account of death were requested. A Critical Event Committee meets at regular intervals to verify the diagnosis or cause of death of the participants of PROCAM. The initial examination was repeated after 6–7 years. Nonfatal myocardial infarction, fatal myocardial infarction, and sudden cardiac death were defined as "major coronary events" and were considered endpoints. This is in contrast to other studies, notably the Framingham study, which also included softer endpoints such as new occurrence of angina pectoris.

In the cohort of 5389 men aged 35–65 years recruited before the end of 1985, 325 major coronary events occurred within 10 years—enough to allow statistically valid longitudinal analysis. This cohort of middle-aged men forms the population in which the various PROCAM risk scores were derived.

2.2. Cox proportional hazards model

In order to extract the maximum information from our study population, we decided to construct our most recent risk algorithm using the Cox proportional hazards model. This model has several advantages over other techniques such as logistic regression: it accounts for variable duration of follow-up, censoring of subjects, proportionality of event occurrence, and time-to-event . Strictly speaking, the Cox model only allows calculation of relative risk. Therefore, in order to convert the results of the Cox model into absolute risk estimates, we calculated survival within our population using Kaplan–Meier statistics [5].

2.3. Scoring scheme

In order to increase the usefulness of the risk algorithm in clinical practice, we simulated it using a simple scoring scheme [4]. Each risk factor was divided into categories and a regression equation was calculated between the logarithm of global risk as calculated using the Cox model in conjunction with the survival curves, and the categories of each risk factor. The coefficients calculated in this manner were then standardized and rounded such that only whole numbers remained. The PROCAM scoring scheme is presented in Tables 1 and 2.

Table 1
The coefficients of the PROCAM scoring scheme

Age (years)	
35–39	0
40–44	6
45–49	11
50–54	16
55–59	21
60–64	26
LDL cholesterol (mg/dl)	
<100	0
100–129	5
130–159	10
160–189	14
≥190	20
HDL cholesterol (mg/dl)	
<35	11
35–44	8
45–54	5
≥55	0
Triglycerides (mg/dl)	
<100	0
100–149	2
150–199	3
≥200	4
Smoker	
No	0
Yes	8
Diabetes mellitus	
No	0
Yes	6
Myocardial infarction in family history	
No	0
Yes	4
Systolic blood pressure (mm Hg)	
<120	0
120–129	2
130–139	3
140–159	5
≥160	8

The categories for the continuous variables in the PROCAM score were based (in the case of age, blood pressure, LDL cholesterol, and HDL cholesterol) on the NCEP III guidelines and (in the case of triglycerides) on the guidelines of the International Task Force for Prevention of CHD.

2.4. Comparison of Cox model with scoring scheme

We compared the performance of our scoring system with that of the full Cox model in calculating the relative risk of an acute coronary event using receiver–operating characteristics (ROC) curve analysis (Fig. 1). While the area under the ROC curve obtained using the Cox function was 82.9%, the area under the ROC curve obtained with the PROCAM

Table 2
Risk of a coronary event associated with each PROCAM score

Number of points	0-year risk of a coronary event (%)
≤20	<1.0
21	1.1
22	1.2
23	1.3
24	1.4
25	1.6
26	1.7
27	1.8
28	1.9
29	2.3
30	2.4
31	2.8
32	2.9
33	3.3
34	3.5
35	4.0
36	4.2
37	4.8
38	5.1
39	5.7
40	6.1
41	7.0
42	7.4
43	8.0
44	8.8
45	10.2
46	10.5
47	10.7
48	12.8
49	13.2
50	15.5
51	16.8
52	17.5
53	19.6
54	21.7
55	22.2
56	23.8
57	25.1
58	28.0
59	29.4
≥60	≥30.0

scoring scheme did not differ significantly at 82.4% ($p=0.251$), indicating that the ability of the PROCAM scoring scheme to predict the relative risk of an acute coronary event was equivalent to that of the full PROCAM Cox algorithm.

2.5. Neural network analysis

A potential drawback of standard models such as the Cox proportional hazards approach or logistic regression analysis is that they are constrained by the mathematical assumptions underlying them, and may therefore fail to completely reflect complex nonlinear relationships that may exist between risk factors. Artificial neural networks

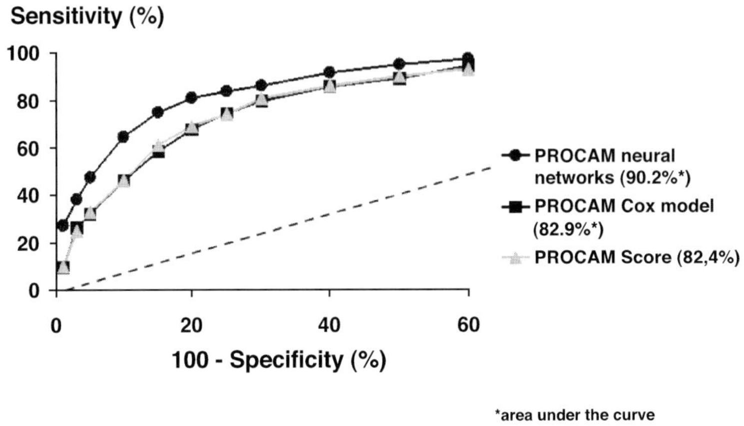

Fig. 1. ROC curve analysis of the performance of a neural network derived from the PROCAM study, a PROCAM Cox proportional hazards model, and a simple risk score derived from this Cox model.

represent a newer technique that has emerged as a potential alternative to logistic regression analysis and other classical statistical techniques. Neural networks are not constrained by a predefined mathematical relationship between dependent and independent variables, and can model any arbitrarily complex nonlinear relationship. Thus, when such complex nonlinear relationships exist in the data, neural network models may provide better generalization than conventional regression techniques.

We therefore used neural network analysis to estimate the risk of major coronary events during the 10-year follow-up among 5159 men aged 35–65 years at recruitment into PROCAM [6]. In this analysis, neural networks proved superior to both the PROCAM Cox model and the PROCAM score, with an area under the ROC curve of 90.2% (Fig. 1). The power of neural network analysis was particularly evident in persons at the extremes of risk. Thus, while the mean 10-year risk of a major coronary event within the top decile

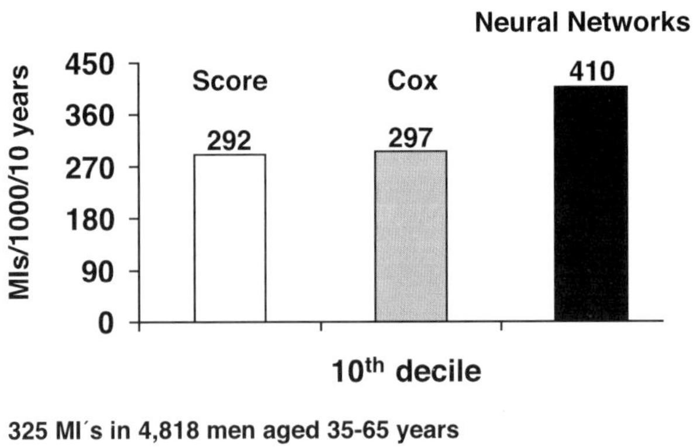

Fig. 2. Observed coronary event risk in the top risk decile as estimated using the PROCAM risk score, the PROCAM Cox model, and a neural network derived from PROCAM.

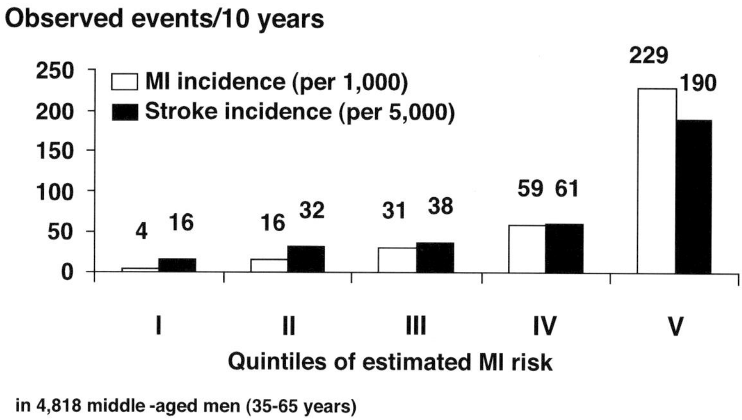

Fig. 3. Observed cases of stroke and myocardial infarction in each of the five quintiles of the PROCAM algorithm (Cox proportional hazards model for risk of myocardial infarction).

of estimated risk was 29% with the PROCAM score and 30% with the PROCAM Cox model, no fewer than 41% of all men in the top decile of risk as defined using neural networks suffered a major coronary event (Fig. 2).

3. Applying the PROCAM algorithms to assessing risk of stroke

Much controversy has surrounded the question as to whether the risk factors for myocardial infarction also apply to risk of stroke. In PROCAM, this appears to be the case, with the progression of 10-year stroke incidence in each of the five quintiles of risk as defined by the PROCAM algorithm very similar to that of major coronary events (Fig. 3). Note that the absolute risk of stroke in PROCAM was about one fifth that of myocardial infarction.

4. Comparison of the PROCAM risk scores with other risk algorithms

Within the last year, three sets of international recommendations have been published for the assessment of coronary risk. The first, published jointly by the International Task Force for Prevention of Coronary Heart Disease and the International Atherosclerosis Society, was based largely on the results of PROCAM [1]. The recommendations of the Third Adult Treatment Panel of the National Cholesterol Education Program (ATP III) were based mainly on the results of the Framingham study, a prospective epidemiological investigation of the residents of Framingham, a mainly blue collar suburb of Boston. The Framingham study was begun in the late 1940s and is still continuing today [2]. The third set of recommendations, the Third Joint European Guidelines, was published by the European Cardiology Societies and other societies on Cardiovascular Disease Prevention and were based on the results of the European SCORE project [7]. In contrast to PROCAM and Framingham, which were prospective studies, SCORE assembled the data of 12 European cohort studies comprising 88,080 women and 117,098 men aged 18–80 years with a total of 2.7 million years of observation. The

Third Joint European Guidelines use a risk of cardiovascular death of at least 5% in 10 years as their basis for deciding on the use of medication, and assumed that this 5% 10-year mortality risk corresponded to the more commonly used definition of high risk, namely a 10-year coronary event risk (morbidity+mortality) of at least 20%. In addition, the Joint European Guidelines differentiated between countries at high risk, such as Germany, and countries at low risk, such as those in the Mediterranean region (Table 3). A source of confusion for German epidemiologists is the fact that while the Joint European Guidelines refer to Germany as a high-risk region, as noted above, the SCORE project itself classifies Germany [in the form of Augsburg cohort of the World Health Organization Monitoring of Trends in Cardiovascular Disease (MONICA) project] as being a low-risk country [7]. We had also commented critically on the approach used in SCORE on other grounds. In particular, we noted that the conflation of coronary and cerebrovascular endpoints (each of which has its own distinct set of risk factors), the exclusive use of mortality data, and the failure to include important risk factors such as triglycerides and family history are major drawbacks [9].

Very recently, von Eckardstein et al. compared the abilities of these three sets of recommendations in predicting coronary risk among the male participants in PROCAM. The recommendations of the International Task Force/International Atherosclerosis Society showed the greatest specificity (94.5%), positive predictive power (32.0%), and diagnostic efficiency (90.5%), while the Third Joint European Guidelines showed the greatest sensitivity (64.6%) but the lowest specificity (77.9%), positive predictive power (17.5%), and diagnostic efficiency (77.0%). The values for the ATP III guidelines were intermediate between these two extremes (Table 3).

The most important criterion for comparing these three sets of recommendations is the predictive power of a positive test; that is, what is the ability of the "high-risk" classification (10-year coronary event risk >20%) to accurately identify those at high risk? Clearly, this was greatest with the ITF/IAS guidelines. It should be noted in this regard, however, that the Von Eckardstein et al. [8] comparison contained an intrinsic bias towards the ITF/IAS guidelines, since these were evaluated in the population in which they had been derived.

The false-positive rate was highest with the Third Joint European Guidelines, the use of which identified no fewer than 25% of all men in PROCAM as being at high risk,

Table 3
Comparison of the guidelines of the International Taskforce for Prevention of Coronary Heart Disease/International Atherosclerosis Society (ITF/IAS) of the Third Adult Treatment Panel of the National Cholesterol Education Panel of the United States of America (ATP III) and of the Third Joint European Guidelines (3JE) in terms of their ability to predict coronary events among the male participants in the PROCAM study

	ITF/IAS (%)	ATP III (%)	3JE (%)	
			Low-risk model	High-risk model
Diagnostic specificity	94.5	91.1	88.4	77.9
Diagnostic sensitivity	35.7	34.5	39.7	64.6
Predictive power of positive test	32.0	21.9	19.8	17.5
Predictive power of negative test	95.3	95.1	95.3	96.8
Diagnostic efficiency	90.5	87.3	85.1	77.0

compared with only 7.5% using the ITF/IAS guidelines. Thus, use of the Third Joint European Guidelines will lead to substantial overtreatment of the population.

5. Conclusions

Powerful tools are now available for the objective assessment of coronary risk. These involve the assessment of global risk using risk scores or algorithms to assess the totality of a person's risk factors. Comparison of recent scores indicates that the recommendations of the International Task Force/International Atherosclerosis Society are most accurate at identifying high-risk individuals and therefore provide the best basis for deciding on the need for intensive therapy. These comparisons highlight the fact that even with a circumscribed geographical region such as continental Europe, significant variation of absolute risk may be seen among persons with similar risk profiles. For this reason, an algorithm derived in one population may give an incorrect estimate of absolute risk when used in another, and may require adjustment before serving as the basis for treatment decisions [10–15].

Finally, even using the ITF/IAS guidelines, the predictive power of a positive test result (i.e., risk estimated to exceed 20% in 10 years) was only 32%, indicating that there is much room for improvement of risk prediction by means of newer biochemical or genetic risk factors or noninvasive imaging.

References

[1] International Task Force for Prevention of Coronary Heart Disease, Pocket Guide to Prevention of Coronary Heart Disease (http://www.chd-taskforce.de/guide.htm).

[2] Executive Summary of the Third Report of the National Cholesterol Education Program (NCEP) Expert Panel on Detection, Evaluation, and Treatment of High Blood Cholesterol in Adults (Adult Treatment Panel III), JAMA 285 (2001) 2486–2497 (http://www.nhlbi.nih.gov/guidelines/cholesterol).

[3] G. De Backer, et al., European guidelines on cardiovascular disease prevention in clinical practice: Third Joint Task Force of European and other Societies on Cardiovascular Disease Prevention in Clinical Practice (constituted by representatives of eight societies and by invited experts), Eur. Heart J. 24 (2003) 1601–1610 (http://www.escardio.org).

[4] G. Assmann, P. Cullen, H. Schulte, Simple scoring scheme for calculating the risk of acute coronary events based on the 10-year follow-up of the prospective cardiovascular Munster (PROCAM) study, Circulation 105 (2002) 310–315.

[5] P.W. Wilson, et al., Prediction of coronary heart disease using risk factor categories, Circulation 97 (1998) 1837–1847.

[6] R. Voss, et al., Prediction of risk of coronary events in middle-aged men in the PROCAM study using neural networks, Int. J. Epidemiol. 31 (2002) 1253–1262.

[7] R.M. Conroy, et al., SCORE project group. Estimation of ten-year risk of fatal cardiovascular disease in Europe: the SCORE project, Eur. Heart J. 4 (2003) 987–1003.

[8] A. Von Eckardstein, H. Schulte, G. Assmann, Vergleich internationaler Konsensus-Empfehlungen zur Erkennung des präsymptomatischen Hochrisikopatienten für den Herzinfarkt in Deutschland, Z. Kardiol. (2004) (in press).

[9] G. Assmann, et al., Response to Conroy et al. SCORE Project, Eur. Heart J. 24 (2003) 2070.

[10] H.W. Hense, et al., Framingham risk function overestimates risk of coronary heart disease in men and women from Germany—results from the MONICA Augsburg and the PROCAM cohorts, Eur. Heart J. 24 (2003) 937–945.

[11] J.P. Empana, et al., Are the Framingham and PROCAM coronary heart disease risk functions applicable to different European populations? The PRIME Study, Eur. Heart J. 24 (2003) 1903–1911.

[12] J. Marrugat, et al., An adaptation of the Framingham coronary heart disease risk function to European Mediterranean areas, J. Epidemiol. Community Health 57 (2003) 634–638.
[13] A. Menotti, P.E. Puddu, M. Lanti, Comparison of the Framingham risk function-based coronary chart with risk function from an Italian population study, Eur. Heart J. 21 (2000) 365–370.
[14] I.U. Haq, et al., Is the Framingham risk function valid for northern European populations? A comparison of methods for estimating absolute coronary risk in high risk men, Heart 81 (1999) 40–46.
[15] A.F. Jones, et al., Comparative accuracy of cardiovascular risk prediction methods in primary care patients, Heart 85 (2001) 37–43.

International Congress Series 1262 (2004) 39–44

www.ics-elsevier.com

Understanding atherothrombosis: from vulnerable plaque to vulnerable patient

Pedro R. Moreno[a,b,*], Roberto Corti[a], Valentin Fuster[a]

[a] *The Zena and Michael Wiener Cardiovascular Institute, Mount Sinai School of Medicine, Mount Sinai Medical Center, P.O. Box 1030, One Gustave L. Levy Place, New York, NY 10029, USA*
[b] *University of Kentucky, Lexington, KY, USA*

Keywords: Atherosclerosis; Thrombosis; Plaque; Remodeling; Neovascularization

1. Introduction

Despite dramatic improvements in diagnosis and therapy, coronary atherothrombosis remains the first cause of death in western countries and will become the first cause of death worldwide within a few years [1,2].

Multiple pathological, angiographic and clinical studies suggest that atherosclerosis, a systemic disease that can be quiescent for years, dramatically changes the natural history when complicated by coronary thrombosis [3]. High-risk plaques (local) and increased thrombogenicity (systemic) interact to precipitate coronary thrombosis. This review presents a mechanistic approach of the current understanding of atherothrombosis.

2. High-risk plaques

Collagenolysis of thin cap fibroatheromas, mediated by macrophage metalloproteinase expression leads to plaque rupture, the main cause of coronary atherothrombosis [4]. More recently, new structural and functional high-risk plaque features have been identified including (1) vascular remodeling; (2) rupture of the internal elastic lamina (IEL); and (3) vasa vasorum neovascularization with lipid core expansion and intraplaque hemorrhage.

2.1. Vascular remodeling

The normal vessel wall is an active, integrated organ composed of endothelial, smooth muscle, and fibroblast cells coupled in a complex autocrine–paracrine set of interactions [5]. In diseased vessels, arterial remodeling allows for plaque growth without significant obstruction of the arterial lumen [6]. Atherosclerotic plaques undergoing remodeling are

* Corresponding author. The Zena and Michael Wiener Cardiovascular Institute, Mount Sinai School of Medicine, Mount Sinai Medical Center, P.O. Box 1030, One Gustave L. Levy Place, New York, NY 10029, USA. Tel.: +1-212-241-3681; fax: +1-212-534-2845.

E-mail address: pedro.moreno@msnyuhealth.org (P.R. Moreno).

0531-5131/ © 2004 Published by Elsevier B.V.
doi:10.1016/j.ics.2004.01.121

characterized by large lipid core, less smooth muscle cells and increased macrophage infiltration [7,8].

2.2. Rupture of internal elastic lamina and vasa vasorum neovascularization

Remodeling is associated with matrix metalloproteinase expression leading to rupture of another important structure, the internal elastic lamina (IEL) [9,10]. This sudden decompression of vessel wall tension may play a role in fibrous cap rupture. Recent studies identified a strong association between rupture of IEL and fibrous cap rupture, along with inflammation in the tunica media and the adventitia [11].

The first step of remodeling is characterized by overexpansion of the vessel wall associated with extensive vasa vasorum neovascularization preceding endothelial dysfunction, the hallmark of early atherosclerosis [12,13]. Multiple studies have also shown that vasa vasorum may have a crucial role in the pathogenesis of early atherosclerosis [13–22].

The vasa vasorum surrounds the adventitia and outer media of large vessels including the aorta, coronary, femoral and carotid arteries. In the coronary arteries, vasa originate from bifurcation segments of epicardial vessels [23]. Their main function is to nurture the vessel wall with a number of vasa vasorum that remains constant throughout life [24]. However, in atherosclerosis, vasa can proliferate leading to extensive neovascularization involving the tunica media and the intima of diseased vessels [25].

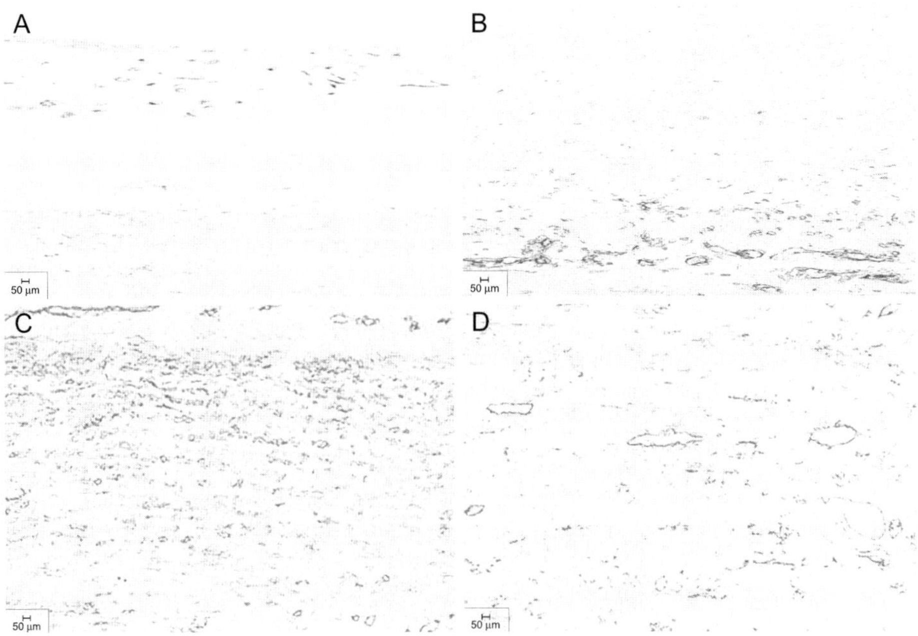

Fig. 1. Histologic examples of plaque and vessel wall neovessels identified by light microscopy in CD-34 immunostained stained sections. (A) Vessels in the fibrous cap, (B) Neovessels in the base of the plaque, (C) Neovessels in the tunica media, (D) Neovessels in the tunica adventitia.

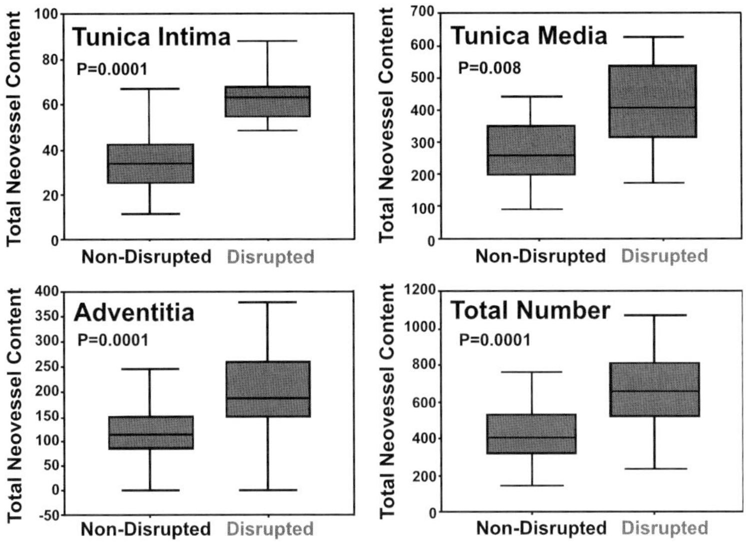

Fig. 2. Box plots showing the median (25th–75th quartile) number of microvessels in nondisrupted (n=55) compared with the number of microvessels in disrupted (n=117) human atherosclerotic plaques. Comparisons of microvessel content within intimal, medial, adventitial, and total vessel wall between nondisrupted and disrupted plaques are presented.

Studies of vasa vasorum in complex atherosclerosis using immunohistochemistry (Fig. 1) have identified increased neovessel content in ruptured plaques from the human aorta (Fig. 2) [26]. High-risk features of plaque vulnerability including inflammation, fibrous cap thickness, lipid core area and neovessel content were studied simultaneously to identify predictors of plaque rupture. Multiple logistic regression analysis identified neovessel content as the most powerful independent predictor of plaque rupture (Fig. 3) [27]. Furthermore, plaques from patients with diabetes mellitus were characterized by increased neovessel content, higher inflammation and intraplaque hemorrhage suggesting a micro-angiopathic process in diabetes atherosclerosis [28].

Independent Predictors for Plaque Disruption Multiple Regression Analysis	*P* Value
Number of Vasa Vasorum at Plaque Base	0.0001
Rupture of Internal Elastic Lamina (%)	0.01
Fibrous Cap Thickness (microns)	0.02
Percent Lipid Area (%)	0.025
Total Intimal Plaque Area (mm2)	0.031

Fig. 3. Multiple logistic regression analysis to identify independent associations with plaque rupture.

Vasa vasorum may also be involved in the process of plaque regression. When compared with lipid-rich plaques, fibrocalcific lesions with reduced lipid area—also known as regression-type lesions—had the lowest microvessel content [29]. Of clinical relevance, this latter observation is in agreement with insightful observations by Corti et al. [30], using sequential MRI testing in patients undergoing aggressive lipid lowering therapy for 24 months. These studies documented for the first time, in vivo the morphological pathway for plaque regression. Plaque area was reduced from the adventitia before improving lumen area. More recently, the Reversal trial confirmed the same inverse Glagovian phenomena for plaque regression after aggressive lipid-lowering therapy in coronary artery disease [31]. Therefore, vasa vasorum may serve as a potential pathway for reverse lipid transport. As cholesterol exits the plaque, neovascularization may also experience regression. This observation, previously validated in experimental animal models may also apply for human disease [32].

3. Increased thrombogenicity: the concept of high-risk blood

In addition to macrophage expression of tissue factor (TF), blood-borne TF may play a critical role in the propagation of thrombosis [33]. Polymorphonuclear leukocytes are involved in the transport of TF to platelets by a CD15-dependent mechanism [34]. Furthermore, circulating TF microparticles have been described in patients with ACS [35], and may be increased in patients with coronary risk factors. To test the hypothesis that diabetes, smoking and hyperlipemia, have increased blood-borne TF, Sambola et al. [38] immunocaptured TF from plasma and quantified factor Xa generation in the presence of factor VIIa. Diabetic patients showed increased circulating TF and increased blood thrombogenicity, assessed as thrombus formation on the Badimon perfusion chamber. Furthermore, both parameters were significantly increased 2 h after smoking two cigarettes. Finally, hypercholesterolemic patients showed higher TF than healthy volunteers suggesting that high levels of circulating TF may play a role in the increased thrombotic complications associated with the presence of cardiovascular risk factors [36].

One major question relates to the source of circulating TF. Corti et al. [37] linked the apoptotic phenomena to atherothrombosis and to the production of TF. Furthermore, Sambola et al. [38] showed that apoptosis of plaque macrophages colocalize with TF expression, suggesting a potential pathogenic mechanism leading to increased plaque thrombogenicity. Apoptotic death of macrophages leads to shedding of membrane microparticles exposing phosphatidylserine and conferring potent procoagulant activity. The shed particles account for almost all the TF activity, activating thrombosis after plaque rupture [39,40].

4. High-risk patient: burden of atherothrombosis

Despite plaque vulnerability and blood thrombogenicity, patient risk stratification is a systemic process that needs careful attention to traditional and novel risk factors for inflammation and thrombosis [41,42]. Quantification of atherosclerotic burden by electron beam computerized planimetry (EBCT), multidetector CT (MDCT) and magnetic resonance angiography are emerging as adjunctive tests in the evaluation of patients at risk for cardiovascular events.

4.1. Coronary calcification

Coronary calcium is only observed in atherosclerotic lesions. Higher calcium scores correlate with older age, increased number of risk factors, and greater extent of atherosclerosis. A metaanalysis [43] of five studies involving asymptomatic persons gave higher calcium scores a relative risk for coronary events of 4.2 (95% confidence interval, 1.6–11). The recent prospective, longitudinal study of 5585 asymptomatic patients showed an incidence of cardiovascular events in 122 patients (0.6%/year). Mean calcium scores were greater in patients with events (584±775 versus 142±381; $P<0.0001$), and predicted cardiovascular events independently from coronary risk factors and the Framingham risk score. Relative risks [95% CI] were 5.9 [3–12] for a score≥0 and 8.0 [5–12) for a score≥600 [44]. Therefore, documenting presence or absence of coronary calcification may offer a unique opportunity for proper risk stratification in clinical practice [45].

4.2. Noninvasive coronary angiography

Assessment of coronary stenosis can be obtained using intravenous contrast with EBCT, with multidetector CT (MD-CT), and with coronary magnetic resonance angiography (CMRA) with sensitivity/specificity of 75–94%. A recent review from our group summarized the advantages of each technique [46]. Magnetic resonance does not use ionizing radiation and does not require contrast. Furthermore, CMRA has been successfully used to study atherosclerotic plaques in human carotid, aortic, and coronary arteries. The superficial location and relative absence of motion in carotid arteries presents less of a technical challenge than coronary arteries, offering excellent soft tissue contrast. Therefore, both MDCT and CMRA are evolving as useful, noninvasive tests to evaluate coronary artery disease. Further improvements will promptly allow for complete evaluation of atherosclerosis noninvasively in the near future.

5. Conclusion

Multiple evolving concepts have emerged in the pathophysiology of atherothrombosis. Plaque neovascularization is now considered a major factor in progression of the disease and may offer potential avenues for stabilization and regression. Circulating tissue factor increases blood thrombogenicity through several pathways including leukocyte–platelet interaction and monocyte apoptosis. Most importantly, increased blood thrombogenicity can be reduced with proper therapy, setting a new therapeutic target for patients with traditional risk factors including diabetes, cigarette smoking and hypercholesterolemia. In addition, novel risk factors for inflammation are now in clinical practice providing better evaluation of ongoing treatment for prevention. Finally, atherosclerotic burden can now be quantified using noninvasive techniques, giving clinicians an additional risk stratification tool in the challenging field of cardiovascular prevention and therapy.

Acknowledgements

Partial support by grants from NIH SCOR HL54469 and NHLBI HL61801 (VF). Dr. Corti was supported by a grant from The Swiss National Research Foundation and is currently working at the University Hospital Zurich, Switzerland.

References

[1] C. Lenfant, N. Engl. J. Med. 349 (2003) 868–874.
[2] V. Fuster, Circulation 99 (1999) 1132–1137.
[3] V. Fuster, et al., J. Thromb. Haemost. 7 (2003) 1410–1421.
[4] P. Libby, Nature 420 (2002) 868–874.
[5] G. Gibbons, V.J. Dzau, N. Engl. J. Med. 330 (1994) 1431–1438.
[6] S. Glagov, et al., N. Engl. J. Med. 316 (1987) 1371–1375.
[7] G. Pasterkamp, et al., J. Am. Coll. Cardiol. 32 (1998) 655–662.
[8] P. Schoenhagen, et al., Circulation 101 (2000) 598–603.
[9] G. Pasterkamp, et al, Atherosclerosis 150 (2000) 245–253.
[10] F. Tronc, et al., Arterioscler. Thromb. Vasc. Biol. 20 (2000) E120–E126.
[11] P.R. Moreno, et al., Circulation 105 (2002) 2504–2511.
[12] S.H. Wilson, et al., Circulation 105 (2002) 415–418.
[13] J. Herrmann, et al., Cardiovasc. Res. 51 (2001) 762–766.
[14] Y. Nakata, et al., Nature 212 (1966) 1258–1259.
[15] A.C. Barger III, et al., N. Engl. J. Med. 310 (1984) 175–177.
[16] R.F.G. Martin, et al., Eur. J. Clin. Investig. 21 (1991) 355–359.
[17] C.I. Stefanadis, et al., Cardiovasc. Res. 27 (1993) 951–956.
[18] S.G.E. Barker, et al., Arterioscler. Thromb. Vasc. Biol. 13 (1993) 70–77.
[19] S.G.E. Barker, et al., Atherosclerosis 105 (1994) 131–144.
[20] G.R.Y. De Mayer, et al, Arterioscler. Thromb. Vasc. Biol. 17 (1997) 1924–1930.
[21] K.S. Moulton, et al., Circulation 99 (1999) 1726–1732.
[22] D.D. Heistad, et al., Blood Vessels 16 (1979) 225–238.
[23] H.M. Kwon, et al., J. Clin. Invest. 101 (1998) 1551–1556.
[24] R.S. Scotland, et al., Cardiovasc. Res. 46 (2000) 403–411.
[25] M. Kumamoto, et al., Human Pathol. 26 (1995) 450–456.
[26] P.R. Moreno, et al., JACC 35 (2000) 275A.
[27] K.R. Purushothaman, et al., JACC 41 (6 Suppl. B) (2003) 352–353.
[28] K.R. Purushothaman, et al., Circulation 108 (IV-98) (2003) 459.
[29] P.R. Moreno, et al., Circulation II-703 (2002) 3468.
[30] R. Corti, et al., Circulation 106 (2002) 2884–2887.
[31] S. Nissen, Reversal Trial. American Heart Association Meeting, http://www.prous.com/aha2003/home.asp.
[32] S.G. Worthley, et al., Circulation 101 (2000) 586–589.
[33] P.L. Giesen, et al., Proc. Natl. Acad. Sci. U. S. A. 96 (1999) 2311–2315.
[34] U. Rauch, et al., Blood 96 (2000) 170–175.
[35] H. Soejima, et al., Circulation 99 (1999) 2908–2913.
[36] Z. Mallat, et al., Circulation 101 (8) (2000) 841–843.
[37] R. Corti, et al., Eur. Heart J., Suppl., (Suppl. 4) (2002) A31–A41.
[38] A. Sambola, et al., Circulation 107 (2003) 973–977.
[39] Z. Mallat, et al., Circ. Res. 88 (10) (2001) 998–1003.
[40] R. Hutter, et al., J. Am. Coll. Cardiol. 37 (2 suppl. A) (2001) 288A.
[41] P.M. Ridker, et al., Circulation 107 (3) (2003 (Jan. 28)) 363–369.
[42] NCEP Panel, JAMA 285 (2001) 2486–2497.
[43] P.G. O'Malley, et al., Am. J. Cardiol. 85 (2000) 945–948.
[44] A.D. Guerci, St. Francis Study, http://www.acc03online.acc.org/ondemand/trials3/sessions.asp?sid=3.
[45] P. Greenland, et al., N. Engl. J. Med. 349 (2003) 465–473.
[46] Z.A. Fayad, et al., Circulation 106 (2002 (Oct.)) 2026–2034.

Symposium

International Congress Series 1262 (2004) 47–50

www.ics-elsevier.com

PPARγ fundamental role in adipogenesis

Terrie-Anne Cock[a], Johan Auwerx[a,b,*]

[a] *Institut de Génétique et de Biologie Moléculaire et Cellulaire, CNRS/INSERM/Université Louis Pasteur, 67404 Illkirch, France*

[b] *Institut Clinique de la Souris, Génopole Strasbourg, 67404 Illkirch, France*

Abstract. The peroxisomeproliferator-activated receptor gamma (PPARγ) is a nuclear receptor that integrates the control of lipid and glucose homeostasis. The actions of PPARγ are mediated by two protein isoforms, the widely expressed PPARγ1 and adipose tissue-restricted PPARγ2 with an additional 28 amino acids in the NH_2-terminus. The effects of the absence of PPARγ has not been extensively characterized in vivo since the PPARγ mice are embryonic lethal, therefore we generated mice that carry a hypomorphic mutation at the PPARγ2 locus, yielding a WAT-specific PPARγ knockdown. The PPARγ$^{hyp/hyp}$ mouse model demonstrates that PPARγ is the master regulator of adipogenesis. Furthermore this model highlights PPARγ fundamental roles in whole body physiology to maintain the metabolic and endocrine functions of white adipose tissue.

Keywords: Peroxisome proliferator-activated receptor gamma; PPARγ; Nuclear receptor; Lipid and glucose metabolism; Mouse model; Adipogenesis; Metabolism

1. Introduction

The peroxisome proliferator-activated receptor gamma (PPARγ) is a prototypical metabolic nuclear receptor involved in the transcriptional control of energy, lipid, and glucose homeostasis. The activity of PPARγ is governed by binding of small lipophilic ligands, mainly fatty acids, derived from nutrition or metabolic pathways, or synthetic agonists, like thiazolidinediones. Docking of these ligands in the ligand-binding pocket alters the conformation of PPARγ resulting in transcriptional activation subsequent to the release of corepressors and the recruitment of coactivators. The actions of PPARγ are mediated by two protein isoforms, the widely expressed PPARγ1 and adipose tissue-restricted PPARγ2, both produced from a single gene by alternative splicing and dif-

* Corresponding author. Institut de Génétique et de Biologie Moléculaire et Cellulaire, Orphan Nuclear Receptors, B.P. 10142, 1 rue Laurent Fries, F-67404 Illkirch, France. Tel.: +33-3-88-65-3425; fax: +33-3-88-65-3200.

E-mail address: auwerx@igbmc.u-strasbg.fr (J. Auwerx).

0531-5131/
doi:10.1016/S0531-5131(03)01767-9

fering only by an additional 28 amino acids in the NH_2-terminus of PPARγ2 (reviewed Ref. [1]).

2. PPARγ the master regulator of adipogenesis

The initial suggestion that PPARγ stimulated adipogenesis was based on the observation that overexpression of PPARγ in cells was by itself sufficient to induce adipocyte differentiation [2]. Targeted mutagenesis of the PPARγ gene in ES cells and knocking down the endogenous PPARγ2 in cell lines confirmed the commanding role of PPARγ in adipocyte differentiation [3,4]. Consistent with this, PPARγ increases the expression of genes that promote fatty acid storage, whereas it represses genes that induce lipolysis in adipocytes. The lipodystrophy in the sole PPARγ$^{-/-}$ mice, rescued by tetraploid aggregation [5], and the characterization of mice chimeric for PPARγ$^{-/-}$ ES cells [3], further underscored the importance of PPARγ in adipose tissue development in vivo.

Human genetic studies further support the important role of PPARγ in adipogenesis. One of the loci with suggestive linkage to obesity in the Pima Indians maps close to the location of *PPARG* on 3p25-p24[6]. Furthermore, subjects with the partial "loss-of-function" Pro12Ala mutation in the PPARγ2-specific B exon have a lower body mass index (BMI), whereas carriers of the dominant negative Pro467Leu and Val290Met mutations or the Phe388Leu mutation that has a reduced affinity to ligand have partial lipodystrophy. Conversely, carriers of the Pro115Gln substitution, that renders PPARγ constitutively active, are extremely obese [7,8]. A final line in favor of a role of PPARγ in adipogenesis comes from pharmacological studies, which demonstrate that PPARγ agonists, such as the thiazolidinediones, invariably increase WAT mass, whereas sub-optimal PPARγ activation, or PPARγ antagonism, is neutral or even reverses weight gain [7].

The effects of the absence of PPARγ has not been extensively characterized in vivo since the PPARγ$^{-/-}$ mice die during intra-uterine development due to defects in cardiac and placental development in vivo [9–11]. Therefore, we generated by homologous recombination, mice that carry a hypomorphic mutation at the PPARγ2 locus, yielding a WAT-specific PPARγ knockdown (PPARγ$^{hyp/hyp}$) [12]. These mice have virtually no expression of PPARγ in the sparse white adipose tissue (WAT), but not in other tissues. One-week-old mice with this WAT-specific PPARγ knockdown display a lipodystrophic phenotype similar to that of humans with congenital generalized lipodystrophy (CGL). In CGL, the adipose deficiency normally is accompanied by severe insulin resistance, hyperglycemia, and fatty liver throughout life [13]. The neonatal PPARγ$^{hyp/hyp}$ phenotype mirrors most of these CGL characteristics, whereas the adult PPARγ$^{hyp/hyp}$ mice overcome some of the complications associated with the absence of WAT. In fact, adult PPARγ$^{hyp/hyp}$ mice do not have a fatty liver or show signs of hyperlipidemia [12]. The PPARγ$^{hyp/hyp}$ mice are furthermore only mildly glucose intolerant, which is distinct from most other lipodystrophy models [14–17]. This suggests that other physiological compensatory mechanisms ameliorate metabolic homeostasis in the PPARγ$^{hyp/hyp}$ mice. Overall the PPARγ$^{hyp/hyp}$ mouse model reveals that the PPARγ locus is the critical regulator of adipogenesis in vivo [12].

3. WAT's place in the scheme of energy metabolism

The comparison of the physiological abnormalities in PPARγ$^{hyp/hyp}$ and PPARγ heterozygote mice provides further insights into how the actions of PPARγ in adipose tissue, liver, muscle and heart coordinate glucose and lipid homeostasis. Ubiquitous reduction of PPARγ in all tissues, such as the PPARγ heterozygote mice, results in normal body weight; these mice are insulin sensitive and resistant to diet-induced obesity [9,11]. In these PPARγ heterozygote mice, circulating lipids can be stored in WAT, which avoids lipid overload in other tissues hence maintaining normal glucose and lipid metabolism [12]. In comparison, the PPARγ$^{hyp/hyp}$ mice with reduced PPARγ levels in WAT have almost no WAT and are mildly glucose intolerant. Our study therefore implicates WAT as an important target tissue for PPARγ activation to maintain glucose tolerance. Treatment with thiazolidinedione PPARγ agonists can overcome the glucose intolerance in PPARγ$^{hyp/hyp}$ mice, although insulin resistance is not corrected. The PPARγ agonist results from our WAT PPARγ$^{hyp/hyp}$ mice together with recent data in liver and muscle specific PPARγ knockout mice indicate that primarily the WAT and not the liver and muscle are crucial for the protective effects of PPARγ agonist on insulin resistance [12,18–20].

4. Selective modulation is the key

The near absence of PPARγ in WAT in adult PPARγ$^{hyp/hyp}$ mice is only causing a slightly abnormal metabolic profile and is rather well tolerated. Taken all together this lends further support to the hypothesis that selective PPARγ modulators (or SPRMs) with a partial agonist or antagonist profile, rather than full agonists (reviewed in Ref. [7]), could be the preferred therapeutic strategy to treat the metabolic disorders associated with obesity, such as the metabolic syndrome, insulin resistance, or type 2 diabetes mellitus. The genetic evidence obtained in the PPARγ$^{hyp/hyp}$ mice arguments that selective PPARγ modulators which have a reduced adipogenic drive, but which maintain agonist activity in other tissues, might maintain glucose homeostasis in such metabolic disorders.

Acknowledgements

This work was supported by grants from CNRS, INSERM, Hôpitaux Universitaires de Strasbourg, European Union, and NIH.

References

[1] J. Auwerx, PPARγ, the ultimate thrifty gene, Diabetologia 42 (42) (1999) 1033–1049.

[2] P. Tontonoz, E. Hu, B.M. Spiegelman, Stimulation of adipogenesis in fibroblasts by PPARγ2, a lipid-activated transcription factor, Cell 79 (1994) 1147–1156.

[3] E.D. Rosen, P. Sarraf, A.E. Troy, et al., PPARgamma is required for the differentiation of adipose tissue in vivo and in vitro, Mol. Cell 4 (1999) 611–617.

[4] D. Ren, T.N. Collingwood, E.J. Rebar, et al., PPARgamma knockdown by engineered transcription factors: exogenous PPARgamma2 but not PPARgamma1 reactivates adipogenesis, Genes Dev. 16 (1) (2002) 27–32.

[5] Y. Barak, D. Liao, W. Hem, et al., Effects of peroxisome proliferator-activated receptor delta on placentation, adiposity, and colorectal cancer, Proc. Natl. Acad. Sci. U. S. A. 99 (1) (2002) 303–308.

[6] R.A. Norman, D.B. Thompson, T. Foroud, et al., Genomewide search for genes influencing percent body fat in Pima indians: suggestive linkage at chromosome 11Q21 Q22, Am. J. Hum. Genet. 60 (1997) 166–173.
[7] F. Picard, J. Auwerx, PPAR(gamma) and glucose homeostasis, Annu. Rev. Nutr. 22 (2002) 167–197.
[8] M. Gurnell, D.B. Savage, V.K. Chatterjee, S. O'Rahilly, The metabolic syndrome: peroxisome proliferator-activated receptor gamma and its therapeutic modulation, J. Clin. Endocrinol. Metab. 88 (6) (2003) 2412–2421.
[9] N. Kubota, Y. Terauchi, H. Miki, et al., PPARg mediates high-fat diet-induced adipocyte hypertrophy and insulin resistance, Mol. Cell 4 (1999) 597–609.
[10] Y. Barak, M.C. Nelson, E.S. Ong, et al., PPARgamma is required for placental, cardiac, and adipose tissue development, Mol. Cell 4 (1999) 585–595.
[11] P.D. Miles, Y. Barak, W. He, et al., Improved insulin-sensitivity in mice heterozygous for PPAR-gamma deficiency, J. Clin. Invest. 105 (3) (2000) 287–292.
[12] H. Koutnikova, T.-A. Cock, M. Wanatabe, et al., Compensation by the muscle limits the metabolic consequences of lipodystrophy in PPARg hypomorphic mice, Proc. Natl. Acad. Sci. U. S. A. (2003).
[13] A. Garg, Lipodystrophies, Am. J. Med. 108 (2) (2000) 143–152.
[14] J. Moitra, M.M. Mason, M. Olive, et al., Life without fat: a transgenic mouse, Genes Dev. 12 (1998) 3168–3181.
[15] I. Shimomura, R.E. Hammer, J.A. Richardson, et al., Insulin resistance and diabetes mellitus in transgenic mice expressing nuclear SREBP-1c in adipose tissue: model for congenital generalized lipodystrophy, Genes Dev. 12 (20) (1998) 3182–3194.
[16] I. Shimomura, R.E. Hammer, S. Ikemoto, et al., Leptin reverses insulin resistance and diabetes mellitus in mice with congenital lipodystrophy, Nature 401 (6748) (1999) 73–76.
[17] J.K. Kim, O. Gavrilova, Y. Chen, et al., Mechanism of insulin resistance in A-ZIP/F-1 fatless mice, J. Biol. Chem. 275 (12) (2000) 8456–8460.
[18] K. Matsusue, M. Haluzik, G. Lambert, et al., Liver-specific disruption of PPARgamma in leptin-deficient mice improves fatty liver but aggravates diabetic phenotypes, J. Clin. Invest. 111 (5) (2003) 737–747.
[19] O. Gavrilova, M. Haluzik, K. Matsusue, et al., Liver peroxisome proliferator activated receptor gamma contributes to hepatic steatosis, triglyceride clearance, and regulation of body fat mass, J. Biol. Chem. 278 (36) (2003) 34268–34276.
[20] A.W. Norris, L. Chen, S.J. Fisher, et al., Muscle-specific PPARgamma-deficient mice develop increased adiposity and insulin resistance but respond to thiazolidinediones, J. Clin. Invest. 112 (4) (2003) 608–618.

International Congress Series 1262 (2004) 51–54

ELSEVIER

www.ics-elsevier.com

Peroxisome proliferator-activated receptor γ—insights from human genetics

V.K.K. Chatterjee*

Department of Medicine, University of Cambridge, Box 157 Addenbrooke's Hospital, Hills Road, Cambridge CB2 2QQ, UK

Abstract. Peroxisome proliferator-activated receptor γ (PPARγ), mediates adipocyte differentiation and is the target for the thiazolidinedione (TZD) group of insulin-sensitising antidiabetic agents. We screened the PPARγ gene in 85 subjects with severe insulin resistance and identified heterozygous, missense mutations in several individuals from different families. Functional studies indicate that the receptor mutants are transcriptionally impaired and inhibit wild-type PPARγ action in a dominant negative manner. The clinical phenotype also includes partial lipodystrophy, dyslipidaemia, hepatic steatosis and early onset hypertension. Diminished fat mass, reduced circulating adiponectin and impaired lipid flux in adipose tissue contribute to severe insulin resistance. Responses to TZD treatment in two subjects mirrored the properties of their mutant receptors in vitro. In a large kindred with five individuals with severe insulin resistance, we have identified frameshift/premature stop mutations in PPARγ and muscle-specific regulatory subunit of protein phosphatase 1 (PPP1R3A) genes. This PPARγ stop mutant exhibits complete loss of function with no dominant negative activity; the PPP1R3A truncation mutant is mislocalised intracellularly. Individuals harbouring either gene defect alone have normal insulin levels, but double heterozygosity for the gene defects co-segregates with severe insulin resistance. This kindred represents the first description of a digenic basis for insulin resistance and suggests that a metabolic dialogue between adipose tissue and skeletal muscle regulates insulin action. © 2003 Elsevier B.V. All rights reserved.

Keywords: PPARγ; Insulin resistance; Partial lipodystrophy; Dominant negative; PPP1R3

1. Peroxisome proliferator-activated receptor γ ligand resistance

1.1. Molecular genetics

Peroxisome proliferator-activated receptor γ (PPARγ) was first characterised as a transcription factor which regulates target gene expression in adipocytes and induces preadipocyte differentiation [1]. The receptor is also the target for thiazolidinediones (TZDs), a novel class of antidiabetic agent which lower blood glucose by enhancing tissue

* Tel.: +44-1223-336842; fax: +44-1223-763401.
E-mail address: kkc1@mole.bio.cam.ac.uk (V.K.K. Chatterjee).

doi:10.1016/j.ics.2003.11.025

sensitivity to insulin in vivo [2]. With the discovery that TZDs act via PPARγ, this candidate gene was screened in a cohort of 85 subjects with severe insulin resistance, defined by the coexistence of extreme hyperinsulinaemia and the skin lesion acanthosis nigricans. Two different heterozygous, missense (P467L, V290M) mutations in the PPARγ ligand binding domain (LBD) were identified in three affected individuals, with autosomal dominant inheritance in one family. Functional studies showed that both mutant receptors exhibited reduced ligand binding and coactivator recruitment, resulting in impaired regulation of target gene transcription. These properties were consistent with modelling based on the crystal structure of the PPARγ LBD which predicted that both mutations destabilise an alpha helix (H12) at the carboxyterminus of the receptor which mediates interaction with both ligand and coactivators [3]. In keeping with this hypothesis, analyses of wild-type or P467L and V290M mutants by fluorescence anisotropy indicated that helix 12 is indeed more unstable in the mutant proteins [4]. Consonant with the dominant mode of inheritance in one family and heterozygosity for the PPARγ defects in affected subjects, the P467L and V290M mutants inhibited the transcriptional activity of coexpressed wild-type PPARγ in a dominant negative manner [3]. Such dominant negative inhibition by the PPARγ mutants is analogous to the properties of thyroid hormone receptor (TRβ) mutants associated with the syndrome of resistance to thyroid hormone [5] or the PML-RARα and Pax8-PPARγ fusion proteins involved in acute promyelocytic leukaemia [6] or follicular thyroid cancer, respectively [7].

Other groups have reported additional loss-of-function mutations in the PPARγ LBD: a female with insulin resistance and early onset type 2 diabetes was heterozygous for an arginine to cysteine mutation (R425C in PPARγ2 or R397C in PPARγ1) [8]; several subjects in three generations of a family were heterozygous for an phenylalanine to leucine codon change (F388L in PPARγ2 or F360L in PPARγ1) which cosegregated with insulin resistance [9].

1.2. Clinical phenotype

In keeping with the critical role of PPARγ in adipogenesis, we now recognize that a central feature of the clinical phenotype in individuals with PPARγ mutations, is a stereotyped pattern of partial lipodystrophy [8–10]. Selective diminution in gluteal and limb adipose tissue is associated with preservation of subcutaneous face, neck and abdominal fat together with the visceral adipose depot. Attendant metabolic abnormalities seen in many subjects include hepatic steatosis and dyslipidaemia (raised circulating triglycerides together with low HDL). Whilst lipodystrophy per se is known to predispose to insulin resistance, detailed metabolic studies of one subject have identified other factors which may also contribute to its pathogenesis. Our studies indicate that subcutaneous adipocytes from an individual with the P467L mutation are relatively metabolically inert, exhibiting both impaired lipogenesis from circulating fatty acids as well as failure to inhibit lipolysis normally following a meal [10]. Together, we suggest that these defects lead to abnormalities in postprandial circulating free fatty acid metabolism which reduce tissue sensitivity to insulin. In addition, circulating levels of adiponectin, a protein secreted by adipocytes which enhances insulin action in skeletal muscle, were strikingly reduced in subjects harbouring PPARγ mutations [11].

All three patients we first described had also developed marked early onset hypertension unrelated to diabetic comorbidity, and this was also a feature in some subjects described by others subsequently [8,9]. Coupled with the knowledge that TZDs inhibit vascular endothelin secretion and calcium channel activity whilst upregulating nitric oxide synthesis suggests an additional role for PPARγ in the regulation of vascular tone. The occurrence of severe pre-eclampsia in both pregnancies in our index case with the P467L mutation may also be highly significant when correlated with the observation that the murine PPARγ gene knockout is embryonic lethal due to impaired trophoblast differentiation and placental vascularisation [12], suggesting an important role for this receptor in placental function.

2. A digenic basis for insulin resistance

Most recently, we have studied a large UK kindred with several subjects exhibiting severe insulin resistance [13]. We identified a heterozygous frameshift/premature stop mutation within the DNA binding domain of PPARγ in seven individuals. Consistent with the location of the mutation, the truncated mutant PPARγ protein was unable to bind to DNA or regulate target gene transcription. In addition, it exhibited negligible dominant negative inhibition of wild-type receptor function when they were coexpressed.

Remarkably, further candidate gene studies in this family revealed that several subjects were heterozygous for a frameshift/premature stop mutation in an unrelated gene (PP1R3A), encoding the regulatory subunit of protein phosphatase 1, which is selectively expressed in skeletal and cardiac muscle and regulates the catalytic activity of protein phosphatase 1 (PP1C). In turn, PP1C mediates the dephosphorylation and activation of glycogen synthase, the rate-limiting enzyme mediating conversion of glucose into glycogen. Functional studies of the truncated mutant PPP1R3A protein, lacking a putative carboxyterminal membrane-spanning domain, showed that it localized aberrantly to the cytosolic rather than membrane compartment when expressed in cells. Correlation of genotype with metabolic parameters in this kindred showed that either gene defect alone was insufficient to mediate the clinical phenotype: thus, subjects who were heterozygous for either the PPARγ or PPP1R3 mutations showed normal insulin sensitivity, whereas individuals who were doubly heterozygous for both gene mutations exhibited marked insulin resistance.

To our knowledge, there is no direct functional interaction between PPARγ and PPP1R3. The two genes are predominantly expressed in different sites (adipose tissue and skeletal muscle, respectively), each of which is an important target for insulin-mediated nutrient storage. This suggests that a combination of modest defects in each tissue and/or a failure of a "metabolic dialogue" between fat and muscle culminates in severe insulin resistance. The mechanism underlying the basis of this digenic cause of insulin resistance remains to be elucidated.

Acknowledgements

This research represents collaboration between several groups including Steve O'Rahilly (University of Cambridge), Ines Barroso and Alan Schafer (Incyte Genetics), John Schwabe (Laboratory of Molecular Biology, Cambridge) and Tim Willson (Glaxo

Smith Kline) together with clinical colleagues referring cases, without whose contribution the work would not have been possible. Our research is supported by the Wellcome Trust, Medical Research Council (UK) and the European Union.

References

[1] P. Tontonoz, et al., Stimulation of adipogenesis in fibroblasts by PPARγ2, a lipid-activated transcription factor, Cell 79 (1994) 1147–1156.

[2] R.R. Henry, Thiazolidinediones, Endocrinol. Metab. Clin. North Am. 26 (1997) 553–573.

[3] I. Barroso, et al., Dominant negative mutations in human PPARγ are associated with severe insulin resistance, diabetes mellitus and hypertension, Nature 402 (1999) 880–883.

[4] B.C. Kallenberger, et al., A dynamic mechanism of nuclear receptor activation and its perturbation in a human disease, Nat. Struct. Biol. 10 (2003) 136–140.

[5] T.N. Collingwood, et al., Spectrum of transcriptional dimerization and dominant negative properties of twenty different mutant thyroid hormone β receptors in thyroid hormone resistance syndrome, Mol. Endocrinol. 8 (1994) 1262–1277.

[6] F. Grignani, et al., Fusion proteins of the retinoic acid receptor-alpha recruit histone deacetylase in promyelocytic leukaemia, Nature 391 (1998) 815–818.

[7] T.G. Kroll, et al., PAX8-PPARγ1 fusion in oncogene human thyroid carcinoma, Science 289 (2000) 1357–1360.

[8] A.K. Agarwal, et al., A novel heterozygous mutation in peroxisome proliferator-activated receptor-gamma gene in a patient with familial partial lipodystrophy, J. Clin. Endocrinol. Metab. 87 (2002) 408–411.

[9] R.A. Hegele, et al., PPARG F388L, a transactivation-deficient mutant, in familial partial lipodystrophy, Diabetes 51 (2002) 3586–3590.

[10] D.B. Savage, et al., Clinical and pathophysiological features of a metabolic syndrome resulting from mutations in the nuclear receptor PPARγ, Diabetes 52 (2003) 910–917.

[11] T.P. Combs, et al., Induction of adipocyte complement-related protein of 30 kilodaltons by PPARγ agonists: a potential mechanism of insulin sensitization, Endocrinology 143 (2002) 998–1007.

[12] Y. Barak, et al., PPARγ is required for placental, cardiac and adipose tissue development, Mol. Cell 4 (1999) 585–595.

[13] D.B. Savage, et al., Digenic inheritance of severe insulin resistance in a human pedigree, Nat. Genet. 31 (2002) 379–384.

International Congress Series 1262 (2004) 55–58

www.ics-elsevier.com

Fatty acids, cholesterol, and sphingolipids: interactive regulators and targets for SREBP processing

Rebecca A. Juliano[a], Richard J. Deckelbaum[a,b,*], Tilla S. Worgall[c]

[a] *Institute of Human Nutrition, Columbia University, College of Physicians and Surgeons, PH 15-1512, 630 West 168th Street, New York, NY 10032, USA*

[b] *Department of Pediatrics, Columbia University, College of Physicians and Surgeons, PH 15-1512, 630 West 168th Street, New York, NY 10032, USA*

[c] *Department of Pathology, Columbia University, College of Physicians and Surgeons, PH 15-74, 630 West 168th Street, New York, NY 10032, USA*

Abstract. Sterol regulatory element-binding protein (SREBPs) have a major role in regulating transcription of many genes involved in lipid biology and pathobiology. In addition to inhibitory effects of cholesterol on cleavage of the precursor of SREBP (pSREBP) to the active mature nuclear form (mSREBP), polyunsaturated fatty acids (PUFA)—but not saturated fatty acids—have a key role in inhibiting formation of the active mSREBP. The ability of PUFA to decrease SREBP-dependent gene transcription is related in part to effects on modulating intracellular cholesterol partitioning and through effects on sphingolipid metabolism. Effects related to sphingolipids are due in part to their higher affinity for free cholesterol, as well as to the ability of PUFA to increase cell sphingomyelinase activity leading to production of ceramide. The inhibitory effects of ceramide on SREBP cleavage are associated with the ability of ceramide to inhibit its own de novo intracellular synthesis, which we hypothesize effects normal SREBP trafficking between the endoplasmic reticulum (ER) and Golgi compartments. Our work indicates that intermediates of sphingomyelin metabolism now join cholesterol and fatty acids as important regulators of SREBP processing, and offer new therapeutic targets for disorders of lipid metabolism including dyslipidemias, steatohepatitis, obesity, and type II diabetes.

Keywords: SREBP; Sphingolipids; Fatty acids; Gene regulation

1. Interactions of cholesterol and fatty acid

Cholesterol and fatty acids (FA) interact in a number of pathways that regulate intracellular and whole body lipid metabolism, as well as membrane structure and function. For example, free FA (FFA) and cholesterol are cosubstrates for sterol esterification via the ACAT reaction. Both cholesterol and FA act independently or interdependently in regulating

* Corresponding author. Institute of Human Nutrition, Columbia University, College of Physicians and Surgeons, PH 15-1512, 630 West, 168th Street, New York, NY 10032, USA. Tel.: +1-212-305-4808; fax: +1-212-305-3079.

E-mail addresses: rj88@columbia.edu (R.A. Juliano), rjd20@columbia.edu (R.J. Deckelbaum), tpw7@columbia.edu (T.S. Worgall).

0531-5131/
doi:10.1016/j.ics.2003.12.094

expression of the LDL receptor. Cholesterol decreases fluidity of cellular membranes, whereas FA increase or decrease fluidity depending on chain length and number of double bonds. Work from our laboratory and others demonstrated that FA and cholesterol also interact in regulation of sterol regulatory element-binding protein (SREBP)-mediated gene transcription [1–6]. Recently, new evidence indicates that sphingolipids are also coregulators of SREBP cleavage and their subsequent effect on gene transcription.

2. Sterol regulatory element-binding protein (SREBP)

Brown, Goldstein, and coworkers first demonstrated that cholesterol regulates gene expression via SREBP binding to sterol regulatory elements (SRE) in the promoter region of genes of lipid and carbohydrate metabolism [7]. The effects of cholesterol on SREs are regulated through distinct proteins that are complexed to each other: SREBP and the SREBP cleavage activating protein (SCAP). The precursor, or inactive, forms of SREBP (pSREBP) contain approximately 1150 amino acids and are located in the endoplasmic reticulum (ER) and nuclear envelope. Under conditions of sterol depletion, the SCAP–SREBP complex translocates to the Golgi, where a two-step proteolytic process releases the transcriptionally active N-terminal fragment, or mature form, of SREBP (mSREBP, approximately 500 amino acids) [5,8].

There are three isoforms of SREBP (SREBP-1a, SREBP-1c, and SREBP-2), which arise from two chromosomal loci. SREBP-1a and SREBP-1c share the same chromosomal location and vary due to differential splicing of their first exon. SREBP-1a is the primary SREBP-1 present in cultured cells, while SREBP-1c is most prevalent in vivo and in mammalian tissues. SREBP-1a and SREBP-1c preferentially regulate pathways related to FA and triglyceride metabolism, whereas SREBP-2 preferentially regulates expression of genes important in sterol-related pathways. Nevertheless, while there is overlap and cross talk between SREBPs in gene regulation, the mechanisms underlying greater responsiveness of SREBP-2 to sterols and SREBP-1 to FA are not defined.

3. Fatty acids, cholesterol and SREBP

Recognizing that cholesterol has a major role in SREBP-dependent gene expression and the multiple interactions of FA and cholesterol, we initially questioned whether FA might regulate SRE-mediated gene transcription via SREBP. Cultured cells (CHO, Hep G2, CV-1), were transfected with an SRE-containing promoter linked to a luciferase reporter and incubated with FA bound to albumin. Unsaturated FA, especially long-chain PUFA decreased SRE-mediated gene transcription and cellular levels of the mSREBP-1 and -2. These effects were observed in the absence of exogenous sterol, and in the presence of sterols, the inhibitory effects of unsaturated FA were additive—or synergistic—to those of sterols. Analyzing SREBP protein, we found that there were marked decreases in cellular levels of mSREBP as well as mRNA levels of SREBP-dependent genes. Experiments using mutant cell lines and other approaches indicated that the effects of FA on inhibiting SREBP cleavage could be modulated, in part, through changing intracellular free cholesterol partitioning between the plasma membrane and other compartments. FA could alter SREBP processing via a number of different pathways, both physical and biochemical.

4. Fatty acids alter properties of cholesterol in model membranes

We questioned whether FFA would affect the physical properties of free cholesterol in the plasma membrane to facilitate transfer to intracellular compartments [9]. To address this "physical" hypothesis, large unilamellar egg yolk phospholipid vesicles (LUV) containing ^{13}C-labeled cholesterol were utilized as a model for the plasma membrane and small egg yolk phospholipid unilamellar vesicles (SUV) as a model for intracellular membrane. FFA effects on cholesterol transfer from LUV to SUV were monitored in real time utilizing novel NMR approaches. FFA markedly enhanced the transfer of free cholesterol from LUV to SUV, an effect linked to FFA increasing both free cholesterol and phospholipid mobilities within the model membranes. Sphingomyelin, a major phospholipid in plasma membrane, was incorporated into LUV and here too FFA increased cholesterol mobility and enhanced transfer to acceptor vesicles. Fatty acyl-CoA has similar effects as FFA, and protonating FFA by lowering pH did not alter cholesterol transfer, demonstrating that FFA effects are due to their hydrocarbon chains and not to their headgroups [9]. While we observed similar effects of saturated and unsaturated FA on membrane fluidity and cholesterol transfer, it is still possible that effects of FFA on SREBP processing may be related, in part, to their ability to change physical properties of cellular membranes.

5. Fatty acids, sphingolipids and SREBP

Knowing that both free cholesterol and now FA would affect maturation of pSREBP to its active transcription form mSREBP, we questioned if this was mediated by a single "essential control pathway" or whether there were multiple levels of control, and if so, what were the interactions between the different pathways? In doing so, we focused on interactions of FFA, cholesterol, and sphingolipids. FFA are known to increase cellular sphingomyelinase activity, and we hypothesized that FFA would decrease sphingomyelin levels within the plasma membrane, the major cellular reservoir of sphingomyelin. Because sphingomyelin has higher affinity for free cholesterol than other phospholipids, this would also result in transfer of free cholesterol intracellularly. Hydrolysis of sphingomyelin produces the second messenger ceramide, and we questioned if ceramide would also affect SRE-mediated gene transcription.

We confirmed that unsaturated FA not only decreased cellular sphingomyelin content but also increased ceramide generation. Adding exogenous ceramides (C2–C8) or their dihydroceramide analogues, we found marked rapid inhibition of SRE-mediated gene transcription. These effects were not associated with effects of ceramide on cell apoptosis, necrosis or toxicity. Increasing intracellular ceramide by incubation with sphingomyelinase or by using agents to decrease cell ceramide catabolism resulted in decreased SRE-mediated gene transcription and cellular levels of mSREBP-1 and -2. Of interest, increasing cell ceramide also increased pSREBP [10].

Based on the above findings, it seemed likely that decreasing cell ceramide by decreasing new ceramide synthesis should increase SRE-mediated gene transcription. In fact, experimental data produced the opposite findings in that inhibition of ceramide de novo synthesis with either myriocin or cycloserine (inhibitors of serine palmityl transferase activity) or with fumonsin B1 (inhibitor of ceramide synthase) decreased SREBP-dependent gene transcription. In experiments monitoring conversion of ^{3}H-serine to ceramide exogenous ceramide inhibited de novo ceramide synthesis. Of note, increasing ceramide synthesis by addition of exogenous sphingosine or inhibitors of sphingosine conversion to sphingosine-1-phosphate increased SRE-mediated gene transcription. These findings raise the hypothesis that the process of ongoing de novo ceramide synthesis may be, in addition to ceramide itself, an important regulatory pathway in the physiological processing of active SREBP. The ceramide synthesis pathway is related to ER–Golgi–nuclear transport, as are other molecules related to ceramide synthesis and thus, the effects of ceramide are likely due to their effects on disrupting ER-Golgi trafficking of SREBP.

6. SREBP as a therapeutic target

FA and sphingolipids join cholesterol as an important regulator of conversion of inactive pSREBP to the active transcription factor, mSREBP. Because of the key regulatory roles of SREBP in modulating pathways of FA, cholesterol, and sterol synthesis in metabolism, we predict that therapeutic modulation of specific steps where FA and sphingolipid metabolism interact with SREBP maturation are likely targets for improving or treating a number of conditions. These include dyslipidemias, obesity and its coconditions such as insulin resistance in type 2 diabetes. Interfering with SREBP-1 processing could aid in conditions leading to fat accumulation in liver or other tissues. An example would be the fatty liver and steatohepatitis now common in obesity and insulin resistance. Likely, other metabolic disorders of lipid metabolism, particularly disorders with increased lipid synthesis could also be improved by modulation by SREBP processing in specific tissues.

References

[1] T.S. Worgall, et al., Polyunsaturated fatty acids decrease expression of promoters with sterol regulatory elements by decreasing levels of mature sterol regulatory element-binding protein, J. Biol. Chem. 273 (40) (1998) 25537–25540.

[2] D.P. Thewke, S.R. Panini, M. Sinensky, Oleate potentiates oxysterol inhibition of transcription from sterol regulatory element-1-regulated promoters and maturation of sterol regulatory element-binding proteins, J. Biol. Chem. 273 (33) (1998) 21402–21407.

[3] H.J. Kim, M. Takahashi, O. Ezaki, Fish oil feeding decreases mature sterol regulatory element-binding protein 1 (SREBP-1) by down-regulation of SREBP-1c mRNA in mouse liver. A possible mechanism for down-regulation of lipogenic enzyme mRNAs, J. Biol. Chem. 274 (36) (1999) 25892–25898.

[4] J. Xu, et al., Sterol regulatory element binding protein-1 expression is suppressed by dietary polyunsaturated fatty acids. A mechanism for the coordinate suppression of lipogenic genes by polyunsaturated fats, J. Biol. Chem. 274 (33) (1999) 23577–23583.

[5] J.D. Horton, J.L. Goldstein, M.S. Brown, SREBPs: activators of the complete program of cholesterol and fatty acid synthesis in the liver, J. Clin. Invest. 109 (9) (2002) 1125–1131.

[6] J. Xu, et al., Dietary polyunsaturated fats regulate rat liver sterol regulatory element binding proteins-1 and -2 in three distinct stages and by different mechanisms, J. Nutr. 132 (11) (2002) 3333–3339.

[7] X. Wang, et al., SREBP-1, a membrane-bound transcription factor released by sterol-regulated proteolysis, Cell 77 (1) (1994) 53–62.

[8] J.D. Horton, J.L. Goldstein, M.S. Brown, SREBPs: transcriptional mediators of lipid homeostasis, Cold Spring Harbor Symp. Quant. Biol. 67 (2002) 491–498.

[9] R.A. Johnson, et al., Free fatty acids modulate intermembrane trafficking of cholesterol by increasing lipid mobilities: novel 13C NMR analyses of free cholesterol partitioning, Biochemistry 42 (6) (2003) 1637–1645.

[10] T.S. Worgall, et al., Unsaturated fatty acid-mediated decreases in sterol regulatory element-mediated gene transcription are linked to cellular sphingolipid metabolism, J Biol Chem. 277 (6) (2002) 3878–3885.

International Congress Series 1262 (2004) 59–62

www.ics-elsevier.com

Detrimental and protective roles of adaptive immunity in atherosclerosis

Göran K. Hansson*, Gabrielle Paulsson Berne, Xinghua Zhou

Department of Medicine, Center for Molecular Medicine L8:03, Karolinska Institute, Karolinska Hospital, SE-17176 Stockholm, Sweden

Abstract. Atherosclerosis is an inflammatory disease elicited by a lipid metabolic disturbance at sites of hemodynamic strain. Careful clinical and histopathological studies in humans as well as investigations in experimental models have identified all these phenomena, i.e. inflammation, metabolism, and hemodynamics, as playing key roles in the initiation and progression of atherosclerotic cardiovascular disease. While in-depth research into the regulation of cholesterol metabolism and blood pressure has led to new therapies against atherosclerotic cardiovascular diseases, our understanding of the inflammatory component of atherosclerosis remains incomplete and will require further research before new therapeutic or preventive strategies can be developed. This brief review will discuss new data regarding the regulation of proatherosclerotic, adaptive immunity, which is a strong driving force for the inflammatory process in the atherosclerotic plaque. © 2004 Published by Elsevier B.V.

Keywords: Atherosclerosis; Cytokines; Immunity; T cells

1. Mobilization of adaptive immunity

During atherogenesis, adaptive immunity is activated when T cells recognize antigens in lesions and also when T and B cells of lymphoid organs respond to disease-associated antigens. These detector steps trigger effector mechanisms that include macrophage activation, cytokine secretion, antibody production, and the development of inflammatory pathology.

T cells participate in the formation of atherosclerotic lesions from their initiation. Indeed, several of the adhesion molecules and chemokines that promote monocyte recruitment also stimulate T cells to enter lesions (e.g., the selectins, VCAM-1, ICAM-1, and MCP-1). In advanced human plaques, T cells constitute approximately 10–20% of the cell population [1] and they often congregate at sites where atheromas rupture and cause fatal thrombosis [2]. Most of the T cells in atherosclerotic lesions bear the CD3 and CD4 markers and the T-cell antigen receptor (TCRαβ+). This pattern of surface molecule expression implies that they recognize protein antigens presented to them by macrophages

* Corresponding author. Tel.: +46-8-51776222; fax: +46-8-313147.
E-mail address: Goran.Hansson@cmm.ki.se (G.K. Hansson).

0531-5131/ © 2004 Published by Elsevier B.V.
doi:10.1016/j.ics.2004.01.052

or dendritic cells after uptake and processing through the endosomal pathway. Such cells represent approximately two-thirds of all CD3+T cells in advanced human lesions [1] and more than 90% of T cells in lesions of apoE KO mice [3].

Recent studies in our laboratory have revealed the presence of yet another cell type in the atherosclerotic plaque: the NKT cell [4]. This cell shares functional properties with orthodox T cells but displays limited variability in its TCR, recognizes antigen in the context of CD1 rather than MHC proteins, and shares several phenotypic properties with natural killer (NK) cells. TCR-Vα14, which is typically expressed by NKT cells, is abundantly expressed in atherosclerotic aortas of apoE−/− mice [5], and CD1 molecules are also present in lesions [6]. We therefore crossed apoE−/− mice with CD1−/− animals. The offspring exhibited significantly reduced atherosclerosis with reduced inflammatory mediators and markers [4]. To test whether this was dependent on CD1-NKT cell interactions, apoE−/− mice were injected with a synthetic CD1 ligand, α-galactosylceramide (aGalCer), which activates NKT cells. This led to an exacerbation of atherosclerosis, with larger lesions containing increased interferon-γ mRNA as well as inflammatory markers [4]. These findings show that CD1-dependent NKT cell activation accelerates early atherosclerosis. They suggest that these cells act in a similar fashion as Th1 cells, i.e. by eliciting an inflammatory signal cascade.

2. Proatherogenic role of Th1 immunity

The role of T cells has been addressed in several experimental models of atherosclerosis. SCID×apolipoprotein $E^{-/-}$ mice, which lack T and B cells, develop less atherosclerosis than immunocompetent apoE−/− mice [7]. Similar but not quite as striking results were obtained in apoE−/− mice crossed with the immunodeficient Rag-1−/− mouse [8]. When SCID×apoE−/− mice were reconstituted with CD4+ T cells from immunocompetent apoE−/− animals, a substantial increase was registered in the size and maturation of atherosclerotic lesions [7]. This implies that the CD4+ subset of T cells carries proatherogenic immunity.

To further elucidate the effector mechanisms involved in proatherogenic adaptive immunity, apoE−/− and LDLR−/− mice have been mated with mice carrying specific defects in cytokine or costimulatory factor genes. ApoE−/− mice deficient in interferon-γ (IFNγ) signalling, interleukin (IL)-18, or CD40L (CD154) exhibit reduced disease development [9–11]. In line with this, administration of blocking anti-CD40L antibodies also inhibits disease development [12].

In conclusion, direct evidence from murine models as well as expression analysis in human lesions therefore point to the Th1 subset of CD4+ T cells as a strongly proatherogenic set of cells. Responses elicited by these cells, mediated through cytokines and cell–cell interactions, probably act by modulating gene expression in target cells. In the macrophage, this can lead to effects such as reduced cholesterol efflux, increased metalloproteinase secretion, expression of tissue factor, production of oxygen and nitrogen radicals, and secretion of several proinflammatory cytokines including TNF-α and IL-1. Endothelial cells respond to these stimuli by expressing several different leukocyte adhesion molecules, changing the fibrinolytic/antifibrinolytic balance, and other reactions. Smooth muscle cells, finally, respond to interferon-γ and other proinflammatory stimuli by inhibition of cell proliferation, expression of cytokine-inducible NO synthase, and down-regulation of α-actin and collagen gene expression. All these modulations in the biological activities of cells present in the atherosclerotic lesion tend to act in the same direction, leading to local inflammation, cholesterol accumulation, and plaque destabilization.

3. Immunoregulatory and anti-inflammatory signals reduce atherogenesis

T-cell activation is controlled by cytokines produced by neighbouring cells. IL-10, which is secreted by macrophages and the Th2 subset of T cells, inhibits secretion of several proinflammatory cytokines by T cells. Another immune regulatory cytokine, transforming growth factor-β (TGFβ), is produced by several different cell types including endothelial and smooth muscle cells, macrophages, platelets, and regulatory T cells (Treg) [13]. Both IL-10 and TGFβ dampen atherosclerosis in mouse models [14–18] and the latter has also been implicated in human disease [19–21].

We hypothesized that proatherogenic T cells are controlled by immunoregulatory TGFβ, which maintains the T-cell population in an inhibited state. To test this, we crossed atherosclerosis-prone E^0 mice with animals carrying dominant-negative transforming growth factor-β receptor-II in T cells. Our data show that E^0 mice with abrogated TGFβ signalling in T cells develop dramatically increased atherosclerosis [22]. At 12 weeks of age, lesions in apoE−/− mice lacking TGFβ receptors in T cells displayed a fivefold increase in lesion size when compared with fully immunocompetent apoE−/− mice. Lesions in the former contained more macrophages, more T cells, increased VCAM-1 and I-A expression, and a 100-fold increase in interferon-γ mRNA [22]. Interestingly, fibrous caps were reduced in these lesions, at the expense of lipid core and inflammatory components, implying that T-cell activity is associated with plaque destabilization. These results show that TGFβ exerts important anti-atherosclerotic activity by inhibiting T-cell activation.

4. Conclusions

Mechanistic studies in gene-targeted animal models have confirmed a proatherogenic role for Th1-type cellular immune responses. They have identified interferon-γ and CD40 ligation as key mediators of the proatherogenic effect and suggest that inflammatory activation of macrophages and vascular cells are important steps in the sequence leading to aggravated atherosclerosis. Recent studies have also identified counterbalancing, anti-inflammatory pathways activated by immune cells. They involve B1 cells producing protective antibodies and also subsets of cells (regulatory T cells, Th3 cells, and others) which secrete T-cell inhibitory cytokines such as IL-10 and TGFβ. The precise balance between proatherogenic and atheroprotective stimuli may determine whether an atherosclerotic lesion will progress into an unstable plaque. The development of therapeutic strategies to promote atheroprotective pathways represents a major challenge for current atherosclerosis research.

Acknowledgements

Research in the authors' laboratory is supported by the Swedish Research Council, the Swedish Heart Foundation, AFA Insurance Fund, Torsten and Ragnar Söderberg Foundation, and King Gustaf V 80th Anniversary Fund.

References

[1] L. Jonasson, et al., Regional accumulations of T cells, macrophages, and smooth muscle cells in the human atherosclerotic plaque, Arteriosclerosis 6 (1986) 131–138.

[2] A.C. van der Wal, A.E. Becker, C.M. van der Loos, P.K. Das, Site of intimal rupture or erosion of thrombosed coronary atherosclerotic plaques is characterized by an inflammatory process irrespective of the dominant plaque morphology, Circulation 89 (1994) 36–44.

[3] X. Zhou, et al., Evidence for a local immune response in atherosclerosis. CD4+ T cells infiltrate lesions of apolipoprotein-E-deficient mice, Am. J. Pathol. 149 (1996) 359–366.

[4] E. Tupin, A. Nicoletti, R. Elhage, M. Rudling, H.G. Ljunggren, G.K. Hansson, G. Paulsson Berne, CD1d-dependent activation of NKT cells aggravates atherosclerosis, J. Exp. Med. (2004) (in press).

[5] G. Paulsson, et al., Oligoclonal T cell expansions in atherosclerotic lesions of apolipoprotein E-deficient mice, Arterioscler. Thromb. Vasc. Biol. 20 (2000) 10–17.

[6] A. Melian, et al., CD1 expression in human atherosclerosis. A potential mechanism for T cell activation by foam cells, Am. J. Pathol. 155 (1999) 775–786.

[7] X. Zhou, et al., Transfer of CD4(+) T cells aggravates atherosclerosis in immunodeficient apolipoprotein E knockout mice, Circulation 102 (2000) 2919–2922.

[8] H.M. Dansky, S.A. Charlton, M.M. Harper, J.D. Smith, T and B lymphocytes play a minor role in atherosclerotic plaque formation in the apolipoprotein E-deficient mouse, Proc. Natl. Acad. Sci. U. S. A. 94 (1997) 4642–4646.

[9] S. Gupta, A.M. Pablo, X.-C. Jiang, N. Wang, A.R. Tall, C. Schindler, IFN-γ potentiates atherosclerosis in apoE knock-out mice, J. Clin. Invest. 99 (1997) 2561–2752.

[10] R. Elhage, et al., Reduced atherosclerosis in interleukin-18 deficient apolipoprotein E-knockout mice, Cardiovasc. Res. 59 (2003) 234–240.

[11] E. Lutgens, et al., Requirement for CD154 in the progression of atherosclerosis, Nat. Med. 5 (1999) 1313–1316.

[12] F. Mach, et al., Reduction of atherosclerosis in mice by inhibition of CD40 signalling, Nature 394 (1998) 200–2003.

[13] L. Gorelik, R.A. Flavell, Transforming growth factor-beta in T-cell biology, Nat. Rev. Immunol. 2 (2002) 46–53.

[14] D.J. Grainger, et al., Tamoxifen elevates transforming growth factor-beta and suppresses diet-induced formation of lipid lesions in mouse aorta, Nat. Med. 1 (1995) 1067–1073.

[15] L.J. Pinderski, et al., Overexpression of interleukin-10 by activated T lymphocytes inhibits atherosclerosis in LDL receptor-deficient mice by altering lymphocyte and macrophage phenotypes, Circ. Res. 90 (2002) 1064–1071.

[16] G. Caligiuri, et al., Interleukin-10 deficiency increases atherosclerosis, thrombosis, and low-density lipoproteins in apolipoprotein E knockout mice, Mol. Med. 9 (2003) 10–107.

[17] E. Lutgens, et al., Transforming growth factor-beta mediates balance between inflammation and fibrosis during plaque progression, Arterioscler. Thromb. Vasc. Biol. 22 (2002) 975–982.

[18] Z. Mallat, et al., Inhibition of transforming growth factor-beta signaling accelerates atherosclerosis and induces an unstable plaque phenotype in mice, Circ. Res. 89 (2001) 930–934.

[19] D.J. Grainger, et al., The serum concentration of active transforming growth factor-β is severely depressed in advanced atherosclerosis, Nat. Med. 1 (1995) 74–79.

[20] T.A. McCaffrey, B. Du, S. Consigli, P. Szabo, P.J. Bray, L. Hartner, B.B. Weksler, T.A. Sanborn, G. Bush, H.L. Bush, Genomic instability in the type II TGF-β1 receptor gene in atherosclerotic and restenotic vascular cells, J. Clin. Invest. 100 (1997) 2182–2188.

[21] T.A. McCaffrey, et al., The expression of TGF-beta receptors in human atherosclerosis: evidence for acquired resistance to apoptosis due to receptor imbalance, J. Mol. Cell Cardiol. 31 (1999) 1627–1642.

[22] A.K.L. Robertson, et al., Disruption of TGF-β signaling in T cells accelerates atherosclerosis, J. Clin. Invest. 112 (2003) 1342–1350.

International Congress Series 1262 (2004) 63–66

www.ics-elsevier.com

The long pentraxin PTX3: from innate immunity to ischemic heart disorders

Barbara Bottazzi[a,*], Giuseppe Peri[a], Cecilia Garlanda[a], Andrea Doni[a], Stefania Baviera[a], Roberto Latini[a], Aldo Maggioni[a], Alberto Mantovani[b]

[a] *Department of Immunology and Cell Biology, Mario Negri Institute for Pharmacological Research, Via Eritrea 62, 2017 Milan, Italy*
[b] *Institute of Pathology, University of Milan, Italy*

Abstract. The long pentraxin PTX3 was originally identified (cDNA and genomic, mouse and human) as an IL-1 inducible gene in endothelial cells. PTX3 is a prototypic long pentraxin consisting of a C-terminal pentraxin domain (with similarity to C-reactive protein, CRP, and serum amyloid P (SAP) component), coupled to an unrelated N terminal portion. Unlike CRP, produced in the liver, it is induced by inflammatory signals mainly in endothelial cells and macrophages. Recent data in gene-targeted mice show that PTX3 is a unique, soluble pattern recognition receptor playing a non-redundant role in innate immunity and female fertility. PTX3 is produced in atherosclerotic lesions and levels increase in ischemic heart disorders. Recent results on the prognostic significance of PTX3 in acute myocardial infarction (AMI) are encouraging. © 2003 Published by Elsevier B.V.

Keywords: Pentraxins; PTX3; Myocardial infarction; C-reactive protein

1. Introduction

Inflammation is a key component of correct paradigms in the pathogenesis of atherosclerosis and its complications. In this general context, the short pentraxin C-reactive protein (CRP) is a widely used biomarker for ischemic vascular pathologies [1].

Pentraxins are a superfamily of conserved proteins characterized by a cyclic multimeric structure [2]. The classical short pentraxins, CRP and serum amyloid P (SAP) component, are acute phase proteins produced in the liver in response to inflammatory mediators [3,4] and involved in the regulation of innate resistance to microbes and scavenging of cellular debris and extracellular matrix components [5].

* Corresponding author. Tel.: +39-2-39014543; fax: +39-2-39014596.
E-mail address: bottazzib@marionegri.it (B. Bottazzi).

0531-5131/
doi:10.1016/S0531-5131(03)01738-2

Long pentraxins are a subfamily of proteins characterized by an unrelated N-terminal domain coupled to the C-terminal pentraxin domain; they differ from classical short pentraxins for gene organization, chromosomal localization, cellular source, inducing stimuli and ligands recognized.

The prototypic long pentraxin PTX3, also called TNF-stimulated gene 14 (TSG14), was originally identified as an IL-1 inducible gene in endothelial cells [6] and as a TNFα inducible gene in fibroblasts [7]. PTX3 is secreted as glycosilated protomers (45 kDa) generally assembled to form 10–20 multimers [8], and is mainly produced by dendritic cells (DC), macrophages and endothelial cells in response to primary inflammatory stimuli and microbial moieties [9–11]. PTX3 does not recognize classical pentraxin ligands, but it binds with the complement component C1q and some selected microorganisms [12,13].

Available information suggests that PTX3 plays an important role in innate resistance against selected pathogens, in female fertility, in the regulation of inflammatory reactions and, possibly, autoimmunity.

2. Normal physiological role

The regulated expression of PTX3 by cells present in peripheral tissues suggests that PTX3, unlike the short pentraxins made in the liver, represents a mechanism of amplification of innate resistance mainly acting locally at sites of infection and inflammation. DCs, in particular, play a key role in the activation and orientation of adaptive immunity. As shown in Table 1, human monocyte-derived DCs produce a significant amount of PTX3 in response to microbial ligands engaging different members of the Toll-Like Receptor family. DC are better producers of PTX3 than monocytes and macrophages and production is restricted to myeloid DC, while plasmacytoid DC do not produce PTX3 [11].

To assess the actual in vivo role of PTX3, defective mice were generated by homologous recombination. These animals showed higher susceptibility to selected pathogens, in particular to *Aspergillus fumigatus*. Susceptibility of ptx3 −/− mice was associated with defective recognition of conidia by alveolar macrophages and DC. Furthermore, ptx3 −/− mice show a severe defect in female fertility [13]. Taken together, the results obtained so far indicate that PTX3 is a soluble pattern recognition receptor playing an important role in innate resistance against selected pathogens.

Table 1
Production of PTX3 by human monocyte-derived DCs following 24-h stimulation with various ligands recognized by TLR

Stimulus	PTX3 (ng/ml in 24 h $\pm$ S.D.)
None	0.5 ± 0.1
LPS	45.6 ± 7.3
Peptidoglycan	13.3 ± 2.9
Poly(I):(C)	26.3 ± 8.5
Candida	5.4 ± 1.7
PAM-1	1.2 ± 0.3

3. PTX3 in ischemic heart disorders

PTX3 plasma levels are very low under normal conditions (≤ 2 ng/ml) but increase in several pathological conditions, including infections [14].

PTX3 is expressed at very high levels in the hearts of rodents after systemic administration of microbial products and inflammatory cytokines or after ligation of the left coronary artery to model acute myocardial infarction [9]. Moreover, we have recently shown that PTX3 is present in atherosclerotic lesions and in small vessel vasculitis in humans [15,16] and it is induced by oxydized, low-density lipoproteins (LDL; M. Klouche and G. Peri, unpublished observations).

The observation that PTX3 is produced in the heart prompted us to investigate PTX3 involvement in acute myocardial infarction (AMI). A pilot study revealed a rapid increase in PTX3 levels in AMI, reaching peak values after 6–8 h compared with 24–48 h for CRP [17]. These preliminary results suggest that PTX3 could be a sensitive and specific prognostic indicator of cardiac injuries. A large study aimed at assessing the prognostic value of PTX3 in ischemic heart disease is currently under analysis. In a representative sample of patients, we will assess whether PTX3 peak levels provide valuable information for risk stratification.

Since PTX3 is mainly produced by the heart and vasculature in response to proinflammatory signals, we hypothesized that locally produced PTX3 may amplify tissue damage: in this context PTX3 could be an acute phase reactant more closely related than CRP to cardiac injuries.

Acknowledgements

This work was supported by the European Commission, MIUR and FIRB.

References

[1] F.C. de Beer, C.R. Hind, K.M. Fox, R.M. Allan, A. Maseri, M.B. Pepys, Measurement of serum C-reactive protein concentration in myocardial ischaemia and infarction, Br. Heart J. 47 (1982) 239–243.
[2] J. Emsley, H.E. White, B.P. O'Hara, G. Oliva, N. Srinivasan, I.J. Tickle, et al., Structure of pentameric human serum amyloid P component, Nature 367 (1994) 338–345.
[3] H. Baumann, J. Gauldie, The acute phase response, Immunol. Today 15 (1994) 74–80.
[4] D.M. Steel, A.S. Whitehead, The major acute phase reactants: C-reactive protein, serum amyloid P component and serum amyloid A protein, Immunol. Today 15 (1994) 81–88.
[5] M.B. Pepys, M.L. Baltz, Acute phase proteins with special reference to C-reactive protein and related proteins (pentaxis) and serum amyloid A protein, Adv. Immunol. 34 (1983) 141–212.
[6] F. Breviario, E.M. d'Aniello, J. Golay, G. Peri, B. Bottazzi, A. Bairoch, et al., Interleukin-1-inducible genes in endothelial cells. Cloning of a new gene related to C-reactive protein and serum amyloid P component, J. Biol. Chem. 267 (1992) 22190–22197.
[7] G.W. Lee, T.H. Lee, J. Vilcek, TSG-14, a tumor necrosis factor- and IL-1-inducible protein, is a novel member of the pentaxin family of acute phase proteins, J. Immunol. 150 (1993) 1804–1812.
[8] B. Bottazzi, V. Vouret-Craviari, A. Bastone, L. De Gioia, C. Matteucci, G. Peri, et al., Multimer formation and ligand recognition by the long pentraxin PTX3—similarities and differences with the short pentraxins C-reactive protein and serum amyloid P component, J. Biol. Chem. 272 (1997) 32817–32823.
[9] M. Introna, V. Vidal Alles, M. Castellano, G. Picardi, L. De Gioia, B. Bottazzi, et al., Cloning of mouse PTX3, a new member of the pentraxin gene family expressed at extrahepatic sites, Blood 87 (1996) 1862–1872.

[10] V. Vidal Alles, B. Bottazzi, G. Peri, J. Golay, M. Introna, A. Mantovani, Inducible expression of PTX3, a new member of the pentraxin family, in human mononuclear phagocytes, Blood 84 (1994) 3483–3493.

[11] A. Doni, G. Peri, M. Chieppa, P. Allavena, F. Pasqualini, L. Vago, et al., Production of the soluble pattern recognition receptor PTX3 by myeloid, but not plasmacytoid, dendritic cells. Eur. J. Immunol. (in press).

[12] A.J. Nauta, B. Bottazzi, A. Mantovani, G. Salvatori, U. Kishore, W.J. Schwaeble, et al., Biochemical and functional characterization of the interaction between pentraxin 3 and C1q, Eur. J. Immunol. 33 (2) (2003) 465–473.

[13] C. Garlanda, E. Hirsch, S. Bozza, A. Salustri, M. De Acetis, R. Nota, et al., Non-redundant role of the long pentraxin PTX3 in anti-fungal innate immune response, Nature 420 (6912) (2002) 182–186.

[14] B. Muller, G. Peri, A. Doni, V. Torri, R. Landmann, B. Bottazzi, et al., Circulating levels of the long pentraxin PTX3 correlate with severity of infection in critically ill patients, Crit. Care Med. 29 (7) (2001) 1404–1407.

[15] M.S. Rolph, S. Zimmer, B. Bottazzi, C. Garlanda, A. Mantovani, G.K. Hansson, Production of the long pentraxin PTX3 in advanced atherosclerotic plaques, Arterioscler. Thromb. Vasc. Biol. 22 (5) (2002) e10–e14.

[16] F. Fazzini, G. Peri, A. Doni, G. Dell'Antonio, E. Dal Cin, E. Bozzolo, et al., PTX3 in small-vessel vasculitides: an independent indicator of disease activity produced at sites of inflammation, Arthritis Rheum. 44 (12) (2001) 2841–2850.

[17] G. Peri, M. Introna, D. Corradi, G. Iacuitti, S. Signorini, F. Avanzini, et al., PTX3, a prototypic long pentraxin, is an early indicator of acute myocardial infarction in man, Circulation 102 (2000) 636–641.

International Congress Series 1262 (2004) 67–70

ELSEVIER

www.ics-elsevier.com

Vascular biology of collagenases in vulnerable atherosclerotic plaques

Masanori Aikawa*

Harvard Medical School, Center for Excellence in Vascular Biology, Cardiovascular Medicine, Brigham and Women's Hospital, 77 Avenue Louis Pasteur, Boston, MA 02115, USA

Abstract. Disruption of the vulnerable atherosclerotic plaque often triggers acute coronary syndromes including acute myocardial infarction, unstable angina, and cardiac sudden death. Interstitial collagen may play a critical role in the mechanical strength of the artery. Members of the matrix metalloproteinase (MMP) family produced by macrophages, particularly interstitial collagenases (MMP-1/collagenase-1, MMP-8/collagenase-2, and MMP-13/collagenase-3), likely contribute to plaque vulnerability. Recent preclinical and clinical studies have suggested that lipid lowering prevents coronary events by reducing plaque vulnerability ("stabilization") rather than merely shrinking the atheroma burden ("regression"). We have shown in hypercholesterolemic rabbits that lipid lowering by either diet alone or statin treatment can reduce a number of features typical of the vulnerable plaque. An inverse relationship between reduced MMP-1/collagenase-1 and increased collagen in rabbit atheromata suggests the important role of collagenase action in collagen metabolism in atheromata. However, further studies are needed to address direct in vivo evidence that links collagenase action with regulation of the plaque collagen, critical to the clinical complications of coronary atherosclerosis. © 2004 Published by Elsevier B.V.

Keywords: Atherosclerosis; MMP; Collagen; Hypercholesterolemia; Acute coronary syndromes; Statins

1. Vascular inflammation induces vulnerability of the plaque

Inflammation plays a fundamental role in the pathogenesis of atherosclerosis and promotes the onset of acute coronary events. Rupture of the atheromatous plaque participates in the pathogenesis of coronary thrombosis and subsequent acute myocardial infarction [1]. Pathological studies have demonstrated that rupture-prone, vulnerable lesions usually contain many inflammatory cells, in particular macrophages, underlying a thin and collagen-poor fibrous cap. Extracellular matrix macromolecules, notably interstitial collagens, confer strength on the plaque's fibrous cap. Macrophage production of proteolytic enzymes including matrix metalloproteinases (MMPs) in atheromata may cause collagen loss in the plaque's protective fibrous cap and promote rupture, which causes the direct contact of blood coagulation factors to tissue factor, a

* Tel.: +1-617-525-4384; fax: +1-617-525-4380.
E-mail address: maikawa@rics.bwh.harvard.edu (M. Aikawa).

0531-5131/ © 2004 Published by Elsevier B.V.
doi:10.1016/j.ics.2003.12.056

potent activator of coagulation cascade overexpressed by lesional macrophages, and may in turn accelerate thrombus formation [1].

2. Collagenases vs. collagen in atheromata

Previous studies including our own demonstrated the expression of interstitial collagenases of the MMP family in experimental and human atherosclerotic lesions [2–8]. Collagenases including MMP-1/collagenase-1, MMP-8/collagenase-2, and MMP-13/collagenase-3 breakdown fibrillar collagens [9], key determinants of the tensile strength of plaques. Interstitial collagen types I and III are major arterial collagens in human atherosclerotic plaques [10]. MMP-family collagenases can initiate degradation of fibrillar collagen at a specific cleavage site, followed by further cleavage of degraded collagen fragments by other members of the MMP family.

3. Plaque stabilization by cholesterol lowering

For the last several decades, a number of preclinical studies addressed the hypothesis that atherosclerotic lesions can be regressed. However, recent clinical trials have suggested that lipid lowering therapy with HMG-CoA reductase inhibitors (statins) effectively prevents the acute coronary events despite no or little reduction in stenoses determined by angiography [11]. This discrepancy suggested the possibility that cholesterol lowering reduces acute thrombotic complications by modifying the nature of vulnerable coronary plaques functionally ("stabilization") rather than by reducing the lesion size ("regression").

Several lines of evidence from preclinical studies including our own support the hypothesis of plaque stabilization. Using rabbit models of atherosclerosis, we demonstrated that cholesterol lowering improves a number of features associated with vulnerable plaques in human coronary arteries such as vascular inflammation, oxidative stress, proteolytic activity, and thrombogenicity [4,7,8,12–14]. Aortic atheromata of hypercholesterolemic rabbits contained MMP-1/collagenase-1, resembling vulnerable plaques in the human coronary artery. However, dietary cholesterol lowering reduced macrophages expressing MMP-1/collagenase-1 and, in parallel, increased interstitial collagen in atheromata (Fig. 1) [4]. This inverse relationship not only suggests a potential mechanism of plaque stabilization by cholesterol lowering but also provides indirect in vivo evidence that collagenases play an important role in collagen metabolism in atheromata. We also reported that cholesterol lowering favors the accumulation of SMCs that exhibit a more mature phenotype and express less MMPs in the fibrous cap of rabbit atheromata compared with those from the baseline lesions [12].

We further demonstrated that cholesterol lowering with statins reduced macrophage-derived MMPs in rabbit atheromata [7,8]. Statins inhibit HMG-CoA reductase, a rate-limiting enzyme in the cholesterol synthesis pathway. Inhibition of HMG-CoA reductase reduces not only the cholesterol biosynthesis but also production of other intermediate metabolites that critically modify protein functions [11]. Although clinical studies suggest that little doubt remains regarding the importance of lipid lowering itself, accumulating preclinical evidence also demonstrates the lipid-independent effects

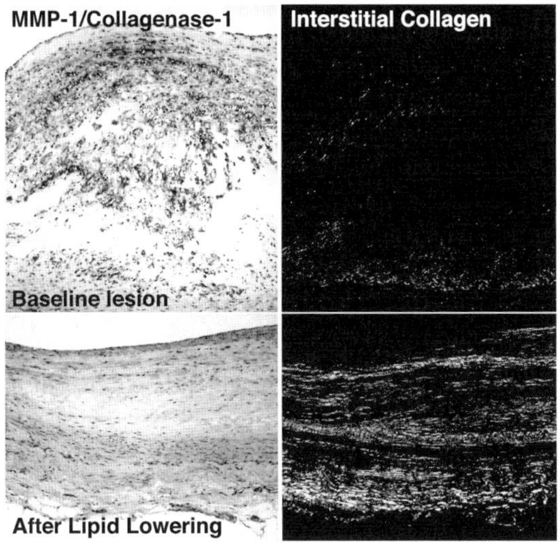

Fig. 1. An inverse relationship between MMP-1/collagenase-1 expression and interstitial collagen content in atheroma of hypercholesterolemic rabbits. The rabbit aortic atheroma after 4 months on a high-cholesterol diet (baseline lesion) contained a number of macrophages expressing high level of MMP-1/collagenase-1. Picrosirius red staining with polarization barely detected accumulation of interstitial collagen on a serial section. Sixteen months of dietary cholesterol lowering reduced MMP-1/collagenase-1 expression and concomitantly increased collagen content, a key determinant of plaque stability. From Ref. [4] with permission.

of statins on vascular inflammation and plaque vulnerability [11]. Statin treatment reduces growth of and MMP expression by human macrophages in vitro [7].

4. The role of collagenases of the MMP family in collagen breakdown in atheromata

This article has discussed accumulating indirect evidence that suggests a role for MMP-family collagenases in the metabolism of plaque collagen. However, no direct in vivo evidence has established that collagenolysis actually regulates the interstitial collagen content of atheromata. Do collagenases of the MMP family really play a critical role in collagen turnover in atheromata? Sukhova et al. [15] from our group demonstrated that human atheromata contain elastinolytic cathepsins K and S. Cathepsin K is also known as a potent interstitial collagenase. The relative contribution between MMP-family collagenases and other non-MMP collagenases such as cathepsin K to collagen breakdown in atheromata remains undetermined. We recently explored direct evidence in vivo for the role of collagenases in the collagen metabolism, employing "knock-in" mice that bear a mutation at the cleavage site of type I collagen shared by collagenases of the MMP family [16]. We introduced this mutation into hypercholesterolemic apoE-deficient mice and found that collagenase resistance increased intimal collagen content (Fukumoto et al., original manuscript, submitted for publication). This study provides unambiguous in vivo evidence for a role of MMP-family collagenases in collagen breakdown. Such preclinical studies substantially increase our mechanistic understanding of the role of collagenolytic activity in plaque vulnerability.

Acknowledgements

We acknowledge our colleagues including Dr. Peter Libby for their invaluable contributions and support to the concepts and experiments described in this paper. We acknowledge Ms. Karen E. Williams for her editorial expertise. The work from our laboratory was supported in part by grants from the NIH (SCOR HL56985 to Drs. Libby and Aikawa and MERIT Award to Dr. Libby) and Japan Heart Foundation to Dr. Aikawa.

References

[1] P. Libby, Molecular bases of the acute coronary syndromes, Circulation 91 (1995) 2844–2850.
[2] Z.S. Galis, G.K. Sukhova, M.W. Lark, P. Libby, Increased expression of matrix metalloproteinases and matrix degrading activity in vulnerable regions of human atherosclerotic plaques, J. Clin. Invest. 94 (1994) 2493–2503.
[3] S.T. Nikkari, K.D. O'Brien, M. Ferguson, T. Hatsukami, H.G. Welgus, C.E. Alpers, A.W. Clowes, Interstitial collagenase (MMP-1) expression in human carotid atherosclerosis, Circulation 92 (1995) 1393–1398.
[4] M. Aikawa, E. Rabkin, Y. Okada, S.J. Voglic, S.K. Clinton, C.E. Brinckerhoff, G.K. Sukhova, P. Libby, Lipid lowering by diet reduces matrix metalloproteinase activity and increases collagen content of rabbit atheroma: a potential mechanism of lesion stabilization, Circulation 97 (1998) 2433–2444.
[5] G. Sukhova, U. Schoenbeck, E. Rabkin, F. Schoen, A. Poole, R. Billinghurst, P. Libby, Evidence of increased collagenolysis by interstitial collagenases-1 and -3 in vulnerable human atheromatous plaques, Circulation 99 (1999) 2503–2509.
[6] M.P. Herman, G.K. Sukhova, P. Libby, N. Gerdes, N. Tang, D.B. Horton, M. Kilbride, R.E. Breitbart, M. Chun, U. Schonbeck, Expression of neutrophil collagenase (matrix metalloproteinase-8) in human atheroma: a novel collagenolytic pathway suggested by transcriptional profiling, Circulation 104 (2001) 1899–1904.
[7] M. Aikawa, E. Rabkin, S. Sugiyama, S.J. Voglic, Y. Fukumoto, Y. Furukawa, M. Shiomi, F.J. Schoen, P. Libby, An HMG-CoA reductase inhibitor, cerivastatin, suppresses growth of macrophages expressing matrix metalloproteinases and tissue factor in vivo and in vivo, Circulation 103 (2001) 276–283.
[8] Y. Fukumoto, P. Libby, E. Rabkin, C.C. Hill, M. Enomoto, Y. Hirouchi, M. Shiomi, M. Aikawa, Statins alter smooth muscle cell accumulation and collagen content in established atheroma of Watanabe heritable hyperlipidemic rabbits, Circulation 103 (2001) 993–999.
[9] R. Visse, H. Nagase, Matrix metalloproteinases and tissue inhibitors of metalloproteinases: structure, function, and biochemistry, Circ. Res. 92 (2003) 827–839.
[10] L.F. Morton, M.J. Barnes, Collagen polymorphism in the normal and diseased blood vessel wall. Investigation of collagens types I, III and V, Atherosclerosis 42 (1982) 41–51.
[11] P. Libby, M. Aikawa, Stabilization of atherosclerotic plaques: new mechanisms and clinical targets, Nat. Med. 8 (2002) 1257–1262.
[12] M. Aikawa, E. Rabkin, S.J. Voglic, H. Shing, R. Nagai, F.J. Schoen, P. Libby, Lipid lowering promotes accumulation of mature smooth muscle cells expressing smooth muscle myosin heavy chain isoforms in rabbit atheroma, Circ. Res. 83 (1998) 1015–1026.
[13] M. Aikawa, S.J. Voglic, S. Sugiyama, E. Rabkin, M.B. Taubman, J.T. Fallon, P. Libby, Dietary lipid lowering reduces tissue factor expression in rabbit atheroma, Circulation 100 (1999) 1215–1222.
[14] M. Aikawa, S. Sugiyama, C. Hill, S. Voglic, E. Rabkin, Y. Fukumoto, F. Schoen, J.L. Witztum, P. Libby, Lipid lowering reduces oxidative stress and endothelial cell activation in rabbit atheroma, Circulation 106 (2002) 1390–1396.
[15] G.K. Sukhova, G.P. Shi, D.I. Simon, H.A. Chapman, P. Libby, Expression of the elastolytic cathepsins S and K in human atheroma and regulation of their production in smooth muscle cells, J. Clin. Invest. 102 (1998) 576–583.
[16] W. Zhao, M.H. Byrne, Y. Wang, S.M. Krane, Osteocyte and osteoblast apoptosis and excessive bone deposition accompany failure of collagenase cleavage of collagen, J. Clin. Invest. 106 (2000) 941–949.

ELSEVIER

International Congress Series 1262 (2004) 71–74

www.ics-elsevier.com

Oxidative stress and inflammation in plaque instability—role of vascular C-reactive protein

Nobutaka Inoue*, Seiichi Kobayashi, Mitsuhiro Yokoyama

Division of Cardiovascular and Respiratory Medicine, Department of Internal Medicine, Kobe University Graduate School of Medicine 7-5-1 Kusunoki-cho, Chuo, Kobe 650-0017, Japan

Abstract. Disruption of vulnerable plaques is the main cause of acute coronary syndrome (ACS). It was reported that reactive oxygen species (ROS) activate matrix metalloproteinases. Therefore, the oxidative stress likely plays an important role in atherogenesis as well as plaque instability. Recent investigations demonstrated the presence of CRP, a potent risk factor of cardiovascular disease, in atherosclerotic vessels, and that CRP has direct pro-inflammatory effects on vascular cells such as induction of adhesion molecules and chemokines. In this review, we discuss the interaction of oxidative stress and inflammatory response in the plaque instability focusing on CRP. © 2004 Published by Elsevier B.V.

Keywords: C-reactive protein; Inflammation; NADH/NADPH oxidase

1. Introduction

Acute coronary syndrome (ACS) is primarily caused by rupture or erosion of atherosclerotic plaques, which give rise to a superimposed thrombosis. According to 'the response to injury theory', endothelial injury is regarded as the initial step of atherogenesis. Various cellular and biological processes contribute to the progression from this first step to acute coronary syndrome, so to speak, the end stage of atherosclerotic vascular disease.

It was demonstrated that the production of superoxide was enhanced in human atherosclerotic coronary arteries [1]. Generated reactive oxygen species (ROS) induce the oxidative modification of LDL, which leads to the formation of oxidized LDL and other deleterious lipids such as lysophosphatidylcholine. These atherogenic lipids have a potent activity to induce endothelial dysfunction and lesion formation [2]. In atherosclerotic lesions, a variety of inflammatory cells accumulate, and various cytokines generated by these cells induce the imbalance between MMP and TIMP. Among these complicated biological processes from endothelial injury to ACS, we can pick up two important key words, that is, oxidative stress and inflammation. In this brief review, we would like to discuss the interaction of oxidative stress and inflammation focusing on CRP.

* Corresponding author. Tel.: +81-78-382-5846; fax: +81-78-382-5859.
E-mail address: nobutaka@med.kobe-u.ac.jp (N. Inoue).

0531-5131/ © 2004 Published by Elsevier B.V.
doi:10.1016/j.ics.2003.12.039

2. Role of vascular NADH/NADPH oxidase and CRP—lessons from directional coronary atherectomy

Although various potential sources have been proposed, it has now become evident that NADH/NADPH oxidase is the most important enzymatic origin in vessel wall. Previously, we demonstrated that NADH/NADPH oxidase p22^{phox} was expressed in all major cellular components of human coronary arteries of autopsied cases: endothelial cells, smooth muscle cells (SMCs), macrophages, and fibroblasts, and this small component was upregulated through the vessel wall with progression of coronary atherosclerosis [3].

Recently, we examined the role of this oxidase system in pathogenesis of coronary artery disease using coronary specimens of angina patients obtained by directional coronary atherectomy (DCA). We observed that the production of ROS was closely associated with the expression of NADH/NADPH oxidase p22^{phox} in coronary arteries of

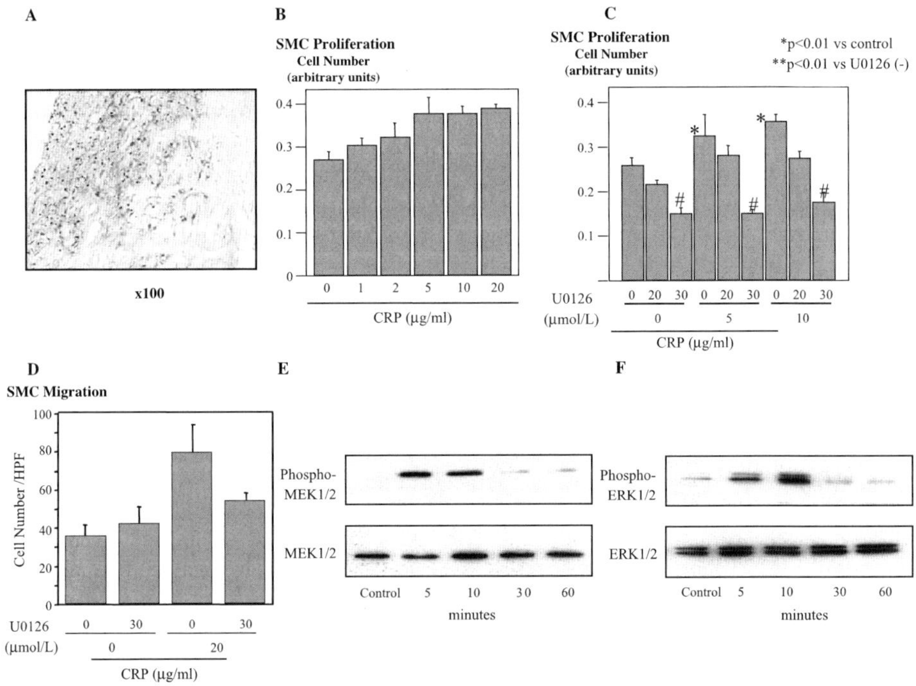

Fig. 1. (A) Immunohistochemical analysis for expression of CRP in human coronary artery of an autopsied case. The intense immunoreactivity of CRP was observed especially in inflammatory cells and medial smooth muscle cells. (B and C) Effect of CRP on proliferation of cultured human coronary artery SMCs (CASMCs) and inhibitory effects of MEK inhibitor. Proliferation was assessed by Cell Titer Non-Radioactive Cell Assay Kit (Promega). CRP stimulated the proliferation in dose-dependent manner, and U0126, an inhibitor of MEK, suppressed this effect (C). (D) Effect of CRP on migration of cultured human coronary artery SMCs (CASMCs) and inhibitory effects of MEK inhibitor. Cell migration was evaluated by chemotaxis chamber. CRP stimulated proliferation as well as migration of CASMCs, and MEK inhibitor suppressed this effect. (E and F) Effect of CRP on the activation of MEK (E) and ERK (F). Phosphorylation of ERK and MEK was determined by immunoblot analysis with phosphospecific antibodies. The same sample was used for immunoblot analysis with anti-MEK and ERK.

Table 1
Biological effect of C-reactive protein on vascular cells

↑ Adhesion molecules (VCAM-1 and E-selection)
↑ Chemokines (MCP-1)
↓Expression of eNOS
↓Release of prostacyclin
↑ Expression of plaminogen activator inhibitor-1
↑ Expression of angiotensin type 1 receptor
↑ LDL uptake by macrophages
Endothelium-independent relaxation of smooth muscle cells
↑ Generation of ROS

angina patients. Furthermore, the generation of ROS was overlapped with the distribution of oxidized LDL and $p22^{phox}$. Although there was no significant difference of angiographic stenosis, the generation of ROS in unstable angina patients was significantly higher compared with stable angina. Thus, the oxidative stress seems to influence the disease state of angina pectoris and vulnerability of plaques rather than the degree of coronary stenosis [4].

Fig. 1A shows the expression of CRP protein in human coronary artery of an autopsied case. Its intense immunoreactivity was observed in inflammatory cells and SMCs. Similarly, we found the expression of CRP in DCA specimens of angina patient [5]. Its immunoreactivity was observed in all DCA specimens. Furthermore, double staining showed a close association of CRP deposition and NADH/NAPDH oxidase $p22^{phox}$ [5]. To clarify its origin, we performed in situ hybridization. It revealed that CRP mRNA was detected in DCA specimens, indicating that vascular cells generated CRP mRNA [5]. On the other hand, we observed that DCA specimens obtained from patients whose serum CRP levels were more than 0.3 mg/dl had more immunoreactivity [5]. From these findings, it is

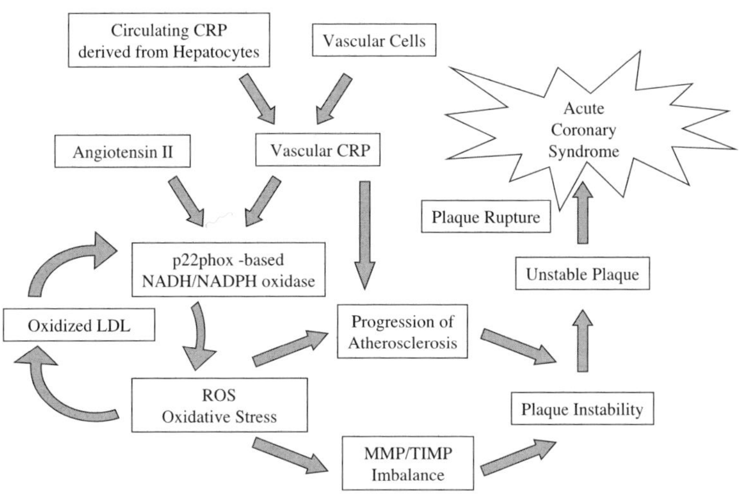

Fig. 2. Possible role of vascular CRP in pathogenesis of coronary artery disease.

likely that CRP in coronary arteries is originated from both the circulating blood and vascular cells themselves. The investigation of characteristics of CRP-expressing vascular cells should provide a new insight into understanding the link of inflammatory process and pathogenesis of atherosclerotic vascular diseases.

3. Direct effect of CRP on coronary artery smooth muscle cells

Recent investigations provide new aspects into the research field with regard to CRP. CRP has been regarded as a maker of inflammation; however, it has now become evident that CRP itself exerts potent biological effects on various cells as shown in Table 1.

To obtain more insight to the direct roles of CRP in atherogenesis, its effects on proliferation and migration of cultured coronary artery SMCs were examined. As shown in Fig. 1B and D, CRP stimulated the proliferation and migration of coronary artery SMCs. Interestingly, an inhibitor of MEK, significantly suppressed CRP-induced proliferation and migration (Fig. 1C and D). Furthermore, CRP activated MEK and ERK in cultured coronary artery SMCs (Fig. 1E and F). Thus, CRP directly promotes the atherogenic process via MEK/ERK-dependent pathway. Furthermore, we reported that CRP increased the expression of $p22^{phox}$ protein as well as ROS production [5].

4. Conclusions

Our hypothesis is shown in Fig. 2. A portion of CRP deposited in vessel wall is generated by vascular cells, and vascular CRP is a direct participant in vascular inflammation and lesion formation via potent biological effects including upregulation of NADH/NADPH oxidase. Given a close association of oxidized LDL and NADH/NADPH oxidase, this oxidase is critical for the oxidative modification of LDL. Since lysophosphatidylcholine, a major atherogenic lipid of oxidized LDL, activates NADH/NADPH oxidase [6], we speculate that there is a vicious circle consisting of NADH/NADPH oxidase, ROS, and oxidized LDL. Thus, CRP, a key molecule linking oxidative stress and inflammation, contributes directly and actively to the pathogenesis of atherosclerotic vascular disease, including ACS.

References

[1] M. Okuda, N. Inoue, et al., Expression of glutaredoxin in human coronary arteries: its potential role in antioxidant protection against atherosclerosis, Arterioscler. Thromb. Vasc. Biol. 21 (2001) 1483–1487.

[2] N. Inoue, K.M. Hirata, et al., Lysophosphatidylcholine inhibits bradykinin-induced phosphoinositide hydrolysis and calcium transients in cultured bovine aortic endothelial cells, Circ. Res. 71 (1992) 1410–1421.

[3] H. Azumi, N. Inoue, et al., Expression of NADH/NADPH oxidase p22phox in human coronary arteries, Circulation 100 (1999) 1494–1498.

[4] H. Azumi, N. Inoue, et al., Superoxide generation in directional coronary atherectomy specimens of patients with angina pectoris: important role of NAD(P)H oxidase, Arterioscler. Thromb. Vasc. Biol. 22 (2002) 1838–1844.

[5] S. Kobayashi, N. Inoue, et al., Interaction of oxidative stress and inflammatory response in coronary plaque instability: important role of C-reactive protein, Arterioscler. Thromb. Vasc. Biol. 23 (2003) 1398–1404.

[6] S. Takeshita, N. Inoue, et al., Lysophosphatidylcholine enhances superoxide anions production via endothelial NADH/NADPH oxidase, J. Atheroscler. Thromb. 7 (2000) 238–246.

International Congress Series 1262 (2004) 75–78

www.ics-elsevier.com

Plaque instability in human coronary atherosclerotic lesions: roles of oxidized LDL and neutrophils

Makiko Ueda[a,*], Shoichi Ehara[b], Yoshiki Kobayashi[b], Takahiko Naruko[c], Nobuyuki Shirai[a], Eishu Hai[a], Yoshihiro Ikura[a], Masahiko Ohsawa[a], Anton E. Becker[d]

[a] *Department of Pathology, Osaka City University Graduate School of Medicine, 1-4-3, Asahi-machi, Abeno, 545-8585, Osaka, Japan*

[b] *Internal Medicine and Cardiology, Osaka City University Graduate School of Medicine, Osaka, Japan*

[c] *Department of Cardiology, Osaka City General Hospital, Osaka, Japan*

[d] *Department of Cardiovascular Pathology, Academic Medical Center, University of Amsterdam, Amsterdam, The Netherlands*

Abstract. Experimental studies have shown that ox-LDL is a key factor in the processes of plaque inflammation. We demonstrated that plasma ox-LDL levels in AMI patients are significantly higher than in patients with UAP or SAP, or in controls. Moreover, our immunohistochemical study showed that culprit lesions of UAP patients contained a significantly higher percentage of ox-LDL-positive macrophages compared with those of SAP patients. These data suggest that increased levels of ox-LDL relate to plaque instability in human coronary atherosclerotic lesions. We have recently demonstrated that neutrophils play an important role in mediating destabilization of human coronary atherosclerotic plaques. Recent studies have demonstrated a strong oxidant, MPO, is capable of oxidizing LDL. We have immunohistochemically studied the expression of MPO in atherectomy specimens obtained from patients with SAP or UAP. Quantitative analysis demonstrated the neutrophil, macrophage, or MPO-positive area in UAP patients was significantly ($P<0.001$) higher than in SAP patients. Immunodouble stainings further revealed that most MPO-positive cells were neutrophils. These observations strongly suggest that MPO-positive neutrophils are actively associated with ACS. Neutrophil infiltration and activation at sites of unstable plaques with thrombosis may play a role in inducing an imbalance between pro-oxidants and antioxidants and promote LDL oxidation.

Keywords: Atherosclerosis; Oxidized LDL; Acute coronary syndrome; Neutrophil; Myeloperoxidase

---

Abbreviations: ox-LDL, oxidized low-density lipoprotein; AMI, acute myocardial infarction; UAP, unstable angina pectoris; SAP, stable angina pectoris; MPO, myeloperoxidase; ACS, acute coronary syndrome.

* Corresponding author. Tel.: +81-6-6645-3740; fax: +81-6-6645-3742.

E-mail address: maki@med.osaka-cu.ac.jp (M. Ueda).

0531-5131/
doi:10.1016/j.ics.2003.12.011

1. Introduction

Evidence has accumulated that activation of the inflammatory response in coronary atherosclerotic lesions relates to rapidly progressive plaque destabilization. Previous in vitro studies have shown that ox-LDL is a key factor in the pathogenesis of these inflammatory processes [1].

Recently, the detection of ox-LDL in circulating plasma has been reported [2]. We developed a new, sensitive method to measure plasma ox-LDL levels, using an anti-ox-LDL monoclonal antibody (DLH3) and an anti-apolipoprotein B (apoB) polyclonal antibody [3]. The monoclonal antibody, DLH3, is specific for ox-LDL and does not react with either native, acetylated, malondialdehyde-treated, or glycated LDL. With the use of this new and highly sensitive method, we investigated plasma levels of ox-LDL in patients with AMI, UAP and SAP.

It is now well recognized that human unstable plaques, such as ruptured plaques or eroded plaques, contain abundant macrophages and T lymphocytes, so-called chronic inflammatory cells. However, thus far, neutrophils in human unstable atherosclerotic lesions have not received much consideration. Moreover, MPO, a strong oxidant and secreted mainly from neutrophils, has been shown to be capable of oxidizing LDL [4]. Therefore, we studied, immnunohistochemically, the presence of ox-LDL, macrophages and neutrophils, and the expression of MPO in the culprit lesion of ACS.

2. Plasma ox-LDL levels relate to the severity of ACS

The measurement of plasma ox-LDL levels was performed using a sandwich ELISA method previously described [3]. The LDL fraction was separated from blood plasma before the ELISA procedure to minimize potential interference with other plasma constituents, such as ox-VLDL, anti-ox-LDL autoantibodies, and anti-phospholipid antibodies. The LDL fractions were obtained from the samples by sequential ultracentrifugation. Diluted LDL fractions (5 μg/well) were added to the microtiter wells precoated with 0.5 μg of the anti-ox-LDL antibody DLH3. After extensive washing, the remaining ox-LDL was detected with a sheep anti-human apoB antibody and an alkaline phosphatase-conjugated anti-sheep IgG antibody. In each ELISA plate, various concentrations of standard ox-LDL, which was prepared by incubating LDL with 5 μmol/l $CuSO_4$ at 37 °C for 3 h, were run simultaneously to determine a standard curve.

Plasma ox-LDL levels were measured in 135 patients with AMI ($n=45$), UAP ($n=45$) and SAP ($n=45$), and in 46 control subjects. In AMI patients, plasma ox-LDL levels were significantly higher than in patients with UAP ($P<0.0005$) or SAP ($P<0.0001$), or in controls ($P<0.0001$) (AMI: 1.95 ± 1.42, UAP: 1.19 ± 0.74, SAP: 0.89 ± 0.48, control: 0.58 ± 0.23 ng/5 μg LDL protein, mean ± S.D.). Serum levels of total, high-density lipoprotein, or LDL cholesterol did not differ among these patient groups. These observations strongly suggest that elevated plasma ox-LDL levels show a positive correlation with the severity of ACS [5].

3. Localization of ox-LDL in the culprit lesion of ACS

Thirty-three atherectomy specimens, obtained from patients with SAP ($n = 10$) and UAP ($n = 23$), were studied immunohistochemically for ox-LDL. For the identification of ox-LDL, the antibody DLH3 was used. The presence of apoB was studied also. In the lesions of UAP patients, abundant ox-LDL-positive cells were found; immunodouble staining for macrophages and ox-LDL revealed distinct ox-LDL positivity in macrophage-derived foam cells. In these lesions, moreover, ox-LDL and apoB colocalized in macrophage-derived foam cells. In contrast, in the atherectomy specimens of SAP patients, ox-LDL positivity was sparse. Morphometric analysis revealed that the number of ox-LDL-positive macrophages in the culprit lesions of UAP patients was significantly higher ($P < 0.0001$) than in those of SAP patients. These findings support the hypothesis that ox-LDL plays a crucial role in the genesis of coronary plaque instability in humans [5].

4. Infiltration of MPO-positive neutrophils in the culprit lesions of ACS

Based on frozen sections and using immunohistochemical single and double staining techniques, we studied the presence of neutrophils in culprit lesions of ACS [6]. Coronary segments were obtained at autopsy from 13 patients with AMI: 8 had a ruptured and 5 an eroded plaque. Coronary segments ($n = 113$), obtained from 45 patients who had died of noncardiovascular diseases, served as reference. Distinct neutrophil infiltration was detected in all specimens with plaque rupture or erosion. Immunodouble staining analysis, moreover, demonstrated that most MPO-positive cells in ruptured or eroded plaques were neutrophils [6].

We further investigated the expression of MPO in coronary atherectomy specimens obtained from patients with SAP ($n = 37$) and UAP ($n = 31$), using frozen sections. Quantitative analysis demonstrated the neutrophil, macrophage, or MPO-positive area in UAP patients was significantly ($P < 0.001$) higher than in SAP patients. Immunodouble staining for MPO and neutrophils, and for MPO and macrophages, revealed that the majority of MPO-positive cells were neutrophils. These findings strongly suggest that MPO-positive neutrophils are actively associated with acute coronary events in humans.

5. Discussion

It was previously believed that ox-LDL was not present in the circulation, since blood plasma has strong anti-oxidative abilities and since experimental studies had shown that ox-LDL injected intravenously was rapidly cleared from the circulation by the liver [7]. Recently, however, it was shown that ox-LDL does occur in blood and that plasma levels of ox-LDL were increased in patients with transplant associated coronary artery disease [2] and patients with AMI [5].

How and where does the oxidation of LDL take place in humans? At present, this is really speculative. Previous in vitro studies have documented that macrophages and lymphocytes are capable of oxidizing LDL [1]. Since the culprit lesions of patients with ACS contain abundant macrophages and T lymphocytes, it is reasonable to assume that these cells contribute to LDL oxidation. The results of our study, moreover, demonstrate that an infiltration of MPO-positive neutrophils is actively associated with acute coronary events in humans [6]. It is well known that neutrophils are an important source of reactive oxygen species. Moreover, recent studies have shown that MPO, a strong pro-oxidant enzyme released from activated neutrophils, induces LDL oxidation [4]. Taken together with our findings, one could hypothesize that neutrophil infiltration and activation and the release of MPO from activated neutrophils may also contribute to LDL oxidation in human coronary unstable plaques.

Our observations that plasma ox-LDL levels show a positive correlation with the severity of ACS [5] strongly suggest that ox-LDL present within unstable plaques may be released into the blood stream in patients with severe endothelial injuries, such as plaque rupture or erosion. Moreover, our results support the hypothesis that neutrophil activation and the release of MPO at sites of coronary unstable plaques with thrombosis may induce a focal imbalance between pro-oxidants and antioxidants and contribute to the enhancement of LDL oxidation, which could cause high levels of plasma ox-LDL in humans.

References

[1] J.L. Witztum, et al., Role of oxidized low density lipoprotein in atherogenesis, J. Clin. Invest. 88 (1991) 1785–1792.

[2] P. Holvoet, et al., Oxidized low density lipoproteins in patients with transplant-associated coronary artery disease, Arterioscler. Thromb. Vasc. Biol. 18 (1998) 100–107.

[3] H. Itabe, et al., Sensitive detection of oxidatively modified low density lipoprotein using a monoclonal antibody, J. Lipid Res. 37 (1996) 45–53.

[4] R. Zhang, et al., Defects in leukocyte-mediated initiation of lipid peroxidation in plasma as studied in myeloperoxidase-deficient subjects: systematic identification of multiple endogenous diffusible substrates for myeloperoxidase in plasma, Blood 99 (2002) 1802–1810.

[5] S. Ehara, et al., Elevated levels of oxidized low density lipoprotein show a positive relationship with the severity of acute coronary syndromes, Circulation 103 (2001) 1955–1960.

[6] T. Naruko, et al., Neutrophil infiltration of culprit lesions in acute coronary syndromes, Circulation 106 (2002) 2894–2900.

[7] T.J. Van Berkel, et al., Different fate in vivo of oxidatively modified low density lipoprotein and acetylated low density lipoprotein in rats. Recognition by various scavenger receptors on Kupffer and endothelial liver cells, J. Biol. Chem. 266 (1991) 2282–2289.

ELSEVIER

International Congress Series 1262 (2004) 79–82

www.ics-elsevier.com

Plasmin activates VEGF-C and VEGF-D

Bradley K. McColl[a], Megan E. Baldwin[a], Sally Roufail[a], Craig Freeman[b], Kari Alitalo[c], Steven A. Stacker[a], Marc G. Achen[a,*]

[a] *Angiogenesis Laboratory, Ludwig Institute for Cancer Research, Royal Melbourne Hospital, P.O. Box 2008, Melbourne, Victoria 3050 Australia*

[b] *Cancer and Vascular Biology Group, Division of Immunology and Genetics, The John Curtin School of Medical Research, The Australian National University, P.O. Box 334, Canberra ACT 2061, Australia*

[c] *Molecular/Cancer Biology Laboratory and Ludwig Institute for Cancer Research, Biomedicum Helsinki, University of Helsinki, P.O. Box 63 (Haartmaninkatu 8), FIN-00014, Helsinki, Finland*

Abstract. Angiogenesis and lymphangiogenesis (growth of lymphatic vessels) are guided by members of the vascular endothelial growth factor (VEGF) family of secreted glycoproteins. In particular, VEGF-C and VEGF-D promote lymphangiogenesis as demonstrated in transgenic animal models and gene delivery studies. VEGF-C and VEGF-D are secreted as full-length forms that require proteolytic activation for high affinity binding to VEGF receptor-2 (VEGFR-2) and VEGFR-3, cell surface receptor tyrosine kinases localised on the endothelial cells of blood vessels and lymphatics. The proteases that activate these lymphangiogenic growth factors are key regulators of lymphatic development but were previously unknown. Here we report identification of the serine protease plasmin as an enzyme capable of activating both VEGF-C and VEGF-D.

Keywords: Lymphangiogenesis; Lymphatics; Proteolysis; Growth factor; Metastasis

1. Introduction—the VEGFs and cancer

The vascular endothelial growth factors (VEGFs) are secreted glycoproteins that drive angiogenesis and lymphangiogenesis. In mammals, five VEGFs have been identified, VEGF, placenta growth factor (PlGF), VEGF-B, VEGF-C and VEGF-D, each containing a VEGF homology domain (VHD) [1]. The VEGFs act via three cell surface receptors, VEGFR-1 and VEGFR-2 (on blood vessel endothelium) and VEGFR-3 (on lymphatic endothelium) [1].

Clinical studies demonstrated a link between VEGF-C or VEGF-D expression and lymph node metastasis in human cancers [2–4]. Animal tumor models overexpressing VEGF-C and VEGF-D exhibit increased lymphatic metastasis relative to controls [5–8]. Furthermore, disrupting ligand binding to VEGFR-3 inhibited lymphatic metastasis in both VEGF-C and VEGF-D tumor models [6,7].

* Corresponding author. Tel.: +61-3-9341-3155; fax: +61-3-9341-3107.
E-mail address: Marc.achen@ludwig.edu.au (M.G. Achen).

0531-5131/
doi:10.1016/j.ics.2003.11.032

VEGFR-3-mediated lymphangiogenesis is therefore an important pathway in the spread of tumor cells, and a target for anti-metastatic agents.

VEGF-C and VEGF-D are secreted as full-length forms with N- and C-terminal propeptides flanking the receptor binding VHD [9,10]. Proteolysis removes the propeptides and generates homodimeric mature forms capable of binding VEGFR-2 and VEGFR-3 with increased affinity relative to unprocessed proteins [9,11]. Proteolysis is therefore a critical regulator of lymphangiogenesis, however, the protease(s) responsible were previously unknown. Here, we report that the serine protease plasmin activates VEGF-D and VEGF-C [12].

2. Plasmin activates VEGF-D

To assay for proteolysis of VEGF-D, a scintillation proximity assay (SPA) was used (Fig. 1A). An N-terminally biotinylated peptide containing the C-terminal cleavage site of VEGF-D was radiolabelled at the C terminus with ^{3}H [13], and treated with a range of candidate proteases. Following digestion, the peptide was bound to streptavidin-coated scintillant beads, and counted. Detectable photons are generated only when the radiolabelled peptide is intact, whereas after proteolysis, the C-terminal peptide fragment in solution is not sufficiently proximal to the scintillant beads to generate photons. Proteolysis of the peptide is therefore detected as a reduction in counts.

Treatment of VEGF-D peptide with plasmin resulted in a substantial reduction in counts detected, indicating digestion of the peptide. Other proteases showed little or no cleavage of the peptide relative to undigested controls (Fig. 1B and data not shown).

To establish if full-length VEGF-D is a substrate for plasmin, purified VEGF-D was digested and analysed by Western blot. Plasmin generated a single 21 kDa species containing the VHD (Fig. 1C), reflecting the size of the previously characterised mature VEGF-D [11]. This indicates that plasmin cleaves both the N- and C-terminal propeptides from VEGF-D.

To ascertain if plasmin-digested VEGF-D is capable of binding and cross-linking VEGFR-2 and VEGFR-3, IL-3 dependent Ba/F3 cell lines expressing chimeric receptor constructs were used. These receptor constructs consist of the extracellular domain of either VEGFR-2 or VEGFR-3 and the cytoplasmic domain of the erythropoietin receptor (EpoR) [10,14,15]. Signalling by the EpoR intracellular domain due to ligand binding and cross-linking of VEGFR-2 or VEGFR-3 extracellular domains allows proliferation in the absence of IL-3. Proliferation is assessed by [^{3}H] thymidine incorporation.

After treatment with plasmin-digested VEGF-D, both VEGFR-2/EpoR and VEGFR-3/EpoR expressing cells showed significantly elevated proliferation relative to cells treated with undigested growth factor (Fig. 1D). Therefore, plasmin digestion generates forms of VEGF-D with enhanced capacity to bind and cross-link VEGFR-2 and VEGFR-3 extracellular domains. Similar results were achieved with plasmin treatment of VEGF-C [12].

3. Plasmin and lymphangiogenesis

Plasmin releases sequestered VEGF from the extracellular matrix or cell surface [16]. The capacity of plasmin to generate mature VEGF-C and VEGF-D from full-length forms is another example of growth factor activation by proteolysis. Plasmin is also responsible

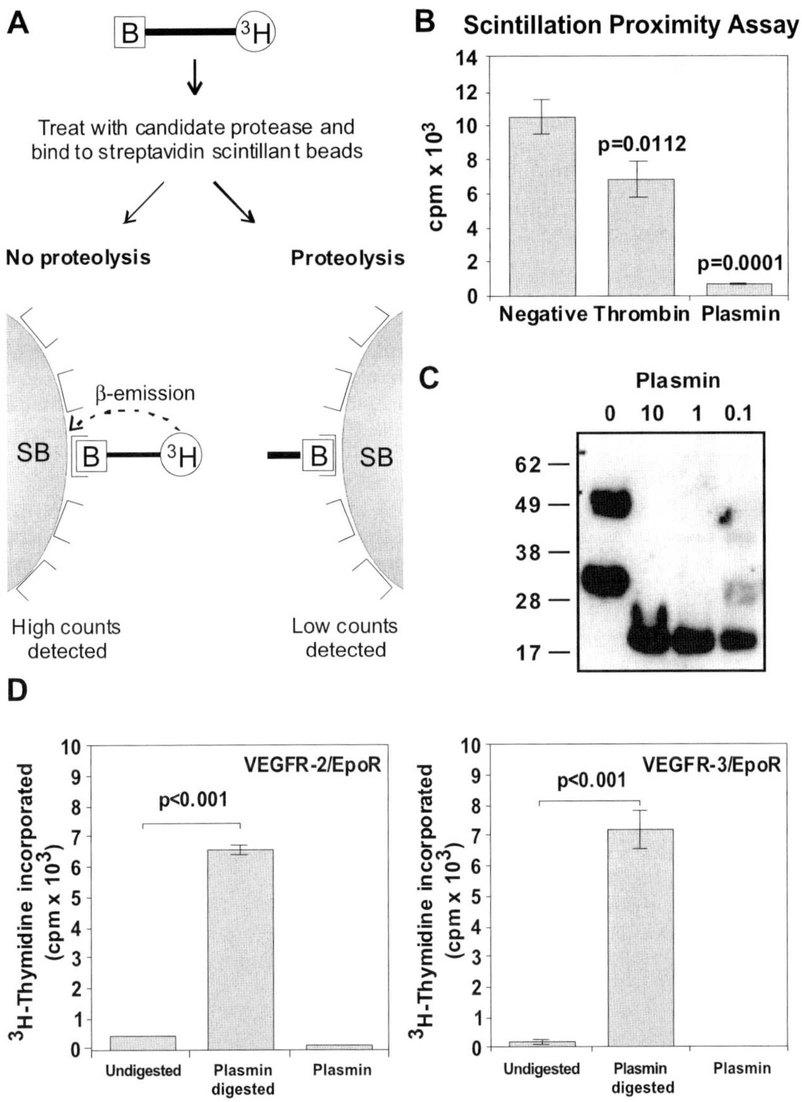

Fig. 1. Plasmin cleavage of VEGF-D. (A) SPA. Black bar represents the biotinylated (denoted B), radiolabelled (^{3}H) VEGF-D peptide. Following protease treatment, the peptide is bound to scintillant beads (SB) via streptavidin conjugated to the beads (brackets). (B) Results of the SPA comparing *plasmin* or *thrombin* digested peptide with undigested control (*Negative*). *P* values comparing protease treated and control samples were calculated with Student's *t*-test. (C) Analysis of plasmin digested VEGF-D. Purified VEGF-D, consisting of full-length (~ 52 kDa) and partially processed forms (~ 31 kDa) was digested with 0, 10, 1 or 0.1 U/ml of plasmin, and Western blotted using anti-VEGF-D (VHD) antibody. Note the 21 kDa species produced following plasmin digestion. (D) Analysis of plasmin digested VEGF-D binding to VEGFR-2 and VEGFR-3 extracellular domains. Ba/F3 cells expressing VEGFR-2/EpoR (left) or VEGFR-3/EpoR (right) chimeric receptors were treated with full-length VEGF-D (*Undigested*), plasmin digested VEGF-D (*Plasmin Digested*) or plasmin without growth factors (*Plasmin*). *P* values comparing digested and undigested samples were calculated using Student's *t*-test.

for the degradation of fibrin clots [17], and may play a central role in vessel formation following wounding by activating growth factors necessary for revascularization of damaged tissue and degrading clots.

Numerous studies have demonstrated the role of plasmin in promoting metastasis [18]. For example, plasminogen-null mice showed fewer lymph node metastases than controls in a tumor model [19]. Manipulation of plasmin and examination of subsequent effects on lymphangiogenesis will provide insights into the role of this enzyme in wound healing and pathological lymphangiogenesis.

References

[1] M.G. Achen, S.A. Stacker, The vascular endothelial growth factor family; proteins which guide the development of the vasculature, Int. J. Exp. Pathol. 79 (1998) 255–265.
[2] Y. Nakamura, H. Yasuoka, M. Tsujimoto, et al, Prognostic significance of vascular endothelial growth factor D in breast carcinoma with long-term follow-up, Clin. Cancer Res. 9 (2003) 716–721.
[3] Y. Nakamura, H. Yasuoka, M. Tsujimoto, et al, Clinicopathological significance of vascular endothelial growth factor-C in breast carcinoma with long-term follow-up, Mod. Path. 16 (2003) 309–314.
[4] J.D. White, P.W. Hewett, D. Kosuge, et al, Vascular endothelial growth factor-D expression is an independent prognostic marker for survival in colorectal carcinoma, Cancer Res. 62 (2002) 1669–1675.
[5] S.J. Mandriota, L. Jussila, M. Jeltsch, et al, Vascular endothelial growth factor-C-mediated lymphangiogenesis promotes tumour metastasis, EMBO J. 20 (4) (2001) 672–682.
[6] S.A. Stacker, C. Caesar, M.E. Baldwin, et al, VEGF-D promotes the metastatic spread of tumor cells via the lymphatics, Nat. Med. 7 (2001) 186–191.
[7] Y. He, K. Kozaki, T. Karpanen, et al, Suppression of tumor lymphangiogenesis and lymph node metastasis by blocking vascular endothelial growth factor receptor 3 signaling, J. Natl. Cancer Inst. 94 (2002) 819–825.
[8] M. Skobe, T. Hawighorst, D.G. Jackson, et al, Induction of tumor lymphangiogenesis by VEGF-C promotes breast cancer metastasis, Nat. Med. 7 (2001) 192–198.
[9] V. Joukov, T. Sorsa, V. Kumar, et al, Proteolytic processing regulates receptor specificity and activity of VEGF-C, EMBO J. 16 (1997) 3898–3911.
[10] M.G. Achen, M. Jeltsch, E. Kukk, et al, Vascular endothelial growth factor D (VEGF-D) is a ligand for the tyrosine kinases VEGF receptor 2 (Flk-1) and VEGF receptor 3 (Flt-4), Proc. Natl. Acad. Sci. U. S. A. 95 (1998) 548–553.
[11] S.A. Stacker, K. Stenvers, C. Caesar, et al, Biosynthesis of vascular endothelial growth factor-D involves proteolytic processing which generates non-covalent homodimers, J. Biol. Chem. 274 (1999) 32127–32136.
[12] B.K. McColl, M.E. Baldwin, S. Roufail, et al, Plasmin activates the lymphangiogenic growth factors VEGF-C and VEGF-D, J. Exp. Med. 198 (2003) 863–868.
[13] A. Brown, S. George, A. Blume, et al, Biotinylated and cysteine-modified peptides as useful reagents for studying the inhibition of cathepsin G, Anal. Biochem. 217 (1994) 139–147.
[14] M.G. Achen, S. Roufail, T. Domagala, et al, Monoclonal antibodies to vascular endothelial growth factor-D block interactions with both VEGF receptor-2 and VEGF receptor-3, Eur. J. Biochem. 267 (2000) 2505–2515.
[15] S.A. Stacker, A. Vitali, C. Caesar, et al, A mutant form of vascular endothelial growth factor (VEGF) that lacks VEGF receptor-2 activation retains the ability to induce vascular permeability, J. Biol. Chem. 274 (1999) 34884–34892.
[16] K.A. Houck, D.W. Leung, A.M. Rowland, et al, Dual regulation of vascular endothelial growth factor bioavailability by genetic and proteolytic mechanisms, J. Biol. Chem. 267 (1992) 26031–26037.
[17] H.R. Lijnen, Elements of the fibrinolytic system, Ann. N.Y. Acad. Sci. 936 (2001) 226–236.
[18] P.A. Andreasen, R. Egelund, H.H. Petersen, The plasminogen activation system in tumor growth, invasion, and metastasis, Cell. Mol. Life Sci. 57 (2000) 25–40.
[19] T.H. Bugge, K.W. Kombrinck, Q. Xiao, Growth and dissemination of Lewis lung carcinoma in plasminogen-deficient mice, Blood 90 (1997) 4522–4531.

International Congress Series 1262 (2004) 83–86

www.ics-elsevier.com

Oxidized lipoprotein regulation of tissue factor in smooth muscle cells

Shu-Ling Liang[a,b], Mei-Zhen Cui[c], Marc S. Penn[b,d], Guy M. Chisolm[b,*]

[a] *Department of Chemistry, Cleveland State University, USA*
[b] *Department of Cell Biology, Cleveland Clinic Foundation, 9500 Euclid Avenue, Cleveland, OH 44195 USA*
[c] *Department of Pathology, University of Tennessee, Knoxville, TN, USA*
[d] *Department of Cardiovascular Medicine, Cleveland Clinic Foundation, Cleveland, OH, USA*

Abstract. Cell surface tissue factor (TF), which can initiate local coagulation, is upregulated in cells within atherosclerotic plaques, including macrophages, endothelial cells (EC) and smooth muscle cells (SMC). TF binds coagulation factors VIIa and Xa to make a catalytically active complex that produces thrombin and ultimately fibrin, leading to inflammation and coagulation. Using rat SMC, we have shown that lipids of low-density lipoprotein (LDL) and oxidized LDL (oxLDL) differentially regulate TF gene expression and TF activity. Unknown lipids of LDL induced the gene, but did not enhance activity. In contrast, oxLDL or its extracted lipids induced both the TF gene and TF activity. Specific lipids of oxLDL, e.g., lipid hydroperoxides, and H_2O_2 increased TF activity without enhancing TF gene or protein. The effects of lipid hydroperoxides were antioxidant-inhibitable. Lysophosphatidic acid (lysoPA) and lysophosphatidylcholine (lysoPC), important lipid mediators of many cellular processes and formed during LDL oxidation, increased TF mRNA, protein and activity. LysoPA induced the TF gene via a Gi-protein-coupled signaling process. Thus, different lipoprotein-borne lipids in atherosclerotic lesions enhance TF gene expression and TF activity through distinct mechanisms. These effects may contribute to lesion development and subsequent complications. © 2003 Published by Elsevier B.V.

Keywords: Atherosclerosis; Lysophospholipids; Oxidized LDL; Smooth muscle cells; Tissue factor

Cell-associated tissue factor (TF) is a 47-kDa glycoprotein expressed on cell surfaces consisting of a transmembrane domain, a short cytoplasmic tail, and a 219-residue extracellular domain. While it has no enzymatic activity, its expression on a cell surface is permissive for the enzymatic production of thrombin. Under appropriate circumstances, e.g., in response to injury or other stimuli, TF binds factor VIIa (FVIIa), which can then cleave FX to FXa, and FIX to FIXa. The TF:FVIIa:FXa complex can cleave prothrombin

* Corresponding author. Tel.: +1-216-4445854; fax: +1-216-4449404.
E-mail address: chisolg@ccf.org (G.M. Chisolm).

0531-5131/ © 2003 Published by Elsevier B.V.
doi:10.1016/j.ics.2003.11.001

to thrombin. Thrombin can cleave fibrinogen to fibrin and amplify the coagulation process by activating factors V, VIII, and XI. TF is thus an initiator of the coagulation cascade. The importance of understanding TF regulation goes beyond the need to understand clotting, since local production of thrombin can elicit multiple potent biological effects, including cell migration and proliferation, cytoskeleton changes and multiple inflammatory responses [1,2].

Enhanced TF expression is closely linked to cardiovascular diseases. In normal blood vessels, the expression of full length TF is limited to adventitia; however, in atherosclerosis, TF is expressed abundantly in lesions [3,4]. Clinical studies have confirmed that increases in TF are detected in plaques from patients with unstable angina, myocardial infarction or coronary thrombosis compared with those from patients with stable angina or uncomplicated coronary lesions [3]. Furthermore, early TF expression predicts subsequent development of cardiac allograft vasculopathy in heart transplantation patients [5]. Therefore, arterial TF expression has been proposed to enhance atherosclerosis risk. Macrophages, smooth muscle cells (SMC), and endothelial cells (EC) are sources of TF in lesions [3,4].

The molecular mechanisms regulating vascular TF expression are becoming better understood. In cultures of monocytes and EC, TF mRNA and TF pathway activity are induced by phorbol esters, TNF-α, lipopolysaccharide, interleukin-1, α-thrombin, and shear. In SMC, TF mRNA and TF pathway activity are induced by various stimuli, including serum, PDGF, EGF, angiotensin-II, α-thrombin, and MCP-1 [2,4]. The mammalian TF promoter contains multiple putative Sp1 sites, which regulate basal expression of the TF gene, one or more Egr-1 sites, two AP-1 sites, and one NF-κB site. Which of these regulates TF induction depends on cell type and stimulus [2].

Oxidized LDL (oxLDL) enhances TF in the three major cell types present in atherosclerotic lesions, i.e., EC, SMC, and macrophages. OxLDL was first shown to induce TF gene expression and TF activity in human EC [6,7]. Reports on the effects of oxLDL on TF expression in various monocytic and macrophage preparations of cells are variable and in apparent contradiction. Some observe enhanced TF by oxLDL in monocyte/macrophage-like cells [8], others find no enhancement [9], and others report only augmentation of the effects of other stimuli [10]. Reasons for the discrepancies are unclear. Species variation, inadvertent lipopolysaccharide contamination, and variations among cell preparations may account for some. The consensus is that oxLDL can induce, or increase induction of, TF in EC or monocyte/macrophages, which could have dramatic effects in vivo.

We have shown that low-density lipoprotein (LDL), oxLDL, or their lipid extracts induced TF gene expression in SMC (unrelated to LPS contamination) [11]. The gene induction was mediated by constitutive Sp1 and induced Egr-1 [11]. Interestingly, oxLDL or its lipids, but not LDL, also enhanced TF activity on SMC surfaces [12]. Seeking the biologically active components of oxLDL responsible for enhanced TF activity, we tested HPLC fractions of oxLDL lipids and some known oxLDL components. Specific lipids of oxLDL were identified that enhanced TF pathway activity in SMC without enhancing TF gene expression, such as 7-β-hydroperoxycholesterol and other lipid hydroperoxides [12]. This suggested that TF mRNA and TF activity can be enhanced through distinct mechanisms, the latter involving a transition from latent TF on the cell surface to TF being a participant in the active TF:FVIIa:FXa complex. The latter depended on oxidative events, since the effects of lipid hydroperoxides were antioxidant inhibitable [12] and since H_2O_2 induced TF activity without inducing the gene [13].

During oxidation of LDL, its various classes of lipids undergo modification, including phospholipid oxidation and the conversion of oxidized phospholipids to lysophospholipids by LDL-associated phospholipase A_2. We have found that lysophosphatidic acid (lysoPA) [14] and lysophosphatidylcholine (lysoPC) (unpublished), which are increased during LDL oxidation and accumulate in lesions, enhance TF gene expression and TF activity in SMC; however, these lysophospholipids induce TF synthesis by distinct mechanisms. Interestingly, lysoPC did not enhance TF in EC [15] or macrophages [16], suggesting that lysoPC's effects on SMC TF may be cell-specific.

The induction of TF expression and the increase in TF activity by lipoproteins, oxidized lipoproteins and certain of their respective lipids in vitro in cell types that reside in vascular lesions, and the presence of these lipids in arterial lesions, invites speculation that these could be among the in vivo stimuli for the marked TF induction observed in arterial lesions. Identification of these stimuli and elucidation of the mechanisms by which they enhance TF may suggest opportunities for therapeutic intervention.

References

[1] M. Riewald, W. Ruf, Orchestration of coagulation protease signaling by tissue factor, Trends Cardiovasc. Med. 12 (2002) 149–154.

[2] N. Mackman, Gene targeting in hemostasis. Tissue factor, Front. Biosci. 6 (2001) D208–D215.

[3] D. Ardissino, P.A. Merlini, R. Arlens, R. Coppola, E. Bramucci, S. Lucreziotti, A. Repetto, R. Fetiveau, P.M. Mannucci, Tissue factor in human coronary atherosclerotic plaques, Clin. Chim. Acta 291 (2000) 235–240.

[4] M.B. Taubman, J.T. Fallon, A.D. Schecter, P. Giesen, M. Mendlowitz, B.S. Fyfe, J.D. Marmur, Y. Nemerson, Tissue factor in the pathogenesis of atherosclerosis, Thromb. Haemost. 78 (1997) 200–204.

[5] M.H. Yen, G. Pilkington, R.C. Starling, N.B. Ratliff, P.M. McCarthy, J.B. Young, G.M. Chisolm, M.S. Penn, Increased tissue factor expression predicts development of cardiac allograft vasculopathy, Circulation 106 (2002) 1379–1383.

[6] J.R. Weis, R.E. Pitas, B.D. Wilson, G.M. Rodgers, Oxidized low-density lipoprotein increases cultured human endothelial cell tissue factor activity and reduces protein C activation, FASEB J. 5 (1991) 2459–2465.

[7] T.A. Drake, K. Hannani, H.H. Fei, S. Lavi, J.A. Berliner, Minimally oxidized low-density lipoprotein induces tissue factor expression in cultured human endothelial cells, Am. J. Pathol. 138 (1991) 601–607.

[8] J.C. Lewis, A.L. Bennett-Cain, C.S. DeMars, G.J. Doellgast, K.W. Grant, N.L. Jones, M. Gupta, Procoagulant activity after exposure of monocyte-derived macrophages to minimally oxidized low density lipoprotein: co-localization of tissue factor antigen and nascent fibrin fibers at the cell surface, Am. J. Pathol. 147 (1995) 1029–1040.

[9] M.M. van den Eijnden, J.T. van Noort, L. Hollaar, A. van der Laarse, R.M. Bertina, Cholesterol or triglyceride loading of human monocyte-derived macrophages by incubation with modified lipoproteins does not induce tissue factor expression, Arterioscler. Thromb. Vasc. Biol. 19 (1999) 384–392.

[10] K. Brand, C.L. Banka, N. Mackman, R.A. Terkeltaub, S.T. Fan, L.K. Curtiss, Oxidized LDL enhances lipopolysaccharide-induced tissue factor expression in human adherent monocytes, Arterioscler. Thromb. 14 (1994) 790–797.

[11] M.Z. Cui, M.S. Penn, G.M. Chisolm, Native and oxidized low density lipoprotein induction of tissue factor gene expression in smooth muscle cells is mediated by both Egr-1 and Sp1, J. Biol. Chem. 274 (1999) 32795–32802.

[12] M.S. Penn, M.Z. Cui, A.L. Winokur, J. Bethea, T.A. Hamilton, P.E. DiCorleto, G.M. Chisolm, Smooth

muscle cell surface tissue factor pathway activation by oxidized low-density lipoprotein requires cellular lipid peroxidation, Blood 96 (2000) 3056–3063.

[13] M.S. Penn, C.V. Patel, M.Z. Cui, P.E. DiCorleto, G.M. Chisolm, LDL increases inactive tissue factor on vascular smooth muscle cell surfaces: hydrogen peroxide activates latent cell surface tissue factor, Circulation 99 (1999) 1753–1759.

[14] M.Z. Cui, G. Zhao, A.L. Winokur, E. Laag, J.R. Bydash, M.S. Penn, G.M. Chisolm, X. Xu, Lysophosphatidic acid induction of tissue factor expression in aortic smooth muscle cells, Arterioscler. Thromb. Vasc. Biol. 23 (2003) 224–230.

[15] N. Sato, K. Kokame, T. Miyata, H. Kato, Lysophosphatidylcholine decreases the synthesis of tissue factor pathway inhibitor in human umbilical vein endothelial cells, Thromb. Haemost. 79 (1998) 217–221.

[16] B. Engelmann, S. Zieseniss, K. Brand, S. Page, A. Lentschat, A.J. Ulmer, E. Gerlach, Tissue factor expression of human monocytes is suppressed by lysophosphatidylcholine, Arterioscler. Thromb. Vasc. Biol. 19 (1999) 47–53.

International Congress Series 1262 (2004) 87–90

www.ics-elsevier.com

Measurement of oxidized LDL present in human plasma and atherosclerotic lesions

Hiroyuki Itabe[a,*], Makiko Ueda[b], Masaaki Uno[c], Tatsuya Takano[a]

[a] *Department of Molecular Pathology, Faculty of Pharmaceutical Sciences, Teikyo University, 1091-1 Suarashi, Sagamiko, Tsukui, Kanagawa 199-0195, Japan*

[b] *Department of Pathology, Osaka City University Graduate School of Medicine, Osaka, Japan*

[c] *Department of Neurosurgery, School of Medicine, The University of Tokushima, Tokushima, Japan*

Abstract. Oxidized low-density lipoprotein (OxLDL) present in circulating plasma and in human atherosclerotic lesions has been measured using a monoclonal antibody recognizing oxidized phosphatidylcholine (OxPC), DLH3. OxLDL levels in patients with acute myocardial and cerebral infarctions were significantly higher than those of controls. Thus, the plasma OxLDL level could be a marker for vascular diseases. Immunohistochemical studies demonstrated the foam cell-associated accumulation of OxLDL in human atherosclerotic lesions. To investigate the intracellular fate of OxLDL in foam cells, OxLDL taken up by J774 macrophages was chased. We found that partially degraded OxLDL particles accumulated in secondary lysosomes. Similarly, apolipoprotein B (apoB) recovered from human carotid plaques was partially degraded, suggesting that OxLDL actually contribute to foam cell formation in atherosclerotic lesions. Minimally modified LDL (MM-LDL) was prepared by dialyzing LDL in the presence of a low concentration of $FeSO_4$. Macrophages did not bind to the MM-LDL effectively, but the DLH3 antibody did bind to MM-LDL as well as with $CuSO_4$-induced OxLDL. Furthermore, MM-LDL appeared to be enriched with aldehyde-containing OxPC. Metabolic dynamics of OxLDL is discussed. © 2003 Elsevier B.V. All rights reserved.

Keywords: Arteriosclerosis; OxLDL; Oxidized phosphatidylcholine; Minimally modified LDL; Foam cells

1. Introduction

It has been widely believed that oxidized low-density lipoprotein (OxLDL) induces foam cell formation as well as inflammatory cellular responses in the vessel wall, which

Abbreviations: OxLDL, oxidized low-density lipoprotein; MM-LDL, minimally modified low-density lipoprotein; OxPC, oxidized phosphatidylcholine; apoB, apolipoprotein B.

* Corresponding author. Tel.: +81-426-85-3739; fax: +81-426-85-3728.
E-mail address: h-itabe@pharm.teikyo-u.ac.jp (H. Itabe).

doi:10.1016/j.ics.2003.11.029

could then lead to lesion formation. We have developed a sandwich-type enzyme-linked immunosorbent assay (ELISA) procedure to determine OxLDL concentrations in human plasma using an anti-OxLDL monoclonal antibody [1]. Using this method, plasma OxLDL levels were found to increase under certain diseased conditions, including acute myocardial and cerebral infarctions [2,3]. Accumulation of OxLDL in atherosclerotic lesions was also demonstrated [2,4]. Thus, studying metabolic features of the OxLDL in atherosclerotic lesions and circulation should be another important key to elucidate the pathological relevance of OxLDL.

2. Measurement of circulating OxLDL levels

A monoclonal antibody, DLH3, binds to OxLDL but not to native or acetylated LDL [5]. Oxidized phosphatidylcholines (OxPC) generated in OxLDL appeared to be recognized by this antibody [6]. We developed a sandwich ELISA procedure to determine the levels of OxLDL that is present in human circulating plasma using the DLH3 antibody [1]. LDL fractions separated from human plasma were added to microtiter wells, which were pre-coated with DLH3. After extensive washing, the amounts of OxLDL bound to the wells were determined using an anti-apolipoprotein B (apoB) polyclonal antibody. Since artificial oxidation of the plasma sample is carefully prevented in the procedure, OxLDL particles present in plasma are detected.

Increased OxLDL levels were observed in patients with vascular diseases. For example, plasma OxLDL levels in patients with acute myocardial infarction were 3.4-fold higher than those of age-matched control subjects [2]. In addition, a 3-fold higher increase in plasma OxLDL levels in patients with cerebral infarction in the cortical regions was observed [3]. These results, together with many other observations, suggest that plasma OxLDL levels provide useful diagnostic information.

3. OxLDL is accumulated in atherosclerotic lesions

The amounts of OxLDL present in human atherosclerotic lesions were compared with those in plasma [4]. The OxLDL content in the lipoprotein fractions extracted from the macrophage-rich plaques, which was obtained by endoarterectomy operations, was 3.6-times higher than those from macrophage-poor plaques. It was noted that lipoprotein fractions from macrophage-rich plaques were highly enriched with OxLDL, and were approximately 100 times higher than those of the plasma LDL fractions from the same patients.

It was observed that OxLDL localized within foam cells in atherosclerotic lesions, especially in the early lesions [2,4,7]. After macrophages take up OxLDL, OxLDL is transferred to lysosomes through endocytic pathways and is eventually degraded in lysosomes [8]. We studied whether OxLDL is concentrated in foam cells by monitoring the actual amounts of OxLDL present in J774 murine macrophages in culture using the sandwich ELISA [7]. Acetylated LDL taken up by the macrophages disappeared completely from the cells within 4 h, whereas OxLDL in the cells decreased by 80% in the first 4 h, but the remaining 20% of OxLDL was present in the cells even after 48 h. The OxLDL accumulated in the macrophages was partially degraded and localized in lysosomal fractions. It is likely that some forms of modified apoB such as OxPC-apoB

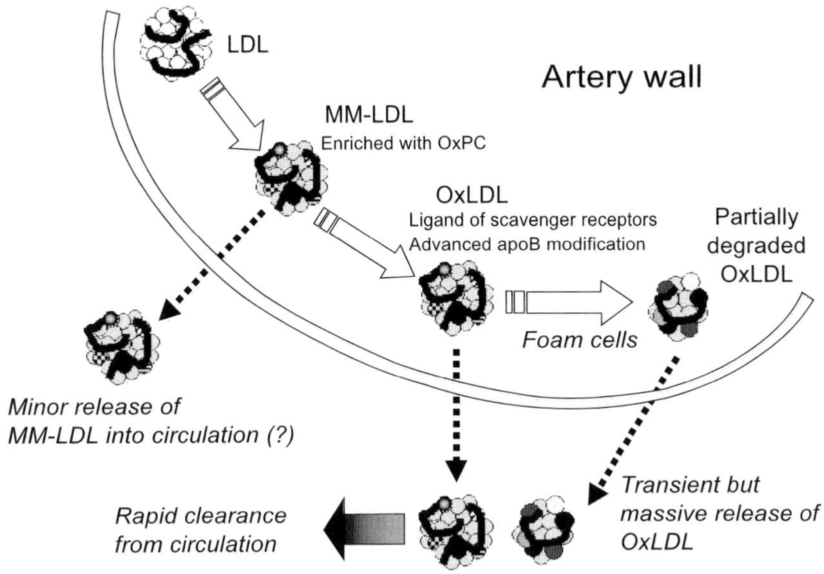

Fig. 1. Possible behavior of heterogeneous types of OxLDL in vivo.

adducts in OxLDL are resistant to lysosomal degradation so that they remain in the cells for a long time [7,8].

4. Searching for in vivo OxLDL

LDL is readily oxidized by incubating at 37 °C with the addition of $CuSO_4$, which is the most popular method of preparing OxLDL in vitro. However, it is unclear whether the OxLDL present in vivo has the same properties as that prepared in vitro.

Minimally modified LDL (MM-LDL), another type of modified LDL first proposed by Berliner et al. [9] has been known for strong stimulatory activities on endothelial cells. MM-LDL can be prepared by several procedures, such as dialysis of LDL in phosphate-buffered saline containing 1 μM $FeSO_4$. MM-LDL prepared with the dialysis procedure did not bind macrophages, while Cu-induced OxLDL did. MM-LDL, however, showed a strong reactivity to DLH3 antibody that was comparable to Cu-induced OxLDL [10]. HPLC analysis revealed that extractable aldehyde-containing OxPC molecules were highly enriched in MM-LDL, rather than in OxLDL. MM-LDL appeared to be a type of oxidatively modified LDL, which is rich in the free forms of OxPC and poor in apoB protein modifications (Fig. 1).

5. Discussion

It should be noted that OxLDL is heterogeneously modified and different types of OxLDL could be present in vivo. OxPC–apoB adducts detected using the DLH3 antibody may be a part of them. Since MM-LDL binds poorly with scavenger receptors [9,10], the clearance of MM-LDL from the circulation may be inefficient. If a small quantity of MM-

LDL-like particles is released into the circulation, it could stay in the circulation for a relatively long period. When OxLDL is formed by further modification of MM-LDL, it is then taken up by macrophages and accumulates in lesion foam cells. This OxLDL, and possibly the partially degraded OxLDL, may be released into the circulation upon vascular events, and they are cleared from the circulation by the liver.

References

[1] H. Itabe, et al., Sensitive detection of oxidatively modified low density lipoprotein using a monoclonal antibody, J. Lipid Res. 37 (1996) 45–53.

[2] S. Ehara, et al., Oxidized low density lipoprotein relates to plaque destabilization in human coronary atherosclerotic lesions, Circulation 103 (2001) 1955–1960.

[3] M. Uno, et al., Elevation of plasma oxidized LDL in acute cerebral infarction, J. Neurol. Neurosurg. Psychiatry, Suppl. 74 (2003) 312–316.

[4] K. Nishi, et al., Oxidized LDL in carotid plaques and plasma associates with plaque instability, Arterioscler. Thromb. Vasc. Biol. 22 (2002) 1649–1654.

[5] H. Itabe, et al., A monoclonal antibody against oxidized lipoprotein recognizes foam cells in atherosclerotic lesions. Complex formation of oxidized phosphatidylcholine and polypeptides, J. Biol. Chem. 269 (1994) 15274–15279.

[6] H. Itabe, et al., Oxidized phosphatidylcholines that modify proteins. Analysis by anti-oxidized low density lipoprotein monoclonal antibody, J. Biol. Chem. 271 (1996) 33208–33217.

[7] H. Itabe, et al., Lysosomal accumulation of oxidized phosphatidylcholine- apolipoprotein B complex in macrophages: intracellular fate of oxidized low density lipoprotein, Biochim. Biophys. Acta 1487 (2000) 233–245.

[8] M. Lougheed, et al., Oxidized low density lipoprotein is resistant to cathepsins and accumulates within macrophages, J. Biol. Chem. 266 (1991) 14519–14525.

[9] J.A. Berliner, et al., Minimally modified low density lipoprotein stimulates monocyte endothelial interactions, J. Clin. Invest. 85 (1990) 1260–1266.

[10] H. Itabe, et al., Minimally modified LDL is an oxidized LDL enriched with oxidized phosphatidylcholines, J. Biochem. 193 (2003) 459–465.

ELSEVIER

International Congress Series 1262 (2004) 91–94

www.ics-elsevier.com

Paraoxonase 1: biochemistry and contribution to atherosclerosis

Bharti Mackness, Mike Mackness*

University Department of Medicine, Manchester Royal Infirmary, Oxford Road, Manchester M13 9WL, UK

Abstract. Serum paraoxonase 1 (PON1) is primarily responsible for the antioxidative activity of high-density lipoprotein (HDL). PON1 protects against the oxidative modification of low-density lipoprotein, apparently by hydrolysing lipid-peroxides. A mechanism for this process is proposed here. In the light of current knowledge, the mechanism has two fundamental requirements. Firstly, that lysolipids are safe to produce on HDL and secondly, that PON1 has two active sites. Data are also presented on the first prospective study of PON1 activity and CHD, showing low PON1 activity to be an independent risk factor for CHD, independent of all other risk factors including HDL.

Keywords: Paraoxonase 1; High-density lipoprotein; Oxidation

1. Introduction

High-density lipoprotein (HDL) has antioxidant and anti-inflammatory properties and retards the oxidation of low-density lipoprotein (LDL), inhibiting the initiation and progression of atherosclerosis [1]. The HDL-associated enzyme, paraoxonase 1 (PON1), is largely responsible for this property of HDL [2]. HDL, which lacks PON1, either naturally or through gene ablation, is unable to retard LDL oxidation [3,4] restoring PON1 to HDL that lacks it, restores its ability to retard LDL oxidation. PON1 activity is lower in diseases prone to the development of premature atherosclerosis [5] and is reduced in inflammatory diseases [6,7]. Despite its potential importance as a natural anti-atherosclerotic agent, most studies seem to concentrate on genetic epidemiological studies of the case control kind. Relatively few studies have tried to determine the basic biochemical mechanisms behind the antioxidant properties of PON1. In this article, more recent advances in PON1 epidemiology and biochemistry will be reviewed.

* Corresponding author. Tel.: +44-1612768633; fax: +44-1612764833.
E-mail address: mike.mackness@cmmc.nhs.uk (M. Mackness).

0531-5131/
doi:10.1016/S0531-5131(03)01736-9

2. PON1 as a risk factor for atherosclerosis

PON1 has two coding region polymorphisms, L55M and Q192R, and several promoter region polymorphisms, all of which to various degrees affect PON1 activity and/or concentration [1], although an added complication is that the Q192R polymorphism is substrate-dependent [8]. Large numbers of case control studies have investigated the relationship of these genetic polymorphisms to the presence of CHD, however, the results have been largely contradictory. A meta-analysis of the genetic studies did show a positive relationship between the PON1 genotype least able to prevent LDL from oxidation and CHD, which was particularly strong in subjects with type 2 diabetes [9]. Those few studies that investigated PON1 activity and concentration found that low activity, and not genotype, was associated with CHD [10,11], giving a confusing picture. For this reason, we conducted the first prospective study of PON1 and CHD. Men in the Caerphilly Prospective Study who had a new coronary event ($n=163$) had significantly lower PON1 activity than those who did not ($n=1190$) ($p=0.039$) [12]. Those in the highest quintile of PON1 activity had a 50% lower odds ratio of having a coronary event than those in the lowest quintile ($p<0.05$) (Fig. 1). Low PON1 activity predicted new coronary events, independent of all other risk factors including HDL.

3. Mechanism of action of PON1

Several groups have shown that various oxidised lipid components of LDL are hydrolysed by PON1, although the exact mechanism of action and products of the

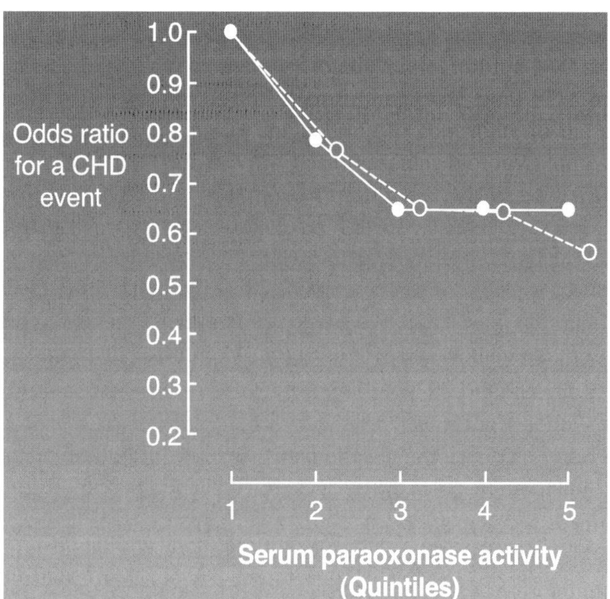

Fig. 1. Odds ratio of having a CHD event by quintile of PON1 activity. Open circles = unadjusted odds, closed circles = adjusted for all other risk factors.

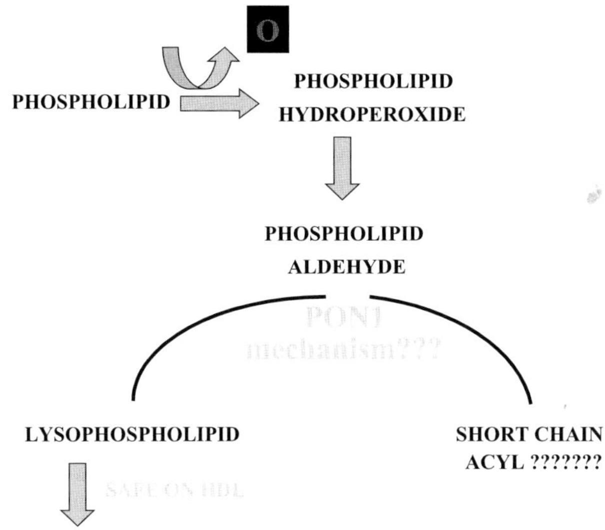

Fig. 2. Putative mechanism of action of PON1 in destroying oxidised lipids in LDL.

reaction remain unknown (reviewed in Ref. [1]). The hydrolysis of oxidised lipids by PON1 prevents reactive aldehydes adducting to apo B, thus preventing interaction with the oxidised LDL receptors [13]. The following scheme summarises current knowledge of the putative mechanism and is a summary of several groups' results [1] (Fig. 2).

There are two important points to note. Firstly, one product of the reaction is probably lysophospholipid, itself a highly cytotoxic compound responsible for many of the effects of oxidised-LDL. However, HDL appears to be a safe place to produce lysophospholipids. Due to the action of LCAT on HDL, gram quantities of lysolecithin are produced daily. Yet, HDL is not cytotoxic and may have a mechanism to dispose of lysophospholipids [2]. Secondly, there is the possibility that PON1 has two active sites, a Ca^{2+}-dependent site which hydrolyses organophosphates and related substrates and a site dependent on the Cys283 residue but not Ca^{2+}, which hydrolyses oxidised lipids [9].

4. Discussion

Recent studies have indicated that PON1 is a strong independent risk factor for CHD and have gone some way in elucidating the mechanism of action of this important anti-atherosclerotic enzyme, however, there is much more to learn. Much more work in this area is required, perhaps at the expense of any further genetic epidemiological studies, unless prospective in nature. Recently, some steps have also been taken to determine nutritional and pharmacological modulations of PON1 [14], but much more research in this area is required to determine the effect of elevating PON1 on atherosclerosis in man.

References

[1] B. Mackness, P.N. Durrington, M.I. Mackness, The paraoxonase gene family and coronary heart disease, Curr. Opin. Lipidol. 13 (2002) 357–362.

[2] M.I. Mackness, P.N. Durrington, High density lipoprotein, its enzymes and its potential to influence lipid peroxidation, Atherosclerosis 115 (1995) 243–253.

[3] B. Mackness, P.N. Durrington, M.I. Mackness, Lack of protection against oxidative modification of LDL by avian HDL, Biochem. Biophys. Res. Commun. 247 (1998) 443–446.

[4] D.M. Shih, L. Gu, Y.-R. Xia, M. Navab, W.-F. Li, S. Hama, L.W. Castellani, C.E. Furlong, L.G. Costa, A.M. Fogelman, A.J. Lusis, Mice lacking serum paraoxonase are susceptible to organophosphate toxicity and atherosclerosis, Nature 394 (1998) 284–287.

[5] M.I. Mackness, P.N. Durrington, B. Mackness, How HDL protects against the effects of lipid peroxidation, Curr. Opin. Lipidol. 11 (2000) 383–388.

[6] B.J. Van Lenten, S.Y. Hama, F.C. de Beer, D.M. Stafforini, T.M. McIntyre, S.M. Prescott, B.N. La Du, A.M. Fogelman, M. Navab, Anti-inflammatory HDL becomes proinflammatory during the acute phase response, J. Clin. Invest. 96 (1995) 2758–2767.

[7] N. Tanimoto, Y. Kumon, T. Suehiro, S. Ohkubo, Y. Ikeda, K. Nishiya, K. Hushimoto, Serum paraoxonase activity decreases in rheumatoid arthritis, Life Sci. 72 (2003) 2877–2885.

[8] H.G. Davies, R.J. Richter, M. Keifer, C.A. Broomfield, J. Sowalla, C.E. Furlong, The effect of the human serum paraoxonase polymorphism is reversed with diazoxon, soman and sarin, Nat. Genet. 14 (1996) 334–336.

[9] P.N. Durrington, B. Mackness, M.I. Mackness, Paraoxonase and atherosclerosis, Arterioscler. Thromb. Vasc. Biol. 21 (2001) 473–480.

[10] G.P. Jarvik, L.S. Rozek, V.H. Brophy, T.S. Hatsukami, R.J. Richter, G.D. Schellenberg, C.E. Furlong, Paraoxonase (PON1) phenotype is a better predictor of vascular disease than is $PON1_{192}$ or $PON1_{55}$ genotype, Arterioscl. Thromb. Vasc. Biol. 20 (2000) 2441–2447.

[11] B. Mackness, G.K. Davies, W. Turkie, W. Lee, D.H. Roberts, E. Hill, C. Roberts, P.N. Durrington, M.I. Mackness, Paraoxonase status in coronary heart disease. Are activity and concentration more important than genotype? Arterioscler. Thromb. Vasc. Biol. 21 (2001) 1451–1457.

[12] B. Mackness, P. Durrington, P. McElduff, J. Yarnell, N. Azam, M. Watt, M. Mackness, Low paraoxonase activity predicts coronary events in the Caerphilly prospective Study, Circulation 107 (2003) 2775–2779.

[13] P. Sangvanich, B. Mackness, S. Gaskill, P.N. Durrington, M.I. Mackness, The effect of HDL on the formation of lipid/protein conjugates during in vitro oxidation of LDL, Biochem. Biophys. Res. Commun. 300 (2003) 501–506.

[14] P.N. Durrington, B. Mackness, M.I. Mackness, The hunt for nutritional and pharmacological modulators of paraoxonase, Arterioscler. Thromb. Vasc. Biol. (2002) 1248–1250.

International Congress Series 1262 (2004) 95–98

ELSEVIER

www.ics-elsevier.com

High-resolution magnetic resonance imaging of carotid atherosclerosis

Thomas S. Hatsukami[a,*], William Kerwin[b], Jian-Ming Cai[b,c], X.J. Kang[b], Nayak Polissar[d], Marina Ferguson[b], Randy Small[e], Xue-Qiao Zhao[f], Chun Yuan[b]

[a] *VA Puget Sound Health Care System, Surgery and Perioperative Care (112), 1660 South Columbian Way, Seattle, WA 98108, USA*

[b] *Department of Radiology, University of Washington, Seattle, WA, USA*

[c] *Department of Radiology, PLA General Hospital, Beijing, China*

[d] *The Mountain-Whisper-Light Statistical Consulting, Seattle, WA, USA*

[e] *Department of Pathology, University of Washington, Seattle, WA, USA*

[f] *Department of Cardiology, University of Washington, Seattle, WA, USA*

Abstract. High-resolution imaging techniques that permit serial, in vivo examination of the atherosclerotic plaque are needed to better understand the mechanisms involved in the progression of stable, early lesions into high-risk plaques in humans. Such an imaging tool would serve as a bridge between what is learned in the laboratory and the clinical setting. Furthermore, it would permit direct assessment of the efficacy of phamacological interventions. Magnetic resonance imaging (MRI) is ideally suited for serial examination of the diseased arterial wall. Studies have shown that MRI is capable of measuring plaque burden, identifying fibrous cap characteristics and lesion types using American Heart Association (AHA) criteria, and quantifying neovasculature within the plaque. Case-control studies have shown an association between thin/ruptured fibrous caps, as identified by MRI, and recent transient ischemic attack (TIA) and stroke, and have shown that prolonged intensive lipid-lowering therapy is associated with decreased plaque lipid content. Thus, MRI is a promising tool for direct, serial assessment of carotid atherosclerosis in vivo. This article will briefly review our previously published work validating the technique.

Keywords: Magnetic resonance imaging; Atherosclerosis; Carotid

1. Introduction

Although much has been learned from studies in animal models of atherosclerosis, translation of basic science findings into improvements in the diagnosis and treatment of human vascular disease has been difficult. The study of human atherosclerosis is hampered by the inability to accurately assess the diseased arterial wall in a serial, non-invasive

* Corresponding author. Tel.: +1-206-764-2245; fax: +1-206-764-2529.
E-mail address: tomhat@u.washington.edu (T.S. Hatsukami).

doi:10.1016/j.ics.2004.01.047

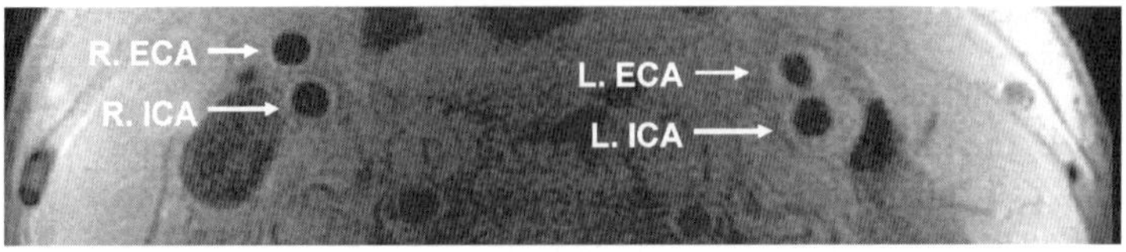

Fig. 1. MRI of right and left internal and external carotid arteries demonstrating good suppression of flow artifact and clear delineation of the lumen and outer boundary of normal (right) and diseased (left) carotid arteries. Note evidence of expansive remodelling on the left side. The cross-sectional area of the lumen is similar on both sides, yet there is significantly greater plaque burden on the left. ICA: internal carotid artery; ECA: external carotid artery.

fashion. Magnetic resonance imaging (MRI) has developed into a highly promising tool for characterizing the morphology and composition of the diseased vessel wall in vivo. Significant improvements in MR image quality have been made possible by a combination of hardware development [1] and novel image acquisition sequences [2,3] (Fig. 1). This article briefly reviews the work performed in this laboratory validating the magnetic resonance imaging (MRI) using examination of corresponding excised carotid endarterectomy (CEA) specimens as a gold standard.

2. Summary of validation studies

2.1. Plaque burden

In a study comparing in vivo carotid MRI with ex vivo MRI of fresh CEA specimens, there was a high level of agreement in area measurements of the disease arterial wall [4], with a mean difference of 13 mm^2 and S.D. of the difference of only 6.5 mm^2. Intra- and inter-observer intraclass correlation coefficient was 0.95 and 0.96, respectively. A follow-up study demonstrated that MRI is capable of detecting a 10% change in volume with 95% confidence [5].

2.2. Fibrous cap status

MRI has been shown to have a high level of agreement with corresponding histological findings for categorizing fibrous caps as thick (>0.25 mm), thin, or ruptured [89% agreement, kappa (95% confidence interval)=0.83 (0.67–1.0)] [6]. Blinded comparison demonstrated a sensitivity of 81% (±6%) and specificity of 90% (±2%) for distinguishing a thick cap from a thin or ruptured cap [7]. Furthermore, fibrous cap status, as identified by MRI, has been shown to have a strong correlation with the clinical status of the patient [8]. Amongst patients undergoing CEA, 70% of those with ruptured fibrous caps on pre-operative carotid MRI had a history of recent TIA or stroke, compared with only 9% of those with thick fibrous caps (p=0.001).

2.3. American Heart Association (AHA) lesion types

For longitudinal studies examining atherosclerosis progression or regression, a standardized classification scheme for describing the characteristics of the lesion at baseline and during follow-up is essential. In a recent study [9], the accuracy of multi-contrast

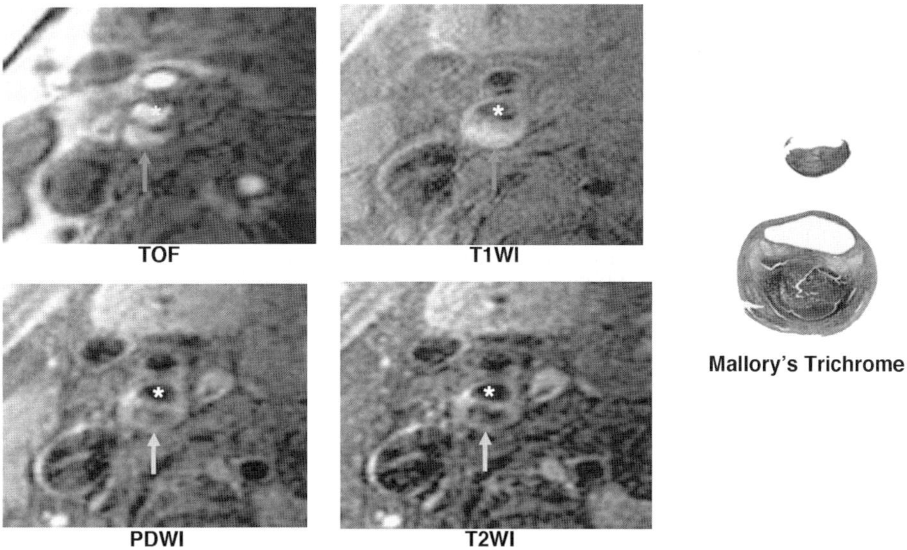

Fig. 2. AHA Type VI (complicated) lesion with acute intraplaque hemorrhage. Asterisks indicate the lumen of the internal carotid artery. Early intraplaque hemorrhage, seen on the corresponding histological cross-section on the right, is identified by a hyperintense (bright) signal on time-of-flight (TOF) and T1-weighted (T1W) MR images, and relatively hypointense (dark) on the proton density- (PDW) and T2-weighted (T2W) images.

weighted MRI for categorizing carotid plaque characteristics was evaluated in 60 CEA patients, using a modified AHA histological classification scheme [10]. Fig. 2 demonstrates the appearance of an AHA Type VI (complicated) lesion, with intraplaque hemorrhage. Overall, there was very good agreement between MRI and findings from the corresponding histological sections [Cohen's kappa (95% CI)=0.74 (0.67–0.82)]. Sensitivity and specificity of MRI for identifying type III–VII lesions ranged from 80% to 84% and from 90% to 98%, respectively.

2.4. Gadolinium contrast enhancement and neovasculature

Studies suggest that neovasculature within the plaque may be a marker for more active lesions that are potentially unstable [11,12]. Recently, Kerwin et al. demonstrated that MRI is able to quantify plaque neovasculature using a dynamic contrast enhanced (DCE) MRI protocol. Images obtained at 15-s intervals following contrast injection were analyzed using a kinetic model [13]. Quantification of plaque neovessels on DCE MRI and on corresponding histology were highly correlated [correlation coefficient=0.80 (p<0.001]. DCE MRI therefore provides an important means for prospectively studying the link between neovasculature and plaque vulnerability [14].

3. Conclusions

MRI provides an important tool for studying mechanisms of human atherosclerosis progression and regression in vivo. In addition to precisely assessing plaque burden, MRI is capable of accurately classifying disease according to established AHA criteria, and identifying critical plaque features such as the fibrous cap and neovasculature. A better understanding of disease mechanisms and associated risk factors will permit identification of high-risk individuals and more selective, appropriate intervention, and potentially lead to the development of novel methods for therapeutic intervention.

Acknowledgements

This work has been supported NIH grants R01-HL60213, R01-HL61851, RO1-HL073401, P01-HL072262, R29-HL56874, Astra-Zeneca Pharmaceuticals, and the Whittaker Foundation.

References

[1] C.E. Hayes, et al., Surface coil phased arrays for high resolution imaging of the carotid arteries, J. Magn. Reson. Imaging 1 (1996) 109–112.
[2] V.L. Yarnykh, C. Yuan, T1-insensitive flow suppression using quadruple inversion-recovery, Magn. Reson. Med. 48 (5) (2002) 899–905.
[3] V.L. Yarnykh, C. Yuan, Multislice double inversion-recovery black-blood imaging with simultaneous slice reinversion, J. Magn. Reson. Imaging 17 (4) (2003) 478–483.
[4] C. Yuan, et al., Measurement of atherosclerotic carotid plaque size in-vivo using high resolution magnetic resonance imaging, Circulation 98 (24) (1998) 2666–2671.
[5] X. Kang, et al., Analysis of the measurement precision of arterial lumen and wall areas using high-resolution MRI, Magn. Reson. Med. 44 (6) (2000) 968–972 (in Process Citation).
[6] T.S. Hatsukami, et al., Visualization of fibrous cap thickness and rupture in human atherosclerotic carotid plaque in vivo with high-resolution magnetic resonance imaging, Circulation 102 (9) (2000) 959–964.
[7] L.M. Mitsumori, et al., In vivo accuracy of multisequence MR imaging for identifying unstable fibrous caps in advanced human carotid plaques, J. Magn. Reson. Imaging 17 (4) (2003) 410–420.
[8] C. Yuan, et al., Identification of fibrous cap rupture with magnetic resonance imaging is highly associated with recent TIA or stroke, Circulation 105 (2) (2002) 181–185.
[9] J.M. Cai, et al., Classification of human carotid atherosclerotic lesions with in vivo multicontrast magnetic resonance imaging, Circulation 106 (11) (2002) 1368–1373.
[10] H.C. Stary, et al., A definition of advanced types of atherosclerotic lesions and a histological classification of atherosclerosis, Circulation 92 (5) (1995) 1355–1374.
[11] A.C. Barger, et al., Hypothesis: vasa vasorum and neovascularization of human coronary arteries. A possible role in the pathophysiology of atherosclerosis, N. Engl. J. Med. 310 (3) (1984) 175–177.
[12] R. Mofidi, et al., Association between plaque instability, angiogenesis and symptomatic carotid occlusive disease, Br. J. Surg. 88 (7) (2001) 945–950.
[13] C.S. Patlak, R.G. Blasberg, Graphical evaluation of blood-to-brain transfer constants from multiple-time uptake data. Generalizations, J. Cereb. Blood Flow Metab. 5 (1985) 584–590.
[14] W. Kerwin, et al., Quantitative magnetic resonance imaging analysis of neovasculature volume in carotid atherosclerotic plaque, Circulation 107 (6) (2003) 851–856.

ELSEVIER

International Congress Series 1262 (2004) 99–102

www.ics-elsevier.com

Angioscopic assessment of vulnerable plaque and therapeutic application—lessons from acute coronary syndrome

Atsushi Hirayama*, Yasunori Yeda, Kazuhisa Kodama

Cardiovascular Division, Osaka Police Hospital, 10-31 Kitayama-cho, Tennoji, Osaka 543-0035 Japan

Abstract. Angioscopic observation revealed occlusive, large amounts of white or mixed thrombus surrounding the ruptured, extensive yellow plaque (YP) or YP with ulceration in most culprit lesions of patients with acute coronary syndrome (ACS), and suggested that YP are vulnerable plaques. These YP were observed at angiographically normal lesions and were graded as grade 0 (white), grade 1 (slight yellow), grade 2 (yellow) and grade 3 (extensive yellow). The thinner the fibrous cap becomes, the brighter the color of YP becomes. This hypothesis is confirmed by the significant, high incidence of thrombus and the positive remodeling determined by the intravascular ultrasound at grade 3 YP. Thus, the angioscopically extensive YP is defined as a clinically unstable plaque. The prevalence of YP is high in the patients with ACS compared with those with other ischemic heart disease, and high-graded YP were frequently observed not only in the infarct-related artery but also non-infarct-related artery without the angiographic stenosis in patients with ACS. These results suggest that ACS represents the pan-coronary process of vulnerable plaque development. It has been recommended that more strict and careful management is necessary for the secondary prevention of ACS, rather than the primary prevention. © 2003 Published by Elsevier B.V.

Keywords: Coronary angioscopy; Acute coronary syndrome; Vulnerable plaque; Lipid lowering therapy

1. Introduction

Acute coronary syndrome (ACS) was caused by plaque rupture and followed by thrombus formation. The plaque susceptible to rupture was called vulnerable plaque, and was characterized by many aspects [1].

The recent advance in intravascular imaging help to understand the atherosclerotic process and identify the vulnerable plaque. Intravascular ultrasound revealed that atherosclerosis is a disease exhibiting at the extra lumen of the artery [2]. Coronary angioscopy revealed yellow plaque (YP) and various kinds of thrombus at the culprit lesion in vivo at the time of the onset [3].

* Corresponding author. Tel.: +81-6-6771-6051; fax: +81-6-6775-2845.
E-mail address: ahirayama@oph.gr.jp (A. Hirayama).

0531-5131/ © 2003 Published by Elsevier B.V.
doi:10.1016/j.ics.2003.11.007

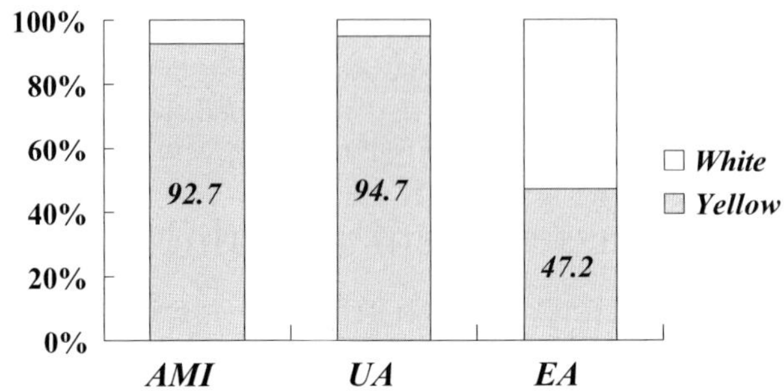

Fig. 1. Prevalence of yellow plaque at the culprit lesion in patients with ACS (AMI: acute myocardial infarction, UA: unstable angina) and Stable effort angina (EA).

In this article, we report the recent coronary angioscopic findings and their application to identify vulnerable plaque.

2. The vulnerability of yellow plaque

The angioscopic findings of the culprit lesion revealed the presence of YP and thrombus. The incidence of YP at the culprit lesion in patients with acute myocardial infarction and unstable angina were 92.7% and 94.7%, respectively, and they were significantly higher than that observed in patients with stable effort angina (47.2%) (Fig. 1) [4].

The YP was not only observed at the culprit lesion but also at the angiographically mild stenotic lesion. As shown in Fig. 2, 94% of 47 lesions with angiographically mild stenotic lesions studied (mean diameter stenosis: 25%) were yellow. The YP observed were classified according to their intensity of color: Grade 0; none, Grade 1; slight yellow, Grade 2; yellow, and Grade 3; extensive yellow. The difference in the color grading may be due to the thickness of the fibrous cup. If the fibrous cup is thin with a large lipid core, its color will be extensively yellow. The significant correlation between the color grade and the incidence of thrombus, and the significant correlation between the vessel

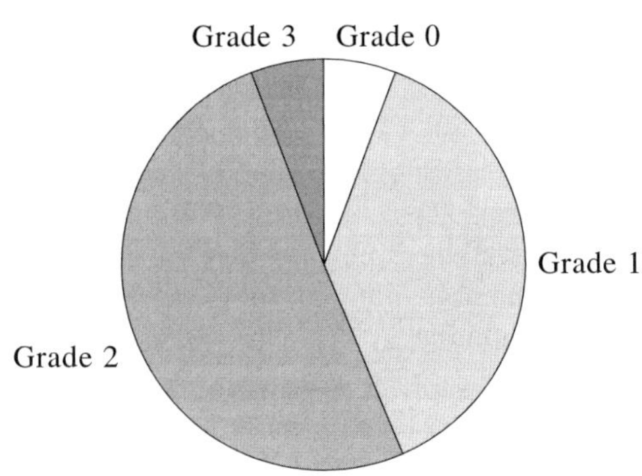

Fig. 2. Prevalence of yellow plaque at the angiographically mild stenotic lesion and their distribution of color grade.

remodeling and the color grade, confirmed this hypothesis; an increased color intensity of YP indicates increased vulnerability. As shown in Fig. 2, 5% of plaque was primarily yellow-colored plaque and confirmed the finding obtained from the angiographic study, which showed the stenosis before the onset of ACS was very mild.

3. ACS as a pan-coronary disease of vulnerable plaque development

Angioscopic observations of all three coronary arteries in patients with myocardial infarction during their recovery period (60 coronary arteries of 20 patients) showed that 95% of coronary arteries had at least one YP somewhere besides in the culprit lesion [5]. The amount of YP in the culprit artery did not differ from that in the non-culprit artery (Fig. 3), which meant that vulnerable plaque developed equally at both coronary arteries. The amount of YP was studied in various coronary heart diseases and showed a significant, high incidence of YP in patients with ACS compared with the patients without ACS. These results indicated that (1) ACS may represent the pan-coronary process of the vulnerable plaque development, and (2) YP may represent the advanced atherosclerotic process.

4. Treatment of patients with previous ACS

Recent clinical trials on cholesterol-lowering therapy by statin showed that the reduction of LCL-cholesterol levels decreased the incidences of cardiac events, and the reduction of the rate of cardiac events has a correlation to the reduction of LDL-cholesterol level. The reduction in cardiac events is magnificent in secondary, rather than primary prevention. Based on the findings, patients with hyperlipidemia were treated by statin, and the angioscopic studies were performed before and after the statin administration. A recent paper [6] showed that statin treatment reduced the yellow color grade in patients with hyperlipidemia, in spite of the increment of plaque color in patients without hyperlipidemia and without statin treatment. Based on the angioscopic findings, statin treatment stabilizes the vulnerable plaque and may reduce the cardiac events.

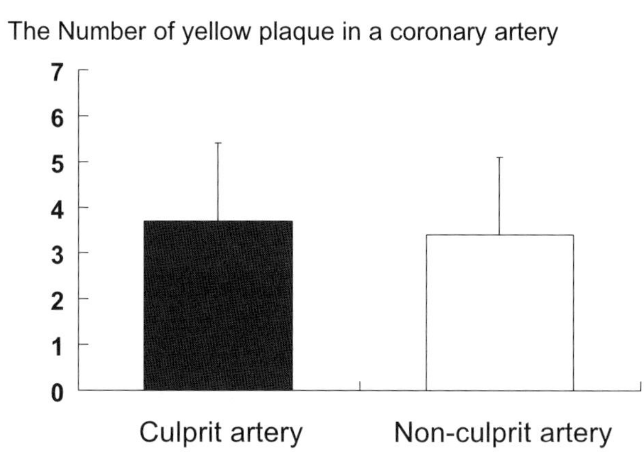

Fig. 3. The number of yellow plaque in a culprit artery or non-culprit in patients with myocardial infarction.

5. Conclusion

In conclusion: (1) vulnerable plaque could be identified by the coronary angioscopy as intensive YP, (2) coronary angioscopy can predict the high-risk patients, and finally (3) coronary angioscopy indicates that plaque stabilization by extensive medical treatment is necessary to prevent cardiac events.

References

[1] P. Libby, Circulation 91 (11) (1995) 2844–2850.
[2] S.E. Nissen, Am. J. Cardiol. 89 (4A) (2002) 24B–31B.
[3] Y. Ueda, et al., J. Am. Coll. Cardiol. 27 (3) (1996) 606–610.
[4] K. Kodama, et al., Intern. Med. 39 (4) (2000) 333–335.
[5] M. Asakura, et al., J. Am. Coll. Cardiol. 37 (5) (2001) 1284–1288.
[6] M. Takano, et al., J. Am. Coll. Cardiol. 42 (4) (2003) 680–686.

International Congress Series 1262 (2004) 103–106

www.ics-elsevier.com

Signal transduction regulating the vascular smooth muscle phenotype and early molecular events of atherogenesis

Kenji Sobue*, Katsushi Shibata, Ken'ichiro Hayashi

Department of Neuroscience (D13), Osaka University Graduate School of Medicine, Yamadaoka 2-2, Suita City, Osaka 565-0871, Japan

Abstract. To study the molecular mechanism underlying the early events of atherosclerosis, we have established a primary culture system of vascular smooth muscle cells (VSMCs) in exhibiting a differentiated phenotype. Using this culture system, we have identified unsaturated lysophosphatidic acids (LPAs) as potent inducers for early atherogenesis *in culture* and in vivo. Unsaturated LPAs also induce the expression of epiregulin, which is involved in early atherogenesis. Thus, unsaturated LPAs and epiregulin may be critical factors in early atherogenesis.

Keywords: Unsaturated lysophosphatidic acid; Epiregulin; Vascular remodeling; Atherosclerosis

1. Introduction

Atherosclerosis is a serious disease that causes heart attack and stroke. The early events of atherosclerosis initiated by the neointimal formation in defined areas and the infiltration of macrophages into the vascular wall result in the progression of atherosclerotic regions [1]. The hallmark is the phenotypic modulation of vascular smooth muscle cells (VSMCs), from a differentiated phenotype to a dedifferentiated one, providing a major constituent of early neointima [2]. The critical factors inducing VSMC dedifferentiation, however, remain unclear, because proper in vitro assay systems have not yet been available. We have established a primary culture system of VSMCs in exhibiting the differentiated phenotype, demonstrated the signaling pathways in regulating the VSMC phenotype [3,4], and identified critical factors involved in early atherogenesis [4–6].

2. Signaling pathways in regulating the VSMC phenotype

Differentiated VSMCs have a spindle-like shape, ligand-induced contractility and SMC molecular marker expression, whereas dedifferentiated VSMCs lose such properties [7].

* Corresponding author. Tel.: +81-6-6879-3680; fax: +81-6-6879-3689.
E-mail address: sobue@nbiochem.med.osaka-u.ac.jp (K. Sobue).

doi:10.1016/j.ics.2003.12.093

Using these typical properties, we have for the first time established a primary culture system of VSMCs in exhibiting the differentiated phenotype [3,4]. Of growth factors and cytokines examined, IGF-I, IGF-II, and insulin maintain the differentiated phenotype. Of these, IGF-I is the most highly potent. One extracellular matrix component, laminin, only inhibits VSMC dedifferentiation. Other growth factors, cytokines, serum, and extracellular matrix components induce VSMC dedifferentiation. Thus, IGF-I and laminin are critical components in exhibiting the differentiated VSMC phenotype.

PDGF, EGF, bFGF, and angiotensin II have been reported to enhance proliferation or hypertrophy of VSMCs through the MAPK cascade in culture and in vitro [8,9], suggesting a close association between the MAPK cascades and vascular disorders. However, the direct involvement of these cascades in regulating the VSMC phenotype had not been demonstrated. Using our VSMC culture system, we demonstrated the signaling pathways in regulating the VSMC phenotype [3,4]. The IGF-I signal via the PI3-kinase/PKB pathway is critically involved in exhibiting the differentiated VSMC phenotype. In contrast, PDGF, EGF, bFGF, and other growth factors trigger the coordinated activation of the ERK and p38MAPK pathways, resulting in the induction of VSMC dedifferentiation. Of these, PDGF triggers both signaling pathways. When the PDGF-activated MAPK pathways are simultaneously blocked by dominant-negative MEK1 and MKK6 or PD98059 and SB203580, PDGF changes, in turn, its function to exhibit the differentiated VSMC phenotype via the PI3-kinase/PKB pathway. Thus, changes in the balance between the strengths of the PI3-kinase/PKB pathway and the ERK and p38MAPK pathways determine the VSMC phenotype.

3. Unsaturated LPA as a VSMC dedifferentiation factor and a potent atherogenic factor in vivo

Human serum, but not plasma, potently induces VSMC dedifferentiation. We isolated the VSMC dedifferentiation factor from human serum and identified unsaturated lysophosphatidic acid (LPA) as a potent factor [4]. The total concentrations of saturated and unsaturated LPAs in human serum are about 20 and 6 μM, respectively (Table 1). Among LPA species, unsaturated LPAs specifically induce VSMC dedifferentiation via the dual

Table 1
LPA species in human serum, moxLDL and atherosclerotic lesion

LPA species	serum (μmol/1 of blood	moxLDL (nmol/mg protein)		atherosclerotic lesions (pmol/mg tissue)	
12 : 0	nd	nd		0.04 ± 0.03	
14 : 0	1.43 ± 0.35	0.05 ± 0.02		0.21 ± 0.12	
16 : 0	11.95 ± 4.04	1.03 ± 0.46		3.53 ± 2.08	
18 : 0	7.93 ± 3.51	0.81 ± 0.58		3.39 ± 2.14	
20 : 0	nd	nd		0.52 ± 0.38	
18 : 1	3.01 ± 0.90	0.37 ± 0.14	1.0μmol/1 of blood	1.04 ± 0.85	1.9μmol/kg wet tissue
18 : 2	2.99 ± 2.47	0.14 ± 0.08		0.77 ± 0.36	
20 : 4	0.37 ± 0.09	0.05 ± 0.02		nd	

The concentrations of LPA were determined by the method as described in Ref. [6].The LDL fraction was mildly oxidized under the presence of 5 μM of $CuSO_4$. nd = not detected.

MAPK pathways. The apparent IC_{50} values of unsaturated LPAs to induce VSMC dedifferentiation range from 20 to 30 nM. Although three types of LPA receptor have been isolated [10], these receptors show affinity for both saturated and unsaturated LPAs that differ only by degree. Thus, another unsaturated LPA-specific receptor may be involved in VSMC dedifferentiation.

The total concentrations of unsaturated LPAs in the human mildly oxidized LDL fraction and atherosclerotic lesions are about 40- and 80-fold higher than the IC_{50} values of VSMC dedifferentiation, respectively (Table 1). We examined the direct effect of LPA on the vasculature [5]. The common carotid arteries (CCAs) treated with unsaturated LPAs show typical neointimal formation, indicating that unsaturated LPA is highly atherogenic in vivo. Unsaturated LPA-induced neointimal formation is also mediated through the dual MAPK pathways. We characterized unsaturated LPA-treated CCAs by histochemical analyses that the phenotypic modulation of VSMCs precedes neointimal formation and macrophage infiltration [5]. Thus, our unsaturated LPA-induced neointimal model faithfully reflects early events of human atherosclerosis [1].

4. Epiregulin as an unsaturated LPA-triggered paracrine factor enhancing early atherogenesis

We have further isolated and identified a paracrine factor involved in the dedifferentiation of surrounding normal VSMCs as epiregulin [6]. Epiregulin potently induces VSMC dedifferentiation and promotes the proliferation and migration of dedifferentiated VSMCs. Interestingly, unsaturated LPA rapidly induces epiregulin expression. Immunohistochemistry reveals that epiregulin is only expressed within the restricted regions of atherosclerotic arteries where the phenotypic modulation of VSMCs actively occurs.

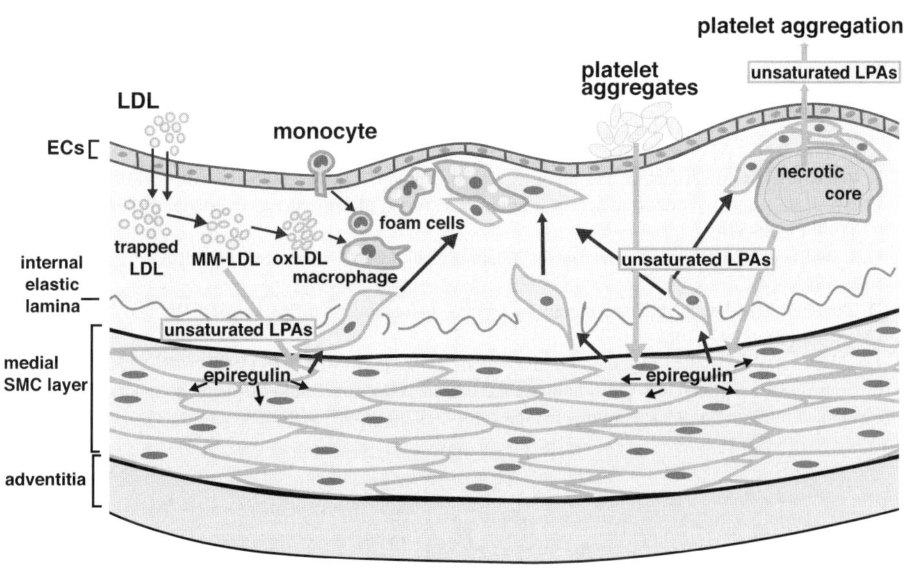

Fig. 1. Unsaturated LPAs and epiregulin trigger the atherogenic cascade. The details are described in the text.

These results suggest that epiregulin expression in VSMCs is an early event in response to atherogenic stimuli such as unsaturated LPAs that promote VSMC dedifferentiation.

5. Conclusions

Oxidation of LDL is highly atherogenic [11]. Platelet activation is also involved in atherogenesis [12]. Since LPA is generated through phospholipase A_2-mediated deacylation of newly generated phosphatidic acid in activated platelets [13], platelet-derived LPAs may be a source of unsaturated LPAs that induce atherogenesis. Taken together, we hypothesize a molecular mechanism for atherosclerosis (Fig. 1). Unsaturated LPAs generated from LDL oxidation and derived from activated platelets act as atherogenic factors that initiate early atherogenesis. Next, unsaturated LPA-primed VSMCs produce and secrete epiregulin, which is involved in the progression of early atherogenesis. Further, unsaturated LPAs released from preformed atherosclerotic regions promote the atherosclerotic cascade. Thus, our VSMC culture and vascular remodeling systems are providing valuable insight into the development and progression of atherosclerosis.

References

[1] H.C. Stary, et al., A definition of advanced types of atherosclerotic lesions and a histological classification of atherosclerosis: a report from the committee on vascular lesions of the council on arteriosclerosis, Circulation 92 (1995) 1355–1374.

[2] R. Ross, The pathogenesis of atherosclerosis: a perspective for the 1990s, Nature 362 (1993) 801–809.

[3] K. Hayashi, et al., Changes in the balance of phosphoinositide 3-kinase/protein kinase B (Akt) and the mitogen-activated protein kinases (ERK/p38MAPK) determine a phenotype of visceral and vascular smooth muscle cells, J. Cell Biol. 145 (1999) 727–740.

[4] K. Hayashi, et al., Phenotypic modulation of vascular smooth muscle cells induced by unsaturated lysophosphatidic acids, Circ. Res. 89 (2001) 251–258.

[5] K. Yoshida, et al., Vascular remodeling induced by naturally occurring unsaturated lysophosphatidic acid in vivo, Circulation 108 (2003) 1746–1752.

[6] M. Takahashi, et al., Epiregulin as a major autocrine/paracrine factor released from ERK- and p38MAPK-activated vascular smooth muscle cells, Circulation 108 (2003) 2524–2529.

[7] K. Sobue, et al., Expressional regulation of smooth muscle cell-specific genes in association with phenotypic modulation, Mol. Cell. Biochem. 190 (1999) 105–118.

[8] T. Force, et al., Growth factors and mitogen-activated protein kinases, Hypertension 31 (1998) 152–161.

[9] Q. Xu, et al., Acute hypertension activates mitogen-activated protein kinases in arterial wall, J. Clin. Invest. 97 (1996) 508–514.

[10] G.B. Mills, et al., The emerging role of lysophosphatidic acid in cancer, Nat. Rev., Cancer 3 (2003) 582–591.

[11] D. Steinberg, A. Lewis, Conner memorial lecture. Oxidative modification of LDL and atherogenesis, Circulation 95 (1997) 1062–1071.

[12] J.A. Ware, et al., Platelet–endothelium interactions, N. Engl. J. Med. 328 (1993) 628–635.

[13] O. Fourcade, et al., Secretory phospholipase A2 generates the novel lipid mediator lysophosphtidic acid in membrane microvesicles shed from activated cells, Cell 80 (1995) 919–927.

ELSEVIER

International Congress Series 1262 (2004) 107–110

www.ics-elsevier.com

KLF5/BTEB2, a Krüppel-like zinc-finger type transcription factor, mediates smooth muscle cell activation as well as cardiovascular remodeling

Ryozo Nagai[a,*], Takayuki Shindo[a], Ichiro Manabe[a], Toru Suzuki[a], Shinsuke Muto[a], Saku Miyamoto[a], Kenichi Aizawa[a], Masahiko Kurabayashi[b]

[a] *Department of Cardiovascular Medicine, University of Tokyo Graduate School of Medicine, 7-3-1 Hongo, 113-8865, Bunkyo, Tokyo, Japan*

[b] *The Second Department of Internal Medicine, Gunma University School of Medicine, Japan*

Abstract. Phenotypic modulation of smooth muscle from the contractile to the synthetic type underlies the pathogenesis of atherosclerosis. We previously isolated a transcription factor, KLF5 (also known as BTEB2 and IKLF), to activate various gene promoters that are activated in phenotypically modulated smooth muscle cells, such as embryonic smooth muscle myosin heavy chain gene (SMemb), plasminogen activator inhibitor-1 (PAI-1), iNOS, PDGF-A, Egr-1 and VEGF receptors. KLF5 is downregulated with vascular development but upregulated in neointima. Chromatin immunoprecipitation assay showed KLF5 to be induced and to bind the promoter of the PDGF-A gene in response to angiotensin II stimulation. To define the role of KLF5 in cardiovascular remodeling, we targeted the KLF5 gene in mice. In response to external stress, arteries of heterozygotes exhibited diminished levels of smooth muscle and adventitial cell activation. We also found that RARα binds KLF5, and that Am80, a potent synthetic RAR agonist, inhibits angiotensin II-induced cardiac hypertrophy. These results indicate that KLF5 is an essential transcription factor that causes not only smooth muscle phenotypic modulation but also cardiac hypertrophy and fibrosis. © 2004 Published by Elsevier B.V.

Keywords: Phenotypic modulation of smooth muscle; KLF5; Cardiovascular remodeling; Cardiac hypertrophy

1. Introduction

Metabolic and/or mechanical stresses induce structural remodeling of blood vessels [1]. However, little is known about the transcriptional regulatory mechanisms underlying them. We recently identified KLF5 as a transcription factor for SMemb/NMHC-B gene [2–5]. KLF5 belongs to the Krüppel-like transcription factor family, which has diverse functions for cell differentiation and embryonic development [6]. Its expression, however,

* Corresponding author. Tel.: +81-3-5800-6526; fax: +81-3-3815-2087.
E-mail address: nagai-tky@umin.ac.jp (R. Nagai).

0531-5131/ © 2004 Published by Elsevier B.V.
doi:10.1016/j.ics.2003.12.030

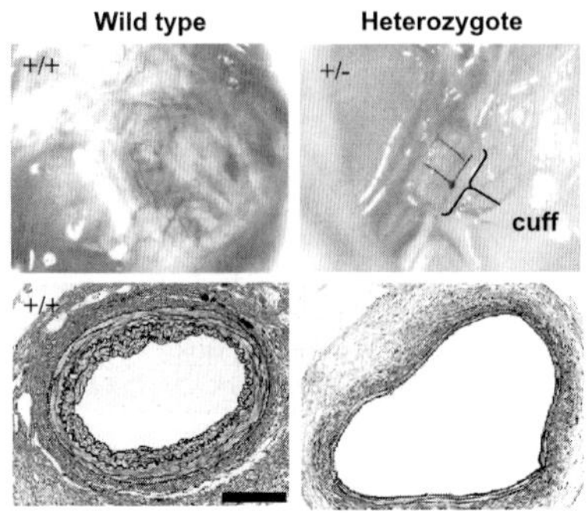

Fig. 1. Vascular injury model entailing placement of a cuff around the femoral artery in KLF5+/+ (wild-type) and KLF5+/ – mice. In wild-type mice, a thick layer of highly vascular granulation tissue surrounded the polyethylene cuff, making it barely visible, whereas KLF5+/ – mice exhibited markedly less granulation tissue, less angiogenesis and less severe fibrosis. Cuff placement also caused intimal hyperplasia in wild-type mice, but not in KLF+/ – .

is strongly upregulated in activated vascular smooth muscle cells in athero- and arteriosclerosis and myofibroblasts in the hypertrophied heart [5]. In the present study, to elucidate the role of KLF5 in the cardiovascular remodeling, we generated KLF5 knockout mice and analyzed the in vivo function of KLF5 [7].

2. Results

The number of pups was significantly reduced when heterozygotes (KLF5+/ –) were intercrossed. Analysis of the embryos from timed KLF5+/ – intercrosses showed that KLF5 – / – homozygotes died prior to E 8.5.

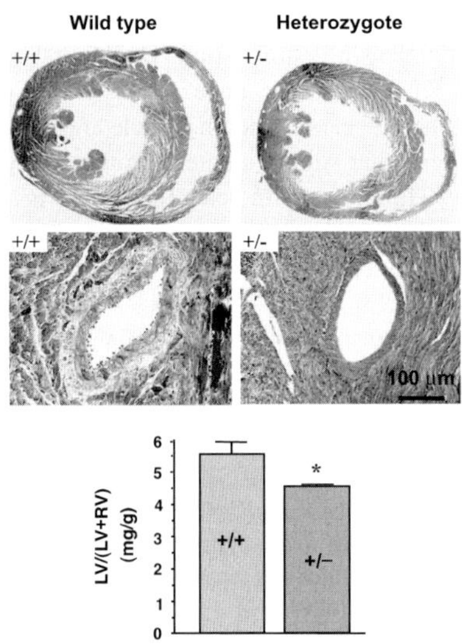

Fig. 2. Cross-sections of heart after 14 days of angiotensin II infusion. Substantial perivascular and interstitial fibrosis were observed in wild-type mice, but such changes were less severe or almost undetectable in KLF5+/ – mice.

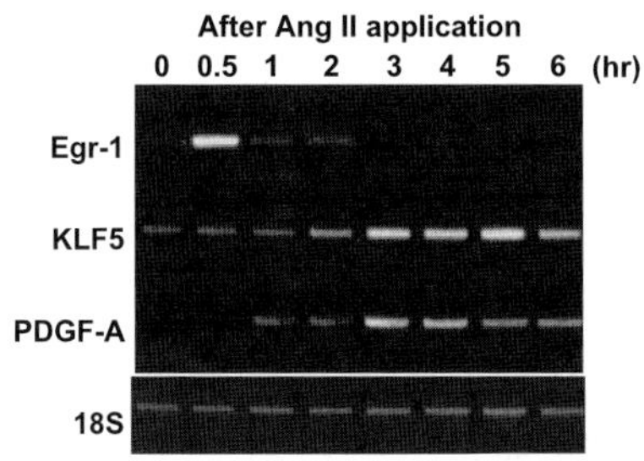

Fig. 3. RT-PCR analyses of KLF5, Egr-1 and PDGF-A expression in angiotensin II-stimulated cardiac fibroblasts. Upregulation of Egr-1 and KLF5 was respectively detected beginning 0.5 and 2 h after angiotensin II application; expression of Egr-1 persisted for only 2 h, while that of KLF5 was sustained for >4 h and was followed by upregulation of PDGF-A expression.

In the femoral arteries injured with a polyethylene tube cuff, we found in KLF5+/+ mice a thick layer of granulation tissue, containing numerous microvessels and inflammatory cells and a large amount of extracellular matrix (Fig. 1).

Following a continuous, 14-day infusion of angiotensin II, the hearts of wild-type mice were found to be significantly heavier than those of heterozygous mice (Fig. 2).

We then examined the molecular mechanisms by which KLF5 controls cardiovascular remodeling. Upregulation of KLF5 was detected within 2 h after the start of angiotensin II stimulation was sustained for >4 h, and was followed by upregulation of PDGF-A (Fig. 3). Overexpression of KLF5 markedly increased PDGF-A promoter activity. Furthermore, angiotensin II was found to clearly increase the binding of KLF5 to the promoter region of the PDGF-A gene as shown by ChIP analysis (data not shown).

We then screened a number of compounds for their ability to modulate KLF5 activity. Am80, a synthetic RAR agonist [11,12], activated PDGF-A promoter activity in cells

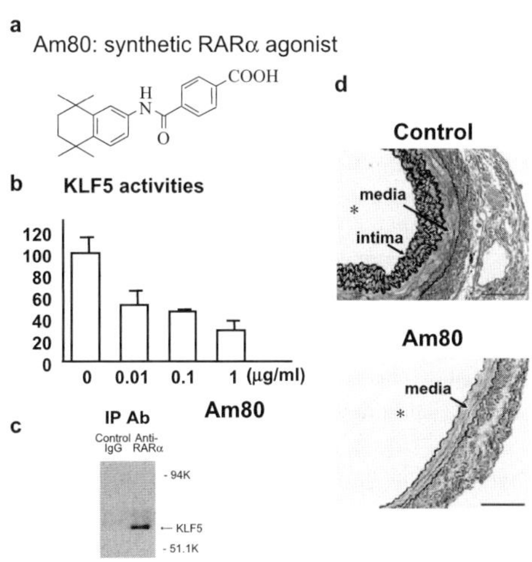

Fig. 4. Am80 which is an RARα agonist inhibits KLF5 activities (a, b). RARα coimmunoprecipitates with KLF5 (c). Am80 reduced angiotensin II-induced cardiac hypertrophy and fibrosis (d).

overexpressing KLF5 and RARα. Furthermore, KLF5 coimmunoprecipitates with RARα. Finally, we found that Am80 reduced development of neointima in wild-type mice until they approximated those seen in KLF5+/− mice and suppressed angiotensin II-induced cardiac hypertrophy (Fig. 4).

3. Discussion

Cardiovascular remodeling is a complex process involving activation of mesenchymal cells, production of extracellular matrix, and angiogenesis, all of which contribute to the pathogenesis of atherosclerosis and heart failure. Following initial activation of mesenchymal cells (e.g., smooth muscle cells and myofibroblasts) by an external stress, several immediate early response genes are activated during the acute phase of the stress response [13]. We originally cloned KLF5 cDNA from a smooth muscle cell cDNA library [6]. Therefore, KLF5 is thought to have a role in the phenotypic modulation and proliferation of dedifferentiated smooth muscle cells. As we expected, neointimal formation was markedly attenuated in KLF5+/− mice, which also showed attenuated interstitial and perivascular fibrosis in cardiac hypertrophy and reduced adventitial thickening in cuff-injured arteries. It is suggested from these data that KLF5 plays an essential role not only in activation of vascular smooth muscle cells, but also activated fibroblasts. Given that KLF5 is induced following activation of immediate early response genes (e.g., Egr-1) [14] and that it, in turn, controls expression of various growth factors (e.g., PDGF-A and TGFβ), KLF5 may be in a position to mediate between the acute response to an external stress and tissue remodeling in general. The present study provides a clear basis for the development of drugs modulating KLF5 function to control cardiovascular remodeling and angiogenesis.

References

[1] P. Libby, Changing concepts of atherogenesis, J. Intern. Med. 247 (2000) 349–358.
[2] M. Kuro-o, et al, Developmentally regulated expression of vascular smooth muscle myosin heavy chain isoforms, J. Biol. Chem. 264 (1989) 18272–18275.
[3] I. Manabe, et al, Isolation of the embryonic form of smooth muscle myosin heavy chain (SMemb/NMHC-B) gene and characterization of its 5′ -flanking region, Biochem. Biophys. Res. Commun. 239 (1997) 598–605.
[4] N. Watanabe, et al, BTEB2, a Kruppel-like transcription factor, regulates expression of the SMemb/Non-muscle myosin heavy chain B (SMemb/NMHC-B) gene, Circ. Res. 85 (1999) 182–191.
[5] I. Shiojima, et al, Embryonic smooth muscle myosin heavy chain SMemb is expressed in pressure-overloaded cardiac fibroblasts, Jpn. Heart J. 40 (1999) 803–818.
[6] J.J. Bieker, Kruppel-like factors: three fingers in many pies, J. Biol. Chem. 276 (2001) 34355–34358.
[7] T. Shindo, et al, Kruppel-like zinc-finger transcription factor KLF5/BTEB2 is a target for angiotensin II signaling and an essential regulator of cardiovascular remodeling, Nat. Med. 8 (2002) 856–863.
[11] H. Umemiya, et al, Regulation of retinoidal actions by diazepinylbenzoic acids. Retinoid synergists which activate the RXR-RAR heterodimers, J. Med. Chem. 40 (1997) 4222–4234.
[12] L. Eyrolles, et al, Retinobenzoic acids: 6. Retinoid antagonists with a heterocyclic ring, J. Med. Chem. 37 (1994) 1508–1517.
[13] B.C. Berk, Vascular smooth muscle growth: autocrine growth mechanisms, Physiol. Rev. 81 (2001) 999–1030.
[14] K. Kawai-Kowase, et al, Transcriptional activation of the zinc finger transcription factor BTEB2 gene by Egr-1 through mitogen-activated protein kinase pathways in vascular smooth muscle cells, Circ. Res. 85 (1999) 787–795.

International Congress Series 1262 (2004) 111–114

www.ics-elsevier.com

Rho and smooth muscle cell phenotype

Nathalie F. Worth, Barbara E. Rolfe, Julie H. Campbell, Gordon R. Campbell*

Centre for Research in Vascular Biology, School of Biomedical Science, University of Queensland, Queensland 4072, Australia

Abstract. This study determined the influence of Rho in regulating phenotype in early passage rabbit aortic smooth muscle cell (SMC) culture. Extended confluence and serum-deprivation induced SMC differentiation, indicated by increased expression of contractile markers (α-SM actin, SM-MHC and SM-2). Activation of Rho by sphingosine-1-phosphate (S-1-P) further enhanced the expression of contractile proteins and their reorganisation such that cells adopted a more 'contractile' phenotype. Inhibition of Rho induced an extreme 'synthetic' morphology including increased vimentin expression. © 2003 Published by Elsevier B.V.

Keywords: Smooth muscle; Phenotype; RhoA; Vascular disease

1. Introduction

Smooth muscle cell (SMC) phenotypic modulation from the 'contractile' state of the healthy adult artery to the less differentiated 'synthetic' state is an early and determining event in development of the atherosclerotic lesion [1,2]. Studies in our laboratory and others have shown that SMC phenotypic modulation involves dramatic changes in expression and organisation of contractile and cytoskeletal proteins [3]. In light of evidence that the cytoskeleton can play an active role in determining cell function, we examined the role of RhoA, a key regulator of the actin cytoskeleton [4], in regulating SMC phenotype. Culture conditions such as confluence and reduced serum affect the rate, degree and reversibility of phenotypic modulation [5]. Thus, the present study investigated the effects of maintaining early passage rabbit aortic SMC under conditions of long-term confluence and serum deprivation in combination with altered RhoA activity.

Abbreviations: FACS, fluorescence-activated cell sorting; GTP, guanosine triphosphate; MHC, myosin heavy chain; SRF, serum response factor; SMC, smooth muscle cell; S-1-P, sphingosine-1-phosphate.

* Corresponding author. Tel.: +61-7-3365-2991; fax: +61-7-3365-2719.
E-mail address: g.campbell@uq.edu.au (G.R. Campbell).

0531-5131/ © 2003 Published by Elsevier B.V.
doi:10.1016/S0531-5131(03)01863-6

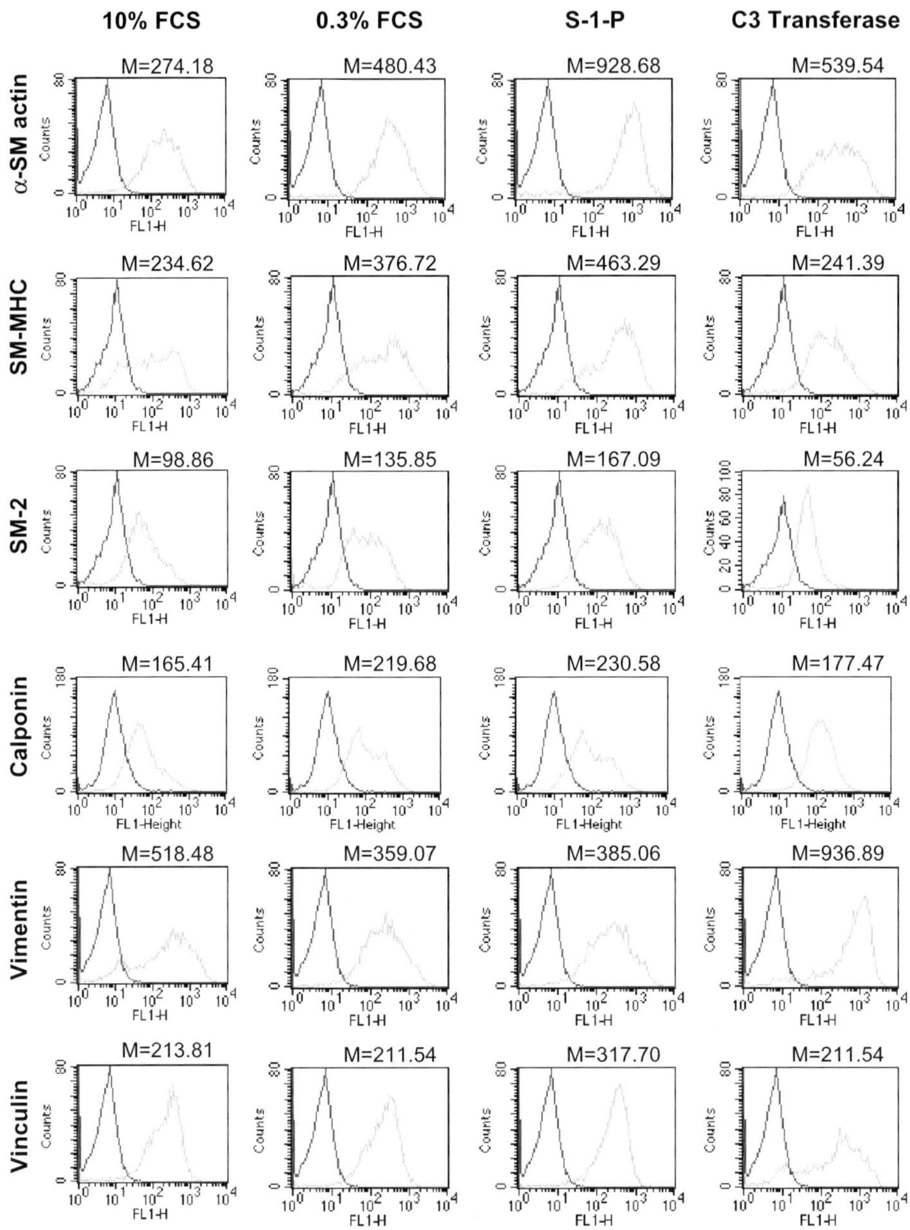

Fig. 1. Flow cytometric analysis of rabbit vascular SMC treated long term at confluence in culture medium containing high serum (10% FCS) or low serum (0.3% FCS) plus additives S-1-P or C3 transferase. Cells are labelled with antibodies specific to either α-SM actin, SM-MHC, SM-2, calponin, vimentin or vinculin. Grey histograms show the fluorescence profile for labelled cells whilst black histograms show the fluorescence profile of negative control cells.

2. Materials and methods

SMC were isolated from the aortic media of New Zealand White rabbits [6]. Cells at passage 1–2 were allowed to reach confluence and then maintained for 12–15 days in M199 containing high (10%) or low (0.3%) FCS with either sphingosine-1-phosphate (S-1-P) (10 μM) to activate, or C3 transferase (10 ng/ml) to inhibit endogenous Rho.

Cells were fixed in 1% formaldehyde, then blocked and permeabilised before incubation with primary antibodies or isotype controls. Cells were incubated with FITC-conjugated anti-mouse Ig, then analysed by flow cytometry.

Cells on coverslips were fixed in 1% paraformaldehyde, permeabilised and blocked. Cells were incubated with primary antibodies followed by biotinylated anti-mouse IgG_1 and Streptavidin-Texas Red, then examined by confocal microscopy.

3. Results

Extended confluence and low serum (0.3% FCS) increased the expression of SMC contractile markers α-SM actin, myosin (SM-MHC, and SM-2) and calponin; activation of Rho by S-1-P further increased their expression (Fig. 1). C3 transferase increased the mean expression of α-SM actin, although heterogeneity of expression was increased. It had no effect on net SM-MHC levels, but decreased expression of the 'contractile'-specific SM-2 isoform [7]. Vimentin expression was lowered by S-1-P treatment and increased by C3 transferase. Only S-1-P increased vinculin expression.

In cells treated with 10% FCS (Fig. 2), α-SM actin was evenly distributed along the stress fibres—typical of 'synthetic' state SMCs. In some cells, serum deprivation and S-1-P caused reorganisation of α-SM actin to concentrate at the centre of the stress fibres—typical of

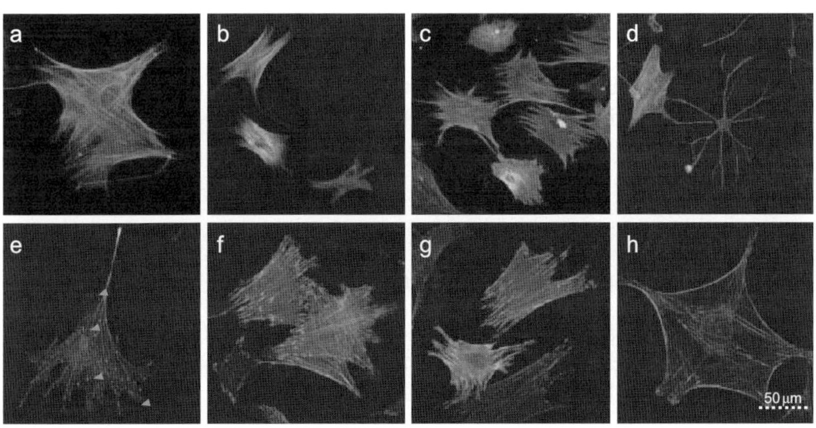

Fig. 2. Immunofluorescence micrographs of rabbit vascular SMC maintained at confluence for 12–15 days in culture medium containing high serum (10% FCS, a,e) or low serum (0.3% FCS, b,f) plus additives S-1-P (c,g) or C3 transferase (d,h). Cells are labelled with antibodies specific to either α-SM actin (green all panels), vimentin (red, a–d) or vinculin (red, e–h).

'contractile' state SMCs [3]. C3 transferase induced an extreme 'synthetic' morphology (stellate and flattened), with an almost complete disruption of stress fibres. These cells were viable and attached and spread on passage. While SM-MHC and calponin followed similar patterns of expression to α-SM actin (not shown), the distribution of vimentin was unaffected by any treatment (Fig. 2a–d). Cells maintained in high serum exhibited small arrowhead-shaped focal adhesions (vinculin, blue arrows) typical of 'synthetic' state SMCs, with many transient focal complexes (pink arrows) at the leading edges (Fig. 2e). Reduced serum and S-1-P increased the size of focal adhesions in some cells (Fig. 2f,g). C3 transferase inhibited the formation of classical focal adhesions, with cells attached to the substratum mainly by focal complexes (Fig. 2h).

4. Discussion

Consistent with Ma et al. [5], we show that extended confluence and serum-deprivation induces SMC differentiation, indicated by increased expression of contractile markers (α-SM actin, SM-MHC and SM-2).

The actions of S-1-P are partly mediated by Rho kinase via activation of serum response factor (SRF) and transcription of SMC-related contractile markers [8]. The present study found that activation of Rho by S-1-P enhanced the expression of contractile markers and induced a population of cells to adopt a more 'contractile' phenotype [3] in which contractile proteins were sorted within the stress fibres. Conversely, specific inhibition of Rho induced an extreme 'synthetic' morphology [3] with increased vimentin expression.

The small guanosine triphosphate (GTP)ases of the Rho family are emerging as potentially important mediators in the cardiovascular system [9]. While the inhibition of Rho alleviates pathogenic effects such as vessel spasm and excessive cell proliferation, the present study identifies the beneficial role for Rho in maintenance of SMC phenotype and highlights the need for selective regulation of its effects.

Acknowledgements

This research was funded by the Heart Foundation of Australia and the Ronald Geoffrey Arnott Foundation. We thank Dr. Ryozo Nagai for the anti-SM-2.

References

[1] G.R. Campbell, J.H. Campbell, Atherosclerosis, vol. II, New York Academy of Sciences, New York, 1990, pp. 143–158.
[2] G.R. Campbell, J.H. Campbell, Exp. Mol. Pathol. 42 (1985) 139–162.
[3] N.F. Worth, B.E. Rolfe, J. Song, G.R. Campbell, Cell Motil. Cytoskelet. 49 (2001) 130–145.
[4] A. Hall, Science 279 (1998) 509–514.
[5] X. Ma, Y. Wang, N.L. Stephens, Am. J. Physiol. 274 (1998) C1206–C1214.
[6] J.H. Campbell, G.R. Campbell, Clin. Sci. 85 (1993) 501–513.
[7] R. Nagai, M. Kuro-o, P. Babij, M. Periasamy, J. Biol. Chem. 264 (1989) 34–37.
[8] C.P. Mack, A.V. Somlyo, M. Hautmann, A.P. Somlyo, G.K. Owens, J. Biol. Chem. 76 (2001) 341–347.
[9] U. Laufs, J.K. Liao, Circ. Res. 87 (2000) 526–528.

International Congress Series 1262 (2004) 115–117

www.ics-elsevier.com

Induction of endothelialization of tissue-engineered cardiovascular constructs via in vivo angiogenesis during post-implant remodeling

Howard P. Greisler*

Loyola University Medical Center, Surgery, 2160 South First Avenue, Bldg. 110-3218, 60153, Maywood, IL, USA

Abstract. In vivo remodeling of implants is absolutely unavoidable. A major focus of tissue engineering should be the utilization of these remodeling processes to (1) induce capillarization to nourish three-dimensional tissue constructs, (2) recruit desired functional cells, (3) recruit supporting matrix components, (4) minimize fibrosis and apoptosis, (5) control cellular phenotype, (6) minimize immunologic reactions to allogeneic or xenogeneic cells, and (7) circumvent practical limitations and time requirements of in vitro utilization of autologous cells. Selected biomolecules can either be induced endogenously by biomaterial characteristics or can be added exogenously as either proteins or as genes. Induction of capillarization of implanted cardiovascular implants may be promoted using novel polymer chemistry, architecture or mechanics, or by application of either naturally occurring or engineered mutations of naturally occurring biologic agents. As an example of the first approach, lactide/glycolide copolymeric vascular grafts induce an angiogenic network, which provides endothelium to the implant surface, phenomena not occurring in clinically used graft materials. This difference is mediated largely by generation of FGF-2 production and angiogenesis. © 2003 Published by Elsevier B.V.

Keywords: Angiogenesis; Remodeling; Growth factors

Site-directed mutagenesis has produced FGF-1-based mutants with biological properties often differing from those of the wild-type protein. Some, such as the cys-free mutant, are more mitogenically active, others, such as the R136K mutant, resist thrombin-induced degradation, while others, including HBGAM containing chimeric constructs, promote endothelial cell specificity. Gene delivery strategies can also provide controlled spatial localization and regulated, delayed bioavailability by use of a variety of gene-activated matrix (GAM) approaches. With these approaches, selected genes may be immobilized and made available to target cells once they have been recruited to that environment. Recent technical advances in the field of tissue engineering have generated enthusiasm and

* Tel.: +1-708-216-8541; fax: +1-708-216-6300.
E-mail address: jacampbell@lumc.edu (H.P. Greisler).

0531-5131/ © 2003 Published by Elsevier B.V.
doi:10.1016/j.ics.2003.11.020

optimism regarding the potential for engineered cardiovascular tissues for use in the replacement of occluded and stenotic arteries and for restitution of functioning myocardium in areas of ischemia. However, several critical issues must still be addressed prior to clinical use. Among these are: (1) cell versatility-regulation of cell function, (2) regulation of post-implantation remodeling processes, and (3) establishment of a stable neovasculature within the engineered tissue constructs.

In vivo remodeling of tissues is absolutely unavoidable. A major focus of tissue engineering should be the utilization of these remodeling processes to (1) induce capillarization to nourish three-dimensional tissue constructs, (2) recruit desired functional cells, (3) recruit supporting matrix components, (4) minimize fibrosis and apoptosis, (5) control cellular phenotype, (6) minimize immunologic reactions to allogeneic or xenogeneic cells, and (7) circumvent practical limitations and time requirements of in vitro utilization of autologous cells.

Our knowledge of mechanisms of angiogenesis has greatly increased in recent years and considerable effort has been made toward the induction of neovascular capillary networks both in vitro and in vivo. However, several critical problems remain unsolved. These include control of the spatial distribution of such neovascular networks, strategies to establish contiguity between these neovascular networks and the host circulation and the need to better understand neovessel regression in order to generate a stable, induced neovasculature persistent over the intended life span of the implant. In most naturally occurring settings of neovascularization, capillary networks are induced by inflammatory processes and are relatively transient in nature.

Many tools are available for generating neovasculatures and include a wide battery of growth factors, induction of growth factor receptor expression, and modulation of extracellular matrix to facilitate neovascular invasion. Selected biomolecules can be either induced endogenously by altering specific chemical or mechanical factors of the material itself in order to selectively activate specific synthetic pathways in vivo post-implantation or the selected biomolecules can be added exogenously. In the latter case, they can be provided either as genes or as proteins. Gene delivery can be achieved via a multitude of gene transfer approaches. Local delivery of genes and proteins is likely more practical than systemic delivery and will be facilitated by improved, engineered scaffold designs.

Utilization of post-implantation remodeling to induce neovascular networks can be achieved by novel polymer chemistry, architecture or mechanics or by application of naturally occurring biological agents or by application of engineered non-naturally occurring biological agents. As an example of the first approach, lactide/glycolide copolymeric vascular grafts induce a transmural angiogenic network, which provides endothelium to the implant surface, phenomena not occurring in clinically used graft materials including Dacron and ePTFE. This difference is largely a result of activation of foreign body giant cells by the lactide/glycolide copolymers resulting in their production of growth factors, approximately 80% of which activity is obliterated by preincubation of conditioned media with neutralizing antibodies to FGF-2.

Utilization of growth factors added exogenously to biomaterials designed to induce angiogenesis should ideally be evaluated in vitro prior to the less controlled and more costly in vivo analyses. Applied angiogens should be assessed for molecular stability within the proposed delivery vehicle, release kinetics in physiologically relevant hemodynamic conditions should be determined and bioassays of endothelial cell migration proliferation and three-dimensional in vitro angiogenesis as well as the cell specificity of responses should be documented. Examples of these analyses may include SDS-PAGE electrophoresis, modified Boyden Chambers, modified under agarose migration assays, cell proliferation assays, and a variety of angiogenesis assays. We have established with these assays fibrin gels to be potentially efficacious for delivery of a variety of growth factors. In the case of fibroblast growth factors, the addition of heparin to the gels is required for the protection of the peptide against thrombin-induced proteolytic degradation. We have further evaluated the angiogenic response in vivo to FGF and a number of FGF-based mutants, which were designed and generated by site directed mutagenesis.

The delivery of FGF-1 via fibrin gels impregnated into the wall of ePTFE grafts induces a post-implant transmural angiogenic response with endothelialization of flow surfaces of 30 cm long thoraco-abdominal grafts implanted into dogs, a response not seen in controls lacking the FGF-1. This neovascularization was accompanied by a transient increase in cell proliferation and by increased thickening of the neointima.

Site directed mutagenesis has produced FGF-1-based mutants with biological properties differing from those of the wild-type protein. Some, most notably the cys-free mutant, are more mitogenically active. Others, including the S130K and the R136K mutants, are relatively resistant to thrombin-induced degradation. Others, including HBGAM-containing chimeric constructs, promote a relative endothelial cell specificity. In vivo evaluation of HBGAM/FGF-1 chimeras reveals the ability of this protein to induce endothelialization without intimal hyperplasia in models of canine carotid artery balloon de-endothelialization injuries.

Gene delivery strategies can also provide controlled spatial localization and regulated delayed bioavailability by use of a number of GAM approaches. With these approaches, selected genes may be immobilized and made available to target cells once they have been recruited to that environment. Among these strategies is the derivitization of surfaces with collagen-1 followed by cross-linking to antibodies directed against adenoviral hexons, the virus containing the gene of choice.

There have been considerable advances in vitro blood vessel engineering as well. Among the difficult issues are cell sourcing vis-à-vis concerns regarding immuno-induction by non-autologous endothelial cells, the most immunogenic cells of the blood vessel wall. The application of endothelial cell-specific angiogens to tissue-engineered arteries devoid of endothelium may logically be expected to promote post-implant endothelialization with a relative diminution in untoward immunologic responses to tissue engineered blood vessels.

International Congress Series 1262 (2004) 118–121

www.ics-elsevier.com

Body cavities as bioreactors to grow arteries

Julie H. Campbell*, Philip Walker, Wai-Leng Chue, Christopher Daly, Hong-Liang Cong, Lina Xiang, Gordon R. Campbell

Centre for Research in Vascular Biology, School of Biomedical Sciences, University of Queensland, Brisbane QLD 4072, Australia

Abstract. 'Artificial blood vessels' were grown in the peritoneal or pleural cavities of the dog for autologous transplantation as arterial interposition grafts. Tubing up to 250 mm long, either bare or wrapped in biodegradable polyglycolic acid (Dexon) mesh, was inserted into the body cavities using minimally invasive techniques. After 3 weeks, the tubes and their tissue capsules were harvested then the inert tubing discarded. The wall of living tissue was uniformly 1–1.5 mm thick and consisted of multiple layers of myofibroblasts that stained for α-smooth muscle actin, and extracellular matrix overlaid by a single layer of mesothelium. The bursting strength of tissue tubes with no biodegradable mesh scaffolds was in excess of 2500 mm Hg and the suture holding strength was 11.5 N. Tissue tubes (5–7 cm) were transplanted as interposition grafts into the femoral artery of the same dog in which they were grown where they remained patent until harvest at 3 to 6.5 months. Endothelial-like cells lined the lumen and the cells of wall stained for α-actin, smooth muscle myosin and smoothelin; a thick 'neo-adventitia' contained vasa vasorum. These studies demonstrate that peritoneal and pleural cavities of large animals can function as a bioreactor to grow tissue tubes for use as autologous vascular grafts. © 2003 Published by Elsevier B.V.

Keywords: Tissue engineering; Artificial blood vessels; Myofibroblasts

1. Introduction

In view of shortfalls in currently available vascular grafts, there is a need to develop an autologous bypass conduit that closely resembles the native artery, not only in its dimensions but also in its cellular constituents, physiological responsiveness, mechanical properties and in its antithrombotic and relaxing factors released at the cellular level. Recently, the peritoneal cavity of rats and rabbits has been used as a bioreactor in which to grow 'arteries' from cells of haemopoietic origin [1,2]. This site not only serves as a humidified, temperature-controlled incubator, but also supplies the cell source, nutrients, growth factors and other components necessary for tissue development. The present study uses minimally invasive techniques for implantation and harvest of tubing in the peritoneal

* Corresponding author. Tel.: +61-7-33654658; fax: +61-7-33652719.
E-mail address: julie.campbell@uq.edu.au (J.H. Campbell).

0531-5131/ © 2003 Published by Elsevier B.V.
doi:10.1016/j.ics.2003.11.022

and pleural cavities of a large animal model (dog) to grow tubes of tissue capsules for use as autologous vascular grafts [3].

2. Materials and methods

2.1. Animal surgery

Following anaesthesia, 23 nonpregnant female mongrel dogs weighing between 20 and 40 kg underwent implantation of 80–250 mm lengths of sterile polymer tubing, either bare or wrapped in biodegradable polyglycolic acid (Dexon) mesh, into the peritoneal (21) or pleural (4) cavity. A three port laparoscopic technique was used consisting of a 10 mm camera port and two other working ports placed laterally.

2.2. Tissue harvest and transplantation

Three weeks after implantation the tubular templates were located in the peritoneal or pleural cavities and harvested using the same minimally invasive techniques. A 5–7 cm length of tissue tube was prepared and an oblique end-to-end anastomosis formed with continuous 6/0 prolene in the severed right femoral artery. Graft pulse and femoral arterial pulse distal to the anastomosis confirmed the patency of the graft. Thereafter, graft patency was monitored by clinical examination, Doppler ultrasound (noninvasive) or angiography on a weekly basis [3].

3. Results

The lengths of polymer tubing inserted into the peritoneal or pleural cavities ranged from 80 to 250 mm with diameter 3–4.5 mm. Upon harvest at 3 weeks, both with and without a mesh scaffold, the tubing was covered by a thick capsule (1–1.5 mm thick) that was homogeneous and consisted of densely packed spindle-shaped cells arranged transversely around the lumen. These stained intensely for α-smooth muscle actin but were negative for both smooth muscle myosin and smoothelin. Extracellular matrix stained intensely for collagen but there was little elastin.

The tubes of tissue that had been grown without a mesh scaffold had their luminal pressure exceed 2500 mm Hg without bursting or leaking and with no aneurysmal swelling ($n=3$). The same occurred when similar lengths of dog carotid or femoral arteries were tested ($n=6$). The suture holding strength of the tubes of tissue was 11.5 N, which was stronger than that of the carotid (8.4 N) or femoral (7.1 N) arteries from the same dogs.

Sixteen myofibroblast tubes were transplanted as interposition grafts into the dog femoral artery, with antithrombotic therapy provided to post-surgery (10 mg/kg body weight aspirin) every second day. Twelve of the grafts remained patent until animal sacrifice between 2 and 6.5 months (Fig. 1A). No vessels had aneurysmal dilatations and the wall thickness was even throughout the graft.

Histologically, all traces of biodegradable Dexon scaffold had disappeared by 2 to 3 months. There was little or no intimal thickening in the region of the anastomoses, and in the four cases where the graft was not patent; this was due to organized thrombus rather

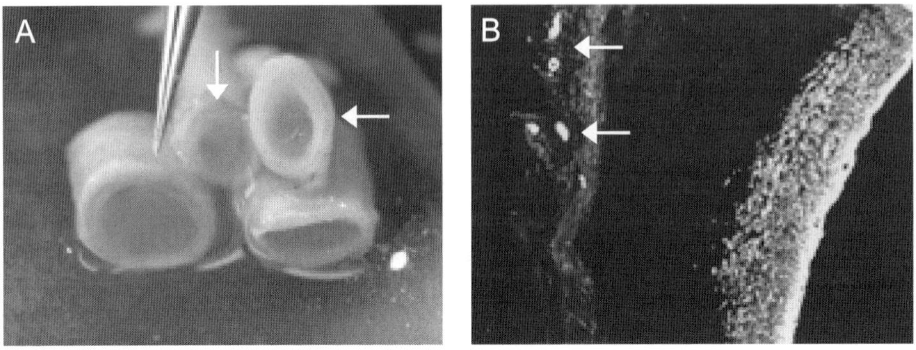

Fig. 1. (A) Four segments including two anastomotic regions (arrows) from a tube of tissue that had grown in the peritoneal cavity of a dog for 3 weeks, 6.5 months after it had been grafted into the femoral artery of the same dog. (B) Immunostaining for smooth muscle myosin of peritoneal cavity-derived tissue 4 months after it had been grafted into the dog femoral artery. Arrows, vasa vasorum.

than intimal hyperplasia. The grafts were about the same thickness as when they were harvested from the peritoneal or pleural cavity. However, while previously the cells were evenly dispersed throughout the full thickness of the wall, now there was clear demarcation between a dense cellular inner region ('media') versus more sparsely cellular outer region ('adventitia'). With immunofluorescence, the cells of the 'media' stained strongly for α-smooth muscle actin, smooth muscle myosin (Fig. 1B) and smoothelin. Also stained were many small blood vessels (vasa vasorum) in the outer part of the 'adventitia'. The cells in the 'media' were usually elongate spindle in shape and separated from each other by collagen bundles with interspersed elastin and other extracellular matrix components. Ultrastructurally, their appearance was that of normal smooth muscle cells.

Lining the lumen of the graft was a flattened layer of cells that stained strongly with an antibody for Ulex lectin, indicating their endothelial-like nature that was confirmed by transmission electron microscopy. These cells had a smooth luminal surface similar to the endothelial lining of native vessels when viewed with scanning electron microscopy.

4. Discussion

This study shows that in large animals (dog), capsules of tissue up to 250 mm in length can be grown in both the peritoneal and pleural cavities over 3 weeks using minimally invasive techniques. Since the tubing is loosely tethered at one end to the ventral surface of the peritoneal wall, the encapsulated tubing can be readily located and laparoscopically retrieved. The harvested tubes of living tissue (without a scaffold) have a bursting strength in excess of 2500 mm Hg, comparable to that of dog femoral and carotid arteries. Following transplantation into the femoral artery, the 5–7 cm long interposition graft differentiates into a structure resembling the native artery with an 'endothelial' lining, a 'media' of smooth muscle-like cells and an 'adventitia' complete with vasa vasorum. If similar tubes of living tissue can be grown in the body cavities of humans, particularly those with conditions such as hypercholesterolemia, diabetes or uremia, then patients in need of coronary artery bypass grafts, below the knee artery replacement or an arteriovenous access fistula for haemodialysis may be able to grow their own vascular grafts.

Why does the tissue capsule form around polymer tubing in the peritoneal and pleural cavities? It has been known for several decades that introduction of a foreign body into the peritoneal cavity initiates an inflammatory response. This, in turn leads to the production of various cytokines that induce the cells of haemopoietic origin (macrophages?) floating in the peritoneal fluid to attach to the foreign body, differentiate into myofibroblasts and form a capsule through their proliferation and production of extracellular matrix [1–5]. Monocyte/macrophages have recently been shown to differentiate into smooth muscle-like cells within the neointima that forms as a result of transplant atherosclerosis or following severe arterial injury [6–8]. Further differentiation into a viable blood vessel is at least partially due to stretching of the wall either by pulsatile flow or intermittent longitudinal tension [9,10].

Acknowledgements

This work was supported by the National Health and Medical Research Council of Australia (JHC, GRC) and Pfizer Australia (W-LC).

References

[1] J.H. Campbell, J.L. Efendy, G.R. Campbell, Circ. Res. 85 (1999) 1173–1178.
[2] J.H. Campbell, J.L. Efendy, C.-L. Han, et al., J. Vasc. Surg. 37 (2000) 364–371.
[3] W.-L. Chue, G. Campbell, N. Caplice, et al., J. Vasc. Surg. (2003) (in press).
[4] G.R. Campbell, G.B. Ryan, Pathology 15 (1983) 253–264.
[5] P.R.L. Mosse, G.R. Campbell, G.B. Ryan, J. Pathol. 17 (1985) 401–407.
[6] C.-L. Han, G.R. Campbell, J.H. Campbell, J. Vasc. Res. 38 (2001) 113–119.
[7] J.H. Campbell, C.-L. Han, G.R. Campbell, Ann. N.Y. Acad. Sci. 967 (2001) 18–25.
[8] A. Bayes-Genis, J.H. Campbell, P.J. Carlson, et al., Atherosclerosis 163 (2002) 89–98.
[9] L.E. Niklason, J. Gao, W.M. Abbott, et al., Science 284 (1999) 489–493.
[10] J.L. Efendy, G.R. Campbell, J.H. Campbell, J. Pathol. 192 (2000) 257–262.

International Congress Series 1262 (2004) 122–125

www.ics-elsevier.com

Critical issues in vascular tissue engineering

Robert M. Nerem*

Parker H. Petit Institute for Bioengineering and Bioscience, Georgia Institute of Technology, 315 Ferst Drive, NW, Atlanta, GA 30332-0363, USA

Abstract. The development of a tissue-engineered small-diameter blood vessel substitute has been the "holy grail" for cardiovascular tissue engineering. Hence, there are a number of critical issues. The chief among these is the issue of providing an "endothelial-like", non-thrombogenic inner lining. The second critical issue is to engineer in the appropriate mechanical properties, including visco-elastic properties that match those of native vessels. Thirdly, when a tissue-engineered blood vessel substitute is implanted into a host, a variety of biological responses will take place. Finally, although the long-term goal must be the engineering of blood vessel substitutes for clinical application, a more realistic short-term goal for tissue engineering is to develop more physiologic models for use in basic vascular biology in vitro studies.

Keywords: Blood vessel substitute; Tissue engineering

1. Introduction

The development of a small-diameter blood vessel substitute has long been a "holy grail" for vascular tissue engineering. The more biological approach of tissue engineering started three decades ago with efforts to reduce thrombosis and thus increase patency by providing a more natural internal lining for a synthetic material vascular graft through the seeding of vascular endothelial cells [1]. Although some success has been achieved, more recently efforts to tissue engineer a blood vessel substitute have moved towards more biological approaches. Many of these have significant potential; however, there are several critical issues facing the field.

2. Cell source

For a tissue-engineered blood vessel substitute to be used in such a manner so as to have a wide impact on patient treatment, it will need to be available off-the-shelf to surgeons. Although there are many who believe that allogeneic smooth muscle cells could be employed without any immune acceptance strategy so as to achieve off-the-shelf availability, the same cannot be said for the vascular endothelial cell, a talented

* Tel.: +1-404-894-2768; fax: +1-404-894-2291.
E-mail address: robert.nerem@ibb.gatech.edu (R.M. Nerem).

0531-5131/
doi:10.1016/j.ics.2003.12.029

antigen-presenting cell needed to create a physiological inner lining. What are possible sources for the vascular endothelial cell that would result in a blood vessel substitute that is available off-the-shelf? There really are only two approaches, and these are as follows: the recruitment of autologous vascular endothelial cells from the host, and the use of an allogeneic source for vascular endothelial cells together with a strategy for immune acceptance. In regard to the former, possibilities for an autologous cell source include adipose tissue, recruitment from the sites of anastomosis, and circulating endothelial progenitor cells. Adipose tissue is a source that does not provide for off-the-shelf availability [2]. As far as recruitment from the sites of anastomosis is concerned, although possible in some animal models, it has never been successfully demonstrated in humans. One is thus left with the circulating endothelial progenitor cells [3,4]. Only if one could recruit these cells directly out of the circulating blood to the surface of a non-endothelialized blood vessel substitute would one be able have a blood vessel substitute with off-the-shelf availability. An alternative, of course, is to use allogeneic cells, in which case one would need to have a strategy for the engineering of immune acceptance. Also, the use of embryonic stem cells is of considerable interest, and some success has been achieved [5]. Finally, it should be noted that there are cases where off-the-shelf availability is not essential, cases where the exact time of surgery is somewhat elective. It is in fact in such cases that initial clinical studies are being conducted.

3. Mechanical properties

There are a variety of approaches being pursued that are aimed at engineering a blood vessel substitute [6–10]. Many of these result in a tubular construct of sufficient strength; however, none have the mechanical properties that mimic those of native blood vessels, and this may be important if one is to optimize patency. This lack of appropriate visco-elastic properties is due to an insufficient amount/assembly of elastin. Several different approaches are being pursued to address this problem. These include the following: (i) use an intact elastin scaffold obtained from a digested animal artery; (ii) employ a scaffold woven from elastin mimetic fibers; and (iii) use genetically engineered cells to exhibit elevated elastin production and assembly. Whether any of these will prove themselves to be viable on a large scale basis remains to be seen. However, they should at least provide model systems that can be used to test how important it may or may not be to have mechanical properties that mimic native blood vessels.

4. Immune acceptance

As noted earlier, if one is to use allogeneic cells, in particular allogeneic endothelial cells, then one will need a strategy for the engineering of immune acceptance. One possibility is lifelong immunosuppression as used for transplanted organs; however, this has never been a desirable strategy. Thus, there is a need for new approaches, both for transplanted organs and tissue-engineered substitutes. In fact, whether one transplants a tissue or organ from a donor to the host or takes tissue, extracts the cells, makes a substitute, and then implants it, the issues are all the same as they both represent allogeneic cell transplantation. A strategy that has been investigated is that of co-stimulatory blockade; however, other strategies will need to be developed. In fact, the ability to manipulate the immune system will have important implications for tissue engineering.

5. Discussion

As already noted, the primary goal for the engineering of a blood vessel substitute is for use in human clinical treatments. This must be viewed as a long-term goal. For existing concepts wide scale clinical trials are at least 5 years away and FDA approval possibly another 5 years. Nevertheless, significant progress is being made, both with endothelial-seeded vascular grafts [11] and with cell-seeded polymeric scaffolds [12]. In the latter case, the applications have been on the pulmonary, low-pressure side of the system.

A more intermediate goal, one that is achievable in the short term, is to engineer models for the in vitro study of vascular biology that are more physiologic. A model that has been developed to better simulate in vitro the in vivo environment of the vascular endothelial cell (EC) is one that includes smooth muscle cells, the natural EC neighbor, in a three-dimensional collagen matrix [13]. Studies of EC biology using this tissue-engineered wall model (TEWM) have included morphology and F-actin localization, cell proliferation, and gene expression. The results indicate that there are major differences between the TEWM substrate as compared with collagen-coated glass. Although the TEWM construct may not be ideal, for investigations designed to increase our understanding of vascular biology, a goal must be made to continue efforts to engineer the in vitro environment so as to make it more physiologic.

In the engineering of a blood vessel substitute, a number of different concepts are being pursued, and at least for a few of these, clinical studies are in progress. Even so, there remain major barriers. These are being addressed and there have been exciting scientific advances. Nevertheless, the development of totally biologic blood vessel substitute is at least 5 years away from clinical trials and even further away from FDA approval. A more realistic, shorter-term goal is for tissue engineering to contribute to the engineering of a more physiologic environment for in vitro basic vascular biology studies.

Acknowledgements

The author acknowledges the Georgia Tech/Emory Center for the Engineering of Living Tissues, an Engineering Research Center that is supported by the National Science Foundation through ERC Award Number EEC-9731643.

References

[1] M.B. Herring, R. Dilley, R.A. Jersild Jr., L. Boxer, A. Gardner, J. Glover, Seeding arterial prostheses with vascular endothelium. The nature of the lining, Ann. Surg. 190 (1979) 84–90.

[2] S.K. Williams, T.F. Wang, R. Castrillo, B.E. Jarrell, Liposuction-derived human fat used for vascular graft sodding contains endothelial cells and not mesothelial cells as the major cell type, J. Vasc. Surg. 19 (1994) 916–923.

[3] Y. Lin, D.J. Weisdorf, A. Solovey, R.P. Hebbel, Origins of circulating endothelial cells and endothelial outgrowth from blood, J. Clin. Invest. 105 (2000) 71–77.

[4] S. Kaushal, G.E. Amiel, K.J. Guleserian, O.M. Shapira, T. Perry, F.W. Sutherland, E. Rabkin, A.M. Moran, F.J. Schoen, A. Atala, S. Soker, J. Bischoff, J.E. Mayer, Functional small-diameter neovessels created using endothelial progenitor cells expanded ex vivo, Nat. Med. 7 (2001) 1035–1040.

[5] S. Levenberg, J.S. Golub, M. Amit, J. Itskovitz-Eldor, R. Langer, Endothelial cells derived from human embryonic stem cells, Proc. Natl. Acad. Sci. U. S. A. 99 (2002) 4391–4396.
[6] C.B. Weinberg, E. Bell, A blood vessel model constructed from collagen and cultured vascular cells, Science 231 (1986) 397–400.
[7] D. Seliktar, R.A. Black, R.P. Vito, R.M. Nerem, Dynamic mechanical conditioning of collagen–gel blood vessel constructs induces remodeling in vitro, Ann. Biomed. Eng. 28 (2000) 351–362.
[8] G.C. Lantz, S.F. Badylak, M.C. Hiles, A.C. Coffey, L.A. Geddes, K. Kokini, et al., Small intestinal submucosa as a vascular graft: a review, J. Invest. Surg. 6 (1993) 297–310.
[9] L.E. Niklason, J. Gao, W.M. Abbott, K.K. Hirschi, S. Houser, R. Marini, et al., Functional arteries grown in vitro, Science 284 (1999) 489–493.
[10] N. L'Heureux, S. Paquet, R. Labbe, L. Germain, F.A. Auger, A completely biological tissue-engineered human blood vessel, FASEB J. 12 (1998) 47–56.
[11] J.G. Meinhart, M. Deutsch, T. Fischlein, N. Howanietz, A. Froschl, P. Zilla, Clinical autologous in vitro endothelialization of 153 infrainguinal ePTFE grafts, Ann. Thorac. Surg. 71 (2001) 327–331.
[12] G. Matsumura, N. Hibino, Y. Ikada, H. Kurosawa, T. Shin'oka, Successful application of tissue engineered vascular autografts: clinical experience, Biomaterials 24 (2003) 2303–2308.
[13] B. Imberti, D. Seliktar, R.M. Nerem, A. Remuzzi, The response of endothelial cells to fluid shear stress using a co-culture model of the arterial wall, Endothelium 9 (2002) 11–23.

International Congress Series 1262 (2004) 126–128

www.ics-elsevier.com

Recent optimization of a tissue engineered blood vessel: the LOEX experience

François A. Auger*, Karina Laflamme, Guillaume Grenier, Murielle Rémy-Zolghadri, Lucie Germain

Laboratoire d'organogénèse expérimentale (LOEX), Centre hospitalier affilié universitaire de Québec-Pavillon Saint-Sacrement, 1050 chemin Sainte-Foy, Québec, Québec, Canada G1S 4L8
Department of Surgery, Laval University, Canada

Abstract. Creating a blood vessel by tissue engineering is one of the most demanding goals in tissue engineering. Our laboratory developed, using the self-assembly approach, the first completely biological tissue engineered blood vessel (TEBV) constituted of living human cells in the absence of any synthetic or exogenous material. The phenotypic and functional variations of smooth muscle cell (SMC) are of paramount importance in TEBV reconstruction. Thus, the phenotype and extracellular matrix (ECM) production of SMC were studied along the whole sequence of TEBV production. The functional and mechanical properties can be greatly enhanced by active cell orientation in the ECM. Accordingly, the method of preparing living tissue engineered sheets was modified to obtain an optimal alignment of SMC before rolling them into a tubular form. These results have allowed us to create a better TEBV. © 2003 Elsevier B.V. All rights reserved.

Keywords: Tissue-engineering; Blood vessel; Regenerative medicine; Smooth muscle cells

1. Introduction

The production of organs by tissue engineering is a novel approach to replace wounded or dead tissues by reconstructed living tissues.

We managed to develop living tissue engineered blood vessels (TEBV) by the self-assembly approach, which did not contain synthetic material, for the replacement of small diameter arteries ($\leq$ 5 mm lumen). Recently, another group [1] has published a two-layered (media and endothelium) blood vessels by using a polyglycolic acid mesh scaffold seeded with bovine smooth muscle cells (SMC). However, in contradistinction, our tissue engineered blood vessel contained all three histological layers: the endothelium, the media and the adventitia from human cells.

* Corresponding author. Laboratoire d'organogénèse expérimentale (LOEX), Centre hospitalier affilié universitaire de Québec-Pavillon Saint-Sacrement, 1050 chemin Sainte-Foy, Québec, Québec, Canada G1S 4L8 Tel.: +1-418-682-7696; fax: +1-418-682-8000.
E-mail address: francois.auger@chg.ulaval.ca (F.A. Auger).

0531-5131/
doi:10.1016/S0531-5131(03)01768-0

Its production was based on a new method, called the self-assembly approach, of tissue engineering in which smooth muscle cells and fibroblasts are cultured in a medium containing serum and ascorbic acid (50 μg/ml). Under these conditions, the cells produce and organize their own extracellular matrix (ECM). The starting materials are only human cells cultured in an enriched medium [6].

2. Blood vessel production

The following steps are necessary to produce a complete blood vessel. Smooth muscle cell sheets were rolled over an acellular inner membrane (dehydrated tubular tissue formed with a fibroblast sheet). After a week of maturation, a fibroblast sheet is then wrapped around the media layer to produce the adventitia after 8 weeks of maturation. Finally, the endothelial cells are seeded in the lumen to be seeded on the inner membrane and form the endothelium [2].

Although it was devoid of biomaterials, this reconstructed human blood vessel was highly resistant with a burst strength of 2500 mm Hg. This improved resistance was likely due to the complex restructuration of the extracellular matrix. Another contributing factor is probably a stable gelatinase activity.

Furthermore, we have shown in our reconstructed blood vessel the presence of elastin fibers [2] absent in other reconstructed models [1]. In addition, we have observed the re-expression of desmin in the human smooth muscle cells present in the TEBV media [2]. Hence, the functionality of these TEBV allows their utilization in pharmacological studies [3,4].

The endothelial cells seeded on the inner membrane formed a confluent and functional endothelium. Endothelial cells expressed von Willebrand factor and incorporated acetylated low-density lipoproteins [2,5].

3. Optimization step of our TEBV

The phenotypic and functional variations of SMC are of paramount importance. Thus, the phenotype and ECM production of SMC were studied along the whole sequence of our TEBV production. Various markers of differentiation such as desmin, calponin and myosin were chronologically observed during the expansion phase and after rolling the SMC sheets into a tubular form. Cell cycle and contractile function were also studied.

As in other tissue engineered reconstruction, the functional and mechanical properties can be greatly enhanced by active cell orientation in the ECM. Thus, the method of preparing ECM sheets was modified to obtain an optimal alignment of SMC before rolling them into a tubular form. Histological and ultrastructural analyses showed that this could be readily attained with an appropriate anchorage of the SMC sheets.

4. Conclusion

Vascular substitutes created by tissue-engineering vessels are a step towards the reconstruction of more complex organs [6]. The advances in tissue engineering will help to provide a therapeutic alternative for human transplantation.

The self-assembly method for organ and tissue reconstruction is a truly different approach in the field of tissue engineering of soft tissues. The integration of various tissues and organs created by such a method should be more rapid and with minimal inflammation. The self-assembly approach is more akin to the physiological phenomenon that occurs in the womb during organogenesis. This may prove to be a distinct advantage for certain types of grafts.

Acknowledgements

This study was funded by the CIHR, FRSQ, Heart and Stroke Foundation of Canada and Fondation de l'Hôpital du Saint-Sacrement. We thank Kathleen Baker and Rina Guignard for their technical assistance. Lucie Germain was recipient of Scholarships from the Canadian Institutes of Health Research (CIHR) and is the holder of the Canadian Research Chair on Stem Cells and Tissue Engineering from CIHR. Karina Laflamme and Guillaume Grenier were recipients of a fellowship from the Fonds FCAR-FRSQ du Québec. Murielle Rémy-Zolghadri was recipient of a fellowship from the Heart and Stroke Foundation of Canada.

For illustrations and extensive LOEX references please refer to www.fmed.ulaval.ca/loex.

References

[1] L.E. Niklason, J. Gao, W.M. Abbott, K.K. Hirschi, S. Houser, R. Marini, R. Langer, Functional arteries grown in vitro, Science 284 (1999) 493–498.

[2] N. L'Heureux, S. Pâquet, R. Labbé, L. Germain, F.A. Auger, A completely biological tissue-engineered human blood vessel, FASEB J. 12 (1998) 47–56.

[3] J.C. Stoclet, R. Andriantsitohaina, N. L'Heureux, C. Martinez, L. Germain, F.A. Auger, Use of human vessels and human smooth muscle cells in pharmacology, Cell Biol. Toxicol. 12 (1996) 223–225.

[4] N. L'Heureux, J.C. Stoclet, F.A. Auger, J.L. Lagaud, L. Germain, A. Andriantsitohaina, A human tissue-engineered vascular media: a new model for pharmacological studies of contractile responses, FASEB J. 15 (2001) 515–524.

[5] N. L'Heureux, L. Germain, R. Labbé, F.A. Auger, In vitro construction of human vessel from cultured vascular cells: a morphologic study, J. Vasc. Surg. 17 (1993) 499–509.

[6] F.A. Auger, M. Rémy-Zolghadri, G. Grenier, L. Germain, The self-assembly approach for organ reconstruction by tissue engineering, e-Biomed: J. Regenerative Med. 1 (2000) 75–86.

International Congress Series 1262 (2004) 129–132

www.ics-elsevier.com

Atheroprotective mechanisms of flow: inhibition of apoptosis

Xinchun Pi, Chen Yan, Bradford C. Berk*

Center for Cardiovascular Research, University of Rochester, Cardiology Unit, Box 679, 601 Elmwood Avenue, Rochester, NY 14642, USA

Abstract. Steady laminar flow is atheroprotective through multiple beneficial effects on endothelial cells (EC). Among these effects, promotion of EC survival by inhibiting apoptosis is particularly important. We discuss the mechanisms by which steady laminar flow inhibits EC apoptosis in this review.

Keywords: Fluid shear stress; Apoptosis; Endothelial cells; Atherosclerosis

1. Introduction

The endothelium, as the inner lining of all blood vessels, plays a critical role in vascular homeostasis and "protects" the vessel from atherosclerosis [1]. An important concept in endothelial cells (EC) atheroprotection is EC survival. EC apoptosis contributes to the initiation of atherosclerosis as well as plaque destabilization and thrombosis.

2. Mechanisms for anti-apoptotic effect of steady laminar fluid shear stress

2.1. PI-3K and Akt pathway

Phosphorylation and activation of Akt was reported to be involved in flow-dependent EC survival [2]. Our group recently showed that shear stress transactivates the VEGF receptor, recruits PI3K and activates Akt, suggesting that the VEGF receptor plays a role in preventing EC apoptosis [3]. Since eNOS inhibitors increase apoptosis in EC induced by serum deprivation, oxidized LDL, hydrogen peroxide and TNF, it is clear that eNOS mediates the apoptosis-inhibiting effect of shear stress through NO production [4]. There are at least three mechanisms by which NO may be anti-apoptotic: (1) NO scavenges O_2^- leading to formation of $ONOO^-$; (2) NO nitrosylates caspase 3 and inhibits its activity [5]; and (3) *S*-nitrosylation of thioredoxin increases its activity and enhances thioredoxin's ability to inhibit the apoptosis signal kinase-1 (ASK1) [6] (Fig. 1).

* Corresponding author. Tel.: +1-585-273-1946; fax: +1-585-273-1497.

E-mail address: Bradford_Berk@urmc.rochester.edu (B.C. Berk).

0531-5131/
doi:10.1016/j.ics.2003.11.036

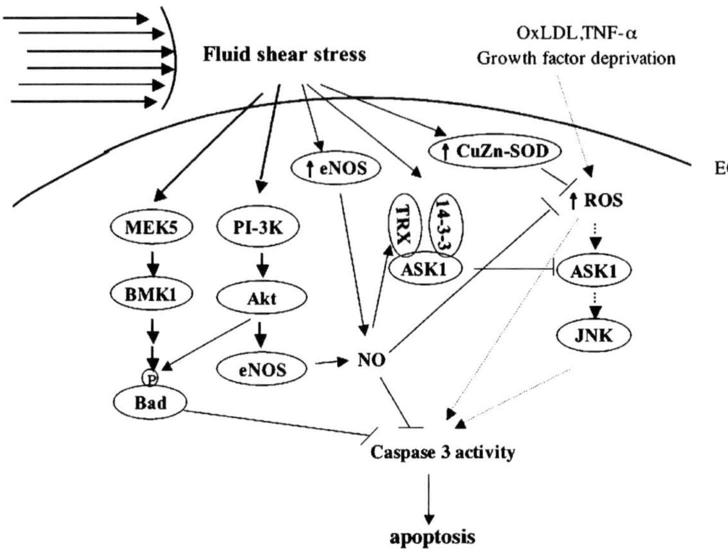

Fig. 1. The major pathways involved in mediating inhibitory effects of flow on endothelial apoptosis.

2.2. ASK1

Published data show that overexpression of ASK1 induced apoptosis through JNK activation, and dominant negative ASK1 inhibited TNF-induced apoptosis [7]. Shear stress inhibited TNF-induced ASK1 and JNK activation by increasing association of ASK1 with its endogenous inhibitor, 14-3-3 [8]. A mutant form of ASK1 lacking the 14-3-3-binding site (ASK1-NS967A) was not inhibited by shear stress and still activated JNK [8]. These data suggest that flow increases binding of 14-3-3 to ASK1 by maintaining phosphorylation of Ser-967. How flow regulates phosphorylation of Ser-967 remains unknown, although Zhang et al. [9] showed that a Ras GTPase-activating protein (Ras-GAP) acts as an ASK1-interacting protein (AIP1) and competes for binding with 14-3-3. AIP1, therefore, represents a new target for regulation by shear stress.

2.3. Anti-oxidant molecules

ROS are endogenously synthesized by NAD(P)H oxidase in EC, or its production is induced by atherosclerotic and proapoptotic stimuli, such as oxidized LDL and TNF. While enhanced ROS are causally involved in apoptosis, antioxidants prevent EC death. TNF-induced activation of ASK1 is inhibited by antioxidants such as *N*-acetylcysteine and thioredoxin, which binds to ASK1 in its reduced form and promotes ASK1 ubiquitination [10]. ROS activate ASK1 by oxidizing thioredoxin to release it from ASK1. The critical cysteines in thioredoxin required for ASK1 binding are cysteines 32 and 35; mutation of either one to serine to prevent oxidation to the disulfide (Trx-S-S) creates a dominant negative thioredoxin that inhibits ASK1-mediated apoptosis [10]. In addition, *S*-nitrosylation of Cys 69 is important to protect EC from apoptosis [6]. Haendeler et al. [6]

showed that mutation of Cys 69 on thioredoxin reduced the anti-apoptotic activity and the anti-apoptotic effect of thioredoxin was dependent on endogenous NO. Other anti-oxidant molecules are involved in the mediation of the anti-apoptotic function of fluid shear stress. Cu/Zn SOD, which scavenges O_2^-, is upregulated by physiological levels of flow in EC and increased the resistance to pro-apoptotic stimuli [4].

2.4. BMK1-Bad pathway

BMK1 (or ERK5) is strongly activated by shear stress [11], and plays an important role in the inhibitory effect of fluid shear stress on EC apoptosis (Pi and Berk, unpublished data). Stimulation of BMK1 by its upstream activator, MEK5, significantly increased EC survival, inhibited caspase 3 activity, and decreased apoptosis induced by serum deprivation. In contrast, inhibiting BMK1 activity by overexpressing a dominant negative BMK1 (DN-BMK1) stimulated apoptosis and blocked the protective effect of shear stress. Analysis of anti-apoptotic mechanisms showed that both shear stress and MEK5 stimulated phosphorylation of the apoptosis mediator Bad on Ser 112 and Ser 136, while DN-BMK1 inhibited phosphorylation. Phosphorylation of Bad maintains 14-3-3 binding and sequesters Bad in the cytoplasm. BMK1-mediated Bad phosphorylation was independent of Akt, protein kinase A or p90RSK kinase, all of which have been shown to phosphorylate Bad in other cells. Of interest, BMK1 null mice display defective EC morphology, blood vessel formation, and cardiac development leading to embryonic lethality [12]. Because the defects in the BMK1 knockout occurred at the onset of blood flow (day 9.5), we speculate that increased apoptosis due to loss of BMK1 may contribute to the BMK1 null phenotype.

3. Summary

This review summarizes the current findings and discusses the potential protective role of fluid shear stress on endothelial cell apoptosis and atherosclerosis. We showed that endothelial progenitor cells are directed to vascular lesion sites to reestablish an intact endothelial layer [13]. The effects of different flow patterns and levels of shear stress on this process should be an area of fruitful investigation. In summary, we believe that understanding the mechanisms for the protective effects of shear stress on EC apoptosis will be helpful in the design of new therapies for the treatment of atherosclerosis.

References

[1] B.C. Berk, W. Min, C. Yan, J. Surapisitchat, Y. Liu, R. Hoefen, Atheroprotective mechanisms activated by fluid shear stress in endothelial cells, Drug News Perspect. 15 (3) (2002) 133–139.

[2] S. Dimmeler, B. Assmus, C. Hermann, J. Haendeler, A.M. Zeiher, Fluid shear stress stimulates phosphorylation of Akt in human endothelial cells: involvement in suppression of apoptosis, Circ. Res. 83 (3) (1998) 334–341.

[3] Z.G. Jin, H. Ueba, T. Tanimoto, A.O. Lungu, M.D. Frame, B.C. Berk, Ligand independent activation of VEGF receptor 2 by fluid shear stress regulates activation of endothelial nitric oxide synthase, Circ. Res. 93 (4) (2003) 354–363.

[4] S. Dimmeler, C. Hermann, J. Galle, A.M. Zeiher, Upregulation of superoxide dismutase and nitric oxide synthase mediates the apoptosis-suppressive effects of shear stress on endothelial cells, Arterioscler. Thromb. Vasc. Biol. 19 (3) (1999) 656–664.

[5] S. Dimmeler, J. Haendeler, M. Nehls, A.M. Zeiher, Suppression of apoptosis by nitric oxide via inhibition of interleukin-1beta-converting enzyme (ICE)-like and cysteine protease protein (CPP)-32-like proteases, J. Exp. Med. 185 (4) (1997) 601–607.
[6] J. Haendeler, J. Hoffmann, V. Tischler, B.C. Berk, A.M. Zeiher, S. Dimmeler, Redox regulatory and anti-apoptotic functions of thioredoxin depend on *S*-nitrosylation at cysteine 69, Nat. Cell Biol. 4 (10) (2002) 743–749.
[7] H. Ichijo, E. Nishida, K. Irie, D.-P. Ten, M. Saitoh, T. Moriguchi, M. Takagi, K. Matsumoto, K. Miyazono, Y. Gotoh, Induction of apoptosis by ASK1, a mammalian MAPKKK that activates SAPK/JNK and p38 signaling pathways, Science 275 (5296) (1997) 90–94.
[8] Y. Liu, G. Yin, J. Surapisitchat, B.C. Berk, W. Min, Laminar flow inhibits TNF-induced ASK1 activation by preventing dissociation of ASK1 from its inhibitor 14-3-3, J. Clin. Invest. 107 (7) (2001) 917–923.
[9] R. Zhang, X. He, W. Liu, M. Lu, J.T. Hsieh, W. Min, AIP1 mediates TNF-alpha-induced ASK1 activation by facilitating dissociation of ASK1 from its inhibitor 14-3-3, J. Clin. Invest. 111 (12) (2003) 1933–1943.
[10] Y. Liu, W. Min, Thioredoxin promotes ASK1 ubiquitination and degradation to inhibit ASK1-mediated apoptosis in a redox activity-independent manner, Circ. Res. 90 (12) (2002) 1259–1266.
[11] C. Yan, M. Takahashi, M. Okuda, J.D. Lee, B.C. Berk, Fluid shear stress stimulates big mitogen-activated protein kinase 1 (BMK1) activity in endothelial cells. Dependence on tyrosine kinases and intracellular calcium, J. Biol. Chem. 274 (1) (1999) 143–150.
[12] S.J. Sohn, B.K. Sarvis, D. Cado, A. Winoto, ERK5 MAPK regulates embryonic angiogenesis and acts as a hypoxia-sensitive repressor of vascular endothelial growth factor expression, J. Biol. Chem. 277 (45) (2002) 43344–43351.
[13] N. Werner, S. Junk, U. Laufs, A. Link, K. Walenta, M. Bohm, G. Nickenig, Intravenous transfusion of endothelial progenitor cells reduces neointima formation after vascular injury, Circ. Res. 93 (2) (2003) e17–e24.

International Congress Series 1262 (2004) 133–136

www.ics-elsevier.com

A molecular mechanism for mechanical activation of endothelial cells

Keigi Fujiwara[a,*], Michitaka Masuda[b], Masaki Osawa[c], Ken-ichi Kusano[a], Feng Shi[a], Tamlyn N. Thomas[a]

[a] *Center for Cardiovascular Research, Aab Institute of Biomedical Sciences, University of Rochester Medical Center, 601 Elmwood Ave. Box 679, Rochester, NY 14642, USA*

[b] *Department of Structural Analysis, National Cardiovascular Center Research Institute, Suita, Osaka 565-8565, Japan*

[c] *Department of Cell Biology, Duke University Medical Center, Durham, NC 27710, USA*

Abstract. In this brief review, we will present evidence that platelet endothelial cell adhesion molecule-1 (PECAM-1) is a mechanoresponsive molecule. When endothelial cells (ECs) are exposed to mechanical stress, PECAM-1 is tyrosine-phosphorylated and recruits SHP-2 and Gab1 to the area of cell–cell attachment. These events are necessary for ERK activation by fluid shear stress (FSS) and cyclic stretch in endothelial cells. Both PECAM-1 tyrosine phosphorylation and ERK activation can be achieved by applying mechanical force directly on PECAM-1, suggesting that PECAM-1 is a mechanotransduction molecule. © 2004 Published by Elsevier B.V.

Keywords: Fluid shear stress; PECAM-1; SHP-2; ERK; Mechanosignal transduction

1. Introduction

There are certain regions within the arterial tree where atherosclerosis is more likely to develop. The most common region is the branch point of large arteries where turbulent flow occurs and the mean fluid shear stress (FSS) is low [1]. Conversely, the areas exposed to steady laminar flow tend to remain plaque-free, suggesting that steady laminar flow promotes normalcy of the endothelium [2]. FSS is known to affect the structure, gene expression, biosynthetic activity, and physiology of endothelial cells (ECs), but our understanding of molecular mechanisms for flow sensing and the subsequent flow-induced signaling is limited. We have recently proposed that platelet endothelial cell adhesion molecule-1 (PECAM-1) is a mechanoresponsive molecule [3]. Here, we will summarize our data on the role of PECAM-1 in mechanosignal transduction in ECs.

* Corresponding author. Tel.: +1-585-273-5714; fax: +1-585-273-1497.
E-mail address: Keigi_Fujiwara@urmc.rochester.edu (K. Fujiwara).

0531-5131/ © 2004 Published by Elsevier B.V.
doi:10.1016/j.ics.2004.01.081

2. Tyrosine phosphorylation of PECAM-1

PECAM-1 is a cell adhesion molecule abundantly expressed in ECs. Its cytoplasmic domain contains five (six for bovine) tyrosine residues, and amino acid sequence data predicted that Tyr663 and Tyr686 were phosphorylatable. Indeed, PECAM-1 tyrosine phosphorylation was detected in ECs exposed to FSS or hyperosmotic and hypoosmotic shocks (OS) [4], in aggregating platelets [5], and in mast cells during IgE receptor aggregation [6]. Subsequently, Masuda et al. [7] and Jackson et al. [5] reported that SHP-2 bound to tyrosine phosphorylated PECAM-1 (pY-PECAM-1).

Tyrosine phosphorylation of PECAM-1 was rapid, detectable within 30 s of flow application [4]. OS also induced PECAM-1 tyrosine phosphorylation whose kinetics was nearly identical to those by FSS. Because OS experiments were easier to perform than flow experiments, many analyses were done using OS. Although PECAM-1 tyrosine phosphorylation by FSS is rapid, there are faster flow-induced responses such as a transient cytoplasmic Ca^{2+}increase [8] and K^+ channel activation [9], and they could trigger PECAM-1 phosphorylation. However, when ECs were treated with Ca-ionophores, thrombin, ATP, histamine, bradykinin, or acetylcholine, all of which are known to increase the cytoplasmic Ca^{2+} concentration, PECAM-1 in these cells was not phosphorylated [4]. Ba^+ and TEA, known K^+ channel inhibitors, failed to block PECAM-1 tyrosine phosphorylation by OS. Furthermore, gadolinium ion, a stretch activated cation channel blocker, failed to inhibit PECAM-1 tyrosine phosphorylation by OS. Activation of protein kinase C did not cause PECAM-1 phosphorylation. These results indicate that tyrosine phosphorylation of PECAM-1 by FSS or OS is not a downstream event of Ca^{2+} mobilization, K^+ channel activation, stretch activated cation channel activity, and PKC activation [10] and suggest that PECAM-1 tyrosine phosphorylation is a part of a novel mechanosignaling pathway in ECs.

Because PECAM-1 does not have a kinase domain, some kinase(s) must be involved in its tyrosine phosphorylation. In an effort for identifying PECAM-1 kinase, we performed coimmunoprecipitation experiments using antibodies against PECAM-1 and found c-Src in the immune complex. Indeed, it binds pY-PECAM-1 in vitro. However, when COS7, HEK293, L, or ECV304 cells were transfected with bovine PECAM-1 and mechanically stimulated, PECAM-1 was not phosphorylated, although PECAM-1 expressed in these cells localized to the cell–cell association area (CCA). GST-tagged bovine PECAM-1 expressed in human ECs was tyrosine-phosphorylated under the same condition, suggesting that ECs but not other cell types had a proper PECAM-1 kinase system. Interestingly, however, human PECAM-1 expressed in HEK293 cells was tyronine phosphorylated when the cells were treated with hydrogen peroxide [11]. Recently, Fer and Fes kinases were shown to tyrosine phosphorylate PECAM-1 in overexpression cell systems [12]. However, this phosphorylation was independent of mechanical stress.

3. PECAM-1 and signal transduction

SHP-2 through its binding to certain types of tyrosine phosphorylated proteins regulates cell signaling [13], and we have found that it binds to pY-PECAM-1 [7]. In mammalian cells, SHP-2 activates the ERK1/2 cascade [14]. Interestingly, flow activates ERK1/2 in ECs [15], and we have shown that OS also activates ERK in ECs [3]. Based on these and other data, we have proposed a mechanosignal transduction pathway initiated by PECAM-1 tyrosine phosphorylation, followed by SHP-2 binding to it and then ERK activation.

There are several lines of evidence that support this hypothesis. FSS-dependent ERK activation was a tyrosine kinase-dependent event [16], and indeed we found that ERK activation by FSS was inhibited in ECs overexpressing phosphatase-negative SHP-2. This mutant SHP-2 can bind to pY-PECAM-1 but due to its lack of enzymatic activity blocks further signaling. When PECAM-1 expression in ECs was downregulated by antisense S-oligonucleotides, ERK activation by OS was significantly reduced. Moreover, when we overexpressed the cytoplasmic tail of PECAM-1 in ECs, ERK activation by FSS but not by VEGF was inhibited. However, this dominant negative effect of the PECAM-1 cytoplasmic domain was lost when Tyr663 and Tyr686 were mutated to phenylalanine. Together, these results suggest that PECAM-1 tyrosine phosphorylation and subsequent activation of SHP-2 are important initial steps for the activation of the ERK pathway by mechanical stress.

4. Direct force application to PECAM-1

We investigated whether direct force application onto PECAM-1 could cause its tyrosine phosphorylation. Magnetic beads coated with antibodies against the external domain of PECAM-1 were applied onto sparsely cultured ECs. A strong magnet was then placed over the culture to apply tugging force to PECAM-1. To our amazement, PECAM-1 bound to beads was tyrosine phosphorylated. pY-PECAM-1 was barely detectable in the absence of a magnetic field, and PECAM-1 not bound to beads was not phosphorylated regardless of magnetic field application. ERK activation was observed only when a magnetic field was applied. When we used polylysine-coated beads instead of those coated with the anti-PECAM-1 to do the same experiment, neither PECAM-1 nor ERK was phosphorylated.

PECAM-1 trapped by the antibody coated magnetic beads was a small fraction of the total PECAM-1 in a cell. To trap a larger fraction of PECAM-1 by the antibody, ECs were plated onto the culture dish coated with the anti-PECAM-1. As controls, cells were plated onto dishes coated with preimmune IgG, polylysine, fibronectin, laminin, or type I collagen. Attached cells were challenged with OS, and the levels of PECAM-1 and ERK phosphorylation were assayed. PECAM-1 and REK were phosphorylated only when cells were plated on the anti-PECAM-1 coated surface. These experiments demonstrate that PECAM-1 is a mechanoresponsive protein.

5. Summary

Our study demonstrates PECAM-1's unique property as a mechanoresponsive molecule. To our knowledge, PECAM-1 is the first molecule in mammalian cells that is shown to be chemically modified by a mechanical force applied directly to it. Our recent results show that PECAM-1 is tyrosine phosphorylated in ECs exposed to cyclic stretch, which also activates ERK. Thus, PECAM-1 is not just a flow sensor but is also a stretch sensor. Although a number of questions remain to be investigated, PECAM-1 tyrosine phosphorylation appears to be a key event in ECs' mechanosignal transduction.

Acknowledgements

Parts of the work described in this review were supported by grants from NIH (HL69041) and American Heart Association (0256265T).

References

[1] M.A. Gimbrone Jr., Endothelial dysfunction, hemodynamic forces and atherosclerosis, Thromb. Haemost. 82 (1999) 722–726.

[2] K. Fujiwara, Mechanical stresses keep endothelial cells healthy: beneficial effects of a physiological level of cyclic stretch on endothelial barrier function, Am. J. Physiol., Lung Cell. Mol. Physiol. 285 (2003) L782–L784.

[3] M. Osawa, et al., Evidence for a role of platelet endothelial cell adhesion molecule-1 in endothelial cell mechanosignal transduction: is it a mechanoresponsive molecule? J. Cell Biol. 158 (2002) 773–785.

[4] M. Osawa, et al., Tyrosine phosphorylation of platelet endothelial cell adhesion molecule-1 (PECAM-1, CD31) in mechanically stimulated vascular endothelial cells, Eur. J. Cell Biol. 72 (1997) 229–237.

[5] D.E. Jackson, et al., The protein-tyrosine phosphatase, SHP-2 binds platelet endothelial cell adhesion molecule-1 (PECAM-1) and forms a distinct signaling complex during platelet aggregation—evidence for a mechanistic link between PECAM-1 and integrin mediated cellular signaling, J. Biol. Chem. 272 (1997) 6986–6993.

[6] K. Sagawa, et al., Aggregation of the high affinity IgE receptor results in the tyrosine phosphorylation of the surface adhesion protein PECAm-1 (CD31), J. Biol. Chem. 272 (1997) 13412–13418.

[7] M. Masuda, et al., Platelet endothelial cell adhesion molecule-1 is a major SH-PTP2 binding protein in vascular endothelial cells, FEBS Lett. 408 (1997) 331–336.

[8] J. Ando, et al., Cytoplasmic calcium response to fluid shear stress in cultured vascular endothelial cells, In Vitro Cell. Dev. Biol. 24 (1988) 871–877.

[9] S.P. Olsen, et al., Hemodynamic shear stress activates a K+ current in vascular endothelial cells, Nature 331 (1988) 168–170.

[10] K. Fujiwara, et al., Tyrosine phosphorylation of platelet endothelial cell adhesion molecule-1 (PECAM-1) and mechanosignal transduction, in: P. Lelkes (Ed.), Mechanical Forces and the Endothelium, Harwood Academic Publishers, Reading, 1999, pp. 55–67.

[11] D.E. Jackson, et al., Characterization of phosphotyrosine binding motifs in the cytoplasmic domain of platelet endothelial cell adhesion molecule-1 (PECAM-1) that are required for the cellular association and activation of the protein-tyrosine phosphatase, SHP-2, J. Biol. Chem. 272 (1997) 24868–24875.

[12] N. Kogata, et al., Identification of Fer tyrosine kinase localization on microtubules as a platelet endothelial cell adhesion molecule-1 phosphorylating kinase in vascular endothelial cells, Mol. Biol. Cell. 14 (2003) 3553–3564.

[13] B.G. Neel, N.K. Tonks, Protein tyrosine phosphatases in signal transduction, Curr. Opin. Cell Biol. 9 (1997) 193–204.

[14] T. Noguchi, et al., Role of SH-PTP2, a protein-tyrosine phosphatase with Src homology 2 domains, in insulin-stimulated Ras activation, Mol. Cell. Biol. 14 (1994) 6674–6682.

[15] T.L. Tang, et al., The SH2-containing protein-tyrosine phosphatase SH-PTP2 is required upstream of MAP kinase for early Xenopus development, Cell 80 (1995) 473–483.

[16] M. Takahashi, B.C. Berk, Mitogen activated protein kinase (ERK1/2) activation by shear stress and adhesion in endothelial cells. Essential role for a hervimycine-sensitive kinase, J. Clin. Invest. 98 (1996) 2623–2631.

International Congress Series 1262 (2004) 137–140

www.ics-elsevier.com

Role of TRP channels in endothelial pathophysiology—evidence for vascular TRPs as a potential target for drug therapy

Annarita Graziani[a], Michael Poteser[b], Christian Rosker[a], Klaus Groschner[a,*]

[a] *Department of Pharmacology and Toxicology, Karl-Franzens-University, Graz, Austria*
[b] *Department of Hygiene and Preventive Medicine, Yamagata University, Japan*

Abstract. Proteins related to the *Drosophila* transient receptor potential (TRP) gene product are key players in Ca^{2+} homeostasis of mammalian cells. TRP proteins form cation channels, which function as sensors for a variety of stimuli including oxidative stress. The canonical TRP proteins TRPC3 and TRPC4 are likely to play a role in endothelial physiology and pathophysiology. Here, we report that overexpression of TRPC3 or TRPC4 generates a redox-sensitive cation conductance in human embryonic kidney cells (HEK293). Redox activation of these TRPC species appears to be due to oxidant-induced promotion of phospholipase C activity and/or sensitisation of TRPC proteins to regulation by phospholipase C. Our results suggest TRPC species as attractive, novel targets for cardiovascular therapy.

Keywords: Endothelial cells; Oxidative stress; Nonselective cation channels; Transient receptor potential

1. Introduction

The function of vascular endothelium is governed by the activity of nonselective cation channels, which are involved in the endothelial response to a variety of stimuli including blood flow-dependent sheer stress, neurotransmitters and oxidative stress [1]. Redox signals are known to determine cellular functions and serve as a switch between apoptotic cell death, differentiation or proliferation [2,3], and excess generation of reactive oxygen species has been recognized as a key event in the pathogenesis of atherosclerosis [4,5]. We tested the hypothesis that canonical transient receptor potential (TRPC) species, which are able to form nonselective cation conductances [6] contribute to the redox sensitivity of the

Abbreviations: Ca_i, intracellular Ca^{2+} concentration; TRP, transient receptor potential; HEK293, human embryonic kidney cells; U73122, 1-[6-((17β-3-methoxyestra-1,3,5(10)-trien-17-yl)-amino)hexyl]-1*H*-pyrrole-2,5-dione.

* Corresponding author. Department of Pharmacology and Toxicology, University of Graz, Universitaetsplatz 2, A-8010, Graz, Austria. Tel.: +43-316-380-5570; fax: +43-316-380-9890.

E-mail address: klaus.groschner@uni-graz.at (K. Groschner).

0531-5131/
doi:10.1016/j.ics.2003.12.034

endothelium. Our initial work suggested TRPC proteins are indeed expressed in vascular endothelium and provided the first evidence that these proteins may serve as primary redox sensors in this tissue [7]. Our recent results suggest that TRPC3 and TRPC4 proteins contribute to the nonselective cation conductance, which depolarizes vascular endothelial cells in the presence of oxidants.

2. Experimental procedures

2.1. Cell culture and cell transfection

Human embryonic kidney cells (HEK293) stably expressing TRPC3 (T3–9) and TRPC4 (T4–60) were kindly provided by M.X. Zhu. Vascular endothelial cells were cultured from pig aorta as described [8].

2.2. Western blot

SDS-PAGE and Western blotting was performed as described [11].

2.3. Electrophysiology

Patch-clamp experiments were performed as described [7,9].

2.4. Materials

1-[6-((17β-3-Methoxyestra-1,3,5(10)-trien-17-yl)-amino)hexyl]-1*H*-pyrrole-2,5-dione (U73122) was purchased from Calbiochem, Germany. The TRPC3 and TRPC4 antibodies were purchased from Alomone Labs, Israel.

3. Results and discussion

3.1. TRPC3 and TRPC4 are coexpressed in pig aortic endothelium

Pig aortic endothelial cells (ECAP) display a prominent redox-sensitive membrane conductance [10], while HEK293 cells are resistant to even strong oxidative stress (unpublished data). As illustrated in Fig. 1, expression of the two candidate cation channel proteins TRPC3 and TRPC4 is evident in pig aortic endothelium, but not in HEK293 cells.

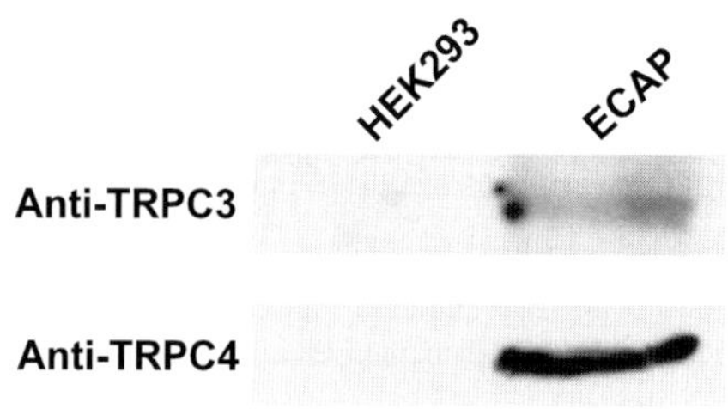

Fig. 1. Expression of TRPC3 and TRPC4 in ECAP cells. A total of 200 μg proteins from HEK and ECAP cell lysates was analyzed by Western blot with the TRPC antibodies shown.

These results prompted us to test whether overexpression of TRPC3 or TRPC4 is able to generate a redox-sensitive cation conductance in HEK293 cells, which resembles that of endothelial cells.

3.2. Overexpression of TRPC species generates a redox-sensitive cation conductance in HEK293 cells

A redox-sensitive cation conductance resembling that of pig aortic endothelium was generated by either overexpression of TRPC3 (T3–9; $N=6$) or TRPC4 (T4–60; $N=6$), while vector-transfected controls ($N=6$) were insensitive to the oxidant (data not shown). Thus, TRPC3 and TRPC4 confer a specific cellular redox-sensitivity, which results in membrane depolarization. Membrane depolarization reduces the driving force for Ca^{2+} entry and may suppress Ca^{2+}-dependent formation of vasoactive mediators. Nonetheless, Na^{+} loading, another consequence of activation of TRPC channels is likely to generate local Ca^{2+} gradients due to reversed mode Na^{+}/Ca^{2+} exchange, which has been demonstrated to promote the formation nitric oxide [11].

3.3. Mechanism of TRPC3 activation by peroxides

The phospholipase C inhibitor U73122 (40 μM) prevented activation of TRPC3-dependent redox-sensitive membrane conductances (data not shown). Phospholipase C, in particular redox-sensitive, TRPC-associated phospholipase Cγ, may therefore be involved in oxidant-induced activation of TRPC channels. Since TRPC3 lacks tight functional coupling to mitochondria [12], this TRPC species may mediate oxidant-induce Ca^{2+} signalling events without promoting mitochondrial dysfunction and apoptosis. TRPC proteins appear to be targeted to signalplexes in caveolae [13]. Thus, it is tempting to speculate that disintegration of caveolae [14] might be involved in redox activation of TRPC species. Indeed, we observed that t-BHP (400 μM; 1 h) distorted cellular localization of caveolin-1 but not that of TRPC3. Recent reports suggest modulation of

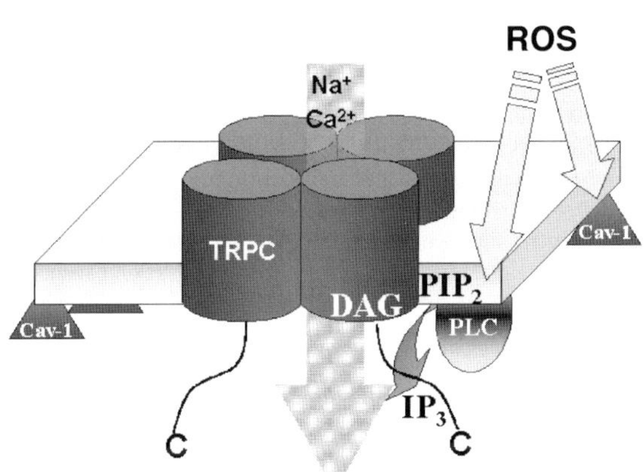

Fig. 2. Reactive oxygen species may activate TRPC channels due to stimulation of phospholipase C activity and alterations in the structure of cholesterol and caveolin-1 (Cav-1)-rich membrane microdomains.

phospholipase Cγ signalling in response to disruption of lipid raft structures [15]. Oxidative disruption of the integrity of cholesterol-rich microdomains is likely to result in alterated phopsholipase C-dependent TRPC signalling (Fig. 2).

3.4. TRPCs represent a novel target for drug therapy

We propose oxidative stress-induced stimulation of phospholipase C activity and oxidant-induced disintegration of cholesterol-rich membrane microdomains as a key signal for activation of endothelial TRPC channels. Endothelial TRPC channels appear as a key signalling component in endothelial pathophysiology and therefore as a potential target for novel cardiovascular drug therapies.

Acknowledgements

This study is supported by the Austrian Research Foundation (FWF), SFB-Biomembranes F715 and FWF-14950.

References

[1] B. Nilius, G. Droogmans, Ion channels and their functional role in vascular endothelium, Physiol. Rev. 81 (2001) 1415.

[2] T. Finkel, N.J. Holbrook, Oxidants, oxidative stress and the biology of ageing, Nature 408 (2000) 239.

[3] J.L. Martindale, N.J. Holbrook, Cellular response to oxidative stress: signaling for suicide and survival, J. Cell. Physiol. 192 (2002) 1.

[4] A. Harris, S. Devaraj, I. Jialal, Oxidative stress, alpha-tocopherol therapy, and atherosclerosis, Curr. Atheroscler. Rep. 4 (2002) 373.

[5] R.W. Alexander, The Jeremiah Metzger Lecture. Pathogenesis of atherosclerosis: redox as a unifying mechanism, Trans. Am. Clin. Climatol. Assoc. 114 (2003) 273.

[6] R. Vennekens, T. Voets, R.J. Bindels, G. Droogmans, B. Nilius, Current understanding of mammalian TRP homologues, Cell Calcium 31 (2002) 253.

[7] M. Balzer, B. Lintschinger, K. Groschner, Evidence for a role of TRP proteins in the oxidative stress-induced membrane conductances of porcine aortic endothelial cells, Cardiovasc. Res. 42 (1999) 543.

[8] B.C. Berk, Redox signals that regulate the vascular response to injury, Thromb. Haemost. 82 (1999) 810.

[9] K. Groschner, S. Hingel, B. Lintschinger, M. Balzer, C. Romanin, X. Zhu, W. Schreibmayer, TRP proteins form store-operated cation channels in human vascular endothelial cells, FEBS Lett. 437 (1998) 101.

[10] S.K. Koliwad, D.L. Kunze, S.J. Elliott, Oxidant stress activates a non-selective cation channel responsible for membrane depolarization in calf vascular endothelial cells, J. Physiol. 491 (Pt. 1) (1996) 1.

[11] M. Teubl, K. Groschner, S.D. Kohlwein, B. Mayer, K. Schmidt, Na(+)/Ca(2+) exchange facilitates Ca(2+)-dependent activation of endothelial nitric-oxide synthase, J. Biol. Chem. 274 (1999) 29529.

[12] B. Thyagarajan, M. Poteser, C. Romanin, H. Kahr, M.X. Zhu, K. Groschner, Expression of TRP3 determines sensitivity of capacitative Ca2+ entry to nitric oxide and mitochondrial Ca2+ handling: evidence for a role of TRP3 as a subunit of capacitative Ca2+ entry channels, J. Biol. Chem. 276 (2001) 48149.

[13] T. Lockwich, B.B. Singh, X. Liu, I.S. Ambudkar, Stabilization of cortical actin induces internalization of transient receptor potential 3 (TRP3)-associated caveolar Ca2+ signaling complex and loss of Ca2+ influx without disruption of TRP3-inositol trisphosphate receptor association, J. Biol. Chem. 276 (2001) 42401.

[14] E.J. Smart, Y.S. Ying, P.A. Conrad, R.G. Anderson, Caveolin moves from caveolae to the Golgi apparatus in response to cholesterol oxidation, J. Cell Biol. 127 (1994) 1185.

[15] I.H. Jang, J.H. Kim, B.D. Lee, S.S. Bae, M.H. Park, P.G. Suh, S.H. Ryu, Localization of phospholipase C-gamma1 signaling in caveolae: importance in EGF-induced phosphoinositide hydrolysis but not in tyrosine phosphorylation, FEBS Lett. 491 (2001) 4.

Featured symposium

International Congress Series 1262 (2004) 143–146
www.ics-elsevier.com

PPARγ signalling and vascular cells in 2003

Dennis Bruemmer, Florian Blaschke, Joey Liu, Ronald E. Law*

Division of Endocrinology, Diabetes and Hypertension, David Geffen School of Medicine, University of California, Los Angeles, CA-90095, USA

Abstract. Peroxisome proliferator-activated receptor γ (PPARγ) is a transcription factor belonging to the nuclear hormone receptor superfamily. PPARγ binds the insulin-sensitizing thiazolidinediones (TZDs) and is prominently upregulated in intimal vascular smooth muscle cells (VSMC) after mechanical injury to the vessel wall. Several TZD PPARγ ligands have been shown to inhibit neointima formation. Suppression of intimal hyperplasia by PPARγ ligands likely results from their activity to inhibit VSMC growth and to promote apoptosis. This review summarizes molecular pathways through which PPARγ regulates the expression and function of multiple cell cycle and apoptosis genes resulting in decreased VSMC proliferation and inhibition of neointima formation.

Keywords: PPARγ; Thiazolidinedione; Vascular smooth muscle; Proliferation; Minichromosome maintenance protein; GADD45

Peroxisome proliferator-activated receptor γ (PPARγ) ligands inhibit growth of vascular cells by interfering with the expression and function of multiple cell cycle regulators [1,2]. In vascular smooth muscle cells (VSMC), we have previously reported that the thiazolidinedione (TZD) PPARγ ligands inhibit exit from G1 into S phase of the cell cycle by attenuating phosphorylation of the retinoblastoma protein [2]. Decreased Rb phosphorylation likely resulted from their effect to elevate levels of the cyclin-dependent kinase inhibitor (CDKI) $p27^{kip1}$ and reduce the activity of cyclin D- and cyclin E-dependent kinases (CDK) [2]. Using DNA microarray analysis, we identified minichromosome maintenance proteins (MCM) 6 and 7 as additional targets mediating the antiproliferative effects of PPARγ ligands [3]. MCM proteins play a central role in the regulation of the initiation of DNA replication [4]. Entry into S phase requires increased phosphorylation of the retinoblastoma protein (Rb), which releases sequestered E2F to permit transcription of genes encoding the replicative machinery for DNA synthesis,

* Corresponding author. UCLA School, Division of Endocrinology, Diabetes and Hypertension, Warren Hall, Suite 24-130, 900 Veteran Avenue, Los Angeles, CA 90095, USA. Tel.: +1-310-794-7555; fax: +1-310-794-7654.
E-mail address: rlaw@mednet.ucla.edu (R.E. Law).

0531-5131/ © 2003 Published by Elsevier B.V.
doi:10.1016/j.ics.2003.11.033

including MCM proteins. The MCM6 and MCM7 promoters contain functional E2F binding sites, suggesting that E2F is responsible for the coordinate expression of MCMs during progression through the cell cycle. Consistent with a central role for E2F in regulating MCM expression, we have found that PPARγ ligands inhibited E2F-dependent MCM transactivation [3].

The precise details of how PPARγ ligands block G1 → S progression and inhibit DNA synthesis are not fully elucidated. Recent findings in PPARγ null stem cells have suggested that PPARγ ligands may have receptor-independent antiproliferative activities [5]. A PPARγ antagonist and overexpression of dominant-negative PPARγ were effective in blocking ligand-mediated repression of MCM7 transcription. Additional evidence that MCMs are targets for PPARγ derives from experiments using an adenovirus to overexpress a constitutively active form of PPARγ in VSMC. Overexpression of constitutively active PPARγ inhibited mitogen-induced MCM7 expression similar to effects observed with the PPARγ ligands. These observations support the conclusion that the inhibitory effects of PPARγ ligands on MCM expression are mediated through a PPARγ-dependent mechanism.

Although many studies have focused on alterations in the regulation of cell growth as a fundamental feature during neointimal hyperplasia after balloon injury, it is becoming increasingly evident that apoptosis may be equally important [6]. Recent studies have shown that TZDs not only inhibit cell growth, but also induce VSMC apoptosis [7]. The molecular pathways by which TZDs induce VSMC apoptosis remain unclear. Again, DNA microarray analysis identified the growth arrest and DNA damage-inducible (GADD) gene GADD45 to be prominently upregulated by PPARγ ligands [8]. Increased GADD45 gene expression has been implicated in growth suppression [9] and apoptosis [10]. GADD45, therefore, may represent a unique target for drugs that induce cell cycle arrest, apoptosis and differentiation such as PPARγ ligands.

Treatment of VSMC with PPARγ ligands and the constitutively active PPARγ induced apoptosis and increased GADD45 mRNA expression. These findings provide evidence that the induction of GADD45 PPARγ ligands is mediated through a PPARγ-dependent mechanism. PPARγ ligands induced GADD45 transcription and 5′-deletions of the promoter revealed that a region harbouring an Oct-1 sequence is essential for the induction of GADD45 transcription by PPARγ. Oct-1 is known to be crucial for regulating GADD45 expression [11–13] and Oct-1 protein levels and DNA binding were induced after stimulation with PPARγ ligands. These findings suggest that activation of PPARγ can lead to apoptosis and growth arrest in VSMC, at least in part, by inducing Oct-1 mediated transcription of GADD45.

PPARγ ligands inhibit intimal hyperplasia in rat models of restenosis after balloon injury in both insulin-resistant and insulin-sensitive animals [1,14–17]. Concomitant with the phenotypic shift from quiescent VSMC resident in the uninjured vessel wall to proliferating VSMC present in the neointima, there is a substantial upregulation of PPARγ expression [7,18]. Increased PPARγ expression in intimal VSMC, therefore, provides an attractive therapeutic target to exploit the antiproliferative and proapoptotic properties of PPARγ ligands. Inhibition of MCM expression and upregulation of GADD45 levels by PPARγ may play a prominent role in limiting neointimal hyperplasia after mechanical injury to the arterial wall. Early clinical trials with troglitazone and pioglitazone have demonstrated an almost 50% reduction in neointimal tissue formation after coronary stent-implantation to treat diabetes-associated macrovascular disease [19,20]. Further identification of novel PPARγ ligands based on their direct vascular activity, as opposed to their portfolio of metabolic effects on glucose and lipids, may yield compounds with even greater efficacy against proliferative vascular diseases.

References

[1] R.E Law, W.P. Meehan, X.P. Xi, K. Graf, D.A. Wuthrich, W. Coats, D. Faxon, W.A. Hsueh, Troglitazone inhibits vascular smooth muscle cell growth and intimal hyperplasia, J. Clin. Invest. 98 (8) (1996) 1897–1905.

[2] S. Wakino, U. Kintscher, S. Kim, F. Yin, W.A. Hsueh, R.E. Law, Peroxisome proliferator-activated receptor gamma ligands inhibit retinoblastoma phosphorylation and G1 → S transition in vascular smooth muscle cells, J. Biol. Chem. 275 (29) (2000) 22435–22441.

[3] D. Bruemmer, F. Yin, J. Liu, J.P. Berger, T. Kiyono, J. Chen, E. Fleck, A.J. Van Herle, B.M. Forman, R.E. Law, Peroxisome proliferator-activated receptor {gamma} inhibits expression of minichromosome maintenance proteins in vascular smooth muscle cells, Mol. Endocrinol. 17 (6) (2003) 1005–1018.

[4] B.K. Tye, MCM proteins in DNA replication, Ann. Rev. Biochem. 68 (1999) 649–686.

[5] S.S Palakurthi, H. Aktas, L.M. Grubissich, R.M. Mortensen, J.A. Halperin, Anticancer effects of thiazolidinediones are independent of peroxisome proliferator-activated receptor gamma and mediated by inhibition of translation initiation, Cancer Res. 61 (16) (2001) 6213–6218.

[6] Y.J. Geng, P. Libby, Progression of atheroma: a struggle between death and procreation, Arterioscler. Thromb. Vasc. Biol. 22 (9) (2002) 1370–1380.

[7] D. Bishop-Bailey, T. Hla, T.D. Warner, Intimal smooth muscle cells as a target for peroxisome proliferator-activated receptor-gamma ligand therapy, Circ. Res. 91 (3) (2002) 210–217.

[8] D. Bruemmer, F. Yin, J. Liu, J.P. Berger, T. Sakai, F. Blaschke, E. Fleck, A.J. Van Herle, B.M. Forman, R.E. Law, Regulation of the growth arrest and DNA damage-inducible gene 45 (GADD45) by peroxisome proliferator-activated receptor gamma in vascular smooth muscle cells, Circ. Res. 93 (4) (2003) e38–e47.

[9] Q. Zhan, K.A. Lord, I. Alamo Jr., M.C. Hollander, F. Carrier, D. Ron, K.W. Kohn, B. Hoffman, D.A. Liebermann, A.J. Fornace Jr., The gadd and MyD genes define a novel set of mammalian genes encoding acidic proteins that synergistically suppress cell growth, Mol. Cell. Biol. 14 (4) (1994) 2361–2371.

[10] M.S. Sheikh, M.C. Hollander, A.J. Fornance Jr., Role of Gadd45 in apoptosis, Biochem. Pharmacol. 59 (1) (2000) 43–45.

[11] S. Takahashi, S. Saito, N. Ohtani, T. Sakai, Involvement of the Oct-1 regulatory element of the gadd45 promoter in the p53-independent response to ultraviolet irradiation, Cancer Res. 61 (3) (2001) 1187–1195.

[12] W. Fan, S. Jin, T. Tong, H. Zhao, F. Fan, M.J. Antinore, B. Rajasekaran, M. Wu, Q. Zhan, BRCA1 regulates GADD45 through its interactions with the OCT-1 and CAAT motifs, J. Biol. Chem. 277 (10) (2002) 8061–8067.

[13] S. Jin, F. Fan, W. Fan, H. Zhao, T. Tong, P. Blanck, I. Alomo, B. Rajasekaran, Q. Zhan, Transcription factors Oct-1 and NF-YA regulate the p53-independent induction of the GADD45 following DNA damage, Oncogene 20 (21) (2001) 2683–2690.

[14] M. Igarashi, Y. Takeda, N. Ishibashi, K. Takahashi, S. Mori, M. Tominaga, Y. Saito, Pioglitazone reduces smooth muscle cell density of rat carotid arterial intima induced by balloon catheterization, Horm. Metab. Res. 29 (9) (1997) 444–449.

[15] E. Shinohara, S. Kihara, N. Ouchi, T. Funahashi, T. Nakamura, S. Yamashita, K. Kameda-Takemura, Y. Matsuzawa, Troglitazone suppresses intimal formation following balloon injury in insulin-resistant Zucker fatty rats, Atherosclerosis 136 (2) (1998) 275–279.

[16] T. Yoshimoto, M. Naruse, H. Shizume, K. Naruse, A. Tanabe, M. Tanaka, K. Tago, K. Irie, T. Muraki, H. Demura, L. Zardi, Vasculo-protective effects of insulin sensitizing agent pioglitazone in neointimal thickening and hypertensive vascular hypertrophy, Atherosclerosis 145 (2) (1999) 333–340.

[17] Y. Aizawa, J. Kawabe, N. Hasebe, N. Takehara, K. Kikuchi, Pioglitazone enhances cytokine-induced

apoptosis in vascular smooth muscle cells and reduces intimal hyperplasia, Circulation 104 (4) (2001) 455–460.

[18] R.E. Law, S. Goetze, X.P. Xi, S. Jackson, Y. Kawano, L. Demer, M.C. Fishbein, W.P. Meehan, W.A. Hsueh, Expression and function of PPARgamma in rat and human vascular smooth muscle cells, Circulation 101 (11) (2000) 1311–1318.

[19] T. Takagi, A. Yamamuro, K. Tamita, K. Yamabe, M. Katayama, S. Mizoguchi, M. Ibuki, T. Tani, K. Tanabe, K. Nagai, K. Shiratori, S. Morioka, J. Yoshikawa, Pioglitazone reduces neointimal tissue proliferation after coronary stent implantation in patients with type 2 diabetes mellitus: an intravascular ultrasound scanning study, Am. Heart J. 146 (2) (2003) E5.

[20] T. Takagi, T. Akasaka, A. Yamamuro, Y. Honda, T. Hozumi, S. Morioka, K. Yoshida, Troglitazone reduces neointimal tissue proliferation after coronary stent implantation in patients with non-insulin dependent diabetes mellitus: a serial intravascular ultrasound study, J. Am. Coll. Cardiol. 36 (5) (2000) 1529–1535.

International Congress Series 1262 (2004) 147–151

www.ics-elsevier.com

Exogenous and endogenous mechanisms of PPAR activation: implications for inflammation and atherosclerosis

Ouliana Ziouzenkova, Jorge Plutzky*

Cardiovascular Division, New Research Building, Brigham and Women's Hospital, 7th Floor, 77 Avenue Louis Pasteur, Boston, MA 02115, USA

Abstract. Peroxisome proliferator-activated receptors (PPARs) are critical transcriptional regulators of key metabolic pathways. Indeed, synthetic PPAR agonists in clinical use improve lipids, like PPAR-α activated fibrates, and decrease insulin resistance, like PPAR-γ activating thiazolidinediones. More recent work implicates PPAR activation in limiting inflammation and atherosclerosis. This body of data suggests that endogenous PPAR ligands may exert effects similar to those seen with synthetic PPAR agonists, improving metabolism, limiting inflammation, and decreasing atherosclerotic responses. Prior evidence regarding endogenous PPAR ligands is considered. More recent studies from our group establishing lipoprotein lipase as an endogenous mechanism for selective PPAR ligand generation are reviewed. © 2004 Published by Elsevier B.V.

Keywords: Peroxisome proliferator-activated receptors; Lipoprotein lipase; TGs; Adhesion molecules; Atherosclerosis; FAs; Endothelium

Peroxisome proliferator-activated receptors (PPARs), like other nuclear receptors, are transcription factors activated by binding to their cognate ligands [1]. PPAR isoforms include PPAR alpha (PPARα), PPAR gamma (PPARγ), and PPAR beta/delta (PPARβ/δ) [2]. Over the past decade, many laboratories established important roles for each PPAR isoform in metabolism [3]. PPARγ is a critical mediator of adipogenesis, lipid metabolism, and glucose control [4]. Chemical screening led to the serendipitous discovery that thiazolidinediones, insulin sensitizers in current clinical use, exert their effects by PPARγ binding [5]. PPARα is an important regulator of fatty acid (FA) metabolism, especially FA beta-oxidation [6]. Fibrates, in clinical use to lower triglyclerides and raise HDL, act at least in part by PPARα binding [7]. PPARδ agonists have yet to reach clinical use [8]. More recently, PPARs have been implicated in inflammation, vascular biology, and atherosclerosis, with evidence suggesting PPAR activation by synthetic agonists may limit inflammation and atherosclerosis [9,10]. These established and emerging PPAR data

* Corresponding author. Tel.: +1-617-525-4360; fax: +1-617-525-4366.
E-mail address: jplutzky@rics.bwh.harvard.edu (J. Plutzky).

0531-5131/ © 2004 Published by Elsevier B.V.
doi:10.1016/j.ics.2004.02.016

suggest a fundamental issue: if synthetic PPAR agonists exert the benefits noted by binding to these nuclear receptors, what endogenous PPAR ligands exist that might replicate the effects of these manufactured drugs? The responses to synthetic PPAR agonists—improved dyslipidemia, lower glucose, less inflammation, and decreased atherosclerosis—suggest that natural PPAR ligands, and the pathways for their generation, might protect against such problems. Despite this potential importance, the nature and generation of endogenous PPAR ligands, especially under physiologic conditions, remain poorly understood.

1. Endogenous PPAR gamma and alpha ligands?

Naturally occurring ligands have been proposed for PPARγ, although this issue remains unresolved. Both 9 and 13 hydroxydecanoic acid (HODE), forms of oxidized linoleic acid, were reported to activate PPARγ [11]. The presence of HODEs in vivo remains unclear, although the enzyme 12/15 lipoxygenase can generate PPARγ-activating HODEs [12]. HODEs also activate PPARα as discussed below [13,14]. The prostaglandin metabolite 15-deoxy-D12, 14-prostaglandin J_2 [15,16] (15d-PGJ_2) may be a PPARγ agonist, but it also acts on IκB kinase [17]. More recent data suggest that 15d-PGJ2 is unlikely to account for significant PPARγ activation in vivo [18]. Like all PPARs, PPARγ can be activated by certain Fas [19–21]. As discussed further, these landmark studies helped define a role for PPARs in lipid metabolism although with some limitations. Both oxidized phospholipids and lysophosphatidiic acid appear to activate PPARγ [22,23]. The association between dominant negative PPARγ mutations and severe insulin resistance supports the importance of endogenous PPARγ ligands [24,25].

In terms of endogenous PPARα ligands, HODEs can also activate PPARα, perhaps even more potently than they do PPARγ [13,14]. As noted, certain long chain FAs are PPARα ligands, at least in vitro. We found that eicospentanoic acid (EPA), an omega 3 FA, could limit endothelial adhesion molecule expression in vitro and monocyte adhesion in vivo in a PPARα-dependent manner [26]. These effects recapitulated reported responses to synthetic PPARα agonists [27,28]. Interestingly, the EPA effects were more pronounced with a mildly oxidized form [26]. These observations suggest that certain diets, like those enriched in fish, may exert their cardiovascular benefits [29] through PPAR ligand generation. Others also find increased PPAR activation with oxidized Fas [13,14,22]. 8(*S*)-Hydroxy-5Z,9E,11Z,14Z-eicosotetraenoic acid [8(*S*)-HETE] have also been reported as an endogenous PPARγ ligand [30,31]. Leukotriene B4 is another endogenous compound reported to activate PPARα; this response may help terminate inflammation [32].

2. New insight into endogenous PPAR ligands

Most prior work into endogenous PPAR ligands considered settings involving inflammation or oxidative stress as opposed to more physiologic conditions. FAs activate PPARα when added to standard assays, although the concentration of FAs required in these in vitro studies was relatively high. Moreover, these studies found FA activation of all three PPAR isoforms. Most existing data would argue for PPAR-isoform specific effects. Equally important, the connection between actual lipoprotein metabolism and subsequent PPAR activation remained undefined. To consider these issues, we took an alternate approach, focusing on pathways that might be involved in endogenous physiologic PPAR activation rather than on specific candidate molecules. We reasoned that more direct, specific links must exist between physiologic pathways of lipid metabolism and activation of PPARs, hypothesizing that lipolysis of TG-rich lipoproteins, especially through lipoprotein lipase (LPL), is a potential mechanism for this.

3. LPL as a pathway to PPAR activation

The hydrolysis of triglyceride (TG)-rich lipoproteins by specific TG lipases releases Fas [33,34]. Beta-oxidation of these FAs is a major energy resource, either to generate ATP or stored in adipose. The TG lipase family, including lipoprotein lipase (LPL), hepatic lipase, and endothelial cell (EC) lipase, figures prominently in lipoprotein metabolism, especially that involving TG and HDL [34]. LPL plays a key role metabolizing TG-rich lipoproteins into FA. LPL, synthesized in adipocytes, myocytes, and macrophages, is transported to the surface of microcapillary ECs where it binds to surface heparan sulfate proteoglycans [35]. There, LPL encounters circulating VLDL and chylomicrons, releasing FAs and monoacylglycerol, leaving behind remanant particles. LPL can also increase lipid uptake nonenzymatically by bridging lipoproteins to lipoprotein receptors.

Multiple lines of evidence now establish LPL as a means of generating PPAR ligands [36,37]. Although treating bovine ECs transfected with PPARα ligand binding domain (LBD) assays with isolated human VLDL, HDL, or LDL induces no response, a different picture emerges after lipoprotein exposure to LPL (Fig. 1) [36]. LPL-treated VLDL robustly activates PPARα, with responses roughly proportional to lipoprotein TG content: VLDLLDL>HDL. Interestingly, these LPL responses depended on intact enzymatic activity and revealed preferential isoform activation: PPARαPPARδ>PPARγ [36]. Direct radioligand assays support these findings and establish LPL generation of PPAR "ligands"

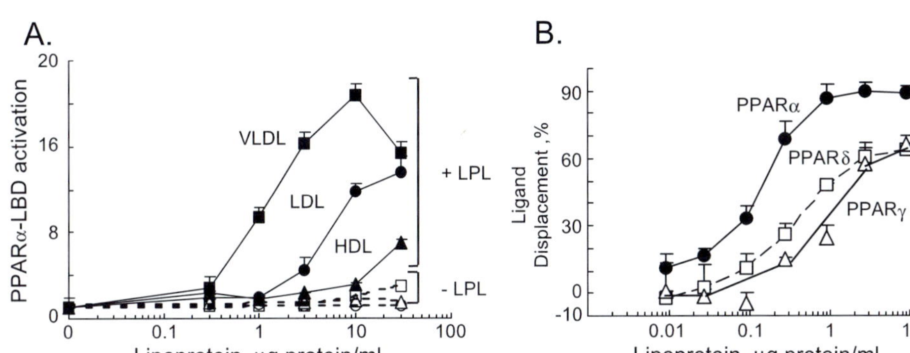

Fig. 1. LPL as a mechanism for PPARα ligand generation. (A) LPL treatment of various lipoproteins activates PPAR LBDs in an isoform-specific manner. Concentration-dependent activation of PPARα-LBD by various lipoproteins in the presence or absence of LPL (30 U/ml) are shown. EC co-transfected with a PPARα-LBD, the luciferase response pUASx4-TK-luc, and β-galactosidase constructs were stimulated as described [33]; relative PPARα-LBD activation by fenofibric acid (100 μM) was 16.2±1.3-fold [33]. (B) LPL-treated VLDL generates PPARα ligands. Cell-free radioligand displacement assays were performed using high specificity PPAR ligands as described [33].

not just "activators" [36]. These findings suggest that lipolysis may lead to distal PPAR responses, including its anti-inflammatory effects. In fact, LPL-treated VLDL inhibited induced VCAM1 expression [36]. The specificity of different lipases may also determine the distal responses seen. Indeed, although treatment of VLDL with either LPL or the pro-inflammatory Group IV secretory phospholipase A2 (sPLA2) releases similar amounts of total FAs, the PPARα activation seen differs markedly, with no apparent sPLA2 effect [36]. In addition to revealing a potential physiologic mechanism for PPAR activation, these observations also suggest that specific pathways of lipoprotein uptake, for example, catalysis versus bridging, may direct distinct transcriptional responses. In fact, we found evidence for this concept by examining LPL-treated LDL activation of PPARα. To study this, we utilized electronegative LDL as a model circulating pro-inflammatory lipoprotein that is also an LPL substrate [38]. Interestingly, the marked augmentation of TNFα-induced VCAM1 expression by electronegative LDL was completely reversed by LPL treatment [14]. Mass spectrometry indicates that LPL-treated electronegative LDL releases HODEs, a known PPARα and -γ ligand [14]. Although electronegative LDL stimulation of ECs overexpressing the LDL receptor increased VCAM1 expression, LDL receptor over-expression had no effect on PPARα responses. This serves as an example of how different mechanisms of lipoprotein uptake can direct different transcriptional responses.

4. Conclusion

No doubt insight into the nature of endogenous PPAR ligands and their generation will continue to evolve, with considerable implications. Natural PPAR ligands may suggest alternative designs for synthetic PPAR therapeutic agonists. Perhaps disease states such as insulin resistance/diabetes or dyslipidemia exist in part due to defects in endogenous ligand generation. Establishing the nature of endogenous PPAR ligands will consider these possibilities while also shedding light on the role of PPARs in cellular function.

References

[1] D. Mangelsdorf, et al., The nuclear receptor superfamily: the second decade, Cell 83 (1995) 835–839.

[2] T.M. Willson, et al., The PPARs: from orphan receptors to drug discovery, J. Med. Chem. 43 (2000) 527–550.

[3] C.H. Lee, et al., Minireview: lipid metabolism, metabolic diseases, and peroxisome proliferator-activated receptors, Endocrinology 144 (2003) 2201–2207.

[4] E.D. Rosen, et al., PPARgamma: a nuclear regulator of metabolism, differentiation, and cell growth, J. Biol. Chem. 276 (2001) 37731–37734.

[5] R.R. Henry, Thiazolidinediones, Endocrinol. Metab. Clin. N. Am. 26 (1997) 553–573.

[6] O. Barbier, et al., Pleiotropic actions of peroxisome proliferator-activated receptors in lipid metabolism and atherosclerosis, Arterioscler. Thromb. Vasc. Biol. 22 (2002) 717–726.

[7] J.C. Fruchart, et al., The role of fibric acids in atherosclerosis, Curr. Atheroscler. Rep. 3 (2001) 83–92.

[8] L. Michalik, et al., Peroxisome proliferator-activated receptors beta/delta: emerging roles for a previously neglected third family member, Curr. Opin. Lipidol. 14 (2003) 129–135.

[9] C.K. Glass, et al., Atherosclerosis. The road ahead, Cell 104 (2001) 503–516.

[10] J. Plutzky, Medicine. PPARs as therapeutic targets: reverse cardiology? Science 302 (2003) 406–407.

[11] L. Nagy, et al., Oxidized LDL regulates macrophage gene expression through ligand activation of PPAR-gamma, Cell 93 (1998) 229–240.

[12] J.T. Huang, et al., Interleukin-4-dependent production of PPAR-gamma ligands in macrophages by 12/15-lipoxygenase, Nature 400 (1999) 378–382.

[13] P. Delerive, et al., Oxidized phospholipids activate PPARalpha in a phospholipase A2-dependent manner, FEBS Lett. 471 (2000) 34–38.
[14] O. Ziouzenkova, et al., Transcriptional PPAR responses to electronegative LDL: dual roles for lipolysis and oxidation, J. Biol. Chem. (2003).
[15] S.A. Kliewer, et al., A prostaglandin J2 metabolite binds peroxisome proliferator-activated receptor gamma and promotes adipocyte differentiation, Cell 83 (1995) 813–819.
[16] B.M. Forman, et al., 15-Deoxy-delta 12, 14-prostaglandin J2 is a ligand for the adipocyte determination factor PPAR gamma, Cell 83 (1995) 803–812.
[17] A. Rossi, et al., Anti-inflammatory cyclopentenone prostaglandins are direct inhibitors of IkappaB kinase, Nature 403 (2000) 103–108.
[18] L.C. Bell-Parikh, et al., Biosynthesis of 15-deoxy-{Delta}12,14-PGJ2 and the ligation of PPAR{gamma}, J. Clin. Invest. 112 (2003) 945–955.
[19] H. Keller, et al., Fatty acids and retinoids control lipid metabolism through activation of peroxisome proliferator-activated receptor-retinoid X receptor heterodimers, Proc. Natl. Acad. Sci. U. S. A. 90 (1993) 2160–2164.
[20] S.A. Kliewer, et al., Fatty acids and eicosanoids regulate gene expression through direct interactions with peroxisome proliferator-activated receptors alpha and gamma, Proc. Natl. Acad. Sci. U. S. A. 94 (1997) 4318–4323.
[21] B.M. Forman, et al., Hypolipidemic drugs, polyunsaturated fatty acids, and eicosanoids are ligands for peroxisome proliferator-activated receptors alpha and delta, Proc. Natl. Acad. Sci. U. S. A. 94 (1997) 4312–4317.
[22] S.S. Davies, et al., Oxidized alkyl phospholipids are specific, high affinity peroxisome proliferator-activated receptor gamma ligands and agonists, J. Biol. Chem. 276 (2001) 16015–16023.
[23] T.M. McIntyre, et al., Identification of an intracellular receptor for lysophosphatidic acid (LPA): LPA is a transcellular PPARgamma agonist, Proc. Natl. Acad. Sci. U. S. A. 100 (2003) 131–136.
[24] M. Ristow, et al., Obesity associated with a mutation in a genetic regulator of adipocyte differentiation, N. Engl. J. Med. 339 (1998) 953–959.
[25] I. Barroso, et al., Dominant negative mutations in human PPARgamma associated with severe insulin resistance, diabetes mellitus and hypertension [see comments], Nature 402 (1999) 880–883.
[26] S. Sethi, et al., Oxidized omega-3 fatty acids in fish oil inhibit leukocyte–endothelial interactions through activation of PPAR alpha, Blood 100 (2002) 1340–1346.
[27] N. Marx, et al., PPARalpha activators inhibit cytokine-induced vascular cell adhesion molecule-1 expression in human endothelial cells, Circulation 99 (1999) 3125–3131.
[28] S.M. Jackson, et al., Peroxisome proliferator-activated receptor activators target human endothelial cells to inhibit leukocyte–endothelial cell interaction, Arterioscler. Thromb. Vasc. Biol. 19 (1999) 2094–2104.
[29] F.B. Hu, et al., Optimal diets for prevention of coronary heart disease, JAMA 288 (2002) 2569–2578.
[30] K. Yu, et al., Differential activation of peroxisome proliferator-activated receptors by eicosanoids, J. Biol. Chem. 270 (1995) 23975–23983.
[31] J. Wigren, et al., Differential recruitment of the coactivator proteins CREB-binding protein and steroid receptor coactivator-1 to peroxisome proliferator-activated receptor gamma/9-*cis*-retinoic acid receptor heterodimers by ligands present in oxidized low-density lipoprotein, J. Endocrinol. 177 (2003) 207–214.
[32] P.R. Devchand, et al., The PPARalpha-leukotriene B4 pathway to inflammation control [see comments], Nature 384 (1996) 39–43.
[33] W. Jin, et al., Lipases and HDL metabolism, Trends Endocrinol. Metab. 13 (2002) 174–178.
[34] H. Wong, et al., The lipase gene family, J. Lipid Res. 43 (2002) 993–999.
[35] I.J. Goldberg, et al., Lipoprotein lipase: physiology, biochemistry, and molecular biology, Front Biosci. 6 (2001) D388–D405.
[36] O. Ziouzenkova, et al., Lipolysis of triglyceride-rich lipoproteins generates PPAR ligands: evidence for an antiinflammatory role for lipoprotein lipase, Proc. Natl. Acad. Sci. U. S. A. (2003).
[37] A. Chawla, et al., PPARdelta is a very low-density lipoprotein sensor in macrophages, Proc. Natl. Acad. Sci. U. S. A. 100 (2003) 1268–1273.
[38] O. Ziouzenkova, et al., Factors affecting resistance of low density lipoproteins to oxidation, Lipids 31 (Suppl.) (1996) S71–S76.

International Congress Series 1262 (2004) 152–155

www.ics-elsevier.com

The role of protein kinase C activation in cardiovascular dysfunctions of diabetes and insulin resistance

Yutaka Yasuda, George L. King*

Joslin Diabetes Center, Vascular Cell Biology, One Joslin Place, Boston, MA 02215, USA

Abstract. A high rate of cardiovascular morbidity and mortality in diabetic patients is caused by metabolic abnormalities due to insulin deficiency or resistance, including hyperglycemia, hyperlipidemia, hyperinsulinemia, and insulin resistance. These metabolic abnormalities have been shown to activate protein kinase C (PKC), enhance the formation of advanced glycation end products, and increase oxidative stress, which are suggested to play a crucial role in the development of cell dysfunctions. Dysfunction of vascular endothelium changes the balance of expression and actions of vasoactive substances in the vascular wall. Imbalance of vasoactive substances toward vasocontraction decreases endothelium-dependent vasodilation and anti-atherogenic function, which promote vasospasm, thrombosis, and occlusion and lead to cardiovascular disease. Recently, the effects of activated PKC have been reported to inhibit insulin-induced production of nitric oxide in endothelial cells. Moreover, activation of PKC in the myocardium has been shown to reduce ventricular performance and promote myocyte hypertrophy and fibrosis, which may lead to cardiac disorder such as congestive heart failure. We have proposed that activation of PKC is a common downstream point of convergence for oxidants, glycation products, and other glycotoxins or lipotoxins to initiate cardiovascular disease in diabetes. © 2004 Published by Elsevier B.V.

Keywords: Protein kinase C; Cardiovascular dysfunction; Diabetes; Insulin resistance

1. Introduction

Diabetic patients are two to three times more likely to have atherosclerotic disease than persons without diabetes [1]. Coronary atherosclerosis in the diabetic state occurs earlier in life and is, especially in women, more severe and diffuse than that in the general population. The Framingham Study also showed that the risk of developing congestive heart failure was increased in patients with diabetes and the relative impact of diabetes on congestive heart failure was even greater than that for coronary heart disease [1]. Although cardiovascular mortality of the overall population has decreased due to advances in risk control and treatments over the past 50 years in the US, diabetes is a rising cause of cardiovascular disease because of its increasing prevalence. In addition, there has not been a reduction in cardiovascular mortality among diabetic patients.

* Corresponding author. Tel.: +1-617-732-2622; fax: +1-617-732-2637.
E-mail address: george.king@joslin.harvard.edu (G.L. King).

0531-5131/ © 2004 Published by Elsevier B.V.
doi:10.1016/j.ics.2003.12.012

2. Activation of PKC in diabetes

Although the mechanisms that are causing diabetic complications are not clear, several theories have been proposed, which include diacylglycerol (DAG)–protein kinase C (PKC) pathway, advanced glycation products (AGE), oxidative-redox stress, the hexosamine pathway and the aldose reductase (AR) pathway. In diabetes, increased glycolytic intermediates, palmitic acid and oleic acid, have been shown to be incorporated into DAG through a de novo pathway and to activate PKC. In addition to this pathway, reactive oxygen spices (ROS) has been shown to activate aldose reductase, induce diacylglycerol, activate PKC, and induce advanced glycation end product formation [2]. AGE can stimulate collagen mRNA expression and the transcriptional upregulation of TGF-β1 in mesangial cells by activating PKC [3]. PKC can be activated by many multiple pathways, inducing extensive cross talks among the many metabolic pathways in the cell. Activation of PKC in diabetes has been postulated to cause multiple cardiovascular dysfunctions, including vascular permeability, cell migration and growth, extracellular matrix production, and expression of several cytokines. Among 12 isoforms of PKC, hyperglycemia and diabetes are reported to activate, preferentially, β2 and δ in the heart and aorta, β2, ε, α, and β1 isoforms in the retina, and β1 and α in the renal glomerulus of diabetic animals [4]. Our laboratory and others have reported that PKC β isoform selective inhibitor, LY333531, could ameliorate abnormal retinal, renal, and neural hemodynamics, decrease albuminuria and extracellular matrix production in diabetic animals [5].

3. Insulin resistance

Insulin resistance is a very important metabolic abnormality in type 2 diabetes and occurs before the onset of overt diabetes, and compensatory hyperinsulinemia exists during glucose intolerance. Insulin-dependent glucose metabolism is regulated by the PI3K–Akt pathway and down-regulation of this pathway has been demonstrated in the skeletal muscle of humans with insulin resistance and type 2 diabetes and in the vasculature of insulin-resistant animal models [6]. In contrast, the MAP kinase pathway has been reported to remain intact in this insulin-resistant animal model [6]. This selective loss of insulin's effects in the PI3K–Akt pathways is postulated to enhance the atherosclerotic risk of diabetic and insulin-resistant patients.

4. Endothelial dysfunction

Endothelial cells secrete both vasoconstrictor and vasodilator to maintain homeostasis, including endothelin-1, thromboxane A2, NO, prostacyclin and endothelium-derived hyperpolarizing factor (EDHF). These vasoactive substances regulate vascular smooth muscle cell contraction, proliferation and migration, platelet aggregation, coagulation, and fibrinolysis. Endothelial cells also regulate the expression of leukocyte adhesion molecules and leukocyte infiltration. Thus, dysfunction of endothelial cells promotes vasospasm, thrombosis, and occlusion and leads to cardiovascular disorder. Endothelial dysfunction is characterized by reduced vasodilatation in response to exogenous acetylcholine, insulin, and reactive hyperemia, which have been demonstrated in both type 1 and type 2 diabetes. Most reports have shown that the vasodilatory response to exogenous nitric oxide donors was normal, as measured by NO's effect of keeping smooth muscle cells intact. Thus, bioavailability of NO is considered to decrease in the diabetic and insulin-resistant state.

5. Decreased NO bioavailability

Expression and activation of the eNOS gene are regulated through the pathway of the PI-3 kinase and Akt in endothelial cells. As the PI-3 kinase pathway is down regulated in insulin-resistant model animal as described above, this may explain the decreased NO production by the endothelium in insulin resistance. Moreover, results from vascular specific insulin receptor KO mice suggested that insulin was necessary to maintain the basal expression level of eNOS in aorta and heart [7]. Activation of PKC by PMA-inhibited, insulin-induced expression of eNOS mRNA and PKC β specific inhibitor increased mRNA expression of eNOS in endothelial cells [8]. Recently, PKC β inhibitor, LY333532, prevented hyperglycemia-induced endothelial dysfunction in patients. Since NO produced by eNOS in endothelial cells can inhibit leukocyte adhesion, platelet aggregation, smooth muscle cell proliferation, and production of plasminogen activator inhibitor-1 and tissue factor beyond its action of vasodilator, reduced bioavailability of NO leads to decreased anti-atherogenic and anti-thrombogenic actions.

6. Reactive oxygen species (ROS)

Superoxide production from NAD(P)H oxidase and mitochondria metabolism may be essential in the physiological response of vascular cells. ROS works as second messengers to activate multiple intracellular signaling pathways in response to angiotensin II, PDGF, TNF, and mechanical forces. Actions of ROS include regulating platelet aggregation, smooth muscle cell proliferation and migration, and modification of the extracellular matrix, and endothelial activation. Excessive superoxide production by NAD(P)H oxidase has been shown to cause vascular dysfunction in human blood vessels and is increased in the presence of many cardiovascular risk factors [9]. Reactive oxygen spices can also react with NO, inactivate and reduce its bioavailability and promote cellular damage. High glucose and fatty acids have been reported to stimulate ROS production through PKC-dependent activation of NAD(P)H oxidase in both vascular smooth muscle cells and endothelial cells [10].

7. Myocardium

An increased occurrence of congestive heart failure has been reported in patients with diabetes, and diabetic cardiomyopathy has been documented in animal models of diabetes and clinical studies. Diabetic cardiomyopathy has been characterized by myocardial hypertrophy and fibrosis, which can increase ventricular stiffness. Though etiology of this condition remains unclear, PKC activation can clearly cause cardiomyopathy. In failed human hearts, expression of PKC β and total activity of PKC were reported to increase [11]. Moreover, myocardium-specific, PKC β2-overexpressing mice showed myocyte hypertrophy, ventricular thickening, multifocal fibrosis, impaired ventricular performance, and increased expression of atrial natriuretic factor, transforming growth factor-β, collagen types IV and VI [12]. A specific inhibitor of PKC β, LY333531, prevented cardiac pathologies in the PKC β-overexpressing transgenic mice and many other vascular changes in diabetic animals [12]. These findings suggested that the activation of the PKCβ2 isoform could cause cardiac cellular and functional changes leading to cardiac hypertrophy and diabetic cardiomyopathy.

8. Conclusion

Diabetes and insulin resistance cause adverse functions and pathologies in the vascular endothelium and myocardium, which leads to the development of cardiovascular disease. Many metabolic pathways are activated by diabetes and insulin resistance in the cardiovascular tissues, but their interactions remain to be clarified. Activation of PKC in diabetes and insulin resistance is suggested to play a key role in cardiovascular dysfunction and diseases.

Acknowledgements

This study was supported by National Institutes of Health grant DK53105, DK59725, and EY 05110-18 (G.L.K), and American Diabetes Association Mentor-based fellowship (Y.Y.).

References

[1] W.B. Kannel, D.L. McGee, Diabetes and cardiovascular disease. The Framingham study, JAMA 241 (19) (1979) 2035–2038.

[2] T. Nishikawa, D. Edelstein, X.L. Du, S. Yamagishi, T. Matsumura, Y. Kaneda, M.A. Yorek, D. Beebe, P.J. Oates, H.P. Hammes, I. Giardino, M. Brownlee, Normalizing mitochondrial superoxide production blocks three pathways of hyperglycaemic damage, Nature 404 (6779) (2000) 787–790.

[3] Y.S. Kim, B.C. Kim, C.Y. Song, H.K. Hong, K.C. Moon, H.S. Lee, Advanced glycosylation end products stimulate collagen mRNA synthesis in mesangial cells mediated by protein kinase C and transforming growth factor-beta, J. Lab. Clin. Med. 138 (1) (2001) 59–68.

[4] D. Koya, G.L. King, Protein kinase C activation and the development of diabetic complications, Diabetes 47 (6) (1998) 859–866.

[5] H. Ishii, M.R. Jirousek, D. Koya, C. Takagi, P. Xia, A. Clermont, S.E. Bursell, T.S. Kern, L.M. Ballas, W.F. Heath, L.E. Stramm, E.P. Feener, G.L. King, Amelioration of vascular dysfunctions in diabetic rats by an oral PKC beta inhibitor, Science 272 (5262) (1996) 728–731.

[6] Z.Y. Jiang, Y.W. Lin, A. Clemont, E.P. Feener, K.D. Hein, M. Igarashi, T. Yamauchi, M.F. White, G.L. King, Characterization of selective resistance to insulin signaling in the vasculature of obese Zucker (fa/fa) rats, J. Clin. Invest. 104 (4) (1999) 447–457.

[7] D. Vicent, J. Ilany, T. Kondo, K. Naruse, S.J. Fisher, Y.Y. Kisanuki, S. Bursell, M. Yanagisawa, G.L. King, C.R. Kahn, The role of endothelial insulin signaling in the regulation of vascular tone and insulin resistance, J. Clin. Invest. 111 (9) (2003) 1373–1380.

[8] K. Kuboki, Z.Y. Jiang, N. Takahara, S.W. Ha, M. Igarashi, T. Yamauchi, E.P. Feener, T.P. Herbert, C.J. Rhodes, G.L. King, Regulation of endothelial constitutive nitric oxide synthase gene expression in endothelial cells and in vivo: a specific vascular action of insulin, Circulation 101 (6) (2000) 676–681.

[9] T.J. Guzik, N.E. West, E. Black, D. McDonald, C. Ratnatunga, R. Pillai, K.M. Channon, UltraRapid communications: vascular superoxide production by NAD(P)H oxidase association with endothelial dysfunction and clinical risk factors, Circ. Res. 86 (9) (2000) 1008.

[10] T. Inoguchi, P. Li, F. Umeda, H.Y. Yu, M. Kakimoto, M. Imamura, T. Aoki, T. Etoh, T. Hashimoto, M. Naruse, H. Sano, H. Utsumi, H. Nawata, High glucose level and free fatty acid stimulate reactive oxygen species production through protein kinase C-dependent activation of NAD(P)H oxidase in cultured vascular cells, Diabetes 49 (11) (2000) 1939–1945.

[11] N. Bowling, R.A. Walsh, G. Song, T. Estridge, G.E. Sandusky, R.L. Fouts, K. Mintze, T. Pickard, R. Roden, M.R. Bristow, H.N. Sabbah, J.L. Mizrahi, G. Gromo, G.L. King, C.J. Vlahos, Increased protein kinase C activity and expression of Ca2+-sensitive isoforms in the failing human heart, Circulation 99 (3) (1999) 384–391.

[12] H. Wakasaki, D. Koya, F.J. Schoen, M.R. Jirousek, D.K. Ways, B.D. Hoit, R.A. Walsh, G.L. King, Targeted overexpression of protein kinase C beta2 isoform in myocardium causes cardiomyopathy, Proc. Natl. Acad. Sci. U. S. A. 94 (17) (1997) 9320–9325.

International Congress Series 1262 (2004) 156–159

www.ics-elsevier.com

Cellular crosstalk under hyperglycemic stress—the diabetic retina as a paradigm

Jihong Lin, Yuxi Feng, Franziska vom Hagen, Hans-Peter Hammes*

Section of Endocrinology, 5th Medical Clinic, Medical Faculty of the University of Heidelberg, Theodor-Kutzer-Ufer 1-3, D-68135 Mannheim, Baden-Wurttemberg 68167, Germany

Abstract. The common denominator of endothelial damage in diabetic complications is mitochondrial overproduction of reactive oxygen species (ROS). ROS partially inhibit the glycolytic enzyme, glyceraldehyde-3-phosphate dehydrogenase, with a subsequent increased availability of the glycolytic metabolites, fructose-6-phosphate and glyceraldehyde-3-phosphate. In contrast to previous concepts, pericyte loss may be the result of an active elimination initiated by endothelial cells. ROS formation and downstream mechanisms have been experimentally addressed by several strategies, including antioxidants and inhibitors of hyperglycemia-induced biochemical pathways. A novel way to prevent vascular damage in diabetes is to divert glycolytic intermediates into the non-oxidative branch of the pentose–phosphate pathway by activating the key enzyme transketolase. Together, in vitro data combined with animal experiments suggest that novel strategies are available for the prevention and treatment of diabetic microvascular damage.

Keywords: Pericyte; Diabetic retinopathy; Biochemistry

1. Introduction

The first discernible morphological change in a diabetic retina observed experimentally is the loss of pericytes. With progressive disease duration, capillary damage cumulates, building up acellular capillaries. They correspond to nonperfused retinal areas, and by this, they are the most important features of progressive vascular damage in the diabetic retina [1]. Microaneurysms, as the initial clinical signs of diabetic retinopathy in patients, cluster around areas of acellular capillaries indicating a secondary process (response to injury) and a direct sign of preceding endothelial cell damage due to diabetes.

2. The function of pericytes during development

The cellular crosstalk between endothelial cells and pericytes during development has been studied using transgenic animals. As described recently in a comprehensive review

* Corresponding author. Tel.: +49-621-383-2663; fax: +49-621-383-2663.
E-mail address: hans-peter.hammes@med5.ma.uni-heidelberg.de (H.-P. Hammes).

0531-5131/
doi:10.1016/S0531-5131(03)01859-4

by Carmeliet [2], the vascular network is elaborated by hemangioblasts, which differentiate into endothelial cells forming tubes via the activity of the VEGF/VEGF-receptor system. Subsequently, vessels expand by sprouting angiogenesis and are stabilized. This process involves an antidromic system in which endothelial cells signal to recruit vessel-stabilizing pericytes, and pericytes signal when they approach the endothelium. The PDGFB/PDGF-beta receptor and the Angiopoietin–Tie system are involved in this stabilization process [3,4]. The final maturation of capillaries requires active TGF-beta. Pericytes have diverse functions ranging from inhibition of endothelial cell growth to precursor attributes for osteoblasts, adipocytes and phagocytes [5]. Work done in the developing rodent retina had generated the concept of a window of plasticity [6]. This denotes that pericytes lag behind the outgrowing endothelium and provide permanent protection against regressive signals, such as VEGF depletion by hyperoxia, when finally attracted to the capillary wall. In turn, when pericytes were defined as the indicators of the end of vessel plasticitiy and of endothelial maturation, and inhibitors of endothelial cell proliferation, pericyte loss would mean facilitation of proliferative retinopathy. New data using advanced morphological technologies and new pericyte markers, however, suggest that pericytes are pioneers of the sprouting process [7]. Both the coordinated and sometimes exclusive expression of pericyte markers, such as NG-2, desmin and SMA, and the various phenotypes of pericytes in the mature retina suggest that different types of pericytes exist in a retina.

3. PDGF-B and the developing retina

If pericytes are pioneers of sprouting angiogenesis, the loss of pericytes and the transition from a resting to an activated endothelium in early diabetes needs reconsideration. PDGF-B knockout mice lack pericytes in brain capillaries and develop microaneurysms and endothelial cell hyperplasia, but are not viable, excluding retinal studies. Heterozygous PDGF-B knockout mice were studied using retinal digest preparation/quantitative retinal morphometry. These mice had fewer pericytes and more acellular capillaries, suggesting that pericytes are protective for the mature endothelium. When chemical diabetes was superimposed in these mice, pericyte loss was aggravated, but endothelial damage as reflected by the numbers of acellular capillaries increased non-linearly. These data suggest that the protective effect of pericytes on endothelial cells in diabetes is partial [8].

4. Mechanisms of pericyte dropout in the diabetic retina

Pericyte loss in the early diabetic retina is currently explained by the accumulation of toxic metabolites [9]. However, the question arises whether pericytes can also be eliminated by an active process, induced by endothelial cells. The Angiopoietin–Tie system, which is involved in pericyte recruitment and vessel maturation during development and in physiological and pathological angiogenesis [4,10], could exert such a function. Hyperglycemia causes upregulation of angiopoetin 2 in the experimental diabetic retina, which precedes the onset of pericyte dropout (Hammes et al., manuscript submitted), and pharmacologic application of angiopoietin 2 induces pericyte loss in the non-diabetic retina. These, and confirmative data, suggest that pericyte loss in the diabetic retina is the result of an active elimination process involving the Angiopoetin–Tie system.

5. Biochemical aspects of hyperglycemic cell damage

Recently, Brownlee suggested that mitochondrial reactive oxygen species (ROS) overproduction is the key component of hyperglycemia-induced endothelial damage, which inhibits the key enzyme of glycolysis leading to an upstream congestion of two intermediates, fructose-6-phosphate and glyceraldehyde-3-phosphate. These intermediates are key substrates of four independent biochemical pathways [11]. The underlying mechanism leading to GAPDH inhibition has now been identified, suggesting that activation of PARP plays a key role in this process [12]. Administration of PARP inhibitors normalizes ADP ribosylation of GAPDH, GAPDH activity and normalized PKC activity, the hexosamine pathway and the formation of AGEs and NF-κ-B activation in bovine aortic endothelial cells. PARP knockout mice are protected from GAPDH inhibition. Together, these data provide additional evidence for the crucial role of mitochondrial ROS overproduction induced by hyperglycemia in endothelial cells as the common denominator of diabetic endothelial damage.

6. Activation of transketolase as a cure for hyperglycemic damage

Activation of transketolase can shift glycolytic intermediates into the nonoxidative branch of the pentose–phosphate pathway. In vitro data indicated that activation of the enzyme by benfotiamine, the lipid-soluble pro-drug of thiamin, reduced all major pathways of diabetic endothelial damage in endothelial cells [13]. Oral benfotiamine, which is 80-fold more potent than thiamin, was administered over 36 weeks to diabetic rats, and retinal hexosamine activity, retinal PKC activity, retinal AGEs and NF-κ-B activation were measured. Benfotiamine inhibited all three pathways and NF-κ-B activation. Structurally, the formation of acellular capillaries, which was increased 2.5-fold, was almost completely inhibited by benfotiamine. Of note, benfotiamine did not inhibit pericyte loss, while proliferation of endothelial cells in areas which were unaffected by the formation of acellular capillaries was significantly reduced towards normal. These data are consistent with the hypothesis that diabetic endothelial cells can survive despite the persistence of pericyte loss and that the endothelium is the primary therapeutic target in diabetes.

In summary, new data from developmental biology have dramatically widened our knowledge about pericyte biology. These advances have also provided techniques and models, which allow us to study cellular crosstalk in the hyperglycemic setting. From these data, it can be summarised at present that the major modulator of vascular damage in diabetes is the endothelium.

Acknowledgements

This work was supported by the Deutsche Forschungsgemeinschaft, the Deutsche Diabetes Gesellschaft, and by grant from the Faculty of Clinical Medicine Mannheim, University of Heidelberg, Germany.

References

[1] E.M. Kohner, P. Henkind, Correlation of fluorescein angiogram and retinal digest in diabetic retinopathy, Am. J. Ophthalmol. 69 (1970) 403–414.
[2] P. Carmeliet, Angiogenesis in health and disease, Nat. Med. 9 (2003) 653–660.
[3] M. Hellstrom, H. Gerhardt, M. Kalen, X. Li, U. Eriksson, H. Wolburg, C. Betsholtz, Lack of pericytes leads to endothelial hyperplasia and abnormal vascular morphogenesis, J. Cell Biol. 153 (2001) 543–553.
[4] G.D. Yancopoulos, S. Davis, N.W. Gale, J.S. Rudge, S.J. Wiegand, J. Holash, Vascular-specific growth factors and blood vessel formation, Nature 407 (2000) 242–248.
[5] D.E. Sims, Diversity within pericytes, Clin. Exp. Pharmacol. Physiol. 27 (2000) 842–846.
[6] L.E. Benjamin, I. Hemo, E. Keshet, A plasticity window for blood vessel remodelling is defined by pericyte coverage of the preformed endothelial network and is regulated by PDGF-B and VEGF, Development 125 (1998) 1591–1598.
[7] H. Gerhardt, M. Golding, M. Fruttiger, C. Ruhrberg, A. Lundkvist, A. Abramsson, M. Jeltsch, C. Mitchell, K. Alitalo, D. Shima, C. Betsholtz, VEGF guides angiogenic sprouting utilizing endothelial tip cell filopodia, J. Cell Biol. 161 (2003) 1163–1177.
[8] H.P. Hammes, J. Lin, O. Renner, M. Shani, A. Lundqvist, C. Betsholtz, M. Brownlee, U Deutsch, Pericytes and the pathogenesis of diabetic retinopathy, Diabetes 51 (2002) 3107–3112.
[9] A.W. Stitt, Y.M. Li, T.A. Gardiner, R. Bucala, D.B. Archer, H. Vlassara, Advanced glycation end products (AGEs) co-localize with AGE receptors in the retinal vasculature of diabetic and of AGE-infused rats, Am. J. Pathol. 150 (1997) 523–531.
[10] D. Hanahan, Signaling vascular morphogenesis and maintenance, Science 277 (1997) 48–50.
[11] T. Nishikawa, D. Edelstein, X.L. Du, S. Yamagishi, T. Matsumura, Y. Kaneda, M.A. Yorek, D. Beebe, P.J. Oates, H.-P. Hammes, I. Giardino, M. Brownlee, Normalizing mitochondrial superoxide production blocks three pathways of hyperglycaemic damage, Nature 404 (2000) 787–790.
[12] X. Du, T. Matsumura, D. Edelstein, L. Rossetti, Z. Zsengeller, C. Szabo, M. Brownlee, Inhibition of GAPDH activity by poly(ADP-ribose) polymerase activates three major pathways of hyperglycemic damage in endothelial cells, J. Clin. Invest. 112 (2003) 1047–1049.
[13] H.P. Hammes, X. Du, D. Edelstein, T. Taguchi, T. Matsumara, Q. Ju, J. Lin, A. Bierhaus, P. Nawroth, D. Hannak, M. Neumaier, R. Bergfeld, I. Giardino, M. Brownlee, Benfotiamine blocks three major pathways of hyperglycemic damage and prevents experimental diabetic retinopathy, Nat. Med. 9 (2003) 294–299.

International Congress Series 1262 (2004) 160–163

www.ics-elsevier.com

Molecular mechanisms of retinal neovascularization in diabetic retinopathy

Hitoshi Takagi*, Hideyasu Oh, Atsushi Otani, Kiyoshi Suzuma, Izumi Suzuma, Hirokazu Ohashi, Daisuke Watanabe, Seiji Kemmochi, Tomonari Ojima, Eri Suganami, Masafumi Kurimoto, Tomoaki Murakami

Department of Ophthalmology and Visual Sciences, Kyoto University Graduate School of Medicine, 54 Shougoin kawara-cho, Sakyou, Kyoto 606-8507, Japan

Abstract. Diabetic retinopathy is a leading cause of visual disturbance in adults. In proliferative diabetic retinopathy, ischemia-induced, pathologic growth of new blood vessels often causes catastrophic loss of vision. Our findings demonstrate that vascular endothelial growth factor (VEGF), angiopoietin2 (Ang2) and neuropilin1 (NP1) are up-regulated and cooperatively promote retinal neovascularization in the ischemic retina. Renin/angiotensin system (RAS) has been reported to be a key factor of development of diabetic retinopathy. Our data indicate that Angiotensin II functions as a potent angiogenic factor and vascular cell survival factor in retinal microvasculature. Our results are indicative of molecular mechanisms underlying RAS involvement in the development of diabetic retinopathy. © 2003 Published by Elsevier B.V.

Keywords: Vascular endothelial growth factor; Angiopoietin; Neuropilin; Angiotensin; Diabetic retinopathy

1. Introduction

Diabetic retinopathy is a leading cause of visual disturbance in adults. In the early stages of retinopathy, abnormal increases in vascular permeability result in diabetic macular edema and, in the late stages, ischemia-induced pathologic growth of new blood vessels causes catastrophic loss of vision. Interactions of vascular cell mediators, including VEGF, angiopoietins and neuropilin1, play a prominent role in promoting retinal neovascularization.

2. Cooperative role of VEGF and angiopoietins in ischemia-induced retinal neovascularization

One primary stimulus for such ocular neovascularization is hypoxia, and recent studies have implicated VEGF as a primary mediator of ocular neovascular diseases.

* Corresponding author. Tel.: +81-75-751-3260; fax: +81-75-751-3258.
E-mail address: hitoshi@kuhp.kyoto-u.ac.jp (H. Takagi).

0531-5131/ © 2003 Published by Elsevier B.V.
doi:10.1016/j.ics.2003.11.017

Suppression of VEGF receptor interaction, VEGF expression and VEGF-induced signaling has been shown to inhibit neovascularization in animal models of retinal ischemia. VEGF itself is able to produce many of the vascular abnormalities common to diabetic retinopathy, and levels of VEGF are elevated in diabetic patients with active ocular neovascularization [1].

Angiopoietin2 has been suggested to suppress interaction between endothelial cells and peri-endothelial components [2]. Our study revealed that both hypoxia and VEGF selectively up-regulate Ang2 expression in bovine retinal endothelial cells and that Ang2 expression is up-regulated in vivo in a mouse model of retinal ischemia [3]. The angiogenic effect of Ang2 might possibly be explained by destabilization of the preexisting vascular tube structure to set up a favorable environment for endothelial cells to migrate or to contact with additional angiogenic cytokines. Alternatively, destabilization of blood vessels by Ang2 may diminish pericyte-dependent inhibition of endothelial proliferation and facilitate subsequent neovascularization.

In human epiretinal membranes surgically obtained from eyes with proliferative diabetic retinopathy, we demonstrated a remarkable concomitant up-regulation of both VEGF and Ang2 compared with those from other ocular proliferative diseases, while Ang1 expression was constant. Intravitreal injection of soluble Tie2 fusion protein (sTie2-Fc), soluble Flt-1 fusion protein (sFlt-1-Fc), and both chimeric proteins suppressed retinal angiogenesis in a murine model of retinal ischemia in the magnitude of sTie2-Fc < sFlt-1-Fc < sTie2-Fc + sFlt-1-Fc [4]. These results reinforce the substantial role of the angiopoietins/Tie2 system as well as the VEGF system in ischemia-induced angiogenesis, as well as in the VEGF system (Fig. 1).

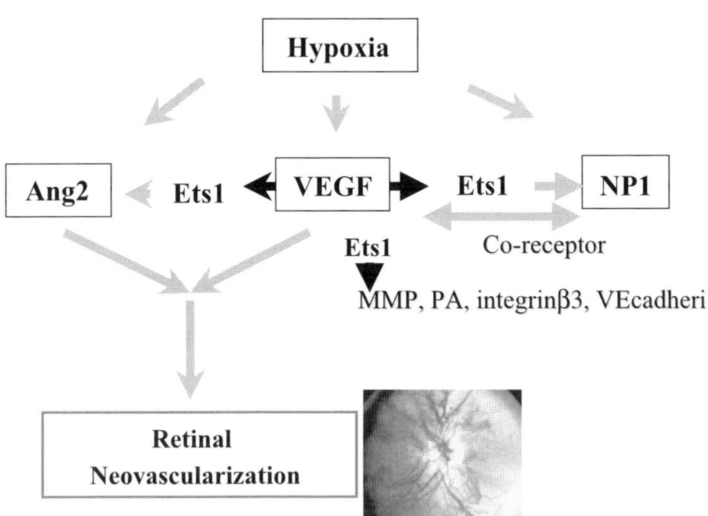

Fig. 1. Interaction of VEGF, angiopoietin2 (Ang2), and neuropilin-1 (NP-1) in ischemia-induced retinal neovascularization.

3. Neuropilin-1-mediated feedback system in retinal neovascularization in diabetic retinopathy

Neuropilin-1 has recently been shown to function also in endothelial cells as an isoform-specific receptor for vascular endothelial growth factor 165 ($VEGF_{165}$) and as a co-receptor in-vitro of VEGF receptor 2 (VEGFR2) [5]. However, its potential role in pathologic angiogenesis remains unknown. We demonstrated that VEGF up-regulates NRP1 via the VEGFR2-dependent pathway. Endothelial proliferation stimulated by $VEGF_{165}$ was significantly inhibited by antibody perturbation of NRP1. In a murine model of VEGF-dependent, angioproliferative retinopathy, intense NRP1 mRNA expression was observed in the newly formed vessels. Furthermore, selective NRP1 inhibition in this model substantially suppressed neovascular formation [6]. These results suggest that VEGF cannot only activate endothelial cells directly but also can contribute to retinal angiogenesis in diabetic retinopathy by a novel mechanism that involves up-regulation of its cognate receptor expression. NP1 could be a therapeutic target for specific inhibition of retinal neovascularization in proliferative diabetic retinopathy (Fig. 1).

4. Role of a VEGF-dependent transcriptional factor in ischemia-induced retinal neovascularization

Since VEGF plays a primary role in retinal neovascularization, we further focused on the regulation of transcriptional factor, which mediates VEGF-dependent angiogenic activities in retinal microvascular endothelial cells. Ets-1, first identified among the Ets gene family, has been shown also to be associated with pathologic angiogenesis. A number of angiogenesis-related molecules, including matrix metalloproteinase-1, -3, -9, urokinase-type plasminogen activator, integrin β3, and VE-cadherin, are reported to be targets of Ets-1 in endothelial cells. Dominant negative Ets-1 inhibited VEGF-induced tube formation and the expression of neuropilin-1 and angiopoietin-2. Intravitreal injection of dominant negative Ets-1 suppressed retinal angiogenesis in a mouse model of retinal ischemia. Ets-1 up-regulation is involved in the development of retinal neovascularization, and inhibition of Ets-1 may be beneficial in the treatment of diabetic retinopathy (Fig. 1).

5. Role of renin/angiotensin system (RAS) in the development of diabetic retinopathy

Previous studies have implicated renin/angiotensin system (RAS) as a key factor in the development of diabetic retinopathy. However, it remains unclear what mechanism underlies the interaction of RAS and the development of diabetic retinopathy. To understand the mechanism, we have determined the impact of AII on two aspects of retinal microvasculature. One is angiogenic aspect and the other is cell survival. First, we demonstrated that AII stimulates VEGF secretion from pericyte, up-regulates VEGFR2 expression in endothelial cells [7] and stimulates Ang2 secretion from endothelial cells [8] (Fig. 2). For the other aspect, we studied potential roles of AII in vascular cell survival, and found that this molecule plays a remarkable anti-apoptotic role in retinal microvascular endothelial cells challenged by serum depri-

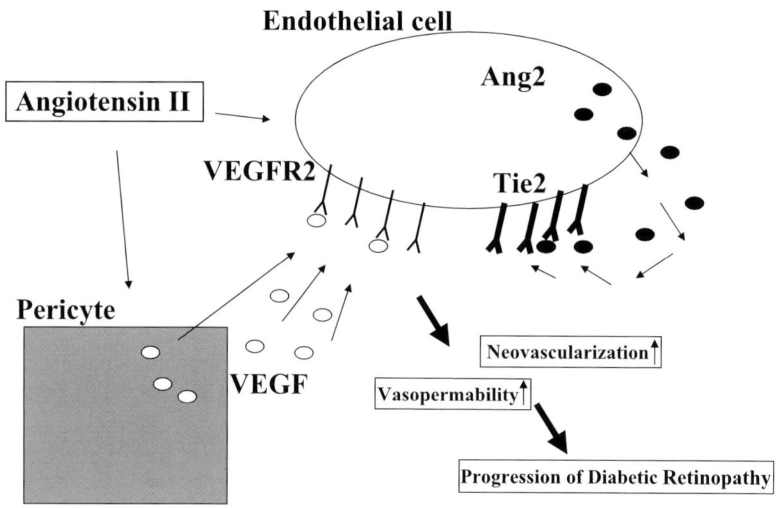

Fig. 2. Role of renin/angiotensin system in diabetic retinopathy.

vation. Our results are indicative of molecular mechanisms that are consistent with beneficial effects of ACE inhibitors for the treatment of retinopathy, such that suppression of AII signaling actually reduces retinal angiogenesis and vascular viability.

References

[1] L.P. Aiello, et al., Vascular endothelial growth factor in ocular fluid of patients with diabetic retinopathy and other retinal disorders, N. Engl. J. Med. 331 (1994) 1480–1487.
[2] P.C. Maisonpierre, et al., Angiopoietin-2, a natural antagonist for Tie2 that disrupts in vivo angiogenesis, Science 277 (1997) 55–60.
[3] H. Oh, et al., Hypoxia and vascular endothelial growth factor selectively up-regulate angiopoietin-2 in bovine microvascular endothelial cells, J. Biol. Chem. 274 (1999) 15732–15739.
[4] H. Takagi, et al., Potential role of the angiopoietin/tie2 system in ischemia-induced retinal neovascularization, Invest. Ophthalmol. Visual Sci. 44 (2003) 393–402.
[5] S. Soker, et al., Neuropilin-1 is expressed by endothelial and tumor cells as an isoform-specific receptor for vascular endothelial growth factor, Cell 92 (1998) 735–745.
[6] H. Oh, et al., Selective induction of neuropilin-1 by vascular endothelial growth factor (VEGF): A novel mechanism contributing to VEGF-induced angiogenesis, Proc. Natl. Acad. Sci. U. S. A. 99 (2002) 383–388.
[7] A. Otani, et al., Angiotensin II potentiates vascular endothelial growth factor-induced angiogenic activity in retinal microcapillary endothelial cells, Circ. Res. 82 (1998) 619–628.
[8] A. Otani, et al., Angiotensin II stimulates expression of angiopoieitin2, a natural antagonist of Tie receptor ligand in bovine retinal endothelial cells, Diabetes 50 (2001) 867–875.

International Congress Series 1262 (2004) 164–167

www.ics-elsevier.com

Nurture vs. nature in diabetic vasculopathy: roles of advanced glycation endproducts and the receptor for them

Yasuhiko Yamamoto[a], Hideto Yonekura[a], Shigeru Sakurai[a], Nobushige Tanaka[a], Hui Li[a], Khin-Mar Myint[a], Chul-Hee Kim[a], Ai Harashima[a], Mari Osawa[a], Masayoshi Takeuchi[b], Takuo Wtanabe[a], Hiroshi Yamamoto[a,*]

[a] *Department of Biochemistry and Molecular Vascular Biology, Kanazawa University Graduate School of Medical Science, 13-1 Takara-machi, Kanazawa 920-8640, Japan*

[b] *Department of Biochemistry, Faculty of Pharmaceutical Science, Hokuriku University, Kanazawa, Japan*

Received 31 October 2003; received in revised form 28 November 2003; accepted 3 December 2003

Abstract. As is diabetes itself, diabetic vasculopathy is a multifactor disease. Studies conducted in this lab revealed advanced glycation endproducts (AGE) as the major environmental account for vascular cell derangement characteristic of diabetes, and the receptor for AGE (RAGE) as the major genetic factor that responds to them. AGE fractions that caused the vascular derangement were proven to be RAGE ligands. When made diabetic, RAGE-overexpressing transgenic mice exhibited the exacerbation of the indices of nephropathy, and this was prevented by the inhibition of AGE formation. We also created RAGE-deficient mice. They showed marked amelioration of diabetic nephropathy. Extracellular signals and nuclear factors that induce the transcription of human RAGE gene were also identified, which would be regarded as risk factors of diabetic complications. Through an analysis of vascular polysomal poly(A)$^+$ RNA, we came across a novel splice variant coding for a soluble RAGE protein, and named it endogenous secretory RAGE (esRAGE). esRAGE was able to capture AGE ligands and neutralize the AGE action on endothelial cells, suggesting that this variant has a potential to protect blood vessels from diabetes-induced injury. The AGE–RAGE system should thus be regarded as a candidate molecular target for overcoming this life- and quality of life (QOL)-threatening disease. © 2004 Published by Elsevier B.V.

Keywords: Diabetes; Diabetic vascular complication; Advanced glycation endproducts; RAGE; esRAGE

* Corresponding author. Tel.: +81-76-265-2182; fax: +81-76-234-4226.
E-mail address: yasuyama@med.kanazawa-u.ac.jp (Y. Yamamoto).

0531-5131/ © 2004 Published by Elsevier B.V.
doi:10.1016/j.ics.2003.12.035

1. Introduction

The number of people who are suffering from diabetes mellitus is steadily increasing. Before being lethal, quality of life (QOL) is greatly impaired in patients with diabetes due to vascular complications like retinopathy and nephropathy. To understand how blood vessels are impaired in the diabetic state is, therefore, crucially important. As is diabetes per se, diabetic complications are caused by multiple environmental and genetic factors, and we should identify such accounts one by one. Those efforts should reveal effective molecular targets for overcoming this life- and QOL-threatening disease.

1.1. Advanced glycation endproducts (AGE) and the receptor for AGE (RAGE)

In 1912, Maillard described that reducing sugars like glucose can react nonenzymatically with the amino groups of proteins to form Schiff bases and then Amadori compounds. These early glycation products undergo further reactions, including dehydration, condensation and cross-linking, yielding irreversible protein derivatives termed advanced glycation endproducts (AGE). AGE formation and accumulation are most accelerated under diabetes. Nonenzymatic pathways that are distinct from the classical Maillard reaction yet can also yield AGE have recently been found [1]. Takeuchi et al. use short-chain carbonyl compounds, such as glyceraldehyde, glyoxal, glycolaldehyde, methylglyoxal and 3-deoxyglucosone, as intermediates. These short-chain aldehydes are more reactive than glucose, taking a shorter time period to accomplish the AGE formation, and do occur in human bodies. Most AGE structures derived from the short-chain carbonyl remain to be defined. Cellular receptors to which AGE can bind have been described. Among them is the receptor for AGE (RAGE), which was initially isolated from bovine lung [2]. It belongs to the immunoglobulin superfamily, having three immunoglobulin-like domains in the N-terminal extracellular segment, one transmembrane region and a short C-terminal intracytoplasmic stretch. RAGE is also known as a multiligand receptor not only for AGE but also for amphoterin, S100 proteins, amyloid-β proteins and transthyretin. We prepared AGE by incubating BSA with glyceraldehyde, glyoxal, glycolaldehyde, methylglyoxal and 3-deoxyglucosone, and tested their abilities to bind purified human RAGE protein using a BIACORE surface plasmon resonance system.

Glyceraldehydes- and glycolaldehyde-derived AGE were found to be associated with the sensor chip, as was the control glucose-derived AGE. Apparent dissociation constant (K_d) values of RAGE interaction with glyceraldehyde-derived AGE and glycolaldehyde-derived AGE were estimated to be ~ 300 nM and ~ 1.4 μM, respectively, when assessed either by the BIACORE assay or by Scatchard analysis with intact cells and ^{125}I-labeled AGE. The results indicated that glyceraldehyde and glycolaldehyde-derived AGE are new RAGE ligands. We thus next examined whether glyceraldehyde and glycolaldehyde-derived AGE inhibit the growth of human pericytes; pericyte loss is a hallmark of diabetic retinopathy. Therefore, glyceraldehyde and glycolaldehyde-derived AGE were found to significantly decrease human brain pericyte synthesis of DNA at lower concentrations than did glucose-derived AGE. On the contrary, when administered to EC, glucose-, glyceraldehyde and glycolaldehyde-derived AGE significantly increased viable cell numbers and upregulated the levels of VEGF mRNA. The results indicate that the RAGE-engaging

AGE fractions occurring in our internal milieu should be regarded as an environmental account for vascular injury in diabetes.

1.2. RAGE transgenic mice

To evaluate in vivo the hypothesis that the AGE–RAGE system may participate in the development of diabetic vascular complications, we created transgenic mice that overexpress human RAGE proteins in vascular cells, and crossbred them with another transgenic mouse line that develops insulin-dependent diabetes early after birth [3]. The resultant double transgenic mice showed statistically significant increases in kidney weight, albuminuria, glomerulosclerosis index and serum creatinine compared with the diabetic control, while blood glucose, hemoglobin A_{1c} and serum AGE levels were essentially invariant between the two groups. The increases in serum creatinine and sclerosis index were effectively prevented with (±)-2-isopropylidenehydrazono-4-oxo-thiazolidin-5-ylacetanilide, an inhibitor of AGE formation. Indices diagnostic of diabetic retinopathy were also most prominent in the double transgenic mice. Thus, this transgenic approach has supported the concept that AGE–RAGE system plays an active role in the development of diabetic complications, and has developed a useful animal model for testing remedies. Furthermore, mice deficient for RAGE showed amelioration of diabetic nephropathy, as evidenced by loss of nephromegaly, significant decrease in albuminuria, improved glomerulosclerosis and no elevation of serum creatinine. This again emphasizes that RAGE is functionally involved in the development of diabetic nephropathy.

1.3. Regulation of human RAGE gene

In light of the findings with RAGE transgenic mice, it is reasonable to assume that upregulation of the endogenous RAGE gene would aggravate diabetic vascular derangement. Accordingly, we screened factors that can influence the EC level of RAGE mRNA. We identified three inducers of RAGE gene transcription: AGE ligands themselves, tumor necrosis factor-α (TNF-α) and 17β-estradiol [4]. TNF-α has been known to be responsible for insulin resistance. The action on RAGE gene unveiled another side of this cytokine; that is, an increased TNF-α level in diabetic patients may worsen diabetic complications through RAGE induction. Between AGE and RAGE, a positive feedback loop may exacerbate diabetic vasculopathy. The RAGE gene activation by estradiol may provide a biochemical basis for the well-known fact that pregnancy worsens diabetic complications.

1.4. esRAGE

We analyzed poly$(A)^+$ RNA isolated from polysomes of human EC and pericytes, and isolated previously undescribed splice variants of RAGE mRNA [5]. Three major variants were identified: the known full-length membrane-bound form, a novel N-terminally truncated membrane-bound form and a novel C-terminally truncated soluble form. The ratio of expression of these variants differed from one cell type to another; C-truncated > full-length = N-truncated in EC; full-length > N-truncated > C-truncated in pericytes. We named the C-truncated form "endogenous secretory RAGE (esRAGE)". esRAGE would be cytoprotective, because it is able to capture AGE outside cells. In effect, this variant was found to effectively neutralize the AGE action on EC and does exist in human circulation. An enzyme-linked immunosorbent assay system for esRAGE has been developed, and, with it, diabetic subjects with or without complications are now being screened.

2. Conclusion

AGE are senescent proteins that accumulate during prolonged diabetic exposure, and can also engage cell surface RAGE; this resulting in the deterioration of vascular functions. The AGE–RAGE system thus should be a candidate target for overcoming this life- and QOL-threatening disease.

Acknowledgements

Authors thank Professor Toshio Doi at Tokushima University, Professor Hiroshi Okamoto, Dr. Shin Takasawa and Dr. Ichiro Kato at Tohoku University for collaboration, and Shin-ichi Matsudaira, Reiko Kitamura and Yoshie Sakurai for assistance.

References

[1] M. Takeuchi, Y. Yanase, N. Matsuura, S. Yamagishi Si, Y. Kameda, R. Bucala, Z. Makita, Immunological detection of a novel advanced glycation end-product, Mol. Med. 7 (2001) 783–791.

[2] M. Neeper, A.M. Schmidt, J. Brett, S.D. Yan, F. Wang, Y.C. Pan, K. Elliston, D. Stern, A. Shaw, Cloning and expression of a cell surface receptor for advanced glycosylation end products of proteins, J. Biol. Chem. 267 (1992) 14998–15004.

[3] Y. Yamamoto, I. Kato, T. Doi, H. Yonekura, S. Ohashi, M. Takeuchi, T. Watanabe, S. Yamagishi, S. Sakurai, S. Takasawa, H. Okamoto, H. Yamamoto, Development and prevention of advanced diabetic nephropathy in RAGE-overexpressing mice, J. Clin. Invest. 108 (2) (2001) 261–268.

[4] N. Tanaka, H. Yonekura, S. Yamagishi, H. Fujimori, Y. Yamamoto, H. Yamamoto, The receptor for advanced glycation endproducts is induced by the glycation products themselves and TNF-α through NF-κB, and by 17β-estradiol through Sp-1 in human vascular endothelial cells, J. Biol. Chem. 275 (33) (2000) 25781–25790.

[5] H. Yonekura, Y. Yamamoto, S. Sakurai, R.G. Petrova, Md.J. Abedin, H. Li, K. Yasui, M. Takeuchi, Z. Makita S. Takasawa, H. Okamoto, T. Watanabe, H. Yamamoto, Novel splice variants of the receptor for advanced glycation endproducts (RAGE) expressed in human vascular endothelial cells and pericytes, and their putative roles in diabetes-induced vascular injury, Biochem. J. 370 (3) (2003) 1097–1109.

International Congress Series 1262 (2004) 168–172

www.ics-elsevier.com

Geoethnic-sensitive and cross-culture differences of dietary patterns and blood pressure among five ethnic populations in China

Longjian Liu[a,b,c,*], Katsumi Ikeda[c,d], Xiaoyan Yin[e,f], Tingzhong Yang[g], Lihong Mu[h], He Zhao[i], Shunsaku Mizushima[c,j], Tomohiro Miki[c], Yasuo Nara[c,k], Yukio Yamori[c]

[a] *Division of Toxicology, University of Arkansas for Medical Sciences, Little Rock, AR 72205, USA*
[b] *Department of Epidemiology, University of Arkansas for Medical Sciences, Little Rock, AR 72205, USA*
[c] *WHO Collaborating Center for Res. on Primary Prevention of Cardiovascular Diseases, Kyoto, Japan*
[d] *Mukogawa Women's University, Nishinomiya, Japan*
[e] *University of Arkansas for Medical Sciences, Little Rock, AR, USA*
[f] *Chongqing Yangtze Navigation Hospital, Chongqing, China*
[g] *Department of Public Health, Zhejiang University, China*
[h] *Chongqing University of Medical Sciences, Chongqing, China*
[i] *Chongqing Jian She Hospital, Chongqing, China*
[j] *International Research Center of Medical Education, University of Tokyo, Japan*
[k] *School of Pharmacy, Shujitsu University, Japan*

Abstract. *Objective*: The present study was aimed to examine the relation of dietary patterns and oxidative DNA damage to blood pressure (BP) among five Chinese national ethnic populations. *Methods*: A random sample of 1901 middle-aged Chinese men and women was collected from five ethnic groups in 11 cooperative study centers in China. *Results*: (1) Significant differences in mean BP, prevalence of hypertension and various dietary markers were observed among the five populations. (2) Na, Na/K ratio and body mass index (BMI) were positively correlated with BP, and magnesium (Mg), 3-methyhistidine (3MH) and taurine were inversely correlated with BP. (3). Factor analyses using eight variables (BMI, Na, K, Na/K ratio, calcium, Mg, 3MH and taurine) yielded three factors that explained 68% of total variance of BP among the five ethnic samples. *Conclusion*: Geoethnic sensitive and cross-cultural differences should partly explain the diet–BP association.

Keywords: Dietary pattern; Blood pressure; Chinese

* Corresponding author. Pharmacology and Toxicology, University of Arkansas for Medical Sciences, UAMS Biomedical Research Center (Room-B320), 4301 West Markham Street, Slot 638, Little Rock, AR 72205, USA. Tel.: +1-501-603-1072; fax: +1-501-603-2278.

E-mail address: Liulongjian@yahoo.com (L. Liu).

0531-5131/ © 2004 Published by Elsevier B.V.
doi:10.1016/j.ics.2004.01.016

1. Introduction

There is continuing interest in links between dietary factors and blood pressure (BP). The individual factors that have been the subject of most intensive investigations are salt, potassium, calcium, magnesium and alcohol consumption. Few studies, however, consider the geographic, ethnic and cross-culture differences in dietary patterns and their association with BP. In the present study, we aimed to further conduct our data analyses by using the database of the WHO Cardiovascular Diseases and Alimentary Comparison (WHO-CARDIAC) Study to examine dietary pattern–BP association among five Chinese national ethnic populations (Han, Uygur, Kazakh, Tibetan and Bouyei).

2. Methods

Data used in the present study were collected from 11 cooperative centers in mainland China, and were categorized into five ethnic groups: the Han people (Beijing, Guangzhou, Shijiazhuang, Shanghai and Chongqing), the Uygur people (Hetian, Tulufan and Urumqi), the Kazakh people (Altai), the Tibetan people (Lhsas) and the Bouyei people (Guiyang). This study is a component of the WHO-CARDIAC study and details of the study design have been published elsewhere [1–4]. Main study variables included BP, body mass index (BMI), urinary excretion of sodium (Na), potassium (K), magnesium (Mg), 3-methylhistidine (a biological marker of animal protein intake) [5,6] and taurine (a biological marker of seafood intake) [7,8]. A 24-h urinary excretion of 8-Hydroxy-2′-deoxyguanosine (8-OHdG, a product of DNA damage following specific enzymatic cleavage after 8-hydroxylation of the guanine base), was measured by using a competitive enzyme-linked immunosorbent assay [9,10].

In statistical analyses, hypertension was defined as those who had a SBP of 140 or higher or a DBP of 90 mm Hg or higher, or those on anti-hypertensive drug therapy. In factor analyses, a principal component analysis was used to extract the initial factors. Only factors with eigen values of more than 1.0 were retained in the analyses [11,12]. In the study, we considered variables with loadings of at least 0.40 on a factor to be heavily loaded on that factor, and variables with loadings of 0.20–0.39 to be moderately loaded. All data analyses were done using SAS version 8.0 (SAS Institute, Cary, NC, USA).

3. Results

3.1. Mean blood pressure and prevalence of hypertension

Significant differences in mean BP and prevalence of hypertension were observed among the five ethnic population samples. The prevalence of hypertension was 40%, 41%, 24%, 21% and 16% for Kazakh, Tibetan, Uygur, Han and Bouyei subjects ($p<0.001$). Age- and gender-adjusted mean (SE) SBP was 130.8 (1.5), 130.1 (1.9), 122.3 (0.9), 122.7 (0.7) and 112.3 (1.5) mm Hg for Kazakh, Tibetan, Uygur, Han and Bouyei subjects, respectively ($p<0.001$). The corresponding adjusted mean DBP was 79.9 (0.9), 83.2 (1.2), 74.1 (0.6), 74.0 (0.5) and 64.8 (0.9) mm Hg, respectively ($p<0.001$). Among the five groups, age- and gender-adjusted mean 24-h urinary sodium (Na) excretion was 213.1 (9.6), 253.7 (10.2), 173.5 (6.0), 198.7 (3.4) and 141.8 (7.1) mmol/

day ($p<0.001$); adjusted 24-h urinary excretion of mean 3-methylhistidine (3MH) was 183.3 (35.7), 172.5 (40.3), 161.4 (23.7), 257.8 (13.8) and 211.1 (8.5) μmol/day ($p<0.001$), respectively. The adjusted-mean values of body mass index (kg/m^2), 24-h urinary excretion of potassium (K) (mmol/day), Na/K ratio, magnesium (mg/day), calcium (mg/day) and taurine (μmol/day) were also statistically different among the five ethnic groups ($p<0.001$).

3.2. Correlation between diet-related factors and blood pressure

Pearson correlation analyses indicated that BMI was positively correlated with SBP and DBP in all five ethnic groups, and statistically significant among the Hans, Uygurs, Kazakhs and Bouyeis. The correlation coefficients (r) of BMI on SBP were 0.21 ($p<0.01$) in the Hans, 0.46 ($p<0.01$) in the Uygurs, 0.47 ($p<0.01$) in the Kazakhs, 0.11 ($p>0.05$) in the Tibetans and 0.26 ($p<0.01$) in the Bouyeis, respectively. The corresponding r on DBP was 0.28 ($p<0.01$), 0.50 ($p<0.01$), 0.54 ($p<0.01$), 0.13 ($p>0.05$) and 0.32 ($p<0.01$) among these five ethnic groups. Increased 24-h urinary Na excretion was positively and significantly correlated with SBP in Han ($r=0.18$, $p<0.01$), Uygur ($r=0.20$, $p<0.01$) and Bouyei subjects ($r=0.25$, $p<0.01$). The corresponding r of Na on DBP was 0.12 ($p<0.01$), 0.23 ($p<0.01$) and 0.25 ($p<0.01$) among the Han, Uygur and Bouyei subjects. A nonsignificant correlation between Na and BP (SBP and DBP) was observed in Kazakh and Tibetan subjects. However, the ratio of Na to potassium (Na/K) was significantly and positively correlated with SBP ($r=0.37$, $p<0.01$) and DBP ($r=0.35$, $p<0.01$) in the Tibetans. A negative and significant correlation between 3-methylhistidine (3MH), and SBP was observed in Han ($r=-0.10$, $p<0.05$) and Uygur ($r=-0.25$, $p<0.01$) subjects and between 3MH and DBP in Han ($r=0.12$, $p<0.01$), Uygur ($r=-0.20$, $p<0.01$) and Tibetan ($r=-0.36$, $p<0.01$) subjects. Magnesium (Mg) was negatively correlated with BP in the five ethnic groups, and a significant correlation between Mg and SBP was observed in the Hans ($r=-0.08$, $p<0.05$) and Tibetans ($r=-0.29$, $p<0.01$), and between Mg and DBP in the Tibetans ($r=-0.30$, $p<0.01$). Negative correlations between taurine and BP were observed among the groups except in the Bouyeis, while none of these correlations showed a statistical significance ($p>0.05$).

3.3. Factor analyses

Factor analyses (Table 1) produced three principal component factors that explained 68% of total variances of BP among the five ethnic population samples. The first factor explained 30% of the variances, with loadings by Na, K, Na/K ratio, Ca and Mg. The second factor, with loadings by BMI, K, Na/K ratio and Mg, explained 23% of the variances. The third factor with loadings by K, Mg, Ca, taurine and 3MH explained 14% of the variances. Across the three factors, K, Na/K ratio and Mg were loaded in both factors 1 and 2. Ca was loaded in both factors 1 and 3. K and Mg were loaded in all three factors.

3.4. Correlation between urinary 8-OHdG and blood pressure and HDL

In the Chongqing center, the results showed that 24-h urinary excretion of 8-OHdG was significantly and positively associated with both SBP and DBP

Table 1
Loadings of eight variables on the three factors rotated and extracted with factor analyses

	Factor 1	Factor 2	Factor 3
Explained variance, %	30	23	14
BMI (kg/m^2)	0.12	0.56**	0.09
Na (mmol/day)	0.84**	0.07	0.06
K (mmol/day)	0.27*	0.85**	−0.26*
Na/K ratio	0.47**	−0.75**	0.14
Mg (mg/day)	0.71**	0.30*	0.38*
Ca (mg/day)	0.74**	−0.08	0.21*
Taurine (μmol/day)	0.07	−0.16	0.86**
3MH (μmol/day)	0.17	0.13	0.86**

* Variables with loadings on factors ≥0.20 and <0.40.
** Variables with loadings on factors ≥0.40.

($p<0.01$), and negatively associated with serum high-density lipoprotein cholesterol ($p=0.03$).

4. Discussion

The present study updated our previous reports [1,13–15]. It showed significant differences in mean BP, prevalence of hypertension and the association between diet-related factors and BP among five different Chinese ethnic populations.

These different associations may be attributed to different dietary habits among the study populations who live in different geographic environment and have different cultures. In the study, for example, the Tibetan sample was collected from Lhasa, the capital of Tibet Autonomous Region of China. Geographically, it rises to 3760 m above sea level. The Tibetans customarily drink a lot of tea with salt and butter. They eat less potassium, particularly because there were fewer vegetables available at such high altitude. Although they showed lower BMI, they had a higher mean BP compared with the other study groups. Bouyeis eat rice, buckwheat, beans and potatoes and they customarily drink oil-tea camellia, but eat less salt. They had the lowest mean BP in the present study.

Significant correlation between 24-h urinary excretion of 8-OHdG and BP, and between 8-OHdG and HDL may indicate a potential mechanism between diet and BP. Similar to this, we found significant association between oxidative stress and hypertension in vivo assessment and a population sample study in Tanzania [16].

In conclusion, increased BMI, Na, and/or Na/K ratio were in general associated with high BP, and K, 3MH and Mg were inversely associated with BP in the Chinese populations. These associations, however, more or less differ among different ethnic populations. Potential geoethnic sensitive and cross-cultural differences may explain these differences.

References

[1] L.J. Liu, et al., Int. J. Epidemiol. 31 (2002) 227–233.
[2] CARDIAC Study Protocol. WHO, Izumo/Geneva, 1986.
[3] Y. Yamori, et al., J. Cardiovasc. Pharmacol. 16 (Suppl. 8) (1990) S43–S47.
[4] Y. Yamori, et al., Hypertens. Res. 24 (2001) 453–457.
[5] C.L. Long, et al., Metabolism 24 (1975) 929–935.
[6] G. Huszar, et al., Br. J. Nutr. 49 (1983) 287–294.

[7] M.A. Petty, et al., Eur. J. Pharmacol. 180 (1990) 119–127.
[8] S.N. Allo, et al., Am. J. Physiol. 273 (1997) H1956–H1961.
[9] S. Loft, et al., Carcinogenesis 13 (1992) 2241–2247.
[10] Y. Yamori, et al., Hypertens. Res. 25 (2002) 559–564.
[11] Cureton, E.E., et al., Factor Analysis: An Applied Approach, Hillsdale, NJ, Lawrence Erlbaum Associates, 1983.
[12] Stevens, J., Hillsdale, NJ, Lawrence Erlbaum Associates, 1986.
[13] L.J. Liu, et al., Hypertens. Res. 24 (2001) 315–322.
[14] L.J. Liu, et al., Hypertens. Res. 3 (2000) 151–157.
[15] L.J. Liu, et al., Hypertens. Res. 25 (2002) 689–695.
[16] H. Negishi, et al., J. Hypertens. 19 (2001) 529–533.

International Congress Series 1262 (2004) 173–175

www.ics-elsevier.com

Homocysteine and folate: from genes to greens

Lale Tokgozoglu*

Department of Cardiology, Hacettepe University Faculty of Medicine, Hacettepe, Ankara 06100, Turkey

Abstract. Several epidemiologic studies have shown correlations between mildly elevated homocysteine levels and cardiovascular disease risk. Hyperhomocysteinemia may be atherogenic or prothrombotic by various mechanisms. Whether mild to moderate hyperhomocysteinemia is a cause, consequence or marker of atherosclerotic vascular disease is still being questioned. The main determinants of plasma homocysteine levels are genetic and nutritional factors. MTHFR 677C>T polymorphism leading to reduced enzyme activity is an important genetic determinant of homocysteine levels. A recent meta-analysis involving more than 23,000 subjects has shown that individuals with the MTHFR 677 TT genotype have 16% higher risk of coronary disease compared with those with the CC genotype. The increase in risk is significant in Europeans but not in North Americans. This discrepancy can be explained by multivitamin intake, ethnic differences and other risk factors showing a typical gene–environment interaction. Folate intake is another determinant of plasma homocysteine levels and dietary supplementation with folic acid, vitamin B12 and B6 can reduce homocysteine concentrations to different extents. However, evidence linking folate and B vitamin levels to cardiovascular disease is inconclusive. Our studies have revealed that patients with the TT genotype and folate levels below the median of the population have the highest homocysteine levels and more extensive atherosclerosis as judged by the coronary angiogram. The important question of whether lowering homocysteine will decrease cardiovascular risk is being addressed by several randomized trials. Meanwhile, two recent trials questioning the effect of lowering homocysteine on restenosis—the Swiss Heart Study and the FACIT trial—have yielded largely discrepant results. Furthermore, a recent trial in patients with stable coronary disease showed that folate supplementation decreased homocysteine levels without having any impact on cardiovascular events. We will have to wait for the results of large randomized trials to see the impact of lowering homocysteine on cardiovascular risk. © 2003 Published by Elsevier B.V.

Keywords: Homocysteine; Folate

In recent years, there has been extensive research on hyperhomocysteinemia and its relation to cardiovascular disease. There are several potential mechanisms by which homocysteine can promote atherosclerosis. Several cross-sectional and retrospective studies have shown an association between plasma homocysteine levels and cardiovas-

* Tel.: +90-312-4683013; fax: +90-312-466-19-06.
E-mail address: latet@bim.net.tr (L. Tokgozoglu).

doi:10.1016/j.ics.2003.11.030

cular risk. A meta-analysis of 27 observational studies of about 4000 subjects showed that hyperhomocysteinemia was an independent, graded risk factor for atherosclerotic vascular disease leading to a significantly increased risk of coronary, cerebrovascular and peripheral vascular disease [1]. This early report showed that a 5 μmol/l increase in homocysteine was associated with a 60% and 80% increase in coronary risk in men and women, respectively. However, prospective studies performed later revealed conflicting results. Although several large studies, including Physicians' Health, BUPA, and AFCAPS/TexCAPS reported a significant association between cardiovascular disease and homocysteine, others such as ARIC, MRFIT, Caerphilly, and the extended follow-up of the Physicians' Health were essentially negative [2]. This prompted skeptics to question whether elevated homocysteine levels were a cause, consequence or marker of cardiovascular disease. Two recent meta-analyses of prospective cohort studies have shown that hyperhomocysteinemia moderately increases the risk of a first cardiovascular event [3,4]. Unlike previous reports, a 5 μmol/l increase in homocysteine was associated with only a 20–30% increase in cardiovascular disease in this meta-analysis of prospective trials. Although the association was weaker than what was originally thought, homocysteine was a cardiovascular risk factor even when adjustment was made for confounding factors, Two of the major determinants of plasma homocysteine are genetics and lifestyle factors such as diet. MTHFR 677C>T polymorphism leading to reduced enzyme activity is an important genetic determinant of plasma homocysteine levels and is a well-studied factor. A recent meta-analysis involving more than 23,000 subjects has shown that individuals with the MTHFR 677 TT genotype have 16% higher risk of coronary disease compared with those with the CC genotype [5]. The increase in risk is significant in Europeans but not in North Americans. This discrepancy can be explained by multivitamin intake, which is significantly higher in North Americans, ethnic differences, linkage disequilibrium with other polymorphisms and distribution of other conventional risk factors showing a typical gene–environment interaction. Plasma homocysteine levels vary in different countries. Higher levels are found in the Irish compared with the French. Furthermore, cardiovascular mortality rates are higher in the Irish despite having similar conventional risk factors with the French [6]. One of the most important determinants is the folate status. In the recent meta-analysis by Klerk, the TT genotype was associated with increased coronary risk only when the folate status was low. We found that in a Turkish population, those with the TT genotype and low folate levels had the highest homocysteine levels. Furthermore, homocysteine and folate were independent predictors of coronary artery disease risk [7]. Similar findings were reported from Japan where the strongest association between TT genotype and homocysteine were found in people with serum concentration of folate and B12 below the median [8].

Several studies have confirmed that folic acid-based supplements lower plasma homocysteine levels. A meta-analysis of randomized trials revealed that a daily dose of at least 0.5 mg folic acid reduced plasma homocysteine about a quarter and the effect would be more pronounced in those with lower folate and higher homocysteine concentrations [9]. Individuals with the MTHFR 677TT genotype do not need higher doses of folate but may need to be supplemented longer than 12 weeks. The PACIFIC study compared folate supplementation at a dose of 0.2 and 2 mg in high-risk individuals [10]. The homocysteine reduction was greater at the higher dose, suggesting that subjects with high risk should get additional supplementation while fortification of foodstuffs should be implemented for the population if lowering homocysteine is proven to decrease cardiovascular risk. Whether folate supplementation will decrease cardiovascular risk has still not been confirmed. Folate supplementation has been shown to improve endothelial function, lower plasma homocysteine and have antioxidant actions. Several population studies have demonstrated that subjects with lower folate intake and levels have higher cardiovascular risk. Recently, the effects of folate supplementation on restenosis following PCI have been assessed. In the Swiss Heart Study, homocysteine-lowering therapy with 1 mg folate, 400 μg B12 and 10 mg pyridoxine per day was shown to decrease the incidence of major cardiovascular events at one year [11]. However, the FACIT trial failed to confirm these results [12]. Another randomized trial that addressed the effects of folate supplementation on clinical outcomes on a secondary prevention setting failed to show a reduction of clinical end points at two years [13]. While current evidence is insufficient to derive conclusions, large ongoing randomized trials such as the NORVIT, WENBIT, VISP, and SEARCH will provide answers about cardiovascular risk reduction. The potential implications for global public health are enormous if hyperhomocysteinemia is a causal risk factor and lowering it can decrease cardiovascular risk.

References

[1] C.J. Boushey, S.A. Beresford, G.S. Omenn, et al., A quantitative assessment of plasma homocysteine as a risk factor for vascular disease, JAMA 274 (1995) 1049–1057.

[2] J.W. Eikelboom, E. Lonn, J. Genest, et al., Homocysteine and cardiovascular disease: a critical view of the epidemiologic evidence, Ann. Intern. Med. 131 (1999) 363–375.

[3] L.E. Bautista, I.A. Arenas, A. Penuela, et al., Total plasma homocysteine level and risk of cardiovascular disease. A meta-analysis of prospective cohort studies, J. Clin. Epidemiol. 55 (2002) 882–887.

[4] The Homocysteine Studies Collaboration, Homocysteine and risk of ischemic heart disease and stroke, JAMA 288 (2002) 2015–2022.

[5] M. Klerk, P. Verhoef, R. Clarke, et al., MTHFR 677C>T polymorphism and risk of coronary heart disease: a meta-analysis, JAMA 288 (2002) 2023–2031.

[6] M.R. Malinow, P. Ducimetiere, G. Luc, et al., Plasma homocysteine and graded risk for myocardial infarction: findings at two populations at contrasting risk for coronary heart disease, Atherosclerosis 126 (1996) 27–34.

[7] S.L. Tokgözoğlu, M. Alikaşifoğlu, İ. Ünsal, et al., MTHFR genotype and the risk and extent of coronary artery disease in a population with low plasma folate, Heart 81 (1999) 518–522.

[8] Y. Moriyama, T. Okamura, K. Kajinami, et al., Effects of serum B vitamins on elevated plasma homocysteine levels associated with the MTHFR gene in Japanese, Atherosclerosis 164 (2002) 321–328.

[9] R. Clarke, J. Armitage, Vitamin supplements and cardiovascular risk: review of the randomised trials of homocysteine lowering vitamin supplements, Semin. Thromb. Hemost. 26 (2000) 341–348.

[10] PACIFIC Study Group, Dose dependent effects of folic acid on plasma homocysteine in a randomised trial conducted among 723 individuals with coronary artery disease, Eur. Heart J. 23 (2002) 1509–1515.

[11] G. Schnyder, M. Roffi, R. Pin, et al., Decreased rate of restenosis after lowering plasma homocysteine levels, N. Engl. J. Med. 345 (2001) 1593–1600.

[12] F. Baker, D. Picton, S. Blackwood, et al., Blinded comparison of folic acid and placebo in patients ischemic heart disese: an outcome trial, Circulation 106 (Suppl. II) (2002) 2–741.

[13] A. Liem, G.H. Reynierse-Buitenwerf, A.H. Zwinderman, et al., Secondary prevention with folic acid: effects on clinical outcomes, J. Am. Coll. Cardiol. 41 (2003) 2105–2113.

International Congress Series 1262 (2004) 176–179

ELSEVIER

www.ics-elsevier.com

Diet, physical activity, childhood obesity and risk of cardiovascular disease

Youfa Wang*

Department of Human Nutrition, University of Illinois at Chicago, 1919 W. Taylor St., Chicago, IL 60612, USA

Abstract. Eating and physical activity (PA) patterns and obesity in childhood have many long-term effects on the risk of cardiovascular disease (CVD). Two-thirds of premature deaths in the US are due to poor nutrition, lack of PA and tobacco use. Obesity, a result of excess energy intake and inadequate PA, is an indicator of unhealthy lifestyles. Currently, over one-third of American children are overweight. Obesity in childhood is associated with dyslipidaemia, elevated blood pressure, and increased future CVD morbidity and mortality. Healthy eating and PA are essential for good health. National representative data show that unhealthy eating and insufficient PA is a serious problem among American children. Efforts should be made to help young people to develop healthy lifestyles at early age.

Keywords: Child; Lifestyle; Diet; Obesity; Cardiovascular disease

1. Introduction

Lifestyles such as eating and physical activity (PA) patterns and obesity in childhood have a long-term effect on risk of cardiovascular disease (CVD). Poor diet and inadequate PA together account for at least 300,000 deaths in the US annually and are second only to tobacco use as the most prominent identifiable contributor to premature death [1]. Obesity, a result of prolonged positive energy balance due to excess energy intake and inadequate PA, is an indicator of unhealthy lifestyles. Currently two-thirds of American adults and over one-third American children are overweight [2,3]. CVD risk factors and atherosclerosis start in childhood [4,5]. In general, cardiovascular events do not happen until middle age. It is challenging to accurately measure people's eating and PA, especially for children. As a result, it has been difficult to study the effects of lifestyles on the risk of CVD in young people. Much of the related research has focused mainly on examining the associations between lifestyles in childhood and the biological risk factors of CVD such as elevated blood pressure and unfavorable blood lipid profile.

* Tel.: +1-312-355-3382; fax: +1-312-413-0319.
E-mail address: youfwang@uic.edu (Y. Wang).

doi:10.1016/j.ics.2003.12.018

2. The influence of childhood lifestyles and obesity on risk of CVD

2.1. Eating patterns and risk of CVD

Healthy eating is critical for good health and numerous studies show that dietary factors such as intakes of dietary fat, cholesterol, sodium, and vegetable and fruit affect the risk of CVD. Diet-related risk factors for CVD include high blood cholesterol, high blood pressure and obesity. These risk factors can be reduced by choosing a healthy diet. It is widely believed that young people having unhealthy eating habits tend to maintain these habits as they age although related findings are inconclusive. Healthy eating with appropriate energy intake, low fat, and adequate vegetable and fruit consumption is essential for the prevention of chronic disease.

2.2. PA patterns and risk of CVD

PA plays an essential role in promoting good health and preventing chronic diseases. Regular PA can help reduce the risk of CVD in the following ways: improve cardiorespiratory fitness; lowers both total cholesterol and triglycerides and increases HDL; lowers the risk of hypertension and obesity; and helps reduce blood pressure in hypertensive patients. However, findings from prospective studies conducted in young people are inconclusive. Twisk et al. [6] reviewed five cohort studies conducted in Europe and North America, and found that high physical fitness during adolescence seems to be predictive of a 'healthy' CVD risk profile, but not high PA. Errors in measuring PA and their small sample sizes are at least partly responsible for this lack of evidence.

2.3. Childhood obesity and risk of CVD

Obesity serves as a good indicator of unhealthy lifestyles such as high-energy and high-fat intake and lack of PA, since obesity is the consequence of a prolonged positive energy balance. Childhood obesity has a number of immediate, intermediate, and long-term health consequences such as dyslipidaemia, elevated blood pressure and hypertension, increased CVD morbidity and morbidity [7–9].

2.4. Possible pathways for the long-term effects of childhood lifestyles on risk of CVD

The long-term impact may be due to both the direct and indirect effects of such factors on the cardiovascular system: (a) these factors have long-lasting effects; (b) clustering of risk factors. Young people who have these unfavorable factors may also have other risk factors such as smoking, social, economic and environmental stress, which may adversely affect health; (c) persistence (tracking) of these factors from childhood into adulthood. Dietary and PA habits developed during childhood are likely to become lifelong habits, and overweight children are likely to remain obese as adults.

2.5. Patterns and trends of children's dietary intake, PA and obesity in North America

2.5.1. Eating patterns

National survey data show that in general American children consume too much fat and sodium, but not adequate fruit, vegetables or calcium [10–12]. On average, they obtain

Table 1
Trends in US adolescents' food intake patterns 1977–1996

	1977	1989-91	1994-96	Trend
Energy (MJ)	8.8	8.8	9.6	⇧
Total fat (%E)	37	34	33	⇩
S_fat (%E)	14	13	12	⇩
CHO (%E)	47	51	54	⇧
Fruits (servings)	1.1	1.2	1.4	⇧
Veg. (servings)	3.0	3.0	3.3	⇧
F&V (servings)	4.1	4.2	4.7	⇧
Soft drink (%E)	3.7	5.7	8.0	⇧

34% of calories from fat and 12% from saturated fat. More than 84% eat too much total fat (%E>30%) and more than 90% eat too much saturated fat (%E>10%). Their vegetable and fruit consumption is very low compared with the recommendations ($\geq$5 servings/day). Only one-fifth meets the recommendations; 51% eat less than one serving of fruit a day. Moreover, studies suggest increased consumption of soft drinks, snack foods and large portion size foods (Table 1).

2.5.2. Physical activity

Compared with the recommendations, American children's PA is far too inadequate. The 2001 US Youth Risk Behavior Surveillance System (YRBSS) data show that 31% do not participate in PA at recommended levels; 9.5% participated in no vigorous or moderate PA [10]. Another recent national survey of children aged 9–13 years shows that 61.5% do not participate in any organized PA during non-school hours while 22.6% do not engage in any free-time PA. On average, American children spend over 4 h a day watching TV or videotapes, playing video games or using a computer. Most of this time (2.8 h) is spent watching TV; 17% watch >5 h of TV a day.

2.5.3. Childhood obesity

National representative data show that the prevalence of overweight (>85th BMI percentile) among American children has more than doubled since the 1970s (increased from 15% in 1971–1974 to 26% in 1988–1994 and 30% in 1999–2000), while the prevalence of obesity (>95th BMI percentile) has increased four-fold, from 4% to 15% [2]. Minority and low-SES groups are disproportionably affected. But the US is not alone; childhood obesity has become a global epidemic. Recently, we found that many countries have experienced the increase of obesity over the past two to three decades (Fig. 1). This may be due to the dramatic changes in young people's lifestyles as a result of social–environmental changes in these countries and the influence of increasing culture exchange and global trade, for example, the westernization of diet in many developing countries.

In conclusion, many biological risk factors of CVD start in childhood. Many factors acting together influence young people's lifestyle. The increasing global obesity epidemic is of great concern as childhood obesity has many immediate and long-term health consequences. At present, our understanding of the long-term impacts of lifestyles and conditions (e.g., obesity) developed during childhood on one's future health is still limited.

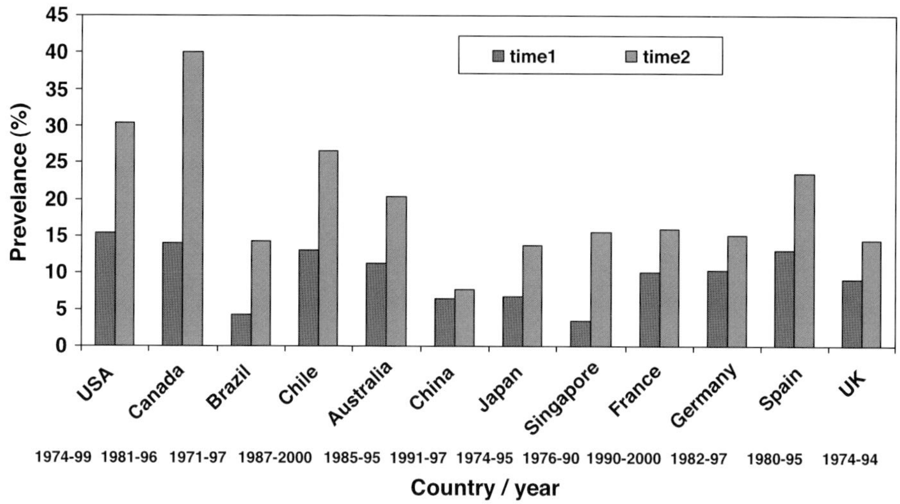

Fig. 1. Trends in the prevalence (%) of childhood overweight in selected countries worldwide. Different classifications of childhood overweight were used in some studies, but were consistent within country over time. The trends presented were based on data collected over different survey periods, from 6 years to 3 decades.

Nevertheless, the development of effective programs and policies for helping young people to develop healthy eating and PA habits at young ages should be a priority for the prevention of chronic disease.

References

[1] J.M. McGinnis, W.H. Foege, Actual causes of death in the United States, JAMA 270 (1993) 2207–2212.
[2] C.L. Ogden, K.M. Flegal, M.D. Carroll, C.L. Johnson, Prevalence and trends in overweight among US children and adolescents, 1999–2000, JAMA 288 (2002) 1728–1732.
[3] K.M. Flegal, M.D. Carroll, C.L. Ogden, C.L. Johnson, Prevalence and trends in obesity among US adults, 1999–2000, JAMA 288 (2002) 1723–1727.
[4] S.R. Daniels, Cardiovascular disease risk factors and atherosclerosis in children and adolescents, Curr. Atheroscler. Rep. 3 (2001) 479–485.
[5] H.C. McGill, Childhood nutrition and adult cardiovascular disease, Nutr. Rev. 55 (1 Pt 2) (1997) S2–S11.
[6] J.W. Twisk, H.C. Kemper, W. van Mechelen, Prediction of cardiovascular disease risk factors later in life by physical activity and physical fitness in youth: general comments and conclusions, Int. J. Sports Med. 23 (Suppl. 1) (2002) S44–S49.
[7] W. Burniat, T.J. Cole, I. Lissau, E. Poskitt, Child and adolescent obesity: causes and consequences, Prevention and Management, Cambridge Univ. Press, New York, 2002.
[8] A. Must, R.S. Strauss, Risks and consequences of childhood and adolescent obesity, Int. J. Obes. Relat. Metab. Disord. 23 (Suppl. 2) (1999) S2–S11.
[9] C. Power, J.K. Lake, T.J. Cole, Measurement and long-term health risks of child and adolescent fatness, Int. J. Obes. Relat. Metab. Disord. 21 (1997) 507–526.
[10] CDC, Youth Risk Behavior Surveillance System (YRBSS), Information and Results, 2001, http://www.cdc.gov.
[11] L. Jahns, A.M. Siega-Riz, B.M. Popkin, The increasing prevalence of snacking among US children from 1977 to 1996, J. Pediatr. 138 (2001) 493–498.
[12] S.J. Nielsen, A.M. Siega-Riz, B.M. Popkin, Trends in food locations and sources among adolescents and young adults, Prev. Med. 35 (2002) 107–113.

International Congress Series 1262 (2004) 180–183

ELSEVIER

www.ics-elsevier.com

The impact of westernization on the risk of atherosclerotic vascular disease among Japanese-American men in Hawaii

Katsuhiko Yano*, Bradley Willcox, Randi Chen, John S. Grove, Beatriz L. Rodriguez, J. David Curb

Pacific Health Research Institute, 846 S. Hotel St., Suite 306, Honolulu, HI 96813, USA

Abstract. *Purpose*: To assess the impact of westernization on the risk of CHD and stroke among first- and second-generation Japanese-American men in Hawaii. *Methods*: The length of time spent in Japan during childhood was used as a negative indicator of westernization. A total of 7479 men, aged 45–68, and free of CHD and stroke were followed up for 33 years (1965–1998). The association of childhood years in Japan with CHD and stroke risk was estimated using the Cox proportional hazards models, adjusted for age, confounding lifestyle variables, and traditional risk factors for CVD. *Results*: Childhood years in Japan were significantly and inversely associated with CHD risk, even after multivariate adjustment. However, there was no significant or consistent association of childhood years in Japan with stroke risk. *Conclusions*: Longer exposure to Japanese traditional culture and lifestyle during childhood reduced the risk of CHD later in life, but did not increase the risk of stroke. This protective effect could not be fully explained by lifestyle variables or traditional CVD risk factors.

Keywords: Childhood; CHD; Stroke; Westernization

1. Introduction

In 1965, the NI-HON-SAN Study began to compare CHD, stroke rates and risk factors among men of Japanese ancestry living in Japan, Hawaii, and California [1]. This study found that the CHD rate was highest in California, lowest in Japan, and intermediate in Hawaii. In contrast, stroke rate was highest in Japan and much lower both in Hawaii and California. There was also a large difference in baseline levels of major risk factors and other lifestyle variables between the native Japanese men and Japanese-American men in the US. These findings may reflect the effect of westernization through migration from Japan to the US. Westernization was defined as changes in lifestyle and cultural patterns from traditional Japanese ones towards those of Caucasian Americans.

* Corresponding author. Tel.: +1-808-524-4411; fax: +1-808-524-4315.
E-mail address: kekrich@phrihawaii.org (K. Yano).

doi:10.1016/j.ics.2003.11.027

In the present study, we attempted to assess the impact of westernization on CHD and stroke risk within the Honolulu Heart Program cohort, which was part of the NI-HON-SAN Study. This cohort included first- and second-generation Japanese-American men who were born in 1900–1919 and living on Oahu in 1965. These men were westernized before entry to the study to varying degrees, depending on their childhood experiences.

Based on the NI-HON-SAN Study findings, we hypothesized that the length of time spent in Japan during childhood and/or adolescence (ages 0–20) was (1) inversely correlated with indicators of westernization measured in mid-life, and (2) inversely associated with CHD risk and positively with stroke risk later in life.

2. Methods

Details of the methods in the Honolulu Heart Program have been described elsewhere [2]. In the present analysis, age-adjusted mean values of baseline characteristics were compared across three subgroups of the cohort, classified by childhood years in Japan (< 1, 1–9, and 10+ years), using analysis of covariance. The association of childhood years in Japan (treated as either a categorical or a continuous variable) with the risk of CHD and stroke was estimated using the Cox proportional hazards model. Age, possible confounding variables closely related to Japanese lifestyle, and traditional risk factors for CVD were included as covariates in separate models.

3. Results

Table 1 shows baseline characteristics for three groups of the cohort classified by childhood years in Japan. As expected, those who spent < 1 year in Japan were most westernized, while those who spent 10+ years in Japan were least westernized. Comparisons of age-adjusted mean values of sociocultural, behavioral, dietary, and physiological variables across the three groups support this presumption.

During 33 years of follow-up through 1998, a total of 1831 cases of CHD and 935 cases of stroke were identified as incident cases. Approximately 2/3 of all CHD (1268 cases) were definite CHD, which included sudden death < 1 h, non-sudden death due to CHD, and nonfatal acute myocardial infarction with ECG evidence or enzyme elevation. Similarly, about 2/3 of all stroke (630 cases) were diagnosed as thromboembolic (TE) stroke, and 65% of the TE cases had CT or MRI evidence.

Age-adjusted incidence rates of all CHD and definite CHD were highest for the most westernized group, lowest for the least westernized group. The difference was significant ($p < 0.001$) only between the two extreme groups. However, when the childhood years in Japan were treated as a continuous variable, it was inversely and significantly ($p < 0.001$) associated with both categories of CHD. In contrast, there was no significant or consistent trend of age-adjusted incidence rate of either all stroke or TE stroke. Although the rate was lowest for the intermediate group (1–9 years in Japan), this U-shaped relationship was not significant when childhood years in Japan were treated as a continuous variable, and quadratic terms were included in the Cox model (Table 2).

The protective effect of childhood years in Japan may be confounded by other variables closely related to Japanese lifestyle and sociocultural characteristics, such as being born in Japan, Japanese language proficiency, preference of Japanese diet, lower education, blue-

Table 1
Baseline characteristics of study subjects

Number of men (%)	Number of childhood years in Japan						p for trend
	<1		1–9		10+		
	5334 (71)		858 (12)		1287 (17)		
	Mean*	S.E.††	Mean	S.E.	Mean	S.E.	
Age (year)	53.3	0.07	54.0	0.18	58.6	0.14	<0.001
% Born in Japan	1.5		9.8		53.7		<0.001
% Read Japanese	22.2		58.1		94.8		<0.001
% High school education	54.0		49.0		30.1		<0.001
% Blue-collar occupation	60.3		57.8		73.9		<0.001
Smoking (pack-years)	23.7	0.34	23.6	0.85	23.8	0.73	>0.1
Alcohol (oz/month)	13.6	0.34	14.8	0.84	15.7	0.73	0.01
Physical activity index	32.7	0.06	32.6	0.15	33.9	0.13	<0.001
Japanese diet index	47.2	0.24	49.4	0.59	54.0	0.57	<0.001
% Eating tofu ≥ 2 × /week	17.2		21.9		36.2		<0.001
% Eating fish ≥ 2 × /week	41.0		47.7		59.7		<0.001
Total energy intake (kcal)	2321	9.9	2290	24.1	2242	20.9	<0.001
% Protein from animal	73.7	0.45	72.7	1.10	70.7	0.94	<0.001
% Calories from fat	33.9	0.13	32.8	0.32	31.8	0.28	<0.001
% Calories from carbohydrates	46.0	0.15	47.0	0.37	47.5	0.32	<0.001
Height (cm)	163.4	0.08	162.8	0.19	160.5	0.16	<0.001
Body mass index (kg/m^2)	23.9	0.04	23.7	0.10	23.4	0.09	<0.001
Diastolic BP (mm Hg)	82.5	0.16	81.9	0.39	80.6	0.34	<0.001
Serum cholesterol (mg/dl)	218.8	0.53	217.9	1.30	214.7	1.12	0.002
Serum triglyceride (mg/dl)	242.1	2.87	243.5	7.07	207.3	6.14	<0.001
Serum glucose (mg/dl)	161.6	0.80	158.5	1.96	159.7	1.69	>0.1

* Age-adjusted mean.
†† Standard error.

collar jobs, etc. However, the protective effect of childhood years in Japan remained significant after adjustment for each of these possible confounders individually, along with age.

After multivariate adjustment for traditional risk factors for CVD such as blood pressure, serum cholesterol, smoking, diabetes, etc., the protective effect of 10 years

Table 2
Age-adjusted incidence rate (per 1000 person-years)

Outcomes	Number of childhood years in Japan								p for trend††
	<1		1–9			10+			
	n	Rate	n	Rate	p*	n	Rate	p*	
All CHD	1368	11.0	204	10.1	>0.1	259	8.0	<0.001	<0.001
Definite CHD	935	7.5	138	6.9	>0.1	195	5.5	<0.001	<0.001
All stroke	646	5.5	100	4.9	>0.1	189	5.1	>0.1	>0.1
TE stroke	439	3.7	58	2.7	>0.05	133	3.5	>0.1	>0.1

*p level for difference in age-adjusted rate compared with <1 year group.
†† p level for the association of childhood years in Japan (as a continuous variable) with each outcome by Cox regression model, adjusted for age.

spent in Japan during childhood on CHD risk remained highly significant (relative risk 0.84, $p < 0.01$), though it reduced, about 30% compared with the effect when adjustment was made only for age.

4. Discussion

The first two of our hypotheses were supported by the study results. The length of time spent in Japan during childhood was inversely correlated with many indicators of westernization measured in mid-life. It was also inversely associated with a long-term risk of CHD, which could not be fully explained by traditional CVD risk factors or other confounding variables measured in mid-life. These findings confirm the earlier report from the Honolulu Heart Program [3] using a larger number of cases and longer follow-up. Although residual confounding by unmeasured variables, and unavailable data on childhood diet and psychosocial conditions may preclude definitive conclusions, the present study results suggest that childhood exposure to anti-atherogenic lifestyle and cultural environment is important to prevent CHD later in life. The public health implications of this study appear to be particularly relevant for countries undergoing rapid westernization.

Acknowledgements

This study was supported by Contract N01-HC-05102 and Grant U01-HL-56274 from the National Heart, Lung, and Blood Institute, Bethesda, MD.

References

[1] A. Kagan, K. Yano, Ni-Hon-San study, in: A Kagan (Ed.), The Honolulu Heart Program. An Epidemiological Study of Coronary Heart Disease and Stroke, Harwoord Academic Publishers, Amsterdam, The Netherlands, 1996, pp. 21–32.
[2] R.M. Worth, J.S. Grove, Methods, in: A. Kagan (Ed.), The Honolulu Heart Program. An Epidemiological Study of Coronary Heart Disease and Stroke, Harwoord Academic Publishers, Amsterdam, The Netherlands, 1996, pp. 5–19.
[3] K. Yano, W.C. Blackwelder, A. Kagan, et al., Childhood cultural experience and the incidence of coronary hearth disease in Hawaii Japanese men, Am. J. Epidemiol. 109 (1979) 440–450.

International Congress Series 1262 (2004) 184–187

ELSEVIER

www.ics-elsevier.com

Global guidelines: national issues

Philip Barter*

The Heart Research Institute, 145 Missenden Road, Camperdown, Sydney, NSW 2050, Australia

Abstract. There are many sets of guidelines for risk assessment and for the prevention and treatment of atherosclerotic vascular disease. Most guidelines have much in common, with a growing recognition that global risk is a function of the interaction between a number of known risk factors. Most guidelines agree on which risk factors are important but differ widely in how they can are used to define global risk. The Australian guidelines represent just one of many possible approaches. However, several principles that were adopted in their development are universal and should be a component of all guidelines. These include simplicity, collective ownership, emphasis on areas of agreement rather than of disagreement, ensure that the guidelines are living documents and emphasise that guidelines are only guidelines that should be promoted as aids to help decision-making and not as rigid prescriptions for management. © 2003 Published by Elsevier B.V.

Keywords: Lipid guidelines; Cholesterol; Cardiovascular disease

Guidelines have undoubtedly brought a degree of consistency and rationality to approaches designed to reduce coronary risk. However, guidelines should not be used blindly, especially when the recommendations are based on data collected in a population that is different from that in which they are being used. There is a strong case for mounting major epidemiological studies of cardiovascular risk in those Asian countries in which cardiovascular disease is now so prevalent.

There are many sets of guidelines for risk assessment and for the prevention and treatment of atherosclerotic vascular disease. Most guidelines have much in common, with a growing recognition that global risk is a function of the interaction between a numbers of known risk factors. Most guidelines agree on which risk factors are important but differ in how they are used to define global risk. Some employ algorithms based on large data sets collected in both the US and Europe. However, there is variation in the weighting given to individual risk factors and also in the recommendations for both initiation triggers and therapeutic targets. In many cases, the differences between guidelines reflect recognition of regional factors and are appropriate. But all too often, guidelines established on the basis of information gathered in one population are adopted without consideration of local factors and in some cases may be inappropriate.

* Tel.: +61-2-95503560; fax: +61-2-95503302.
E-mail address: p.barter@hri.org.au (P. Barter).

0531-5131/ © 2003 Published by Elsevier B.V.
doi:10.1016/j.ics.2003.11.021

This paper will first summarise the approach used in Australia and then outline issues that should be considered in the development of guidelines anywhere in the world.

The Australian guidelines represent a joint venture of the National Heart Foundation of Australia and the Cardiac Society of Australia and New Zealand. They were endorsed by the Australian Association for Exercise and Sports Science, the Australian Atherosclerosis Society, the Australian Kidney Foundation, Diabetes Australia, the Dietician's Association of Australia, the Internal Medicine Society of Australia and New Zealand, the Royal College of General Practitioners of Australia and the National Stroke Foundation of Australia.

The guidelines were based on the available evidence that low-density lipoproteins (LDL) are atherogenic and high-density lipoproteins (HDL) have a direct protective effect against the development of atherosclerosis and stroke. The guidelines emphasise, however, that abnormalities of plasma lipids are only one of several risk factors for CHD. The importance of plasma lipids is greatest when combined with other risk factors.

The guidelines stress the importance of lifestyle measures both as a cause of atherosclerosis and as interventions designed to prevent and reverse the process. Lifestyle measures considered to be important include smoking, physical inactivity and excess weight.

The main focus of the guidelines is the management of subjects at high global risk. The guidelines aim to simplify risk assessment and management of those identified at high risk. Whereas previous guidelines included reference to highest, high and lower risk categories, the current guidelines identify a single high-risk group of individuals whose risk approximates those with manifest coronary heart disease. Previous guidelines defined a variety of lipid targets defined according to risk categorization. The current guidelines identify only one set of targets for the single high-risk group. While emphasizing targets, the guidelines also state that any movement towards the targets will be beneficial even if they are not reached.

The target levels for total cholesterol, LDL-C and HDL-C and plasma triglyceride have been developed from information obtained from population studies and intervention studies, recognizing that none of reported intervention studies to date have been designed specifically to determine what the LDL-C, HDL-C or triglyceride targets should be.

The new Australian guidelines recognise the particularly high CHD risk of patients with pre-existing atherosclerotic disease, including those with manifest CHD, ischaemic cerebrovascular disease and peripheral artery disease. However, the role of lipid modification in the prevention of stroke is not resolved. The new guidelines recognise others who are particularly at high risk of CHD including those with diabetes, renal disease and multiple risk factors. Of particular importance is the new emphasis on Aboriginal peoples and Torres Strait Islanders who have an exceedingly high age-standardised mortality from CVD, which has not shown the downward trend seen in the rest of the Australian community in the past 20 years.

1. Summary of recommendations in the Australian guidelines

Most of what follows has been extracted directly from the summary of recommendations in the published Australian guidelines of which I was the lead author. For the complete guideline, see Ref. [1].

2. Definition of higher absolute risk of CHD for treatment initiation

1. Known CHD; or
2. Other known manifestations of atherothrombotic disease: peripheral arterial disease (lower limb atherosclerosis), ischaemic cerebrovascular disease, abdominal aortic aneurysm; or
3. Diabetes mellitus; or
4. Chronic renal failure/renal transplant; or
5. Aboriginal peoples and Torres Strait Islanders; or
6. Familial hypercholesterolemia; or
7. Familial combined hyperlipidaemia; or
8. Absolute risk of 5–10% or higher in next 5 years according to the New Zealand cardiovascular risk calculator; or
9. Increased absolute risk judged by LDL-C>4.0 mmol/l or total cholesterol>6.0 mmol/l, plus:

Any two (or more) other risk factors: HDL-C < 1.0 mmol/l, significant family history, hypertension, overweight, smoking, impaired fasting glucose or glucose intolerance, microalbuminuria with renal impairment, age ≥ 45.

Treatment initiation

- For those considered to be at higher absolute risk and above target levels
  (a) Monitor diet fortnightly for 6 weeks, then retest lipid levels. If still above target levels consider commencing lipid-modifying therapy (taking into account PBS criteria).
  (b) Retest fasting lipids every 2 months until a satisfactory and stable response has been achieved.
- In those who are known to have CHD and who have total cholesterol of 4.0 mmol/l or above, it is appropriate to consider commencement of drug treatment without awaiting assessment of the effects of dietary intervention.

Lipid targets

Important caveat: Less evidence exists for target levels than for populations in whom treatment should be initiated. The target levels may be higher in lower risk individuals, e.g. LDL-cholesterol < 3.0 mmol/l. It should be emphasised that any lowering of plasma total cholesterol and LDL-cholesterol and any raising of HDL-cholesterol is likely to be beneficial even if the recommended target is not achieved.

LDL-cholesterol < 2.5 mmol/l
Total cholesterol < 4.0 mmol/l
HDL-cholesterol > 1.0 mmol/l
Triglycerides < 2.0 mmol/l
Encourage smoking cessation
Encourage physical activity
Encourage weight reduction
Lipid modifying therapy

- Statins are the agents of choice for LDL-C lowering
- Fibrates are effective triglyceride-lowering/HDL-C raising agents.
- A statin and fibrate combination should be considered in high-risk people whose lipid profile remains unacceptable after a trial on monotherapy, recognizing that there is an increased risk of myositis in people taking a statin and fibrate combination.

Adherence

- When relevant, commence lipid-modifying therapy in patients with CHD while patients are still in hospital.
- When possible, consider ancillary measures (e.g. special clinics, telephone support) to assist the patient to achieve and maintain target lipid levels.
- Assess patient's adherence to medications at each visit.

3. General principles in the development of guidelines

The Australian guidelines outlined above represent just one of many possible approaches. However, several principles that were adopted in their development are universal and should be a component of all guidelines. These include:

- *Simplicity*: unless guidelines are simple, they will not be used. It may sometimes be necessary to compromise slightly on accuracy in the interest of a set of recommendations that can be understood and easily applied.
- *Collective ownership*: The wider the ownership of the guidelines, the more likely they are to be promoted and adopted.
- *Emphasise areas of agreement rather than of disagreement*: Where the opinions of two professional expert groups differ, much more is achieved by identifying points of agreement than having public (and sometimes hostile) disagreements that may undermine the credibility of both professional groups.
- *Ensure that the guidelines are living documents*: Guidelines are based on currently available knowledge and must be flexible enough to accommodate new knowledge as it becomes available without undermining the credibility of the recommendations.
- *Emphasise that guidelines are only guidelines*: Guidelines should be promoted as aids to help decision-making and not as rigid prescriptions for management.

4. Conclusion

For guidelines to be useful, they must be a blend of accuracy and simplicity. They must have as wide an ownership as possible to ensure that they will be promoted rather than attacked. And they must be clearly seen as a living document that will be updated and modified as new evidence becomes available.

Reference

[1] The National Heart Foundation of Australia and the Cardiac Society of Australia and New Zealand, The Lipid Management Guidelines—2001, Med. J. Aust. 175 (2001) S57–S88.

International Congress Series 1262 (2004) 188–192

www.ics-elsevier.com

Japan Atherosclerosis Society (JAS) guidelines for diagnosis and treatment of atherosclerotic cardiovascular diseases

Hiroshi Mabuchi*

Molecular Genetics of Cardiovascular Disorders, Division of Cardiovascular Medicine, Kanazawa University Graduate School of Medical Science, Takahara-machi 13-1, Kanazawa, Japan

Abstract. Japan Atherosclerosis Society (JAS) published Guidelines for Diagnosis and Treatment of Atherosclerotic Cardiovascular Diseases 2002. According to the global risk, the patients are categorized into six groups in the guidelines. The global risks in ATP III is 5–10 times higher than JAS guidelines. For this reason, clinical guidelines for prevention of Coronary heart disease (CHD) must be adapted and modified according to national and regional requirements. © 2004 Published by Elsevier B.V.

Keywords: Guideline; Cholesterol; Coronary heart disease; Relative risk; Absolute risk

1. Japan Atherosclerosis Society (JAS) Guidelines for Diagnosis and Treatment of Atherosclerotic Cardiovascular Disease 2002

The JAS Epidemiology and Treatment Committee published JAS Guidelines for Diagnosis and Treatment of Atherosclerotic Cardiovascular Diseases 2002 [1]. The guidelines are designed for the management of hypercholesterolemia, but emphasize that atherosclerosis is a multiple-risk disease and the treatment of this disorder must be based on the idea of comprehensive risk reduction.

1.1. Serum lipid values for screening

It has been shown in Japan as well as in western countries that a higher incidence of myocardial infarction is observed among those with a higher serum cholesterol level and a lower incidence among those with lower cholesterol levels [2]. In the current JAS guidelines, hypercholesterolemia was defined as total cholesterol 220 mg/dl or higher and LDL-C 140 mg/dl or higher, and the value less than 40 mg/dl as low HDL-C, and the value above 150 mg/dl as hypertriglyceridemia.

* Tel.: +81-76-265-2000; fax: +81-76-234-4251.
E-mail address: mabuchi@med.kanazawa-u.ac.jp (H. Mabuchi).

0531-5131/ © 2004 Published by Elsevier B.V.
doi:10.1016/j.ics.2003.12.109

Table 1
Japanese Atherosclerosis Society management goals by patient category for primary and secondary prevention of atherosclerotic diseases

Risk category	Coronary Heart Disease*	Major coronary risk factors other than LDL-C**	Lipid management goal (mg/dl)				Management of Other CHD Risk		
			TC	LDL-C	HDL-C	TG	Hyper-tension	Diabetes mellitus	Cigarette smoking
A	Absent	0	<240	<160	≧40	<150	Follow the guidelines by the Japanese Society of Hypertension	Follow the guidelines by the Japan Diabetes Society	Smoking cessation
B1		1	<220	<140					
B2		2							
B3		3	<200	<120					
B4		>4							
C	Present		<180	<100					

TC:total cholesterol; LDL-C:LDL-cholesterol, HDL-C:HDL-cholesterol, TG:triglyceride.

* Coronary heart disease is myocardial infarction and angina pectoris.

** Major coronary risk factors other than LDL-C: age (≧45 years for men, 55 years for women), hypertension, diabetes mellitus (including impaired glucose tolerance), cigarette smoking, family history of coronary heart disease, Low HDL-cholesterolemia (HDL-C<40mg/dl).

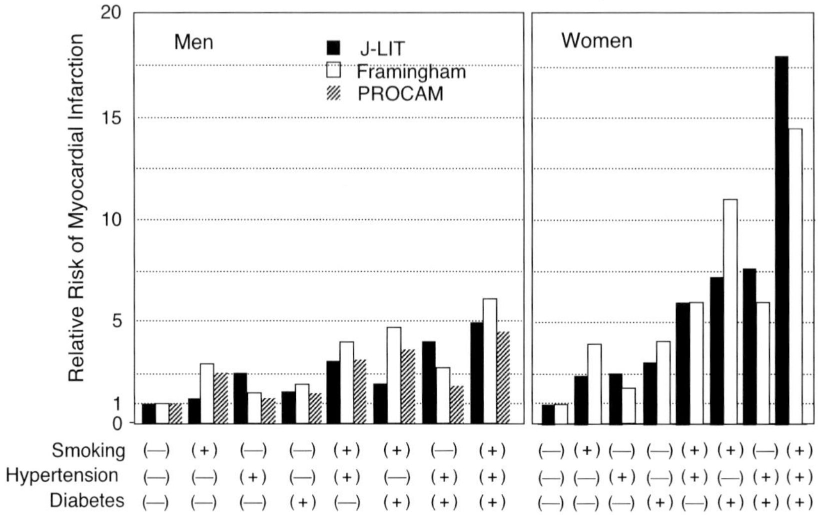

Fig. 1. Relative risk of myocardial infarction calculated by the equations of J-LIT, Framingham Heart Study, and PROCAM. Relative risks are similar among these assessments.

1.2. Risk assessment for categorization of patients and their management goals

A major issue about direct application of the NCEP guidelines [3] to Japanese guidelines was the significant difference in the overall prevalence of coronary heart disease (CHD) between Japanese and Americans/Europeans; the CHD incidence in Japan is approximately 1/4 of western levels [4]. Prevalence of CHD and its association with risk factors among Japanese were evaluated in the Japan-Lipid Intervention Trial (J-LIT), a

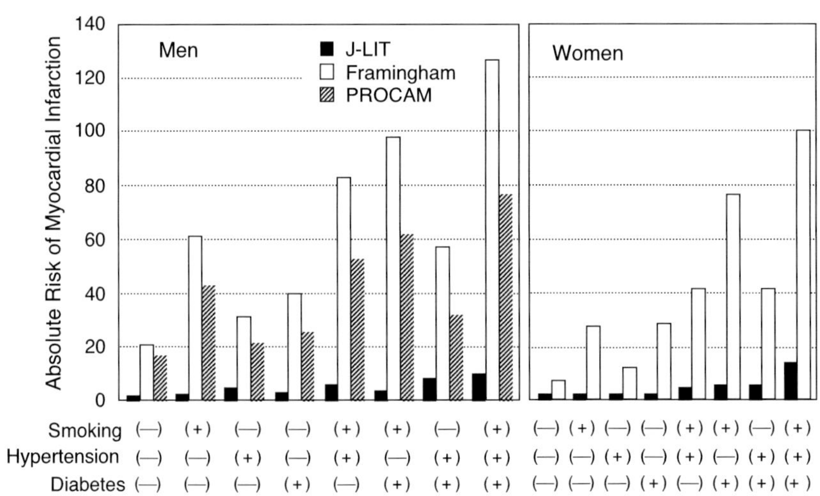

Fig. 2. Absolute risk of myocardial infarction calculated by the equations of J-LIT, Framingham Heart Study, and PROCAM. Absolute risks are quite different among these assessments.

Table 2
Comparison between Japanese Atherosolerosis Society (JAS) guidelines and NCEP-ATP III

	JAS guidelines				NCEP-ATPIII			
	CHD	Other coronary risk factors	Absolute risk (%)*	Goal of LDL-C management (mg/dl)	Goal of LDL-C management (mg/dl)	CHD	Other coronary risk factors	Absolute risk (%)*
A	–	0		<160	<160	–	0	
B1	–	1	0.5	<140			1	
B2	–	2	1		<130	–	2+	<10
B3	–	3	2.1	<120				10–20
B4	–	>4	4.4		<100		CHD-Eq	>20
C	+		12.2	<100		+		

*Incidence of coronary heart disease (%)/10 years.
CHD: coronary heart disease, CHD-Eq: CHD-equivalent.

prospective observation of 51,321 patients who were administered a low dose of simvastatin since 1992 [5,6]. Definite risk factors other than LDL-C (total cholesterol) used in this categorization are age, hypertension, diabetes mellitus (including glucose intolerance), CHD family history, and low HDL-C. The relative CHD risk in primary prevention increases exponentially as 2-, 4-, 8-, 15-, and 31-fold, those without any risk as the number of risks increases as 1, 2, 3, 4, and 5 [5,6]. According to the global risk, the patients are categorized into six groups in the guidelines (Table 1) [1]. For primary prevention of those without other risks (category A), LDL-C should be kept below 160 mg/dl (corresponds to a total cholesterol of 240 mg/dl). The goals are set for LDL-C below 140 mg/dl (corresponds to a total cholesterol of 220 mg/dl) in the patients with one (category B1) or two risk factors (category B2), LDL-C below 120 mg/dl (total cholesterol 200 mg/dl) in patients with three (category B3) or more risk factors (category B4). For the secondary prevention (category C), the treatment goal for LDL-C is set below 100 mg/dl (corresponds to a total cholesterol of 180 mg/dl). The goals for triglyceride, below 150 mg/dl, and for HDL-C, above 40 mg/dl, are set for all the groups. Primary prevention must be attempted first by improvement of lifestyle. If patients do not respond well to the treatment to achieve the target levels, then appropriate drug treatment must be considered.

2. Comparison of JAS guidelines and ATP III guidelines, and international harmonized guidelines

In Japan, there are very few prospective studies, but several Japanese cross-sectional epidemiological data coincide with those of MRFIT [2]. Therefore, relative risks of CHD are the same throughout the world. However, the absolute incidences of CHD death among various countries are quite different [4]. To assess the absolute risk of developing CHD, most of the European and American guidelines use algorithms developed by the Framingham Heart Study [8]. However, Framingham risk scoring cannot be applied to Japanese and other east Asian people. Comparisons among Framingham Heart Study, PROCAM study [9], and J-LIT [5,6] have shown that number of coronary events per 1000-persons-year in each study were 5.8, 7.0, and 1.0, respectively. Relative risks of MI were calculated by J-LIT, Framingham, and PROCAM equations. Relative risks are almost same in any assessment (Fig. 1). However, the absolute risks are quite different, and those of J-LIT are much smaller than PROCAM and Framingham (Fig. 2).

Comparison between JAS guidelines [7] and ATP III [2] showed apparent differences. In both guidelines, the patients were separated into six categories according to the number of risk factors and global risk within 10 years (Table 2). However, the global risks in ATP III is 5–10 times higher than JAS guidelines. For this reason, clinical guidelines for prevention of CHD must be adapted and modified according to national and regional requirements.

3. Conclusions

Relative risks are similar in different countries, and the benefits of risk-factor modification are universal, even though the absolute incidence of CHD is the highest in northern and eastern European countries, and lowest in Japan and eastern Asia. JAS has to make guidelines according to the data of Japanese people.

References

[1] H. Mabuchi, S. Biro, G. Egusa, M. Eto, et al., JAS Committee for Epidemiology and Clinical Management of Atherosclerosis, Japan Atherosclerosis Society (JAS) guidelines for diagnosis and treatment of atherosclerotic cardiovascular diseases, J. Atheroscler. Thromb. (2002) (in press).

[2] J. Stamler, D. Wentworth, J.D. Neaton, Is relationship between serum cholesterol and risk of premature death from coronary heart disease continuous and graded? Findings in 356,222 primary screenees of the Multiple Risk Factor Intervention Trial (MRFIT), JAMA 256 (1986) 2823–2828.

[3] Expert Panel on Detection, Evaluation, and Treatment of High Blood Cholesterol in Adults, Executive summary of the third report of The National Cholesterol Education Program (NCEP) expert panel on detection, evaluation, and treatment of high blood cholesterol in adults (Adult Treatment Panel III), JAMA 285 (2001) 2486–2497.

[4] W.M. Verschuren, D.R. Jacobs, B.P. Bloemberg, et al., Serum total cholesterol and long-term coronary heart disease mortality in different cultures. Twenty-five-year follow-up of the seven countries study, JAMA 274 (1998) 131–136.

[5] M. Matsuzaki, T. Kita, H. Mabuchi, et al., J-LIT Study Group, Japan Lipid Intervention Trial. Large scale cohort study of the relationship between serum cholesterol concentration and coronary events with low-dose simvastatin therapy in Japanese patients with hypercholesterolemia, primary prevention cohort study of the Japan Lipid Intervention Trial (J-LIT), Circ. J. 66 (2002) 1087–1095.

[6] H. Mabuchi, T. Kita, M. Matsuzaki, et al., J-LIT Study Group, Japan Lipid Intervention Trial. Large scale cohort study of the relationship between serum cholesterol concentration and coronary events with low-dose simvastatin therapy in Japanese patients with hypercholesterolemia and coronary heart disease: secondary prevention cohort study of the Japan Lipid Intervention Trial (J-LIT), Circ. J. 66 (2002) 1096–1100.

[7] T. Okamura, T. Kadowaki, T. Hayakawa, et al., Nippon Data80 Research Group, What cause of mortality can we predict by cholesterol screening in the Japanese general population? J. Intern. Med. 253 (2003) 169–180.

[8] P.W. Wilson, R.B. D'Agostino, D. Levy, et al., Prediction of coronary heart disease using risk factor categories, Circulation 97 (1998) 1837–1847.

[9] G. Assmann, P. Cullen, H. Schulte, Simple scoring scheme for calculating the risk of acute coronary events based on the 10-year follow-up of the prospective cardiovascular Munster (PROCAM) study, Circulation 105 (2002) 310–315.

International Congress Series 1262 (2004) 193–199

www.ics-elsevier.com

Low HDL-C: lessons learned from the Turkish Heart Study

U. Hodoğlugil[a], D. Williamson[a], R.W. Mahley[a,b,*]

[a] *Gladstone Institute of Cardiovascular Disease, University of California, San Francisco, P.O. Box 419100, San Francisco, CA 94141-9100, USA*

[b] *Departments of Pathology and Medicine, University of California, San Francisco, P.O. Box 419100, San Francisco, CA 94141-9100, USA*

Abstract. Low levels of high-density lipoprotein cholesterol (HDL-C) are highly prevalent in Turks. Analysis of approximately 10,000 Turkish men and women revealed the lowest HDL-C levels of any previously characterized population (~10–15 mg/dl lower than in western Europeans or Americans). These low HDL-C levels are primarily of genetic origin. A survey of the activities of candidate enzymes and transfer proteins showed that Turks have uniquely elevated hepatic lipase mass and activity, and their hepatic lipase levels are 25–30% higher than in non-Turkish American controls. As in other populations, Turkish newborns of both sexes have low total cholesterol and HDL-C levels (~30 mg/dl), and 8–9-year-old boys and girls have virtually identical HDL-C levels (50–60 mg/dl) similar to those in other populations. After puberty, however, HDL-C levels decrease markedly to typical adult levels, 36–37 mg/dl in males and 40–43 mg/dl in females. The mechanism for these striking reductions is unknown. Recent studies have shown that polymorphisms in the ATP-binding cassette A1 protein (ABCA1) and cholesterol ester transfer protein (CETP) are associated with altered HDL-C in Turks. Furthermore, a polymorphism in acyl CoA:diacylglycerol acyltransferase (DGAT) is associated with altered body mass index (BMI), HDL-C, and blood pressure in Turks.

Keywords: HDL; Hepatic lipase; ATP-binding cassette A1; Cholesterol ester transfer protein; Acyl CoA:diacylglycerol acyltransferase

1. Introduction

Analysis of risk factors for coronary heart disease conducted as part of the Turkish Heart Study revealed that low levels of high-density lipoprotein cholesterol (HDL-C) are highly prevalent in Turks [1]. Lipid studies of approximately 10,000 Turkish adult men and women living in six different regions of Turkey demonstrated that the Turks have

* Corresponding author. Gladstone Institute of Cardiovascular Disease, University of California, San Francisco, P.O. Box 419100, San Francisco, CA 94141-9100, USA. Tel.: +1-415-826-7500; fax: +1-415-285-5632.

E-mail address: rmahley@gladstone.ucsf.edu (R.W. Mahley).

0531-5131/
doi:10.1016/j.ics.2004.01.098

some of the lowest HDL-C levels of any population in the world (~ 53% of men and 26% of women had HDL-C levels <35 mg/dl). Turks living in Germany and the United States also had low HDL-C levels, suggesting that the condition is at least partly of genetic origin [2,3]. Low HDL-C was associated with an increase in hepatic lipase (levels 25–30% higher than in non-Turkish American controls) [2]. The prevalence of low HDL-C levels in Turks is not explained by hypertriglyceridemia or the metabolic syndrome [1–7]. The observations related to the unique lipid profile of Turks have been confirmed and extended by Onat et al. [4,5].

2. Discussion

2.1. Characterization of HDL subclasses

To define more precisely the factors associated with low HDL in Turks, we have characterized the HDL subclasses [6]. Turks have low levels of HDL_2, LpAI, and preβ-1 HDL and increased levels of LpAI/AII particles (potentially an atherogenic lipid profile). The frequency distributions of HDL-C and LpAI levels were skewed toward bimodality in Turkish women but were unimodal in Turkish men. The apolipoprotein (apo) E genotype affected HDL-C and LpAI levels in women only. In women, but not men, the ε2 allele was strikingly more prevalent in those with the highest levels of HDL-C and LpAI than in those with the lowest levels [6]. The higher prevalence of the ε2 allele in these subgroups of women was not explained by plasma triglyceride or total cholesterol level, age, or body mass index (BMI). The modulating effects of apoE isoforms on lipolytic hydrolysis of HDL by hepatic lipase (apoE2 prevents efficient hydrolysis) or on lipoprotein receptor binding (apoE2 interacts poorly with the LDL receptor) may account for differences in HDL-C levels in Turkish women (the ε2 allele is associated with higher HDL levels). In Turkish men, who have substantially higher levels of hepatic lipase activity than women, the modulating effect of apoE may be overwhelmed. The gender-specific effect of the apoE genotype on HDL-C and LpAI levels in association with elevated levels of hepatic lipase provides new insights into the metabolism of HDL.

2.2. Effect of puberty on plasma lipids

Our most recent studies were designed to determine if HDL-C levels are unusually low throughout life in Turks and to assess the effect of puberty on plasma lipids in Turks [7]. The plasma lipids of cord blood of healthy newborns (n=105) and 8–10-year-old school children (n=225) have been analyzed in ethnic Turks [7]. Lipid values in typical western European populations and in Turks are shown in Table 1. Typically, newborns have very low total cholesterol and HDL-C levels that are virtually identical in males and females. Both total cholesterol and HDL-C levels rise with age, and there are no gender differences before puberty. The HDL-C levels of 8–9-year-old western European children were 50–60 mg/dl and were virtually identical in both males and females. Turkish newborns and prepubescent children have somewhat lower total cholesterol levels, but have similar HDL-C levels (mean for the prepubescent group, ~ 50 mg/dl) (Table 1).

After puberty, however, HDL-C levels in western European males decrease to typical adult levels (~ 47 mg/dl) and in females decrease much less to typical adult levels (~ 55–

Table 1
Plasma lipid levels change with age

	Western Europeans		Turks	
	Total cholesterol (mg/dl)	HDL-C (mg/dl)	Total cholesterol (mg/dl)	HDL-C (mg/dl)
Newborns	<100	~ 30	~ 60	~ 30
Male/female differences	none	none	none	none
Children	135–165	55–60	~ 140	50–60
Male/female differences	none	none	none	none
Young adults	>160	47–57	>160	37–43
Male/female differences	M>F	M: 66–60→47 F: 55–60→55	M>F	M: 58→37* F: 55→43

* Values shown here are for Turks in the upper socioeconomic groups whose diets are similar to those of western European populations.

57 mg/dl) (Table 1) (for reviews, see Refs. [7–9]). On the other hand, the HDL-C levels in Turkish boys drop from a mean of ~ 58 to 37 mg/dl and then the levels remain at 36–37 mg/dl during adulthood [7]. The HDL-C levels in Turkish girls decrease from ~ 55 to 43 mg/dl and remain at an average of 40–43 mg/dl in adulthood [7]. The changes in HDL-C levels in Turks are illustrated in Fig. 1.

The mechanism for the striking reduction in HDL-C levels after puberty in Turks is unknown. We hypothesize that androgen production plays a major role in modulating HDL-C levels at puberty. Consistent with this hypothesis is the observation from Hergenç et al. [10], suggesting that Turks have lower levels of sex hormone-binding globulin, which should result in increased levels of free bioactive testosterone in both males and females. Hepatic lipase production is regulated by androgens, and high levels of androgens are associated with increased levels and activity of hepatic lipase. Thus, high levels of free

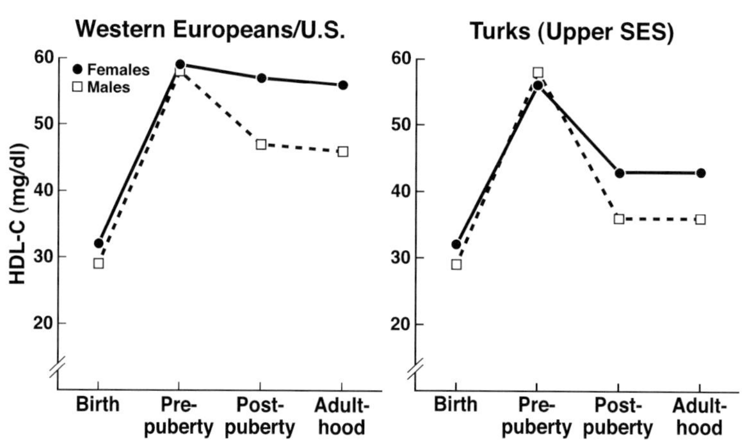

Fig. 1. Changes in HDL-C levels with age. There is a dramatic difference in the magnitude of the decrease in HDL-C levels post puberty in the western European versus Turkish males and females. Values for the Turkish children are those from upper socioeconomic status (SES) groups since the diet of this group closely resembles the European diets with respect to carbohydrate and fat.

testosterone may explain the high levels of hepatic lipase activity and protein mass that are characteristic of Turkish males and females.

We have begun to explore single nucleotide polymorphic sites that may be associated with lipid abnormalities and coronary artery disease in the Turkish population. To date, we have examined polymorphic sites in acyl CoA:diacylglycerol acyltransferase (DGAT), cholesterol ester transfer protein (CETP), and the ATP-binding cassette A1 protein (ABCA1).

2.3. DGAT polymorphisms

Studies characterizing DGAT promoter polymorphisms were undertaken using genomic DNA from Turkish Heart Study participants [11]. Plasma lipid and lipoprotein profiles in Turks have demonstrated lower plasma HDL-C levels and increased triglyceride levels. Turks also have slightly higher systolic and diastolic blood pressures than other populations. In addition, as in other populations, obesity has become a major health issue for Turkish people. About 50% of Turkish men and women were overweight (BMI>25 kg/m^2), and 11% of men and 22% of women were obese (BMI>30 kg/m^2). A more recent study has shown an increase in the prevalence of obesity in Turks, with 38% of Turkish women being obese [12]. These observations suggested that studies of the enzymes involved in triglyceride metabolism and adipose tissue biology might be revealing.

DGAT catalyzes the synthesis of triglyceride from fatty acyl CoA and diacylglycerol, and DGAT deficiency in mice is associated with leanness and resistance to diet-induced obesity [13–15]. In a recent study, we identified five polymorphisms within the human DGAT promoter and 5′ noncoding sequence [11]. One common variant, a C to T transition 79 bases 3′ of the transcriptional start site was associated with lower BMI, higher HDL-C, and lower systolic and diastolic blood pressures (p=0.003, 0.058, 0.020,

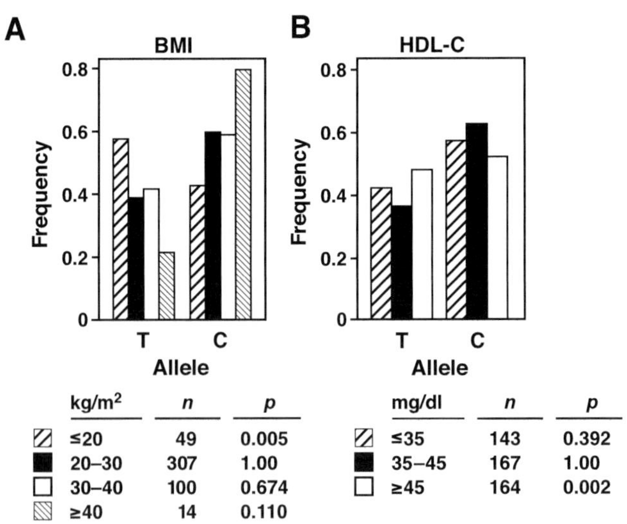

Fig. 2. Distributions and frequencies of the C79T alleles according to BMI and HDL-C in women. All p values were determined by chi-square test for independence. (A) Each group was compared with the control group (BMI>20 to <30 kg/m^2). (B) The low and high HDL-C groups were compared with the moderate HDL group.

and 0.015, respectively) in randomly selected Turkish women (n=476). In a subsequent case-control study, the 79TT genotype and 79T allele were significantly associated with lower BMI (p=0.0003 and 0.0001, respectively), higher HDL-C levels (p=0.0039 and 0.0016), lower diastolic (p=0.0057 and 0.0034), and lower systolic blood pressure (p=0.0144 and 0.0077) in Turkish women (Fig. 2). Functional analysis of the C79T polymorphism in the DGAT promoter by transient transfection experiments in cultured adipocytes, hepatocytes, and intestinal cells revealed a 20–33% decrease in promoter activity for the 79T allele compared with the 79C allele. Our data indicate that, in Turkish women, the DGAT C79T polymorphism is associated with alterations in three parameters that are features of the metabolic syndrome—body weight, HDL-C level, and blood pressure—and suggest that this polymorphism may contribute to these effects.

2.4. Cholesterol ester transfer protein

CETP facilitates the transfer of cholesterol esters and neutral lipids between HDL and apoB-containing lipoproteins (for a review, see Ref. [16]). High levels of CETP activity result in low HDL-C levels. Several groups have shown that the *Taq*IB polymorphism in CETP affects HDL-C levels [17–19]. Genotyping of 1219 Turkish males and 792 Turkish females revealed that the B2 polymorphism was associated with significantly higher HDL-

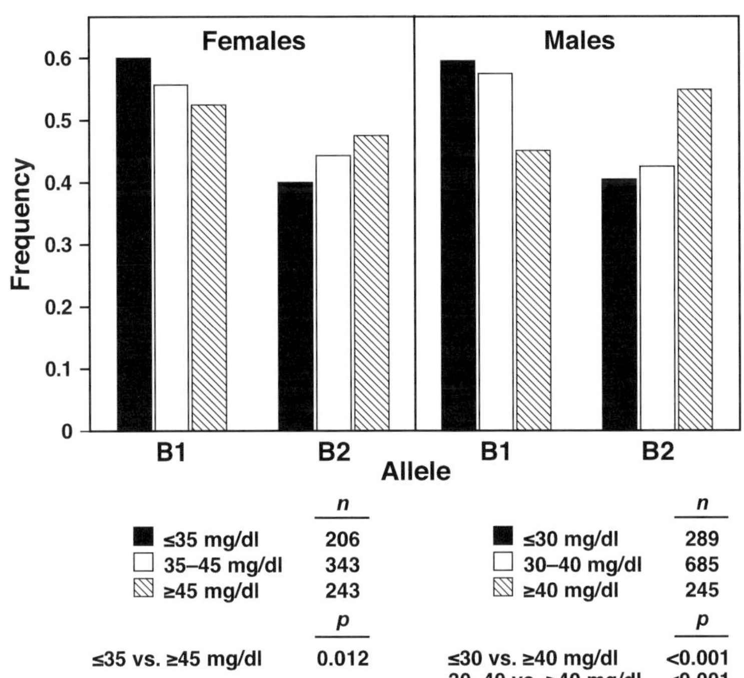

Fig. 3. Frequencies of the CETP *Taq*IB variation in a random male and female Turkish population. Alleles are defined as B1 (common) and B2 (rare). Allele frequencies are stratified by HDL-C level. Statistical significance was determined by chi-square analysis. n, number of subjects for each group.

C levels (Fig. 3). Individuals with the CETP B2B2 genotype had lower plasma CETP activity and higher HDL-C levels than those with the B1B1 genotype.

2.5. ATP-binding cassette A1 protein

ABCA1, which transports free cholesterol and phospholipid across plasma membranes to form HDL-C in the plasma (for a review, see Ref. [20]), represents an ideal target to study in this Turkish population with low HDL-C. Thus far, two polymorphic sites, one in the promoter region and the other in the coding sequence, have proven to be of interest.

In a random Turkish population of ~2700 men and women, the C−14T promoter polymorphism was associated with variable HDL-C levels. In men, the less frequent −14T (~38% in the Turkish population) allele was associated with significantly higher HDL-C levels (~5.5% increase) than the −14C allele. There was no association between the C−14T polymorphism and HDL-C levels in Turkish females. In cultured Cos-7, Chinese hamster ovary, and HepG2 cells expressing a luciferase construct encoding the −14T promoter polymorphism, luciferase activity increased by 25–75%.

The V771M variant in exon 16 was also associated with significantly higher HDL-C levels in Turkish males but not in females. We have begun to analyze haplotypes to demonstrate the effect of other ABCA1 polymorphic sites on V771M, especially in Turkish females. These studies are likely to reveal the importance of ABCA1 polymorphisms on HDL-C levels in Turks.

3. Summary

Continued studies of the Turkish population will shed light on the multiple genetic factors that modulate HDL-C levels. Undoubtedly, the interaction between genes and environment plays a key role in determining the lipid profile characteristic of Turks.

Acknowledgements

We are indebted to our associates at the American Hospital, Istanbul, especially Guy Pépin and Sibel Tanir in the Gladstone Institute (Istanbul), and Dr. K. Erhan Palaoğlu at the American Hospital (Istanbul). We thank Sylvia Richmond and Theresa Hashim for manuscript preparation and Stephen Ordway and Gary Howard for editorial assistance. We acknowledge the generous support of the American Hospital, especially Mr. George Rountree, and the J. David Gladstone Institutes. This work was supported in part by R01 grant HL71027 from the National Institutes of Health.

References

[1] R.W. Mahley, et al., Turkish Heart Study: lipids, lipoproteins, and apolipoproteins, J. Lipid Res. 36 (1995) 839–859.

[2] T.P. Bersot, et al., Elevated hepatic lipase activity and low levels of high density lipoprotein in a normotriglyceridemic, nonobese Turkish population, J. Lipid Res. 40 (1999) 432–438.

[3] S. Lüttmann, et al., Electrophoretic screening for genetic variation in apolipoprotein C-III: identification of a novel apoC-III variant, apoC-III(Asp45→Asn), in a Turkish patient, J. Lipid Res. 35 (1994) 1431–1440.

[4] A. Onat, et al., Plasma lipoproteins and apolipoproteins in Turkish adults: overall levels, associations with

other risk parameters and HDL's role as a marker of coronary risk in women (in Turkish), Arch. Turk. Soc. Cardiol. 27 (1999) 72–79.
[5] A. Onat, Risk factors and cardiovascular disease in Turkey, Atherosclerosis 156 (2001) 1–10.
[6] R.W. Mahley, et al., Low levels of high density lipoproteins in Turks, a population with elevated hepatic lipase: high density lipoprotein characterization and gender-specific effects of apolipoprotein E genotype, J. Lipid Res. 41 (2000) 1290–1301.
[7] R.W. Mahley, et al., Plasma lipids in Turkish children: impact of puberty, socioeconomic status, and nutrition on plasma cholesterol and HDL, J. Lipid Res. 42 (2001) 1996–2006.
[8] C.M. Loughrey, et al., Race and gender differences in cord blood lipoproteins, Atherosclerosis 148 (2000) 57–65.
[9] L.S. Webber, et al., Tracking of serum lipids and lipoproteins from childhood to adulthood. The Bogalusa Heart Study, Am. J. Epidemiol. 133 (1991) 884–899.
[10] G. Hergenç, et al., Associations of obesity markers, insulin, and sex hormones with HDL-cholesterol levels in Turkish and German individuals, Atherosclerosis 145 (1999) 147–156.
[11] E.H. Ludwig, et al., DGAT1 promoter polymorphism associated with alterations in body mass index, high density lipoprotein levels and blood pressure in Turkish women, Clin. Genet. 62 (2002) 68–73.
[12] A. Onat, et al., Indices of obesity and central obesity in Turkish adults: distinct rise in obesity in 1990–98 more pronounced among men, (in Turkish). Arch. Turk. Soc. Cardiol. 27 (1999) 209–217.
[13] S.J. Smith, et al., Obesity resistance and multiple mechanisms of triglyceride synthesis in mice lacking DGAT, Nat. Genet. 25 (2000) 87–90.
[14] S. Cases, et al., Identification of a gene encoding an acyl CoA: diacylglycerol acyltransferase, a key enzyme in triacylglycerol synthesis, Proc. Natl. Acad. Sci. U. S. A. 95 (1998) 13018–13023.
[15] R.V. Farese Jr., S. Cases, S.J. Smith, Triglyceride synthesis: insights from the cloning of diacylglycerol acyltransferase, Curr. Opin. Lipidol. 11 (2000) 229–234.
[16] A. Ritsch, J.R. Patsch, Cholesteryl ester transfer protein: gathering momentum as a genetic marker and as drug target, Curr. Opin. Lipidol. 14 (2003) 173–178.
[17] M. Corbex, et al., Extensive association analysis between the CETP gene and coronary heart disease phenotypes reveals several putative functional polymorphisms and gene=environment interaction, Genet. Epidemiol. 19 (2000) 64–80.
[18] J.M. Ordovas, et al., Association of cholesteryl ester transfer protein–*Taq*IB polymorphism with variations in lipoprotein subclasses and coronary heart disease risk. The Framingham Study, Arterioscler. Thromb. Vasc. Biol. 20 (2000) 1323–1329.
[19] M.E. Brousseau, et al., Cholesteryl ester transfer protein TaqI B2B2 genotype is associated with higher HDL cholesterol levels and lower risk of coronary heart disease end points in men with HDL deficiency. Veterans Affairs HDL Cholesterol Intervention Trial, Arterioscler. Thromb. Vasc. Biol. 22 (2002) 1148–1154.
[20] A.D. Attie, J.P. Kastelein, M.R. Hayden, Pivotal role of ABCA1 in reverse cholesterol transport influencing HDL levels and susceptibility to atherosclerosis, J. Lipid Res. 42 (2001) 1717–1726.

ELSEVIER

International Congress Series 1262 (2004) 200–202

www.ics-elsevier.com

Nonfasting serum triglycerides and risk of ischemic heart disease among Japanese men and women

Hiroyasu Iso[a,*], Akihiko Kitamura[b], Shinichi Sato[b], Yoshihiko Naito[b], Noriyuki Imano[b], Tetsuya Ohira[b], Kazumasa Yamagishi[a], Takeshi Tanigawa[a], Takashi Shimamoto[b]

[a] *Department of Public Health Medicine, Institute of Community Medicine, University of Tsukuba 1-1-1, Tennodai, Tsukuba, Ibaraki, 305-8575 Japan*

[b] *The Osaka Medical Center for Health Science and Promotion, Osaka, Japan*

Abstract. To examine the relation of triglycerides with ischemic heart disease (IHD) among populations with low mean total cholesterol, we conducted a 16-year prospective study of 11,068 Japanese aged 40–69 (4452 men and 6616 women with mean total cholesterol=4.73 and 5.03 mmol/l, respectively), initially free of IHD or stroke. We documented 236 IHD events comprising 133 myocardial infarctions, 68 angina pectoris and 44 sudden cardiac deaths. Median values of serum triglycerides were higher among IHD incident cases than among controls in each of subgroups of time since last meal <2, 2, 3–7 and 8 h or more. Median difference was particularly large in the subgroup of 3–7 h since last meal (0.90 mmol/l for men and 0.75 mmol/l for women). The IHD incidence was greater in a dose-response manner across increasing quartiles of nonfasting triglycerides for both sexes. The multivariate relative risk of CHD adjusting for coronary risk factors and time since last meal was 2.81 (95% CI, 1.56–5.05) for men and 2.76 (1.34–5.68) for women. The multivariate relative risk associated with 1 mmol/l greater triglycerides was 1.29 (1.09–1.53) for men and 1.42 (1.15–1.75) for women. The trend was similar for myocardial infarction, angina pectoris and sudden cardiac death. The relation of triglycerides with IHD was not influenced materially by total cholesterol levels or in a subsample analysis (51% of total sample) by HDL cholesterol levels. Nonfasting serum triglycerides predict the incidence of IHD among Japanese men and women, who possess low mean values of total cholesterol.

Keywords: Triglyceride; Total cholesterol; Ischemic heart disease; Follow-up study

1. Introduction

Contributions of high total cholesterol, high LDL cholesterol and low HDL cholesterol concentrations to the development of ischemic heart disease (IHD) are well established, but the role of triglycerides is controversial [1]. To partially solve this methodological

* Corresponding author. Department of Public Health Medicine, Institute of Community Medicine, University of Tsukuba 1-1-1, Tennodai, Tsukuba, Ibaraki, 305-8575, Japan. Tel./fax: +81-298-53-2695.

E-mail address: fvgh5640@infoweb.ne.jp (H. Iso).

0531-5131/
doi:10.1016/j.ics.2004.01.014

problem in epidemiologic studies, several prospective studies have conducted subgroup analyses stratifying on levels of total, LDL cholesterol or HDL cholesterol, but the results has been inconsistent [2]. A study of populations with low cholesterol levels, such as Japanese men and women living in Japan, may be valuable to examine the relation between triglycerides and risk of IHD. Our a priori hypothesis was that serum triglycerides would be positively associated with risk of IHD, and the association would be similar in subgroups divided by medians of total and HDL cholesterol levels.

2. Material and methods

The surveyed population was residents aged 40–69 years in four communities who participated in cardiovascular risk surveys between 1975 and 1980 in a northeast rural community and a southwest rural community, and between 1981 and 1986 in a central rural community, and between 1975 and 1984 in a southwest urban suburb [3]. Persons with a history of IHD (n=61) and persons with missing values of triglycerides (n=241) were excluded, and the data of 11,068 persons (4452 men and 6616 women) were used for the analyses. Subjects were followed up on the average 16 years to determine IHD endpoints occurring by the end of 1997. The IHD endpoint was ascertained under systematic surveillance and the criteria for IHD were modified from those of a WHO Expert Committee.

At baseline, nonfasting blood was drawn and the serum was separated. The distribution of time since last meal was 39% for <2 h, 43% for 2 h, 9% for 3–7 h and 9% for 8 h and over. Serum triglycerides were measured by an enzymatic method and serum total cholesterol by the Liebermann–Burchard direct method using the Autoanalyzer II (Technicon, Terrytown, USA). For 51% of total sample (n=5641), HDL cholesterol was measured after heparin–manganese precipitation using the Libermann–Burchard method.

Person years were calculated as the sum of individual follow-up time until the occurrence of incident IHD, death, emigration, or the end of 1997. The relative risk of IHD incidence and its 95% confidence interval were calculated with reference to the risk of persons with the lowest quartile of serum triglycerides, using the Cox proportional hazards model.

3. Results

During the 16-year follow-up, there were 236 IHD events (135 in men and 101 in women), comprising 133 myocardial infarctions (86 in men and 47 in women), 68 angina pectoris (35 in men and 33 in women), and 44 sudden cardiac deaths (19 in men and 25 in women).

When stratified by time since last meal, there were consistent case control differences in medians of triglyceride levels for both men and women. The median difference was particularly large in the subgroup of 3–7 h since last meal: 0.90 mmol/l for men and 0.75 mmol/l for women. There was a dose-response relation between serum triglycerides and the risk of IHD; the multivariate relative risk in the highest vs. lowest quartiles of triglycerides was 2.81 (95%CI, 1.56–5.05) for men, and 2.76 (1.34–5.68) for women. The respective multivariate relative risks associated with a 1 mmol/l greater triglycerides were 1.29 (1.09–1.53) and 1.42 (1.15–1.75), while for women the relative risk associated with total serum cholesterol levels did not reach statistical significance.

The relation between triglycerides and IHD was similarly observed for persons with total cholesterol levels lower vs. higher than the median for men and women combined.

We conducted a subanalysis with further adjustment for HDL cholesterol (sample n=5641). For men and women combined, the multivariate relative risk of IHD remained significant, with some attenuation of the association. When examined by sex, the multivariate relative risk was of borderline significance for men (p=0.09) and remained significant for women (p=0.04). When stratified by HDL cholesterol levels above vs. below the median, we found a similar relation between triglycerides and risk of IHD. The interaction term between HDL cholesterol and triglycerides was not statistically significant for men and women combined, or either sex.

4. Discussion

Nonfasting serum triglycerides were positively associated with the incidence of IHD for Japanese men and women, whose mean serum total cholesterol was low by Western standards. For women, serum total cholesterol was not significantly associated with risk of IHD. The positive relation with triglycerides was similarly observed for men and women after adjustment for age, serum total cholesterol levels, serum glucose category, other coronary risk factors and time since last meal.

The relation between triglycerides and risk of IHD was not influenced by serum total cholesterol levels and this result was consistent with our hypothesis. Our study showed that even in a subgroup with lower cholesterol levels or higher HDL cholesterol levels, triglycerides were associated with increased risk of IHD, which strengthens the implication that triglyceride level is predictive of IHD with populations of low total cholesterol levels.

Because over 80% of the participants were nonfasting with a large case control difference in median triglycerides in postprandial state, our findings were primarily for postprandial triglycerides and IHD. A high triglyceride level postprandially is closely linked with delayed clearance of chylomicron remnants, which are taken up by the arterial wall by means other than the LDL cholesterol receptor, and thus are as atherogenic as LDL cholesterol. Furthermore, high triglyceride levels in either the postprandial or fasting state are associated with atherogenic small, LDL particles, which may be more atherogenic than larger LDL particles because of increased susceptibility to oxidation. High triglyceride levels are also associated with increased concentrations of factor VII and plasminogen activator inhibitor, increased insulin resistance, and increased blood leukocyte counts, all of which may accelerate atherosclerotic and thrombotic processes.

In conclusion, serum triglycerides predict the risk of IHD, independent of total cholesterol and HDL cholesterol, among Japanese men and women who possess low mean values of total cholesterol. A clinical trial is necessary to examine whether the lowering of triglycerides reduces risk of IHD among Japanese.

References

[1] M.A. Austin, Plasma triglyceride as a risk factor for IHD. The epidemiologic evidence and beyond, Am. J. Epidemiol. 129 (1989) 249–259.

[2] S.B. Hulley, R.H. Rosenman, R.D. Bawol, et al., Epidemiology as a guide to clinical decisions. The association between triglyceride and IHD, N. Engl. J. Med. 302 (1980) 1383–1389.

[3] H. Iso, Y. Naito, S. Sato, et al., Serum triglycerides and risk of coronary heart disease among Japanese men and women, Am. J. Epidemiol. 153 (2001) 490–499.

International Congress Series 1262 (2004) 203–206

www.ics-elsevier.com

Hypercholesterolemia and hypertriglyceridemia—greatest cardiac risk in subjects with high apoB/apoA-I levels

Göran Walldius[a,b,*], Are Aastveit[c], Ingmar Jungner[d]

[a] *King Gustaf V Research Institute, Karolinska Institute, Stockholm, Sweden*
[b] *AstraZeneca, SE-431 83 Molndal, Sweden*
[c] *Department of Mathematical Sciences, Agricultural University of Norway, As, Norway*
[d] *CALAB Research, Stockholm and Karolinska Institute, Stockholm, Sweden*

Abstract. Hypercholesterolemia and hypertriglyceridemia are risk factors for cardiovascular disease. The potentially atherogenic very low-density lipoprotein (VLDL), intermediate-density lipoprotein (IDL), large buoyant, and small dense low-density lipoprotein (LDL) particles are all transported by apolipoprotein (apo) B, one protein per particle. The anti-atherogenic HDL contains apoA-I. In the apolipoprotein-related mortality risk (AMORIS) study, 98,722 males and 76,831 females aged 20–80 years were investigated at health check-ups. They were followed for 98 months, and 1267 males and 586 females died from myocardial infarction. The aim of the study is to investigate if apoB and apoA-I are more closely related to cardiac risk than lipids. The most common lipid phenotype in those who died was combined hypercholesterol- and hypertriglyceridemia (type IIB, 48%), followed by isolated hypercholesterolemia (type IIA, 40%). However, irrespective of lipid phenotype, and also in subjects with normal lipids, the highest CV risk was seen in those with a high apoB/apoA-I (>0.9 in males, >0.8 in females) compared with those with values below these cut-points. It is concluded that the balance of apoB/apoA-I is a simple and precise indicator strongly reflecting CV risk irrespective of lipid levels or combinations of lipids. © 2004 Published by Elsevier B.V.

Keywords: Apolipoprotein B; Apolipoprotein A-I; Cholesterol; Triglycerides; Myocardial infarction

1. Introduction

Hypercholesterolemia due to high levels of low-density lipoprotein (LDL) cholesterol (C), hypertriglyceridemia often associated with low values of high-density lipoprotein (HDL)-C, and especially combined hyperlipidemias are all associated with increased risk of cardiovascular morbidity and mortality. The potentially atherogenic lipoprotein particles very low density (VLDL), intermediate density (IDL), large buoyant LDL, and small

* Corresponding author. AstraZeneca, SE-431 83 Molndal, Sweden. Tel.: +46-31-776-2678; fax: +46-31-776-3802.

E-mail address: goran.walldius@astrazeneca.com (G. Walldius).

0531-5131/ © 2004 Published by Elsevier B.V.
doi:10.1016/j.ics.2003.12.033

dense LDL all contain one apolipoprotein (apo) B per particle, whereas the anti-atherogenic HDL particles contain apoA-I, the major apolipoprotein that can remove excess cholesterol from peripheral tissues and transport it back to the liver in the reverse cholesterol transport. New data from our apolipoprotein-related mortality risk (AMORIS) study [1] and other prospective data [2], as well as results from lipid-lowering trials, indicate that the higher the values for the ratio, i.e., the balance between apoB/apoA-I, the greater is the risk of suffering from a cardiac event [2]. The objective of the present AMORIS report is to analyse if an abnormal apoB/apoA-I balance can identify those at greatest risk of a fatal acute myocardial infarction (AMI) irrespective of their lipid levels and their lipid phenotypes.

2. Materials and methods

In the AMORIS study, we have followed prospectively 98,722 males and 76,831 females from under 20 to above 80 years of age at entry for in average 98 months. The subjects were investigated at health check-ups, and no patients were hospitalized or investigated in acute situations. All details on the design, laboratory, and statistical methods have been described previously [1,3].

In the present report, the results from the cohort of individuals above 40 years of age at entry are presented. The subjects were classified in different lipid phenotypes based on TC cut levels of 5.0 mmol/l and TG cut levels of 1.5 mmol/l. Thus, isolated hypercholesterolemia is indicated as type IIA subjects, isolated hypertriglyceridemia as type IV subjects, and combined hyperlipidemias as type IIB subjects. Normal individuals (N) had lipid levels below both cut values. Prevalence numbers for the different lipid phenotypes are given. The subjects were also categorized according to their apoB/apoA-I ratio. The cut values chosen were 0.9 for males and 0.8 for females. These cut-points were chosen based on the cumulative curves for apoB/apoA-I values corresponding to about the 25th percentile of those dying from an AMI.

3. Results

At entry into the study, the most common lipid phenotype was type IIA, which occurred in about 45% of the males and in 58% of the females. The corresponding numbers for type IIB were 39% and 25%, respectively. Isolated hypertriglyceridemia, i.e., type IV, was uncommon—below 5% in both genders.

At the follow-up, 1243 males and 586 females died from AMI. A total of 48% of all subjects suffering a fatal AMI had type IIB hyperlipidemia, and above 40% had type IIA hypercholesterolemia. Type IV occurred only in 2–4% of the subjects and in only 8% of males and 6% of females with normal TC and TG levels. The highest risks were seen in subjects with type IIB hyperlipidemia, similar in both genders with $p<0.0001$, compared with subjects having normal lipid levels. AMI risk was also higher in type IIA subjects, $p<0.0001$ for both genders, as well as for subjects with type IV hypertriglyceridemia, $p<0.004$ for males, and $p<0.005$ for females.

In all subjects, males and females pooled, irrespective of their lipid phenotype, the risk was significantly greater in those having a high apoB/apoA-I value with a mean value of about 1 or higher, compared with those with a low value, $p<0.0001$ for all phenotypes

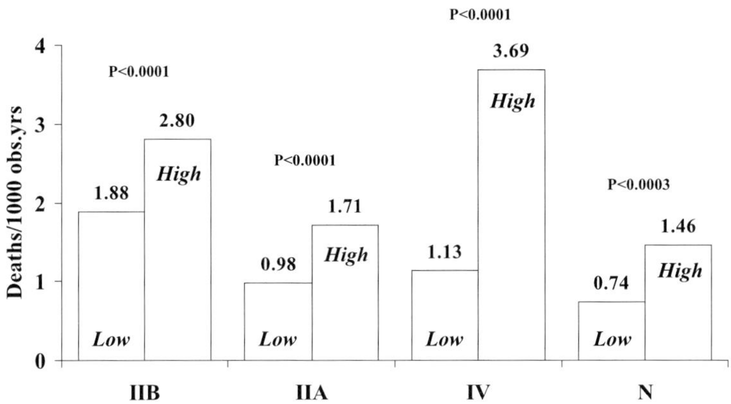

ApoB/apoA-I	0.75	1.25	0.69	1.07	0.70	1.06	0.63	0.99
ApoB, g/L	1.18	1.65	1.11	1.47	0.95	1.18	0.88	1.12
ApoA-I, g/L	1.60	1.35	1.63	1.39	1.38	1.13	1.42	1.15
TC, mmol/L	6.09	6.91	5.98	6.59	4.55	4.67	4.50	4.62
TG, mmol/L	2.34	2.66	0.91	1.08	2.22	2.47	0.83	0.98
AMI	100	784	242	510	18	43	91	41
Prevalence	7074	35232	31171	33983	2145	1520	14951	2962

Fig. 1. Cardiac risk (deaths/1000 obs.yrs.) in relation to lipid phenotypes and levels of apoB/apoA-I.

(Fig. 1). Also in subjects with normal lipids, those with a high apoB/apoA-I ratio had a greater risk, $p<0.0003$. However, although they were comparatively few, the greatest risk was observed in type IV subjects having a high ratio, $p<0.0002$ vs. normals with a high ratio. The greatest number of AMI cases ($n=784$) was found in subjects with a high apoB/apoA-I and type IIB. Their risk factor was double that of normals with a high apoB/apoA-I, $p<0.0001$. Notably, subjects with type IIA and a high ratio did not have a greater risk than normals with a high ratio despite 2-mmol/l higher TC values in type IIA subjects. In fact, many of type IIA subjects had a high apoA-I and a fairly normal apoB (Fig. 1), indicating a proportionally high contribution of HDL-C in this cohort.

4. Discussion

Although isolated hypercholesterolemia was more prevalent in the population, combined hyperlipidemia of type IIB was the most common abnormality in those suffering a fatal AMI. The difference in the risk of dying from AMI was somewhat bigger for subjects with type IIA hypercholesterolemia than for those with normal lipids, but the difference was not as big as that for individuals with combined hyperlipidemia or isolated hypertriglyceridemia. Although few individuals had isolated hypertriglyceridemia, they experienced a great risk, especially those with a high apoB/apoA-I ratio.

The greatest risk of dying from AMI, irrespective of lipid phenotype, was obtained in subjects having a high ratio apoB/apoA-I compared with those having a low ratio. In addition, in those with normal lipid levels, the risk was greater in those with a high apoB/apoA-I ratio than those having a low ratio. Notably, individuals with type IIA and a high ratio did not differ in risk vs. those with normal lipids and a high ratio.

The present findings confirm and extend our previous AMORIS results showing that the apoB/apoA-I ratio has additional predictive value above that of TC and TG irrespective of age and gender [1,2]. The present results show that apoB/apoA-I has a superior predictive value not only above the lipid levels as such, but also in subjects with different, and commonly occurring lipid phenotypes. This is further illustrated in those with normal lipid levels and a high apoB/apoA-I ratio.

In conclusion, our results indicate that the balance in apoB/apoA-I is a simple and informative risk indicator that is valid in both genders of all ages and largely independent on the lipid levels and lipid profiles or phenotypes. Since apoB and apoA-I methods are internationally standardized [3] and can be measured with low errors, CV 3–5%, they are cheap and insensitive to the nutritional state; these risk indicators should be used also in the clinical routine. In fact, new international guidelines now recognize these apolipoproteins as new important cardiovascular risk markers [4]. In addition, cut levels, at least for apoB, have been proposed [5]. Since apoB and apoA-I are also at least as good or, in fact, better markers of lipid-lowering treatment by statins [2], apoB, apoA-I, and especially the balance of apoB/apoA-I will become important predictors of cardiac risk and targets for lipid-lowering therapy.

References

[1] G. Walldius, I. Jungner, I. Holme, A.H. Aastveit, W. Kolar, E. Steiner, High apolipoprotein B, low apolipoprotein A-I, and improvement in the prediction of fatal myocardial infarction (AMORIS study): a prospective study, Lancet 358 (2001) 2026–2033.

[2] A.D. Sniderman, C.D. Furberg, A. Keech, J.E. Roeters van Lennep, J. Frohlich, I. Jungner, G. Walldius, Apolipoproteins versus lipids as indices of coronary risk and as targets for statin treatment, Lancet 361 (2003) 777–780.

[3] I. Jungner, S.M. Marcovina, G. Walldius, I. Holme, W. Kolar, E. Steiner, Apolipoprotein B and A-I values in 147 576 Swedish males and females, standardized according to the World Health Organization—International Federation of Clinical Chemistry First International Reference Materials, Clin. Chem. 44 (1998) 1641–1649.

[4] International Atherosclerosis Society, Harmonized clinical guidelines on prevention of atherosclerotic vascular disease, Executive Summary, 2003, 1–23, http://www.info@athero.org.

[5] S.M. Grundy, Low-density lipoprotein, non-high density lipoprotein, and apolipoprotein B as targets of lipid lowering therapy, Circulation 106 (2002) 2526–2529.

International Congress Series 1262 (2004) 207–210

www.ics-elsevier.com

Are plasma triglycerides a good predictor of CHD risk?

Philippa J. Talmud[a,*], Emma Hawe[a], George J. Miller[b], Steve E. Humphries[a]

[a] *Division of Cardiovascular Genetics, British Heart Foundation Laboratories, Department of Medicine, Rayne Building, Royal Free and University College Medical School, 5 University St., London WC1E 6JF, UK*

[b] *Wolfson Institute of Preventive Medicine, Charterhouse Square, London, UK*

Abstract. We investigated which of the established lipid risk traits were the best risk predictors in a large prospective study. In multivariate analysis apoB and triglycerides (TG) gave the best risk prediction. Since very low density (VLDL) and low density lipoproteins (LDL) have one apoB molecule/particle, and VLDL is cleared faster than LDL, apoB levels reflect LDL *number* and TGs over 1.5 mmol/l are correlated with LDL size. From a genetic viewpoint we examined which of the genes in *APOA5-A4-C3* cluster, using haplotype analysis, determined TG levels and coronary heart disease (CHD) risk. While *APOA5* and *APOC3* variants defined the major TG-raising haplotypes, *APOA4* variants defined CHD risk haplotypes. Thus, TG per se is not the best risk predictor from both a phenotypic and genetic viewpoint. These data confirm the complex multifactorial nature of CHD risk. © 2003 Published by Elsevier B.V.

Keywords: *APOA5-A4-C3*; Triglycerides; ApoB; Small dense LDL; ApoAIV; CHD risk

1. Introduction

The aim of this study was to examine, from two viewpoints, how good risk predictor plasma triglycerides (TGs) are. First, we compared the efficacy of TG as a risk predictor with other lipid, lipoprotein and apolipoprotein parameters, in a large prospective study of healthy middle-aged men in the UK. Then in the same study we used haplotype analysis, specifically of the *APOA5-A4-C3* gene cluster, to see if haplotypes predicting TG levels correlated with CHD risk.

* Corresponding author. Tel.: +44-2076-796968; fax: +44-2076-796212.
E-mail address: p.talmud@ucl.ac.uk (P.J. Talmud).

doi:10.1016/S0531-5131(03)01733-3

2. Study

The Northwick Park Heart Study is a study of 3052 healthy men aged 50 to 61 years, recruited for prospective surveillance [1]. In addition DNA samples were genotyped for nine SNPs within the gene cluster [2].

3. Best phenotypic predictors of CHD risk

3.1. TG and apoB together are the best risk predictor in NPHSII

The pair-wise relative risk ratios for CHD by quartiles of the TG and cholesterol and TG and apoB are presented in Fig. 1. Overall, TG and apoB above the 50th percentile for both, appeared to be a better predictor of risk compared with the combination of TG and cholesterol at equivalent percentiles [3].

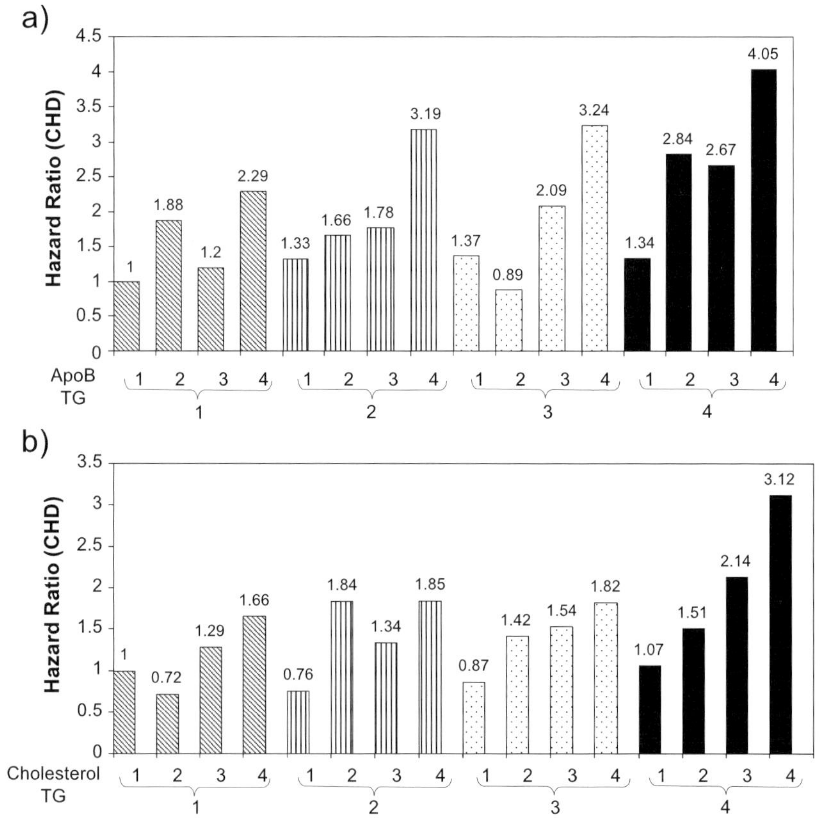

Fig. 1. Stratification of proportion of events by quartiles of apoB (g/l) and TG (a) (mmol/l) and TG (mmol/l) and cholesterol (mmol/l) (b). Quartile cut-offs for: TG (mmol/l)—1 < 1.25; 2,1.74; 3 < 2.59; 4>2.60. ApoB (g/l)—1 < 0.72; 2 < 0.85; < 1.01; >1.02. cholesterol (mmol/l)—1 < 5.0; 2 < 5.7; 3 < 6.4; 4>6.5.

3.2. Mechanism for the TG/apoB risk association

The mechanism by which raised apoB and TG in combination increase risk of CHD is as yet uncertain. There is only one apoB molecule for each very low density (VLDL) and LDL particle [4], and since VLDL particles are cleared much faster than LDL [5], apoB levels essentially reflect LDL *number*. Increased TG levels also reflect the extent of cholesterol depletion of LDL. In a recent meta-analysis, Austin identified a 60% increase in risk for CHD for every 10Å decrease in LDL size [6].

4. Contribution of variant of the APOA5-A4-C3 gene cluster to TG levels and CHD risk

The involvement of variation in the *APOA4* and *APOC3* in determining independent difference in lipid levels is well documented (reviewed by Groenendijk et al. [7]). The newest identified member of this gene cluster is *APOA5*. In contrast to apoCIII, where

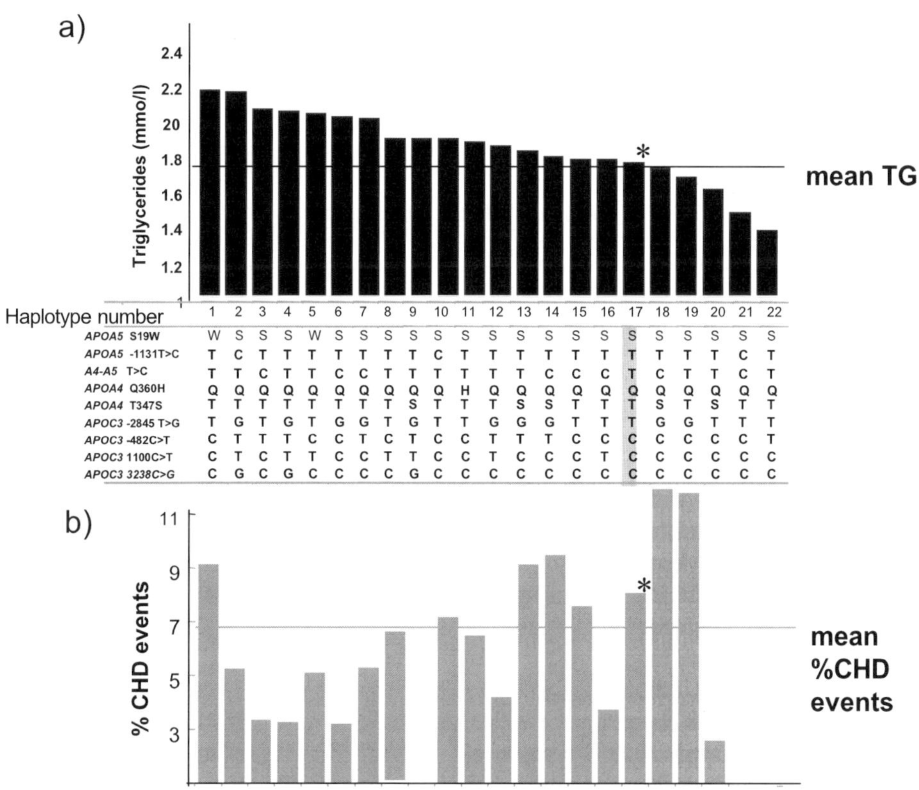

Fig. 2. (a) Ranking of the haplotypes derived from the nine SNPs according to triglyceride levels. The mean TG level for the sample is represented by a horizontal line. (b) The proportion of events by haplotypes, ranked in the same order as the above. The mean proportion of events for the sample is represented by a horizontal line. The common alleles are shaded and marked with an asterisk.

high plasma levels are associated with high TG levels [8], apoAV appears to be *inversely* related to TG levels.

Using haplotypes defined by nine variants spanning the *APOA5-A4-C3* gene cluster, *APOA5* (S19W, -1131T>C, 1259T>C) *APOA4* (T347S, Q360H), and *APOC3* (2845T>G, -482C>T, 1100C>T, 3238C>G) we examined the relative contribution of these variants to plasma TG levels [2] and CHD risk [9]. The outcome was surprising.

The major TG-raising alleles were defined by *APOA5* W19 and *APOC3*–482T (Fig. 2a). Thus, variation in *APOA5* is associated with difference in TGs in healthy men, *independent* of those previously reported for *APOC3*. The highest CHD risk-estimate haplotypes carried *APOA4* S347 and rare alleles of the two flanking intergenic markers [9] (Fig. 2b).

5. Conclusion

From these initial studies, we conclude that TGs alone are *NOT* a strong independent CHD risk factor. However, together with apoB, TGs are the best risk predictors and define the number and LDL particle size. Haplotype analysis of the *APOA5-A4-C3* gene cluster, showed that there was not a good correlation between haplotypes determining TG levels and those determining CHD risk. These data confirm the multifactorial and complex genetic inter-relationships that determine both CHD risk factors and CHD risk itself.

Acknowledgements

This work is supported by the British Heart Foundation.

References

[1] G.J. Miller, et al., The effects of quality and timing of venipuncture on markers of blood coagulation in healthy middle-aged men, Thromb. Haemost. 73 (1995) 82–86.
[2] P.J. Talmud, et al., Relative contribution of variation within the APOC3-A4-A5 gene cluster in determining plasma triglycerides, Hum. Mol. Genet. 11 (2002) 3039–3046.
[3] P.J. Talmud, et al., Nonfasting apolipoprotein B and triglyceride levels as a useful predictor of coronary heart disease risk in middle-aged UK men, Arterioscler. Thromb. Vasc. Biol. 22 (2002) 1918–1923.
[4] J. Elovson, Plasma very low density lipoproteins contain a single molecule of apolipoprotein B, J. Lipid Res. 29 (1988) 1461–1473.
[5] A. Sniderman, et al., Effect of moderate hypertriglyceridemia on the relation of plasma total and LDL apo B levels, Atherosclerosis 89 (1991) 109–116.
[6] M.A. Austin, Triglyceride, small, dense low-density lipoprotein, and the atherogenic lipoprotein phenotype, Curr. Atheroscler. Rep. 2 (2000) 200–207.
[7] M. Groenendijk, et al., The *apoAI-CIII-AIV* gene cluster, Atherosclerosis 157 (2001) 1–11.
[8] C.C. Shoulders, et al., Variation at the *apo AI/CIII/AIV* gene complex is associated with elevated plasma levels of apo CIII, Atherosclerosis 87 (1991) 239–247.
[9] W.R. Wong, et al., Apolipoprotein AIV gene variant is associated with increased risk of coronary heart disease and lower ApoAIV plasma concentrations, Circ. Res. 92 (2003) 969–972.

International Congress Series 1262 (2004) 211–214

www.ics-elsevier.com

The role of atypical PKCs in insulin-resistant states

Robert V. Farese*

Department of Internal Medicine, College of Medicine, University of South Florida, Research Service, James A. Haley Veterans Hospital, 13000 Bruce B. Downs Blvd. VAR 151, Tampa, FL 33612, USA

Abstract. Insulin-stimulated glucose transport requires IRS1/PI3K, atypical PKCs (aPKCs) and PKB, but mechanisms underlying clinical insulin-resistance in humans are unclear. We and others recently reported that activation of IRS1/PI3K and aPKCs, but not PKB, is defective in muscles of obese/glucose-intolerant and type 2 diabetic humans. Defects in activation of aPKCs, but not IRS1, PI3K or PKB, have also been found in muscles of glucose-tolerant obese women and, to a greater degree, obese women who have polycystic ovary syndrome (PCOS). In each condition, there were defects in aPKC activation by both insulin in vivo and the PI3K lipid product, PIP_3, in vitro. Conclusions: (a) insulin resistance in muscle in states of obesity, PCOS, the metabolic syndrome, impaired glucose tolerance and type 2 diabetes is at least partly due to defective activation of aPKCs; and (b) defective aPKC activation is partly due to poor responsiveness to PIP_3, which may precede defects in IRS1/PI3K activation. © 2003 Published by Elsevier B.V.

Keywords: Diabetes mellitus; Insulin resistance; Glucose transport; Skeletal muscle; Obesity; Metabolic syndrome; Adipocytes; Atypical protein kinase C; Protein kinase C-zeta

1. Introduction

Type 2 diabetes mellitus results from defects in insulin action and secretion. Defects in insulin action occur in subjects who have obesity and other features of the metabolic syndrome long before they develop impaired glucose tolerance (IGT) or overt diabetes. Insulin resistance is present in each of these conditions and contributes importantly to the development of the hyperlipidemia, hypertension and atherosclerosis that is prevalent in these conditions.

Resistance to insulin occurs in muscle and adipose tissues. Muscle is the major organ for insulin-stimulated glucose disposal, and insulin-stimulated glucose transport into muscle is diminished in obesity and type 2 diabetes. Defective insulin action in adipose tissue is attended by release of free fatty acids, which causes insulin resistance in muscle and increases hepatic lipogenesis and gluconeogenesis. Adipocytes also release leptin, resistin, TNF-α and adiponectin, which modulate insulin action in adipocytes, muscle and liver.

* Tel.: +1-813-972-7662; fax: +1-813-972-76923.
E-mail address: rfarese@hsc.usf.edu (R.V. Farese).

0531-5131/ © 2003 Published by Elsevier B.V.
doi:10.1016/S0531-5131(03)01860-0

Of insulin-sensitive tissues, muscle is most resistant to insulin. Accordingly, resistance to insulin in muscle may be attended by normal or excessive responses to insulin in other tissues, e.g., increases in hepatic lipid production (favoring hyperlipidemia), renal salt/water retention (favoring hypertension) and endothelial and vascular smooth muscle hyper-responsiveness and proliferation (favoring hypertension and atherosclerosis). In short, certain features of the metabolic syndrome may be caused by muscle insulin resistance.

2. Signaling factors controlling insulin-stimulated glucose transport

Following insulin binding, the insulin receptor tyrosine phosphorylates IRS-1, IRS-2 and Cbl, which, via tyrosine-phosphorylated pYXXM motifs, activate SH2 groups in the p85 subunit of phosphatidylinositol (PI) 3-kinase (3K) and Crk. Atypical PKCs (aPKCs) and PKB/Akt are thereupon activated by lipid products of PI3K, most notably PI-3,4,5-$(PO_4)_3$ (PIP_3) and 3-phosphoinositide-dependent protein kinase-1 (PDK1), and in turn activate the machinery that translocates Glut4 glucose transporters to the plasma membrane, thereby increasing glucose transport. Small G-proteins Rab, Rac, Cdc42 and other trafficking/docking factors are needed to translocate Glut4. In 3T3/L1 adipocytes, there are requirements for factors operating: (a) upstream of Cbl, APS, CAP and flotillin; and (b) downstream of Cbl, Cbl-dependent PI3K, Crk, C3G, TC10 and other factors in caveolin-rich lipid rafts of the plasma membrane. It is debated if Cbl/Crk/C3G/TC10-dependent factors are important in muscle.

Like insulin, exercise and AICAR, which activates AMPK, stimulate Glut4 translocation/glucose transport, independently of PI3K, most likely through increases in phosphatidic acid (PA) generated by phospholipase D (PLD) operating downstream of ERK or other factors.

3. Defects in insulin signaling in skeletal muscle in insulin-resistant states

3.1. IRS1/PI3K

Activation of IRS1/PI3K is defective in muscle in type 2 diabetes [1], but not necessarily at earlier times. Tendencies toward diminished IRS1/PI3K activation are seen in obese/glucose-tolerant [2], but, in some cases, this may reflect hyperinsulinemia-induced increase in basal activity with no decrease in total IRS1/PI3K activation. In obese women, polycystic ovary syndrome (PCOS) and obese IGT subjects [3], we have not observed significant decreases in insulin-stimulated IRS1/PI3K activity.

3.2. PKB

Although defective PKBα activation was seen in incubations of muscle strips of lean type 2 diabetic subjects, no such defect in activation of either PKBα or PKBβ was observed in muscle obtained during hyperinsulinemia/euglycemic clamp studies of obese type 2 diabetic subjects [1,3] or obese glucose-tolerant women (unpublished).

3.3. aPKCs

In contrast to PKB, marked defects in muscle aPKC activation were observed during euglycemic/hyperinsulinemic clamp studies of type 2 diabetics [2,3]. The level of PKC-ζ, the major aPKC, was diminished by 35–40% in diabetic muscle [2,3], but PKC-ζ mRNA levels were increased, and decreases in aPKC levels did not account for the decreases in aPKC enzyme activity [3]. Interestingly, aPKCs immunoprecipitated from diabetic muscle failed to respond to the direct addition of PIP_3 [3]. Thus, defective aPKC activation in diabetic muscle emanates from three sources, viz., defective IRS1/PI3K activation, poor aPKC responsiveness to PIP_3 and diminished PKC-ζ levels.

Importantly, muscle aPKC activation is similarly defective in IGT and type 2 diabetes [3] and therefore does not appear to be due to hyperglycemia. Moreover, defects in aPKC activation were surprisingly profound in diabetics who were excellently controlled [3]. This may explain unabated cardiovascular disease in 'well-controlled' diabetics.

Defects in insulin-stimulated glucose disposal and muscle aPKC activation are also present in glucose-tolerant obese men [2] and women (unpublished). Defects in aPKC activation in obese subjects are not as pronounced as those observed in IGT and type 2 diabetes and are not attended by significant defects in IRS1/PI3K or PKB activation, or decreases in PKC-ζ levels. As in IGT and type 2 diabetes, aPKCs immunoprecipitated from muscles of obese glucose-tolerant subjects failed to respond normally to PIP_3 (unpublished). Obese/PCOS women have lower glucose disposal rates and greater defects in muscle aPKC activation to both insulin and PIP_3 than simply obese women (unpublished).

4. Prevention and treatment of defects in aPKC activation in insulin-resistant states

In euglycemic/hyperinsulinemic clamp studies of monkeys, we followed the emergence and progression of a defect in muscle aPKC activation as these monkeys passed from a lean to an obese insulin-resistant pre-diabetic state and finally to type 2 diabetes [4]. Importantly, if obesity was avoided by caloric restriction, monkeys remained glucose-tolerant and failed to develop defects in aPKC activation.

Dietary weight loss improved insulin-stimulated aPKC activity in some, but not all, obese humans [2]. In diabetic subjects, however, we have not seen improvement in aPKC activation with comparable weight loss. Thus, defects in muscle aPKC activation may be reversible in some but not all cases.

Treatment of type 2 diabetes with the thiazolidinedione (TZD), rosiglitazone, improves the defect in muscle aPKC activation and insulin-stimulated glucose disposal, at least partly through increases in IRS1/PI3K activation [3]. TDZs may improve insulin-signaling mechanisms through decreases in plasma levels of free fatty acids, resistin and TNF-α, or increases in adiponectin.

Physical exercise was found to activate aPKCs better than insulin in muscles of diabetic subjects, albeit not as great as exercise or insulin in non-diabetic muscle [3]. Accordingly, exercise is an important adjunct in the treatment of type 2 diabetes.

5. Concluding remarks

Common to all states of insulin resistance, i.e., from simple obesity and the metabolic syndrome through IGT and type 2 diabetes, there are defects in aPKC activation by both insulin in intact cells and PIP_3 in vitro. Defects in aPKC activation in intact cells in diabetes may be partly due to defects in the activation of upstream activators, e.g., IRS1/PI3K, but such defects are not always evident in earlier states. The defect in aPKC responsiveness to PIP_3 is observed in all states, which suggests that there are defects in factors that operate downstream of PI3K/PDK1 and directly regulate/modulate aPKC activity/activation. Accordingly, there is an urgent need to elucidate the mechanisms for downregulation of aPKC activity/activation. In the meantime, aPKCs are logical targets for the development of agents that should be useful for treating the clinical insulin resistance in type 2 diabetes, and its precursors, IGT, obesity and the metabolic syndrome.

References

[1] Y.-B. Kim, S.E. Nikoulina, T.P. Ciaraldi, R.R. Henry, B.B. Kahn, Normal insulin-dependent activation of Akt/protein kinase B, with diminished activation of phosphoinositide 3-kinase in muscle in type 2 diabetes, J. Clin. Invest. 104 (1999) 733–741.

[2] Y.-B. Kim, K. Kotani, T.P. Ciaraldi, R.R. Henry, B.B. Kahn, Insulin-stimulated PKC-λ/ζ activity is reduced and PDK-1 activity is normal in muscle of insulin resistant humans, Diabetes 52 (2003) 1936–1942.

[3] M. Beeson, M.P. Sajan, M. Dizon, D. Grebenev, J. Gomez-Daspet, A. Miura, Y. Kanoh, J. Powe, G. Bandyopadhyay, M.L. Standaert, R.V. Farese, Activation of protein kinase C-ζ by insulin and phosphatidylinositol-3,4-5-$(PO_4)_3$ is defective in muscle in type 2 diabetes and impaired glucose tolerance, Diabetes 52 (2003) 1926–1934.

[4] M.L. Standaert, H.K. Ortmeyer, M.P. Sajan, Y. Kanoh, G. Bandyopadhyay, B.C. Hansen, R.V. Farese, Skeletal muscle insulin resistance in obesity-associated type 2 diabetes mellitus in monkeys is linked to a defect in insulin activation of protein kinase C-ζ/λ/ι, Diabetes 51 (2002) 2936–2943.

International Congress Series 1262 (2004) 215–219

www.ics-elsevier.com

PPARα controlling HDL metabolism and atherosclerosis

Réjane Paumelle, Daniel Duran-Sandoval, Jean-Charles Fruchart, Bart Staels*

U.R. 545 INSERM, Département d'Athérosclerose, Institut Pasteur de Lille, 1, Rue du Professeur Calmette BP245, 59019, Lille, France
Faculté de Pharmacie, Université de Lille 2, 59006, Lille, France

Abstract. Low serum high-density lipoprotein (HDL) cholesterol concentrations are a feature of the metabolic syndrome that is increasingly being recognized as an important risk factor for cardiovascular disease. HDL is a key mediator of reverse cholesterol transport (RCT), a pathway transporting cholesterol from extrahepatic cells and tissues to the liver for excretion. HDL metabolism is controlled by the interaction of its protein constituents, the apolipoproteins, such as apoA-I and apoA-II, with different enzymes (LCAT, HL, LPL), transfer proteins (CETP, PLTP,...) and lipoprotein receptors (ABCA-1, SR-BI,...). The level of expression of most of these proteins is partly controlled at the level of transcription by transcription factors, among which are the nuclear receptors. Nuclear receptors are activated by small lipophilic signalling molecules. Among these nuclear receptors, peroxisome proliferator-activated receptors were first identified to play a role in the control of lipid metabolism. In this paper, we will focus on the role of PPARα in HDL metabolism, its molecular action mechanism and its potential as pharmacological targets for future drug discovery. © 2004 Published by Elsevier B.V.

Keywords: Nuclear receptors; PPARα; HDL metabolism; Atherosclerosis; Reverse cholesterol transport

1. HDL and the reverse cholesterol transport pathway

The control of HDL metabolism occurs at both quantitative (synthesis/catabolism) and qualitative (functionality of HDL particles) levels. HDL mediate cholesterol efflux from peripheral tissues (such as lipid-laden macrophages in atherosclerotic lesions) promoting its transport back to the liver, resulting in cholesterol secretion into bile, either directly or after conversion to bile acids, a process termed the reverse cholesterol transport (RCT) pathway.

The first step of the RCT pathway lies in the mobilization of cholesterol from intracellular pools to the cytoplasmic membrane and its transfer to nascent discoidal HDL particles (pre-β HDL), which are generated either directly in the liver and intestine or

* Corresponding author. U.R. 545 INSERM, Département d'Athérosclerose, Institut Pasteur de Lille, 1, Rue du Professeur Calmette BP245, 59019, Lille, France. Tel.: +33-3-20-87-73-88; fax: +33-3-20-87-71-98.
E-mail address: bart.staels@pasteur-lille.fr (B. Staels).

0531-5131/ © 2004 Published by Elsevier B.V.
doi:10.1016/j.ics.2003.12.046

as a product of lipoprotein lipase (LPL)-mediated lipolysis of triglyceride-rich lipoproteins [1]. Cholesterol transfer to nascent pre-β-HDL requires interaction of HDL apolipoproteins, such as apoA-I, with transporters of the ABC superfamily, such as ABCA-1 or ABCG-1 [2]. The importance of ABCA-1 in this process is illustrated by the fact that mutations in the ABCA-1 gene are responsible for Tangier disease as well as familial HDL deficiency and are associated with an increased risk of CVD. The expression of several ABC transporters and cholesterol efflux are induced by cholesterol loading of human macrophages as a counterregulatory mechanism preventing the accumulation of cholesteryl esters in the atherosclerotic lesion [2,3]. Studies demonstrating that the rate of cholesterol efflux mediated by HDL or serum is correlated with cellular scavenger receptor-BI (SR-BI)/CLA-1 expression levels [4] suggest that cholesterol removal from peripheral cells, including macrophages, may occur also via this receptor.

Cholesterol in these nascent particles is subsequently esterified by the action of the enzyme lecithin:cholesterol acyl transferase (LCAT). HDL cholesteryl esters are cleared from plasma either through selective uptake by the liver via the SR-BI pathway [5] or after phospholipid transfer protein (PLTP) and cholesteryl ester transfer protein (CETP) mediated HDL remodeling, resulting in the exchange of lipids between HDL and VLDL-LDL particles. Hepatic cholesteryl ester uptake from HDL is enhanced by LPL and hepatic lipase (HL) [6]. Once internalized in the liver, cholesterol can be excreted into bile, either directly or after conversion to bile acids. It is important to note that fecal excretion of cholesterol and bile acids is quantitatively the most important way for the body to eliminate cholesterol excess. The initial and rate-limiting step in the synthesis of bile acids from cholesterol is catalysed by the liver-specific enzyme cholesterol 7α-hydroxylase (CYP7A1), which converts cholesterol into 7α-hydroxycholesterol.

2. Peroxisome proliferator-activated receptors (PPARs)

PPARs were first identified in 1990 when the α isoform (PPARα) was shown to be the receptor for xenobiotics inducing peroxisome proliferation in rodent liver. Subsequently, two other PPAR genes, PPARγ and PPARβ/δ, have been identified. PPARα is mainly expressed in tissues in which fatty acids (FA) are catabolized, whereas PPARγ is present in adipose tissue, mammary glands and numerous other tissues and PPARβ/δ is ubiquitously expressed (see review [7]). PPARs bind as heterodimers with RXR and regulate gene expression after recognition of specific DNA sequences so-called 'peroxisome proliferator response elements' (PPREs) composed of a direct repeat of the hexanucleotide AGGTCA sequence separated by one or two spacers (DR1 or DR2) (Fig. 1). A wide range of compounds have been identified as PPAR ligands. FAs and FA-derived compounds such as leukotriene B4 (LTB4) and prostaglandin J2 (PGJ2) are natural ligands for PPARα, PPARγ and PPARβ/δ [8]. Fibrates are synthetic PPARα activators (Fig. 1).

3. PPARα and the control of HDL metabolism

In humans, fibrates increase plasma HDL-cholesterol levels (10–15%) in patients with hypertriglyceridemia, combined hyperlipidemia and hypercholesterolemia (see review [9]). The increase in HDL-cholesterol levels is associated with significant increases in the levels of apoA-II and, depending on the fibrate used, apoA-I. PPARα activators

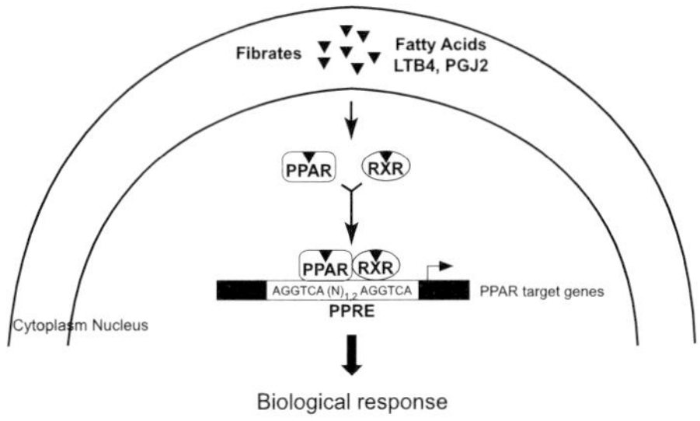

Fig. 1. Mechanism of transcriptional regulation by PPARs.

increase the production of pre-β-HDL particles by increasing apoA-I and apoA-II synthesis via a functional PPRE present in the promoters of human ApoA-I and ApoA-II. By contrast, PPARα activation in rodents leads to a decrease of circulating HDL as well as apoA-I and apoA-II levels. Three nucleotide substitutions in the rat apoA-I promoter render this gene unresponsive to PPARα in rodents. Furthermore, Rev-erbα, an orphan nuclear receptor, inhibits apoA-I transcription through a negative response element situated next to the TATA box in the rat, but not in the human promoter. Rev-erbα that is induced by PPARα could thus be responsible for the repressive effect of fibrates on rat apoA-I expression. In addition, PPARα increases also the activity and gene expression of LPL via a functional PPRE present in the promoter of the human LPL (see review [10]).

In human macrophages, PPARα activators also enhance cholesterol efflux by increasing the expression of ABCA-1 and SR-BI/CLA1 [11]. PPARα induces the expression of ABCA-1 by an indirect mechanism via induction of the Liver X receptor alpha (LXRα), another nuclear receptor [11].

More recently, it has been shown that PPARα agonists induce the expression and the activity of PLTP in mice leading to a marked enlargement of HDL [12]. In addition, clinical studies have shown that fenofibrate treatment of normolipidemic patients increases lecithin:cholesterol acyl transferase (LCAT) activity. But in rodents, PPARα agonists decrease LCAT expression and activity [9]. Thus, although fibrates influence the expression of HDL-remodeling enzymes, such as PLTP and LCAT, in rodents, little is known about the regulation of these proteins in humans.

Conversion of cholesterol to bile acids in the liver is quantitatively the most important pathway for elimination of cholesterol from the body. The role of PPARα in the control of bile acid synthesis and composition is still unclear and controversial. Whereas PPARα has been shown to induce the hepatic expression of LXRα, which subsequently upregulates the expression of cholesteryl 7α-hydroxylase (CYP7A1) in rodents, fibrates reduce the activity of this enzyme in rodents and humans. By contrast, PPARα has been reported as a positive regulator of murine and human CYP7A1 promoter activity [10]. Thus, the role of PPARα on CYP7A1 expression and activity is not completely understood. However, activated PPARα induces the expression of cholesterol 12α-hydroxylase (CYP8B1), an enzyme that determines the lithogenic index (ratio of cholic acid/chenodeoxycholic acid) of bile [13].

In summary, PPARα activators influence both HDL production by increasing apoA-I and apoA-II expression and HDL remodeling by influencing the expression of LPL and, in rodents, the expression of PLTP. PPARα activators influence also cholesterol efflux by

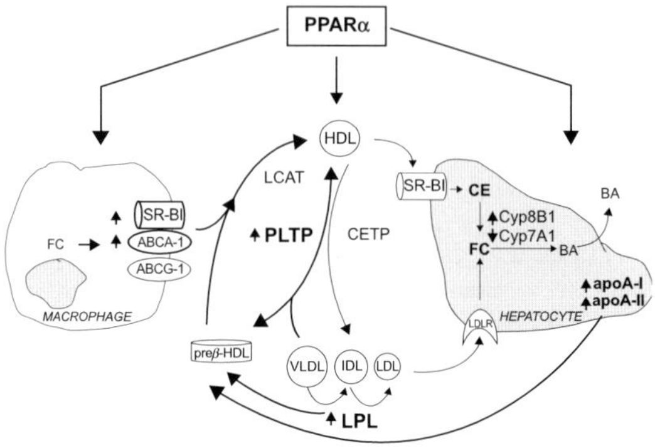

Fig. 2. PPARα-mediated regulation of RCT (FC = free cholesterol; CE = cholesteryl ester; BA = bile acid).

regulating HDL receptors such as ABCA-1 and SR-BI/CLA1 (Fig. 2). Therefore, by increasing both HDL synthesis and cellular cholesterol efflux, PPARα activators probably increase RCT and reduce atherogenesis, as suggested from clinical trials showing a reduction in the progression of atheroma in atherosclerotic patients treated with fibrates [9].

4. Conclusions

The identification of the nuclear receptor PPARα as target for the fibrates opened new avenues for the development of new therapeutics acting via nuclear receptors to control lipid metabolism. Over the last few years, several other nuclear receptors, such as the Retinoid X receptor (RXR), Liver X receptor (LXR) and Farnesoid X receptor (FXR), have also been identified to regulate lipid metabolism. Identification of such highly specific chemical ligands provided invaluable tools to understand the function of these different nuclear receptor pathways.

Acknowledgements

This work was supported by grants from Fondation Leducq (to R. P.), the ministerio de Hacienda del Gobierno de Chile (to D. D. S) and the European community (grant QLRT-1999-01007).

References

[1] J.G. Strauss, S. Frank, D. Kratky, G. Hammerle, A. Hrzenjak, G. Knipping, et al., Adenovirus-mediated rescue of lipoprotein lipase-deficient mice. Lipolysis of triglyceride-rich lipoproteins is essential for high density lipoprotein maturation in mice, J. Biol. Chem. 276 (39) (2001) 36083–36090.

[2] T. Burris, P. Eacho, G. Cao, Genetic disorders associated with ATP binding cassette cholesterol transporters, Mol. Genet. Metab. 77 (1–2) (2002) 13–20.

[3] G. Schmitz, W.E. Kaminski, E. Orso, ABC transporters in cellular lipid trafficking, Curr. Opin. Lipidol. 11 (5) (2000) 493–501.

[4] Y. Ji, B. Jian, N. Wang, Y. Sun, M.L. Moya, M.C. Phillips, et al., Scavenger receptor BI promotes high density lipoprotein-mediated cellular cholesterol efflux, J. Biol. Chem. 272 (34) (1997) 20982–20985.

[5] S. Acton, A. Rigotti, K.T. Landschulz, S. Xu, H.H. Hobbs, M. Krieger, Identification of scavenger receptor SR-BI as a high density lipoprotein receptor, Science 271 (5248) (1996) 518–520.

[6] F. Rinninger, T. Kaiser, W.A. Mann, N. Meyer, H. Greten, U. Beisiegel, Lipoprotein lipase mediates an increase in the selective uptake of high density lipoprotein-associated cholesteryl esters by hepatic cells in culture, J. Lipid Res. 39 (7) (1998) 1335–1348.
[7] B. Desvergne, W. Wahli, Peroxisome proliferator-activated receptors: nuclear control of metabolism, Endocr. Rev. 20 (5) (1999) 649–688.
[8] T.M. Willson, W. Wahli, Peroxisome proliferator-activated receptor agonists, Curr. Opin. Chem. Biol. 1 (2) (1997) 235–241.
[9] B. Staels, J. Dallongeville, J. Auwerx, K. Schoonjans, E. Leitersdorf, J.C. Fruchart, Mechanism of action of fibrates on lipid and lipoprotein metabolism, Circulation 98 (19) (1998) 2088–2093.
[10] V. Bocher, I. Pineda-Torra, J.C. Fruchart, B. Staels, PPARs: transcription factors controlling lipid and lipoprotein metabolism, Ann. N.Y. Acad. Sci. 967 (2002) 7–18.
[11] G. Chinetti, F.G. Gbaguidi, S. Griglio, Z. Mallat, M. Antonucci, P. Poulain, et al., CLA-1/SR-BI is expressed in atherosclerotic lesion macrophages and regulated by activators of peroxisome proliferator-activated receptors, Circulation 101 (20) (2000) 2411–2417.
[12] M. Bouly, D. Masson, B. Gross, X.C. Jiang, C. Fievet, G. Castro, et al., Induction of the phospholipid transfer protein gene accounts for the high density lipoprotein enlargement in mice treated with fenofibrate, J. Biol. Chem. 276 (28) (2001) 25841–25847.
[13] M.C. Hunt, Y.Z. Yang, G. Eggertsen, C.M. Carneheim, M. Gafvels, C. Einarsson, et al., The peroxisome proliferator-activated receptor alpha (PPARalpha) regulates bile acid biosynthesis, J. Biol. Chem. 275 (37) (2000) 28947–28953.

International Congress Series 1262 (2004) 220–223

ELSEVIER

www.ics-elsevier.com

Genetic and genomic studies of type 2 diabetes in mice

Alan D. Attie*

Department of Biochemistry, University of Wisconsin-Madison, 433 Babcock Dr., Madison, WI 53706, USA

Abstract. Most people with type 2 diabetes mellitus (DM2) are obese. However, most obese people do not develop diabetes. Genetic factors are thought to make a major contribution to diabetes susceptibility. To identify DM2 susceptibility genes, we have developed a mouse model in which strain background determines diabetes susceptibility of obese mice. C57BL/6 (B6) *ob/ob* mice are not diabetic. In contrast, BTBR *ob/ob* mice develop severe DM2. We have mapped three quantitative trait loci for glucose and insulin traits in F2 *ob/ob* mice derived from the B6 and BTBR strains. We are using interval-specific congenic strains to positionally clone the genes responsible for these traits. We profiled gene expression in lean and obese B6 and BTBR strains. Adipose tissue from obese mice shows a global downregulation of lipogenic and adipogenic genes, most notably the master regulator SREBP-1c. In contrast, the expression of SREBP-1c and its target lipogenic genes are upregulated in the liver of obese mice. The diabetes-resistant B6 *ob/ob* mice have a much higher level of expression of liver SREBP-1c and its target genes than the diabetes-susceptible BTBR *ob/ob* mice. Hence, increased hepatic lipogenic capacity correlates with diabetes resistance.

Keywords: Diabetes; Obesity; SREBP; Genetics; QTL; Positional cloning; Microarrays; Gene expression

1. Introduction

More than 80% of people with type 2 diabetes mellitus (DM2) are obese. Yet, most people who are obese never develop diabetes. An important unmet need in this field is to understand the difference between non-diabetic obese individuals fated to become diabetic vs. obese individuals who will never develop diabetes.

There is a consensus in the field that genetic factors play a major role in determining whether or not an obese individual will develop DM2 [1]. However, despite numerous large-scale studies, there have been relatively few genes identified that confer diabetes diathesis. Diabetes is what geneticists describe as a "complex trait." Very likely, modest allelic variations at numerous loci combine to confer disease susceptibility. Even more complex, these changes may require environmental interactions. These include nutrition,

* Tel.: +1-608-262-1372; fax: +1-608-263-9609.
E-mail address: attie@biochem.wisc.edu (A.D. Attie).

doi:10.1016/j.ics.2003.12.107

obesity, and, possibly, inflammation. This contrasts with the success in identifying six loci for maturity onset diabetes of the young (MODY) where the disease is due to single-gene mutations acting in a dominant fashion; 'clean' Mendelian genetics [2].

2. Strain background determines disease susceptibility

The pioneering studies of Douglas Coleman first showed that diabetes in a genetically obese mouse is determined by strain background. Coleman showed that whereas the C57BL/6 (B6) *db/db* mouse has mild transient hyperglycemia, the C57BL/Ks *db/db* mouse develops severe diabetes [3]. This finding begged the question, what genes differ in the two strains that are responsible for this dramatic difference in diabetes susceptibility? The answer is still not known in this particular case, but several important developments have made it feasible to answer these types of questions.

3. The BTBR mouse strain

The BTBR strain is a *Mus musculus* strain originally inbred by Dobrovolskaia-Zavadskaia. The strain was transferred to L.C. Dunn and maintained at Columbia University, then transferred to several laboratories over a period of about fifty years. It is currently in the Jackson Laboratory collection. Several years ago, our laboratory discovered that male BTBR mice are mildly insulin resistant and develop fasting hyperinsulinemia on a high fat diet [4]. The animals have impaired insulin stimulated glucose transport in adipose tissue [5]. Recent in vivo studies show impaired transport of glucose into adipose tissue under hyperinsulinemic clamp conditions (Byers and Attie, unpublished).

4. Mapping diabetes susceptibility QTL

We bred the BTBR strain to B6 mice heterozygous for the null allele of the *leptin* locus, *ob/+* mice. The offspring were backcrossed to the BTBR strain for eight generations with marker assisted selection to generate a congenic strain consisting of the BTBR background with approximately 20 cm surrounding the *leptin* locus on chromosome 6 coming from the B6 strain. When the mice were bred to generate *leptin*$^{ob/ob}$ homozygotes, we obtained mice that developed severe diabetes beginning at about 6 weeks of age [6].

We performed a genome scan on F2 *ob/ob* mice derived from the B6 and BTBR backgrounds. Three loci emerged with Lod scores exceeding the conservative $p<0.05$ Lod threshold of 4.3 defined by Lander and Kruglyak [7]. One locus, on chromosome 16, gave a significant Lod peak for glucose and a suggestive peak for fasting insulin. As expected, the diabetogenic allele was derived from the BTBR strain. The other two loci, on chromosomes 2 and 19, yielded significant Lod scores for the fasting insulin trait. Interestingly, the low insulin and presumably pro-diabetes allele on the chromosome 19 locus comes from the diabetes-resistant strain, B6. This phenomenon, termed transgression, is not uncommon in QTL studies and reflects the fact that phenotypes emerge in F2 animals not found in parentals because they are unique mosaics of alleles from both parental strains.

The three diabetes susceptibility QTLs are presently in varying stages of positional cloning. Our approach is the use of interval-specific congenic strains [8]. It is encouraging that thus far, all the loci for which we have developed congenic strains retain the predicted phenotype. This indicates that each allele can express the phenotype in the absence of isogenic alleles at other loci.

5. Gene expression profiles in obesity

We surveyed gene expression using Affymetrix arrays in lean and obese B6 and BTBR animals. Our initial study was conducted on adipose tissue [9]. That study yielded the unexpected result that lipogenic and adipogenic gene expression is decreased in adipose tissue from obese mice. Of special interest to us was the collection of genes necessary for fatty acid synthesis. All are regulated by the transcription factor SREBP-1c. Accordingly, SREBP-1c expression is also decreased in adipose tissue from obese animals. This result has been replicated in several studies of human obese subjects [10–12]. In fact, in obese humans undergoing weight loss, SREBP-1c levels rise [13].

6. Gene expression in DM2

We surveyed gene expression in adipose tissue, muscle, liver, and pancreatic islets from B6 and BTBR lean and obese mice [14]. In an extension of the foregoing studies, we observed that in both mouse strains, obesity is associated with increased expression of SREBP-1c and its target genes in the liver. We have proposed that this amounts to a shift in the lipogenic burden from adipose tissue to the liver [15]. Interestingly, when we compared the *ob/ob* mice of the two mouse strains, B6 with BTBR, we found that there was a much higher expression of SREBP-1c and genes for lipogenic enzymes in the B6 *ob/ob* mice, suggesting that increased lipogenesis may actually be protective against diabetes even though it is associated with hepatic steatosis.

Acknowledgements

The work described in this review was supported by grants from NHLBI, NIDDK, American Heart Association, American Diabetes Association, and Xenon Genetics.

References

[1] P. Bougneres, Genetics of obesity and type 2 diabetes: tracking pathogenic traits during the predisease period, Diabetes 51 (Suppl. 3) (2002) S295–S303.

[2] S.S. Fajans, G.I. Bell, K.S. Polonsky, Molecular mechanisms and clinical pathophysiology of maturity-onset diabetes of the young, N. Engl. J. Med. 345 (2001) 971–980.

[3] D.L. Coleman, K.P. Hummel, The influence of genetic background on the expression of the obese (Ob) gene in the mouse, Diabetologia 9 (1973) 287–293.

[4] T. Ranheim, C. Dumke, K.L. Schueler, G.D. Cartee, A.D. Attie, Interaction between BTBR and C57BL/6J genomes produces an insulin resistance syndrome in (BTBR×C57BL/6J) F1 mice, Arterioscler. Thromb. Vasc. Biol. 17 (1997) 3286–3293.

[5] S.T. Nadler, J.P. Stoehr, M.E. Rabaglia, K.L. Schueler, M.J. Birnbaum, A.D. Attie, Normal Akt/PKB with reduced PI3K activation in insulin-resistant mice, Am. J. Physiol.: Endocrinol. Metab. 281 (2001) E1249–E1254.

[6] J.P. Stoehr, S.T. Nadler, K.L. Schueler, M.E. Rabaglia, B.S. Yandell, S.A. Metz, A.D. Attie, Genetic obesity

unmasks nonlinear interactions between murine type 2 diabetes susceptibility loci, Diabetes 49 (2000) 1946–1954.

[7] E. Lander, L. Kruglyak, Genetic dissection of complex traits: guidelines for interpreting and reporting linkage results, Nat. Genet. 11 (1995) 241–247.

[8] A. Darvasi, Interval-specific congenic strains (ISCS): an experimental design for mapping a QTL into a 1-centimorgan interval, Mamm. Genome 8 (1997) 163–167.

[9] S.T. Nadler, J.P. Stoehr, K.L. Schueler, G. Tanimoto, B.S. Yandell, A.D. Attie, The expression of adipogenic genes is decreased in obesity and diabetes mellitus, Proc. Natl. Acad. Sci. U. S. A. 97 (2000) 11371–11376.

[10] F. Diraison, E. Dusserre, H. Vidal, M. Sothier, M. Beylot, Increased hepatic lipogenesis but decreased expression of lipogenic gene in adipose tissue in human obesity, Am. J. Physiol.: Endocrinol. Metab. 282 (2002) E46–E51.

[11] P.H. Ducluzeau, N. Perretti, M. Laville, F. Andreelli, N. Vega, J.P. Riou, H. Vidal, Regulation by insulin of gene expression in human skeletal muscle and adipose tissue. Evidence for specific defects in type 2 diabetes, Diabetes 50 (2001) 1134–1142.

[12] H. Oberkofler, N. Fukushima, H. Esterbauer, F. Krempler, W. Patsch, Sterol regulatory element binding proteins: relationship of adipose tissue gene expression with obesity in humans, Biochim. Biophys. Acta 1575 (2002) 75–81.

[13] M. Kolehmainen, H. Vidal, E. Alhava, M.I. Uusitupa, Sterol regulatory element binding protein 1c (SREBP-1c) expression in human obesity, Obes. Res. 9 (2001) 706–712.

[14] H. Lan, M.E. Rabaglia, J.P. Stoehr, S.T. Nadler, K.L. Schueler, F. Zou, B.S. Yandell, A.D. Attie, Gene expression profiles of nondiabetic and diabetic obese mice suggest a role of hepatic lipogenic capacity in diabetes susceptibility, Diabetes 52 (2003) 688–700.

[15] S.T. Nadler, A.D. Attie, Please pass the chips: genomic insights into obesity and diabetes, J. Nutr. 131 (2001) 2078–2081.

International Congress Series 1262 (2004) 224–229

www.ics-elsevier.com

Genetics of the metabolic syndrome and implications for therapy

Robert I. Hughes[a,*], Timothy J. Aitman[b]

[a] Department of Experimental Medicine and Toxicology, Imperial College London (ICL), Hammersmith Campus, Ducane Rd, London W12 ONN, UK
[b] Physiological Genomics and Medicine Group, MRC Clinical Sciences Centre, Faculty of Medicine, ICL UK

Abstract. Insulin resistance (IR) is a key feature of several major risk factors for coronary heart disease, including type 2 diabetes, essential hypertension, combined hyperlipidaemia and obesity. These coronary risk factors have been brought together under the term "Metabolic Syndrome". Despite their high prevalence in Western populations, the molecular basis of these risk factors, and their pathogenic relationship to insulin resistance, remain poorly understood. We studied the genetics of insulin resistance in a rodent model of cardiovascular disease, the spontaneously hypertensive rat (SHR) and identified a defective SHR gene, *Cd36* or fatty acid translocase, which causes defects in insulin action and fatty acid metabolism in this rat model. Cd36 is a transmembrane transporter of long-chain fatty acids and a receptor for oxidised, low-density lipoproteins and has been proposed to play a key part in foam cell formation. Cd36 is induced by peroxisome proliferator-activated receptor γ (PPARγ), the target of the thiazolidinedione insulin-sensitising drugs. Deficiency of Cd36 is associated with reduced action of thiazolidinediones and marked protection against atherosclerosis. Elucidation of the mechanisms through which Cd36 influences insulin action and atherogenesis may lead to new insights into the pathogenesis of these common causes of cardiovascular disease and, ultimately, to new therapeutic approaches for their management.

Keywords: Metabolic syndrome; Insulin resistance; Cd36; Thiazolidinedione; Atherogenesis

1. Insulin resistance and the metabolic syndrome

Insulin resistance (IR) has a central role in the development of hypertension, dyslipidaemia, and type 2 diabetes mellitus (T2DM) (Fig. 1), and is a contributory factor in 40–60% of cases of premature coronary heart disease [1–3]. Since the original description of the metabolic syndrome, its component features have expanded to include microalbuminuria, central obesity, and raised levels of plasminogen activator inhibitor-1 (PAI-1) and uric acid. However, the mechanisms underlying these associations and their influence in the pathogenesis of cardiovascular disease are incompletely understood. It is

* Corresponding author. Tel.: +44-20-8383-4829; fax: +44-20-8383-2066.
E-mail address: r.hughes@imperial.ac.uk (R.I. Hughes).

doi:10.1016/j.ics.2003.12.005

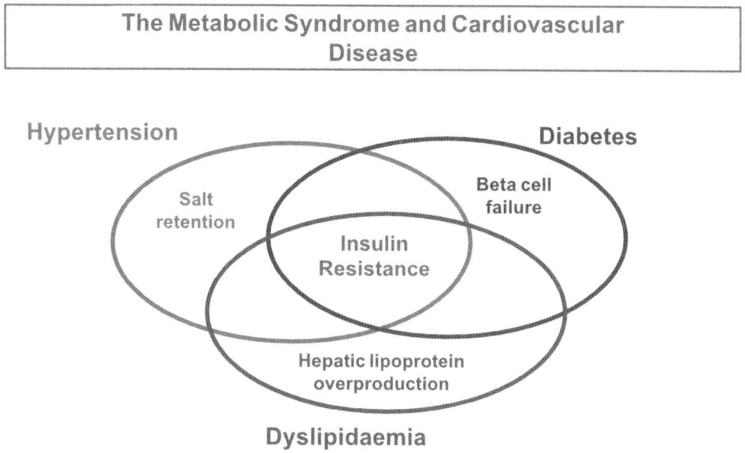

Fig. 1. Insulin resistance and the development of major cardiovascular risk factors. Insulin resistance alone has subtle effects that can be detected biochemically, but when combined with pancreatic beta cell failure, renal salt retention or hepatic overproduction of lipoproteins, leads to clinically overt diabetes, hypertension and dyslipidaemia. These are amongst the strongest and most prevalent risk factors for coronary heart disease.

likely that genetic and environmental influences act in concert to bring together this cluster of risk factors recognised as the metabolic syndrome.

2. Genetics of human insulin resistance

Despite significant insights gained from the study of rare familial cases of insulin resistance, the varying phenotypes of the highly prevalent IR syndromes suggest that these disorders are most usefully considered as genetically complex traits. Family and twin studies have consistently detected insulin resistance in non-diabetic subjects with a family history of diabetes, and formal segregation analyses in several population groups have found evidence of multiple major genes having effects on insulin action.

Genetic associations have been shown in case-control studies, although many of these still require replication and mechanistic explanation. The most consistent of these associations is that of the peroxisome proliferator-activated receptor γ (PPARγ) polymorphism Pro12Ala with T2DM and insulin sensitivity [4]. However, identification of the individual genes that underlie most genetic linkages reported to date in family studies has been prevented by the genetic complexity of the human phenotypes. We sought to simplify and accelerate the genetic study of IR by harnessing the power of linkage studies in rodent inbred strains, seeking confirmation of our results in gene targeting experiments.

3. Cd36 deficiency as a cause of insulin resistance in the spontaneously hypertensive rat (SHR)

The SHR was recognised as a model for studying defective insulin action 10–15 years ago when insulin resistance was identified in this model organism at the whole body level and in individual tissues. Since then, the coexistence of other features such as central obesity and dyslipidaemia have suggested the SHR as a valuable model for the human metabolic syndrome. Using the genome screen approach, a proximal area of SHR chromosome 4 was found to contain a quantitative trait locus (QTL) for both defective insulin action and catecholamine-mediated lipolysis [5,6]. QTLs for hypertriglyceridaemia and hypertension also mapped to the same region of chromosome 4.

Through an approach that combined use of DNA microarrays with positional information from their genetic linkage studies, Aitman et al. [6] identified a defect in an SHR gene, *Cd36* or fatty acid translocase, that was found to reside at the peak of linkage to the chromosome 4 QTL. Multiple variants were detected by cDNA sequencing in the SHR Cd36 coding sequence and western blot analysis showed that the Cd36 protein was undetectable in SHR adipocyte membranes. These data suggested that SHR is functionally deficient in Cd36. Since Cd36 is a cell-surface transporter of long chain fatty acids [7,8] whose expression is induced by the nuclear transcription factor PPARγ [9–11], it was concluded that the defective *Cd36* gene is a cause of insulin resistance, defective fatty acid metabolism and hypertriglyceridaemia in the NIH-derived strain of SHR [6].

Subsequent studies in *Cd36* knockout mice, compared with controls, revealed high levels of triglyceride (TG) and non-esterified fatty acid (NEFA) [12]. Knockout mice were furthermore shown to be insulin resistant and glucose intolerant, although this required the environmental stress of a high fructose diet to bring out this phenotype [13]. Most definitively, insulin resistance and dyslipidaemia were improved by introgressing wild type *Cd36* into the SHR genome by transgenic rescue [14].

4. Cd36 biology and its deficiency in humans

Cd36 is a multi-functional protein with a diverse tissue distribution and wide range of ligands. It belongs to the scavenger receptor family typified by SrB1 and mediates the specific uptake of long chain free fatty acids by adipocytes and muscle cells. Cd36 is also a high affinity receptor for oxidised low-density lipoproteins [8], a role that has been suggested to play a part in macrophage foam cell formation and atherosclerosis [9,10]. In macrophages and in fat cells, the Cd36 gene is transcriptionally induced by PPARγ [9–11].

Varying rates of prevalence of CD36 deficiency in different ethnic groups have been documented–the null allele is particularly common in Africans and far-Eastern Asians, in whom the heterozygous and homozygous frequency is 10–15% and 1%, respectively. The deficiency state is virtually non-existent in Caucasians. Despite the high frequency in certain populations, only the haematological consequences have been definitively established [16].

Miyaoka et al. [17] reported that Japanese subjects with CD36 deficiency have increased levels of triglycerides, increased fasting plasma glucose, hypertension and reduced insulin action. While CD36-deficient subjects consistently demonstrate impaired utilisation of free fatty acids, the regulation of glucose homeostasis in these individuals is less certain. For example, Furuhashi et al. [18] reported no significant increase in the frequency of insulin resistance in a CD36-deficient Japanese group (28% vs. 20% in the control group); although their study population had a 20% prevalence of diabetes (cf. 2–5% of the general population). Together, these data suggest that diabetes and IR are more common in CD36-deficient Japanese than in the wider Japanese population.

5. Cd36, the TZDs and atherogenesis

The thiazolidinedione group of drugs (TZDs) is attractive not only because of their effects on insulin resistance but also because they lower blood pressure, reduce inflammatory markers, and increase reverse cholesterol transport. They may also lower cardiovascular risk (see Fig. 2), although this is as yet unsubstantiated in long-term clinical trials.

Cd36 deficiency in rodents leads to development of a pro-atherogenic metabolic milieu with insulin resistance and dyslipidaemia. However, the expected consequence of premature, accelerated atherosclerosis does not occur—Cd36 knockout mice have a six-fold reduction in atheroma compared with controls [15]. This may be explained by reduced foam cell and atheroma formation due to interruption of the chain of events proposed by Tontonoz and Nagy (Fig. 2 and Refs. [9,10]). If Cd36 deficiency protects against atherosclerosis in mice, in part through decreased activation of PPARγ, the question arises whether PPARγ activation by the TZDs may promote atherogenesis. Currently, in vivo evidence supports a predominantly anti-atherogenic influence of these drugs. Treatment with the TZD, rosiglitazone, reduced atheroma formation in LDL-receptor deficient mice [19], while pioglitazone reduced carotid artery intima-media thickness in humans over treatment periods of 3 and 6 months [20].

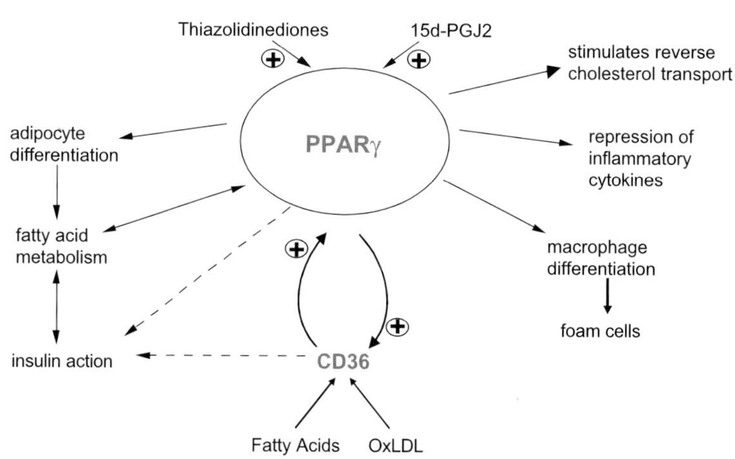

Fig. 2. PPARγ, CD36, insulin action and atherogenesis. Thiazolidinediones activate the nuclear receptor PPARγ, which has multiple actions including induction of CD36 expression. CD36 is a high-affinity ligand for long-chain fatty acids and for oxidised low-density lipoproteins (OxLDL), which are transported by CD36 across the plasma membrane by CD36. Inside the cell, fatty acid derivatives of OxLDL activate PPARγ, setting up a possible positive feedback loop between CD36 and PPARγ. The mechanism by which CD36 deficiency inhibits atherogenesis may be through inhibition of foam cell formation via PPARγ (15d-PGJ2, 15deoxy-prostaglandin J2).

6. Cd36 deficiency and TZD action

The close relationship of Cd36 to PPARγ, and the demonstration of Cd36 as an insulin resistant gene, raises a further question as to the role of Cd36 in TZD action on insulin resistance. To date, this has only been addressed in rat models. Cd36-deficient rats were found to be resistant to TZD effects on insulin resistance and lipid metabolism when compared with Cd36-replete strains [21,22]. These data suggest a key role for Cd36 in mediating TZD action, but the effect of CD36 deficiency in humans is unknown and warrants further investigation.

7. Summary

Cd36 deficiency is a cause of varying phenotypic features of the metabolic syndrome in rodents and humans. Animal models deficient in Cd36 are protected against atherosclerosis probably through prevention of foam cell formation. Cd36 deficient rodents are resistant to the effects of PPARγ activation by TZDs, although the efficacy of TZD action in CD36-deficient humans remains to be determined.

References

[1] G.M. Reaven, Role of insulin resistance in human disease (Banting Lecture), Diabetes 37 (1988) 1595–1607.

[2] P.M. McKeigue, J.E. Ferrie, T. Pierpoint, M.G. Marmot, Association of early-onset coronary heart disease in South Asian men with glucose intolerance and hyperinsulinemia, Circulation 87 (1) (1993) 152–161.

[3] D.M. Nathan, J. Meigs, D.E. Singer, The epidemiology of cardiovascular disease in type 2 diabetes mellitus: how sweet it is ... or is it? Lancet 350 (Suppl. 1) (1997) SI4–SI9.

[4] D. Altshuler, J.N. Hirschhorn, M. Klannemark, C.M. Lindgren, M.C. Vohl, J. Nemesh, C.R. Lane, S.F. Schaffner, S. Bolk, C. Brewer, T. Tuomi, D. Gaudet, T.J. Hudson, M. Daly, L. Groop, E.S. Lander, The common PPARγ Pro12Ala polymorphism is associated with decreased risk of type 2 diabetes, Nat. Genet. 26 (2000) 76–79.

[5] T.J. Aitman, T. Gotoda, A.L. Evans, H. Imrie, K.E. Heath, P.M. Trembling, H. Truman, C.A. Wallace, A. Rahman, C. Doré, J. Flint, V. Kren, V. Zidek, T. Kurtz, M. Pravenec, J. Scott, Quantitative trait loci for cellular defects in glucose and fatty acid metabolism in hypertensive rats, Nat. Genet. 16 (2) (1997) 197–201.

[6] T.J. Aitman, A.M. Glazier, C.A. Wallace, L.D. Cooper, P.J. Norsworthy, F.N. Wahid, K.M. Al-Majali, P.M. Trembling, C.J. Mann, C.C. Shoulders, D. Graf, E.S. Lezin, T.W. Kurtz, V. Kren, M. Pravenec, A. Ibrahimi, N.A. Abumrad, L.W. Stanton, J. Scott, Identification of *Cd36* (*Fat*) as an insulin-resistance gene causing defective fatty acid and glucose metabolism in hypertensive rats, Nat. Genet. 21 (1999) 76–83.

[7] N.A. Abumrad, M.R. El-Maghrabi, E.-Z. Amri, E. Lopez, P.A. Grimaldi, Cloning of a rat adipocyte membrane protein implicated in binding or transport of long chain fatty acids that is induced during preadipocyte differentiation, J. Biol. Chem. 268 (1993) 17665–17668.

[8] G. Endemann, L.W. Stanton, K.S. Madden, C.M. Bryant, R.T. White, A.A. Protter, CD36 is a receptor for oxidized low density lipoprotein, J. Biol. Chem. 268 (16) (1993) 11811–11816.

[9] P. Tontonoz, L. Nagy, J. Alvarez, V. Thomazy, R. Evans, PPARγ promotes monocote/macrophage differentiation and uptake of oxidized LDL, Cell 93 (1998) 241–252.

[10] L. Nagy, P. Tontonoz, J. Alvarez, H. Chen, R. Evans, Oxidized LDL regulates macrophage gene expression through ligand activation of PPARγ, Cell 93 (1998) 229–240.

[11] G. Chinetti, S. Lestavel, V. Bocher, A.T. Remaley, B. Neve, I.P. Torra, E. Teissier, A. Minnich, M. Jaye, N. Duverger, H.B. Brewer, J.-C. Fruchart, V. Clavey, B. Staels, PPAR-α and PPAR-γ activators induce cholesterol removal from human macrophage foam cells through stimulation of the ABCA1 pathway, Nat. Med. 7 (2001) 53–58.

[12] M. Febbraio, N.A. Abumrad, D.P. Hajjar, K. Sharma, W. Cheng, S.F.A. Pearce, R.L. Silverstein, A null

mutation in murine CD36 reveals an important role in fatty acid and lipoprotein metabolism, J. Biol. Chem. 274 (1999) 19055–19062.

[13] T. Hajri, X.X. Han, A. Bonen, N.A. Abumrad, Defective fatty acid uptake modulates insulin responsiveness and metabolic responses to diet in CD36-null mice, J. Clin. Invest. 109 (10) (2002) 1381–1389.

[14] M. Pravenec, V. Landa, V. Zidek, A. Musilova, V. Kren, L. Kazdova, T.J. Aitman, A.M. Glazier, A. Ibrahimi, N.A. Abumrad, N. Qi, J.-M. Wang, E.M. St. Lezin, T.W. Kurtz, Transgenic rescue of defective Cd36 ameliorates insulin resistance in spontaneously hypertensive rats, Nat. Genet. 27 (2) (2001) 156–158.

[15] M. Febbraio, E.A. Podrez, J.D. Smith, D.P. Hajjar, S.L. Hazen, H.F. Hoff, K. Sharma, R.L. Silverstein, Targeted disruption of the class B scavenger receptor CD36 protects against atherosclerotic lesion development in mice, J. Clin. Invest. 105 (2000) 1049–1056.

[16] B.R. Curtis, S. Ali, A.M. Glazier, D.D. Ebert, T.J. Aitman, R.H. Aster, Isoimmunization against CD36 (glycoprotein IV): description of four cases of neonatal isoimmune thrombocytopenia and brief review of the literature, Transfusion 42 (2002) 1173–1179.

[17] K. Miyaoka, T. Kuwasako, K. Hirano, S. Nozaki, S. Yamashita, Y. Matsuzawa, Human CD36 deficiency is associated with insulin resistance, Lancet 357 (2001) 686–687.

[18] M. Furuhashi, N. Ura, T. Nakata, K. Shimamoto, Insulin sensitivity and lipid metabolism in human CD36 deficiency, Diabetes Care 26 (2003) 471–474.

[19] A.C. Li, K.K. Brown, M.J. Silvestre, T.M. Willson, W. Palinski, C.K. Glass, Peroxisome proliferator-activated receptor γ ligands inhibit development of atherosclerosis in LDL receptor-deficient mice, J. Clin. Invest. 106 (2000) 523–531.

[20] H. Koshiyama, D. Shimono, N. Kuwamura, J. Minamikawa, Y. Nakamura, Rapid communication: inhibitory effect of pioglitazone on carotid arterial wall thickness in type 2 diabetes, J. Clin. Endocrinol. Metab. 86 (2001) 3452–3456.

[21] N. Qi, L. Kazdova, V. Zidek, V. Landa, V. Kren, H.A. Pershadsingh, E.S. Lezin, N.A. Abumrad, M. Pravenec, T.W. Kurtz, Pharmacogenetic evidence that *Cd36* is a key determinant of the metabolic effects of pioglitazone, J. Biol. Chem. 277 (2002) 48501–48507.

[22] O. Seda, L. Kazdova, D. Krenova, V. Kren, Rosiglitazone fails to improve hypertriglyceridemia and glucose tolerance in CD36-deficient BN. SHR4 congenic rat strain, Physiol. Genomics 12 (2003) 73–78.

International Congress Series 1262 (2004) 230–233

www.ics-elsevier.com

Unraveling the role of phospholipid transfer protein (PLTP) in lipoprotein metabolism and atherogenesis

Sarah Siggins, Minna Kärkkäinen, Vesa M. Olkkonen, Matti Jauhiainen, Christian Ehnholm*

Department of Molecular Medicine, National Public Health Institute, Biomedicum, P.O. Box 104, FIN-00251, Helsinki, Finland

Abstract. Plasma phospholipid transfer protein (PLTP) plays an essential role in HDL metabolism. Its role in the transfer of surface remnants from triglyceride-rich particles to HDL during lipolysis is of importance for the maintenance of HDL levels. It also modulates the size and composition of HDL particles, a function important for the reverse cholesterol transport process. Two forms of PLTP exist in plasma, one catalytically active and the other inactive. A new PLTP ELISA, has been developed whereby pre-treatment of the samples with the detergent SDS leads to the efficient detection of both forms of the protein. The new ELISA is an essential tool when addressing the mechanisms by which PLTP is converted from one form to the other. In addition to its central role in lipoprotein metabolism, a role for PLTP in macrophage cholesterol metabolism has been revealed. Differentiated macrophages produce PLTP, and during foam cell formation production of PLTP is markedly increased. As foam cells are a hallmark of early atherosclerotic lesions, further studies on the intra- and extracellular role of macrophage-derived PLTP will advance our knowledge on the function of PLTP in atherogenesis. © 2003 Published by Elsevier B.V.

Keywords: Atherosclerosis; Phospholipid transfer protein; Cholesterol efflux; Reverse cholesterol transport; High-density lipoproteins

1. Introduction

The ability of HDL to protect against the development of atherosclerotic coronary artery disease (CAD) is well documented and although the exact molecular mechanism(s) behind this finding remain unsolved, its role in the pathway of reverse cholesterol transport is well recognised [1]. Today the focus is directed towards three important areas: HDL-

Abbreviations: HDL, high-density lipoproteins; PLTP, phospholipid transfer protein; HA-PLTP, high-activity form of PLTP; LA-PLTP, low-activity form of PLTP; ELISA, enzyme-linked immunosorbant assay; SDS, sodium dodecyl sulphate.

* Corresponding author. Tel.: +358-9-4744-8258; fax: +358-9-4744-8960.

E-mail address: christian.ehnholm@ktl.fi (C. Ehnholm).

0531-5131/ © 2003 Published by Elsevier B.V.
doi:10.1016/j.ics.2003.11.004

associated apolipoproteins, HDL-modifying enzymes, and cellular proteins involved in HDL metabolism. The present review deals with the role of phospholipid transfer protein (PLTP) in HDL metabolism and the function of PLTP in atherogenesis.

2. PLTP function

The regulatory role of PLTP in HDL metabolism is achieved via its two main functions, phospholipid transfer activity [2] and its capability to modulate HDL size and composition [3]. In HDL conversion the generation of preβ-HDL particles enhances cholesterol efflux from peripheral cells, suggesting that PLTP is important for the prevention of atherosclerosis [4].

3. PLTP in animal models

The importance of PLTP-mediated phospholipid transfer in vivo is illustrated by studies using PLTP knock out (KO) mice. The plasma of homozygous PLTP KO-mice shows a total absence of ability to transfer phospholipids in vitro and in vivo [5]. The consequence of PLTP deficiency is a 60–70% reduction in HDL lipid and apoA-I levels, resulting from hypercatabolism of phosphatidylcholine-depleted HDL particles.

The physiological role of PLTP in human lipoprotein metabolism is still far from resolved, yet the in vivo overexpression of PLTP either with adenovirus or by transgene results in a marked reduction of HDL levels [6,7]. The increased capacity of mice overexpressing PLTP to produce pre β-HDL has been demonstrated [6]. Plasma from these animals prevents accumulation of intracellular cholesterol in macrophages more efficiently than plasma from wild-type mice, indicating that PLTP is mediating an increase in cholesterol efflux [6]. However, PLTP-deficient mice display decreased atherosclerosis due to lowered secretion of circulating apoB-containing lipoproteins and a decreased oxidation potential [8,9]. Furthermore, PLTP overexpression in hyperlipidemic mouse strains also increases the tendency for developing lesions [9]. These mice provide evidence for the importance of PLTP-mediated lipid transfer in the maintenance of lipoprotein levels.

4. Catalytically active and inactive forms of PLTP in human plasma

The development of the PLTP mass ELISA revealed the presence of two forms of PLTP in plasma, one catalytically active, high-activity PLTP (HA-PLTP) and the other inactive, low-activity PLTP (LA-PLTP) [10]. We have isolated and partially characterised these forms [11]. A similar HA-PLTP form was characterised from HepG2 cells [12]. The LA-PLTP is complexed with apoA-I, whereas HA-PLTP co-purifies with apoE. We suggest a model in which nascent PLTP enters plasma as a high activity form not associated with apoA-I. During or after the transfer of lipolytic surface remnants to HDL, PLTP is transferred to apoA-I, containing HDL particles and thereby becomes part of the low activity complex. Further characterisation of these complexes will clarify the physiological implications of the distribution of PLTP between the two forms and the mechanism behind PLTP inactivation.

A new PLTP ELISA, to accurately quantitate LA-and HA-PLTP has been developed so that a pre-treatment of the samples with SDS detergent is used to reveal epitopes, thus leading to the efficient detection of both forms of the protein. The new ELISA is an essential tool for addressing the mechanisms by which PLTP is converted from one form to another.

5. Regulation of PLTP synthesis and secretion

The central role of nuclear hormone receptors in the control of HDL-associated factors and the reverse cholesterol transport process is evident [13]. The promoter of the human PLTP gene contains peroxisome proliferator-activated receptor (PPAR)-responsive element-like sequences, which are apparently responsible for the fibrate-induced down-regulation of PLTP expression observed in HepG2 cells [14]. PLTP gene expression is also activated by bile acids through a mechanism involving the farnesoid X-activated receptor (FXR) [15] and by a specific liver X-activated receptor (LXR) agonist [16].

6. PLTP in HepG2 cells

We have used the human hepatoma cell line, HepG2, as a model to study hepatic PLTP secretion [12]. HepG2-derived PLTP: (i) was enriched by Heparin-Sepharose affinity chromatography and eluted in size-exclusion chromatography at a position corresponding to 160 kDa; (ii) co-eluted with apoE but not with apoB-100 or apoA-I; (iii) was partially retained by an anti-apoE immunoaffinity column together with apoE, suggesting an interaction between these two proteins and finally; (iv) antibodies against apoE, but not those against apoB-100 or apoA-I-inhibited PLTP activity. These results show that the HepG2-derived PLTP resembles the plasma HA counterpart.

7. PLTP in other tissues

In addition to a central role in plasma lipoprotein metabolism, recent studies suggest a role for PLTP in macrophage cholesterol metabolism. PLTP is a target for LXR regulation not only in the liver but also in macrophages [16]. Moreover, PLTP is highly expressed by macrophages in human atherosclerotic lesions [17]. Furthermore, loading of macrophages with acetylated LDL induces a marked increase in PLTP mRNA and protein expression [17]. Differentiated macrophages and foam cells are a hallmark of early atherosclerotic lesions. The observation that PLTP, as well as apoE, are produced by macrophages and that their production is markedly increased during foam cell formation indicates that the role of locally produced macrophage-derived PLTP in atherogenesis is an important topic for investigation.

Acknowledgements

This work was supported by the International HDL Research Awards Program (to C.E., M.J., and V.M.O), Finska Läkaresällskapet (to S.S.), Magnus Ehrnrooths Stiftelse (to S.S.), Wihuri Research Foundation (to M.K.), Finnish Foundation for Cardiovascular Research (to M.K. and M.J.), and Sigrid Juselius Foundation (to M.J.).

References

[1] K.-A. Rye, M.A. Clay, P.J. Barter, Atherosclerosis 145 (1999) 227–238.
[2] R. Rao, J.J. Albers, G. Wolfbauer, H.J. Pownall, Biochemistry 36 (1997) 3645–3653.

[3] M. Jauhiainen, J. Metso, R. Pahlman, S. Blomqvist, A. van Tol, C. Ehnholm, J. Biol. Chem. 268 (1993) 4032–4036.

[4] M. Lee, J. Metso, M. Jauhiainen, P.T. Kovanen, J. Biol. Chem. 278 (2003) 13539–13545.

[5] X.C. Jiang, C. Bruce, J. Mar, M. Lin, Y. Ji, O.L. Francone, A.R. Tall, J. Clin. Invest. 103 (1999) 907–914.

[6] R. van Haperen, A. van Tol, P. Vermeulen, M. Jauhiainen, T. van Gent, P. van den Berg, S. Ehnholm, F. Grosveld, A. van der Kamp, R. de Crom, Arterioscler. Thromb. Vasc. Biol. 20 (2000) 1082–1088.

[7] S. Ehnholm, K.W. van Dijk, B. van't Hof, A. van der Zee, V.M. Olkkonen, M. Jauhiainen, M. Hofker, L. Havekes, C. Ehnholm, J. Lipid Res. 39 (1998) 1248–1253.

[8] X.C. Jiang, S. Qin, C. Qiao, K. Kawano, M. Lin, A. Skold, X. Xiao, A.R. Tall, Nat. Med. 7 (2001) 847–852.

[9] X.P. Yang, D. Yan, C. Qiao, R.J. Liu, J.G. Chen, J. Li, M. Schneider, L. Lagrost, X. Xiao, X.C. Jiang, Increased Arterioscler. Thromb. Vasc. Biol. (2003) (In Press).

[10] T. Oka, T. Kujiraoka, M. Ito, T. Egashira, N.M. Nanjee, N.E. Miller, J. Metso, V.M. Olkkonen, C. Ehnholm, M. Jauhiainen, H. Hattori, J. Lipid Res. 41 (2000) 1651–1657.

[11] M. Karkkainen, T. Oka, V.M. Olkkonen, J. Metso, H. Hattori, M. Jauhiainen, C. Ehnholm, J. Biol. Chem. 277 (2002) 15413–15418.

[12] S. Siggins, M. Jauhiainen, V.M. Olkkonen, J. Tenhunen, C. Ehnholm, J. Lipid Res. 44 (2003) 1698–1704.

[13] J.J. Repa, S.I. Turley, J.-M.A. Lobaccaro, J. Medina, L. Li, K. Lustig, B. Shan, R.A. Heyman, J.M. Dietschy, D.J. Mangelsdorf, Science 289 (2000) 1524–1529.

[14] A.-Y. Tu, J.J. Albers, Biochem. Biophys. Res. Commun. 264 (1999) 802–807.

[15] N.L. Urizar, D.H. Dowhan, D.D. Moore, J. Biol. Chem. 275 (2000) 39313–39317.

[16] B.A. Laffitte, S.B. Joseph, M. Chen, A. Castrillo, J. Repa, D. Wilpitz, D. Mangelsdorf, P. Tontonoz, Mol. Cell. Biol. 23 (2003) 2182–2191.

[17] C.M. Desrumaux, P.A. Mak, W.A. Boisvert, D. Masson, D. Stupack, M. Jauhiainen, C. Ehnholm, L.K. Curtiss, J. Lipid Res. 44 (2003) 1453–1461.

ELSEVIER

International Congress Series 1262 (2004) 234–238

www.ics-elsevier.com

Effect of hormone replacement therapy on the reverse cholesterol transport

Carlos Calvo*

Department of Clinical Biochemistry and Immunology, University of Concepción, Casilla 237, Correo 3, Concepción, Chile

Abstract. Hormone replacement therapy (HRT) in healthy postmenopausal women modifies the HDL lipid composition, selectively increases the HDL subpopulation that only contains apolipoprotein A-I (LpA-I) and decreases the activity of phospholipid transfer protein (PLTP), a key protein regulating HDL levels. In addition, HRT increases the plasma capacity to promote cholesterol efflux in vitro. These findings demonstrate that HRT not only increases HDL-cholesterol levels, but also modifies HDL physiochemical properties, possibly optimising its function in the reverse cholesterol transport. © 2004 Elsevier B.V. All rights reserved.

Keywords: Hormone replacement therapy; Antiatherogenesis; HDL; Reverse cholesterol transport

1. Introduction

In spite of the fact that estrogenic substitution in postmenopausal women has failed to demonstrate protection from cardiovascular disease, the beneficial effects of estrogens on the mechanisms leading to atherogenesis are evident [1].

The beneficial effects of hormone replacement therapy (HRT) may in part result from increases in HDL-cholesterol. Furthermore, as HRT constitutes a potent method for raising HDL levels [2], it may be useful for exploring the mechanisms that regulate HDL metabolism.

A major hypothesis to explain the antiatherogenic properties of HDL is related to its role in the reverse cholesterol transport (RCT), a pathway by which excess cholesterol is removed from the peripheral cells and transported to the liver for elimination in bile [3]. The first step of RCT begins with cholesterol efflux from cell membranes to pre-β1-HDL, which are the first acceptors of cell-derived free cholesterol. Thereafter, lecithin–cholesterol acyltransferase (LCAT) catalyses the cholesterol esterification in these particles and HDL-cholesterol ester may be transferred to triglyceride-rich lipoproteins by cholesterol ester transfer protein (CETP) with subsequent metabolism and hepatic uptake or removed by a selective uptake in liver or other tissues involving the scavenger receptor (SR-B1).

* Tel./fax: +56-41-207086.
E-mail address: ccalvo@udec.cl (C. Calvo).

doi:10.1016/j.ics.2003.12.086

In addition, the plasma contains another lipid transfer protein known as phospholipid transfer protein (PLTP). It has been proposed that PLTP might exert a dual beneficial effect on RCT through the concomitant generation of pre-β-HDLs and large cholesteryl ester-rich α-HDLs, which can carry large amounts of cholesterol back to the liver [4]. Furthermore, PLTP transports postlipolytic surface remnants, mainly phospholipids, to the HDL fraction, and via this function participates in the maintenance of plasma HDL levels [5].

This report shows the effect of sequential combined estrogen–progestin replacement therapy on lipid composition of HDL, concentration of apolipoprotein A-I (LpA-I) and LpA-I:A-II particles, plasma capacity to carry out cholesterol efflux from Fu5AH cells, and the activities of PLTP and LCAT (two key proteins regulating HDL levels), in a group of healthy postmenopausal women.

2. HDL lipid composition

The HDL lipid composition consisting of HDL-cholesterol ester, HDL-free cholesterol, HDL-phospholipids, and HDL-triglycerides showed significant variation during HRT.

The HDL content of cholesterol increased rapidly at 15 days of therapy and reached a mean increase of 12.2% above baseline at day 71. This increment was due almost exclusively to the increase of HDL-free cholesterol. The cholesterol ester remained unchanged.

Phospholipids and triglycerides of HDL also showed a significant increase after 71 days of HRT in comparison to baseline. No significant differences were observed in HDL lipids in the placebo group.

3. HDL-lipoparticles

It is well known that HDL is a heterogeneous entity containing two main lipoparticle subpopulations. These subfractions are identified as those containing both apolipoproteins (apo) A-I and A-II, called LpA-I:A-II, and those that only contain apo A-I, called LpA-I [6]. Since premenopausal women have higher levels of LpA-I than age-matched men [7] it is possible to speculate that estrogen could selectively increase these lipoparticle levels. In vitro studies have concluded that the apoA-I and apoA-II content of HDL is one determinant in its ability to promote cholesterol efflux from cell membranes [8]. In addition, a higher association between cholesterol efflux and plasma LpA-I than LpA-I:A-II was demonstrated, suggesting that LpA-I is a better cholesterol acceptor from cell membranes [9].

HRT produced selective increase in LpA-I particles at 15 days post-therapy, and this effect was maintained during the evaluation period. No significant differences were observed in the placebo group. The intergroup comparison revealed a significantly higher value in the HRT group than in the placebo group. There was not a significant difference in the LpA-I:A-II concentration in either the HRT or placebo group.

Another study supporting our finding demonstrated in six surgically postmenopausal women that oral estrogen replacement therapy selectively raised LpA-I levels [10]. The increase in LpA-I as a consequence of HRT is in agreement with previous in vitro findings using HepG2 cells, where it was demonstrated that estradiol stimulates a selective increase in ^{3}H-Leu incorporation into LpA-I but not LpA-I:A-II particles and also stimulates transcription of hepatic apoA-I mRNA without affecting its half-life [11]. Since LpA-I appears to be a better cholesterol acceptor in some in vitro systems [8], increased levels could explain to a certain extent the antiatherogenic effect of HRT. However, epidemiologic insights concerning LpA-I and LpA-I:A-II lipoparticles as protective HDL subfractions are still controversial. Some cross-sectional epidemiologic studies have suggested that LpA-I is apparently more antiatherogenic than LpA-I:A-II [12,13]. However, a recent prospective study showed that LpA-I and LpA-I:A-II were both reduced in male survivors of myocardial infarction, suggesting that a decrease in both particles is a risk marker of CHD [14]. Therefore, the question if LpA-I is or is not more protective than LpA-I:A-II still remains unanswered.

4. Cholesterol efflux

The basal values of cholesterol efflux did not display significant differences between HRT and placebo. There was a significant difference in the response of cholesterol efflux between the two groups starting at day 15 of HRT, which remained constant through the entire period. While the HRT group significantly increased the cholesterol efflux at day 71, the placebo group did not show significant modifications during treatment.

The increase in cholesterol efflux was very close to the mean increase of HDL-cholesterol during HRT, a result that agrees with the correlation found between HDL and cholesterol efflux [9].

Positive correlations were found between cholesterol efflux and LpA-I lipoparticles, HDL-phospholipids, HDL-free cholesterol and apoA-I. The other HDL lipids did not demonstrate significant correlations with cholesterol efflux.

The positive relationship between LpA-I lipoparticles and cholesterol efflux suggests that HRT may optimize the cholesterol efflux in vivo. The positive relationship between cholesterol efflux and phospholipid from HDL agrees with previous in vitro studies reporting a strong positive correlation between both variables [15]. It has been postulated that the cholesterol efflux from plasma membranes to HDL could be accomplished by two mechanisms. First, if HDL is rich in lipids (α-HDL), it is believed that free cholesterol from membranes enter into HDL by an aqueous diffusion, a mechanism by which LCAT generates a concentration gradient favourable to cholesterol efflux. Second, if there are apoA-I particles poor in lipids (pre-β1-HDL), there could be a simultaneous micro-solubilization of free cholesterol and phospholipids from plasma membranes with both lipids being directly incorporated into the particle rich in apoA-I and poor in lipid. This theory, together with our findings that HRT increases apoA-I, LpA-I, HDL-phospholipids, and HDL-free cholesterol, and that all of these parameters are positively correlated between themselves, suggests that HRT may generate a high concentration of lipid-poor apoA-I, which could increase the phospholipid efflux driving cholesterol efflux from plasma membranes to HDL.

5. LCAT activity

LCAT activity evaluated with exogenous substrates (liposomes) was unchanged by hormonal substitution. Although these findings suggest that this enzyme was not increased, the possibility that LCAT could be more active with its natural substrate, endogenous HDL, cannot be excluded. These findings appear to be contradictory to a previous report from our group that demonstrated an increase in LCAT activity with HRT [16]. However, in that study, the blood was collected in the combined estrogen–progestin period, whereas in this study it was done at the end of unopposed estrogenic period.

6. PLTP activity

PLTP activity was significantly decreased after 71 days post-therapy and this modification was also significant when compared with the placebo group. No significant changes were observed early on, at 15 or 43 days post-HRT.

Negative correlations between PLTP activity and LpA-I:A-II, LpA-I and apoA-I were found.

PLTP activity showed a behavior different from all other parameters. A late significant decrease was evident only after 71 days of HRT. Since it has been demonstrated that PLTP shows a positive relationship with blood glucose levels [17] and that the promoter of the human PLTP gene possesses five consensus sequences for the transcription factor Sp1 which is considered a glucose-responsive element, it has been suggested that PLTP is related to glucose metabolism [4]. Taking this information into consideration, the late PLTP decrease could be explained as a secondary effect to the improvement in glucose tolerance that appears to be produced by HRT [18]. On the other hand, the possibility that the hormonal effect launched by estrogen–progestin treatment itself might affect and reduce PLTP activity is not excluded. Interpretation of these results should be made with caution due to the fact that the PLTP decrease was seen only after 71 days (i.e., at one time point); however, this finding is in agreement with a recent study [19] done in normolipidemic Finnish women aged 25–34 and 35–44 years with normal female hormone status and which results showed that PLTP activity was significantly lower compared with that seen among postmenopausal women aged 55–64 years. Since PLTP has been implicated as one of the key factors that mediates pre-β1-HDL formation, the present decline in PLTP activity suggests that other mechanisms to generate pre-β-HDL along with PLTP might be involved here. Furthermore, estrogen–progestin treatment may generate HDL subpopulations with increased substrate properties for PLTP function, like the present increment of HDL particle triglyceride content. It has been demonstrated that when HDL is enriched with triglycerides, the PLTP-mediated HDL conversion and thus pre-β-HDL generations is enhanced [20]. However, further studies are needed to elucidate the mechanism by which estrogens appear to diminish the PLTP activity and its consequences on lipid metabolism.

References

[1] The Women's Health Initiative Investigators, Risks and benefits of estrogen plus progestin in healthy postmenopausal women, JAMA 288 (2002) 321-333.

[2] B. Walsh, H. Li, F. Sacks, Effects of postmenopausal hormone replacement with oral and transdermal estrogen on HDL metabolism, J. Lipid Res. 35 (1994) 2083–2093.

[3] C. Fielding, P. Fielding, Molecular physiology of reverse cholesterol transport, J. Lipid Res. 36 (1995) 211–218.

[4] L. Lagrost, C. Desrumaux, D. Masson, et al., Structure and function of the plasma phospholipid transfer protein, Curr. Opin. Lipidol. 9 (1998) 203–209.

[5] K. Kawano, S. Qin, M. Lin, et al., Cholesteryl ester transfer protein and phospholipids transfer protein have nonoverlapping functions in vivo, J. Biol. Chem. 275 (2000) 29477–29481.

[6] P. Bustos, N. Ulloa, C. Calvo, et al., Monoclonal antibodies to human apolipoproteins: application to study of high density lipoprotein subpopulations, Clin. Chim. Acta 299 (2000) 151–167.
[7] H. Parra, H. Mezdour, N. Ghalim, et al., Differential electroimmunoassay of human LpA-I lipoprotein particles on ready-to-use plates, Clin. Chem. 36 (1990) 1431–1435.
[8] L. Lagrost, C. Dengremont, A. Athias, et al., Modulation of cholesterol efflux from Fu5AH hepatoma cells by the apolipoprotein content of high density lipoprotein particles, J. Biol. Chem. 270 (1995) 13004–13009.
[9] M. De la Llera Moya, V. Atger, J. Paul, et al., A cell culture system for screening human serum for ability to promote cellular cholesterol effux. Relations between serum components and efflux, esterification and transfer, Arterioscler. Thromb. Vasc. Biol. 14 (1994) 1056–1065.
[10] E. Brinton, Oral estrogen replacement therapy in postmenopausal women selectively raises levels and production rates of lipoprotein A-I and lowers hepatic activity without lowering the fractional catabolic rate, Arterioscler. Thromb. Vasc. Biol. 16 (1996) 431–440.
[11] F. Jin, V. Kamanna, M. Kashyap, Estradiol stimulates apolipoprotein A-I but not A-II containing particles synthesis and secretion by stimulating mRNA transcription rate in Hep G2 cells, Arterioscler. Thromb. Vasc. Biol. 18 (2000) 999–1006.
[12] P. Puchois, A. Kandoussi, P. Fievet, Apolipoprotein A-I containing lipoprotein in coronary artery disease, Atherosclerosis 68 (1987) 35–40.
[13] C. Calvo, A. Olmos, N. Ulloa, P. Bustos, Lipoprotein particles LpA-I, LpA-II and LpB in coronary artery disease, Rev. Med. Chile 128 (2000) 9–16.
[14] C. Luc, J. Bard, A. Evans, et al., The relationship between apolipoprotein containing lipoprotein fractions and environ metal factors: the PRIME study, Atherosclerosis 152 (2000) 399–405.
[15] N. Fournier, M. De la Llera Moya, B. Burkey, et al., Role of HDL phospholipids in efflux of cell cholesterol to whole serum: studies with human apoA-I transgenic rat, J. Lipid Res. 37 (1996) 1704–1711.
[16] N. Ulloa, C. Verdugo, M. Ríos, J. Sepúlveda, R. Naveas, C. Calvo, Increased activity of lecithin: cholesterol acyltransferase during a short term oral estrogen-progestative replacement therapy in a group of postmenopausal women, Metabolism 47 (1998) 297–300.
[17] S. Murdoch, M. Carr, J. Makanson, et al., PLTP activity in premenopausal women: relationship with lipoprotein lipase, HDL, LDL, body fat, and insulin resistance, J. Lipid Res. 41 (2000) 237–244.
[18] F. Cucinelli, P. Paparello, L. Soranna, et al., Different effect of transdermal strogen plus progestagen replacement therapy on isulin metabolism in post-menopausal women: relation to their insulinemic secretion, Eu. J. Endocrinol. 140 (1999) 215–223.
[19] J. Huuskonen, M. Ekstrom, E. Tahvanaivien, et al., Quantification of human plasma phospholipid transfer protein (PLTP): retalionship between PLTP mass and phospholipid transfer activity, Atherosclerosis 151 (2000) 451–461.
[20] K. Rye, M. Jauhiainen, P. Barter, et al., Triglyceride-enrichment of high density lipoproteins enhances their remodelling by phospholipid transfer protein, J. Lipid Res. 39 (1998) 613–622.

International Congress Series 1262 (2004) 239–242

www.ics-elsevier.com

Bridging the decades: new era is open for preclinical and clinical trials Introductory remarks—"looking back the past decades"

Akira Yamamoto *

Health Care Facilities for the Aged, Minoh Life Plaza, and National Cardiovascular Center Research Institute, 5-8-2 Kayano, Minoh, Osaka 562-0014, Japan

Abstract. The last three decades of the 20th century were the decades of statins in the prevention and treatment of atherosclerotic diseases. Statins not only gave strong support to the lipid hypothesis in atherogenesis but also broke down the idea that lowering serum cholesterol might be harmful. Results obtained by intervention studies using statins fundamentally changed the interpretation of the ideal cholesterol level in Europe and America. Probucol made a great contribution to understanding the role of oxidative LDL in atherogenesis and developing the idea of "beyond cholesterol". The term "pleiotropic effect" is now very popular. Among many lipid-lowering drugs, it is the fibrate which most deserves this expression through its multiple effects including those on lipids, fibrinogen and glucose tolerance. However, it took 20–30 years from the appearance of the first fibrate for such multiple effects to be explained by their function through a nuclear receptor, PPAR. Development of new drugs has often promoted the creation of a novel academic theory in medical and biological sciences, but it sometimes has taken a long time to meet such a chance. Elucidation of genes will accelerate this process. While the complexity of factors related to atherogenesis will make it more difficult to prove the effectiveness of a drug by clinical trials, the drug will be a useful tool to determine the real function of genes. © 2003 Published by Elsevier B.V.

Keywords: Antilipidemic drug; Statin; Fibrate; Probucol; ACAT inhibitor

1. Decades of statins

It is 30 years since Akira Endo discovered compactin in the culture extract of penicillium citrinum. In 1978, the first application of compactin in patients with familial hypercholesterolemia was carried out. Soon after the appearance of simvastatin and pravastatin, two important intervention studies, 4S and WOSCOP, were designed and started in Europe. Around that time, the fear of the harmful effects of lowering cholesterol

* Tel.: +81-72-727-9530; fax: +81-72-727-3598.
E-mail address: ymmt-a@juno.dti.ne.jp (A. Yamamoto).

0531-5131/ © 2003 Published by Elsevier B.V.
doi:10.1016/S0531-5131(03)01858-2

arose and a sensation was created by an essay written by Thomas Moore entitled "Cholesterol Myth" published in the Atlantic Monthly. The results of 4S and WOSCOP broke down the idea that lowering cholesterol was risky.

The safety of statins has been assured by the knowledge that their cholesterol lowering effect is mediated by the upregulation of LDL receptors. In fact, the development of the statin in its early stage has advanced in favor of the progress in research on the homeostasis of cholesterol carried out by Goldstein and Brown. Recently, more powerful statins, which can suppress cholesterol synthesis efficiently in the liver, have appeared on the market, and choosing the proper antilipidemic agent for the purpose of achieving the goal of the ideal cholesterol level has become a matter of great discussion.

2. Forty years since the appearance of the first fibrate

Statins also led to the popularization of the term "pleiotropic effect". However, it might be the fibrate, which most deserves this phrase. It is already 40 years since the appearance of clofibrate, the first fibrate compound. Early experiences of clofibrate have shown that (1) it decreases triglyceride and increases HDL-cholesterol, (2) decreases free fatty acid, (3) improves glucose tolerance, (4) suppresses platelet aggregation, (5) decreases fibrinogen and enhances fibrinolysis and (6) decreases uric acid.

Several intervention studies using fibrates, such as, the Helsinki Heart Study, Veterans Administration-HDL-Cholesterol Intervention Trial (VA-HIT), Bezafibrate Infarction Prevention (BIP), Bezafibrate Coronary Atherosclerosis Intervention Trial (BECAIT), and Diabetes Atherosclerosis Intervention Study (DAIS) showed that fibrates were effective in preventing the progression of coronary atherosclerosis and decreasing coronary events.

Understanding of the particular features of fibrates showed great progress through the discovery of PPAR, which regulates the intracellular utilization of both lipids and glucose, and encouraged the development of new drugs that are effective in the treatment of metabolic syndrome.

3. Probucol—an inhibitor of LDL-oxidation

An important finding obtained in the 20th century on the mechanism of atherosclerosis was the role of macrophages. About 20 years ago, an interesting drug named probucol, which was originally developed as an antioxidant to protect rubber from oxidation, was brought on the market as a cholesterol-lowering agent. It soon attracted attention of lipidologists as the drug caused rapid regression of skin and tendon xanthomas in homozygous familial hypercholesterolemia. Probucol became a useful tool for Daniel Steinberg in developing his theory that oxidative LDL plays an important role in atherogenesis and creating a catchphrase "beyond cholesterol".

Although an intervention trial targeted to the regression of femoral arteries failed to produce satisfactory results, clinical studies are still continuing to re-examine the effect of probucol by angiographical assessment, especially targeting the prevention of restenosis after balloon angioplasty [1]. Sawayama et al. compared the effects of probucol and pravastatin on the intima-media thickness of carotid arteries in asymptomatic patients with hypercholesterolemia with an average serum LDL-cholesterol level of 166 mg/dl. After 2 years, both drugs succeeded in preventing an increase in intima-media thickness. The total number of coronary events was much less in the probucol group, despite the reduction of LDL-cholesterol in the probucol group being significantly less than in the pravastatin group [2].

Probucol did not receive a high evaluation in the market in Europe and America because it decreased HDL. However, evidences have been obtained that suggest that probucol enhances the transport of cholesterol. A recent report from Monte Krieger's laboratory showed that probucol prevented early coronary death in the SR-B1/apolipoprotein E double knockout mouse [3].

4. Inhibitors of cholesterol absorption

Inhibition of cholesterol absorption has also been a matter of interest. Sitosterol and other plant sterols have been used as a cholesterol-lowering agent and their presence in vegetable oil is thought to be beneficial in keeping healthy. Sterol glycoside is also known to inhibit cholesterol absorption. Recently, an interesting drug named ezetimibe has been approved in the United States and some European countries. The drug is useful in combination therapy with statins or fibrates. The mechanism of the effect of ezetimibe will serve well in the elucidation of the mechanism of cholesterol absorption.

5. Multifarious effects of ACAT inhibitors

The first ACAT inhibitor produced by Sumitomo Pharmaceuticals had also been developed as an inhibitor of cholesterol absorption. Later on, ACAT inhibitors were intensively researched in the last two decades of the 20th century targeting the prevention of the lipid storage in macrophages. An ACAT inhibitor, which seems promising at present, is avasimibe [4]. This drug is now undergoing a long-term clinical trial using intravascular ultrasound to examine whether avasimibe can prevent the progression of coronary atherosclerosis. Although there is a discrepancy in cholesterol lowering potency between animal experiments and the Early Phase II Study, the reduction in triglycerides and VLDL-cholesterol observed in clinical cases seems important.

Interesting results obtained by the use of ACAT inhibitors including avasimibe are an increase in expression of SR-B1 and an increase in bile acid synthesis in cultured hepatocytes. In view of the limited conversion of cholesterol to bile acid in humans, the effect of ACAT inhibitors on the metabolic sequence of cholesterol in humans seems very important.

An important issue regarding the development of the ACAT inhibitor is that there are two enzymes: ACAT 1 which is distributed in many tissues including macrophages and the adrenal glands and ACAT 2 which is specific to the liver and intestine. The specific inhibition of ACAT in macrophages is a matter of particular interest with regard to the anti-atherogenic activity. However, specific care must be taken with regard to serious side effects due to the accumulation of free cholesterol in various tissues. Disturbances in adrenal function were especially a matter of concern in preclinical studies.

6. CETP inhibitor: increasing HDL-cholesterol

Suppression of cholesterol ester transfer protein (CETP) has been a target for elevating HDL-cholesterol and treating atherosclerosis, because small dense LDL particles produced by the effect of CETP are more atherogenic than ordinary LDL particles. JTT-705 has been shown to attenuate atherosclerosis in preliminary animal experiments. But, further studies on cholesterol-fed, hypercholesterolemic rabbits suggested a relatively minor favorable effect of HDL-elevating treatment as compared with decreases in non-HDL-cholesterol levels [5]. An early phase II trial was carried out in Europe to test efficacy and safety in humans and the results showed its effectiveness in increasing HDL-cholesterol with minor side effects. Further studies are needed to investigate whether the observed increase in HDL-cholesterol translates into a concomitant reduction in coronary artery disease risk.

References

[1] H. Daida, Y. Kuwabara, H. Yokoi, and the PART Investigators, Effects of probucol on repeat revascularization rate after percutaneous transluminal coronary angioplasty (from the Probucol Angioplasty Restenosis Trial (PART)), Am. J. Cardiol. 86 (2000) 550–552.

[2] Y. Sawayama, C. Shimizu, N. Maeda, M. Tatsukawa, N. Kinukawa, S. Koyanagi, S. Kashiwagi, J. Hayashi, Effects of probucol and pravastatin on common carotid atherosclerosis in patients with asymptomatic hypercholesterolemia: Fukuoka Atherosclerosis Trial (FAST), J. Am. Coll. Cardiol. 39 (2002) 610–616.

[3] A. Braun, S. Zhang, H.E. Miettinen, S. Ebrahim, T.M. Holm, E. Vasile, M.J. Post, D.M. Yoerger, M.H. Picard, J.L. Krieger, N.C. Andrews, M. Simons, M. Krieger, Probucol prevents early coronary heart disease and death in the high-density lipoprotein receptor SR-B1/apolipoprotein E double knockout mouse, Proc. Natl. Acad. Sci. U. S. A. 100 (2003) 7283–7288.

[4] G. Llaverias, J.C. Laguna, M. Alegret, Pharmacology of the ACAT inhibitor avasimibe, Cardiovasc. Drug Rev. 21 (2003) 33–50.

[5] Z. Huang, A. Inazu, A. Nahara, T. Higashikata, H. Mabuchi, Cholesteryl ester transfer protein inhibitor (JTT-705) and the development of atherosclerosis in rabbits with severe hypercholesterolemia, Clin. Sci. 103 (2002) 587–594.

ELSEVIER

International Congress Series 1262 (2004) 243–246

www.ics-elsevier.com

Ezetimibe: first in a new class of cholesterol absorption inhibitors

Harry R. Davis*

Department of CNS and Cardiovascular Research, Schering-Plough Research Institute, K-15-2/2600, 2015 Galloping Hill Rd., Kenilworth, NJ 07033, USA

Abstract. Ezetimibe is a selective cholesterol absorption inhibitor, which potently inhibits the absorption of biliary and dietary cholesterol from the small intestine without affecting the absorption of fat-soluble vitamins, triglycerides or bile acids. Ezetimibe reduces the small intestinal enterocyte uptake and absorption of cholesterol, which keeps the cholesterol in the intestinal lumen for excretion. Ezetimibe undergoes glucuronidation to a single metabolite and localizes at the intestinal wall, where it prevents cholesterol absorption. Enterohepatic recirculation of ezetimibe and/or its glucuronide ensures repeated delivery to the site of action and limited peripheral exposure. Ezetimibe has no effect on the activity of major drug metabolizing enzymes (CYP450), which reduces any potential drug–drug interactions with other medications. Ezetimibe (10 mg/day) was found to inhibit cholesterol absorption by an average of 54% in hypercholesterolemic individuals ($p<0.001$). Ezetimibe alone reduced plasma total and LDL-C (18%) levels ($p<0.001$) in patients with primary hypercholesterolemia. When ezetimibe was added to ongoing statin treatment, an additional 25% reduction in LDL-C was found in patients with primary hypercholesterolemia and an additional 21% reduction in LDL-C in homozygous familial hypercholesterolemia ($p<0.001$). Ezetimibe, in combination with a statin, produces additional reductions in plasma cholesterol levels and allows for more patients to achieve their LDL-C goals. © 2003 Published by Elsevier B.V.

Keywords: Cholesterol absorption inhibitor; Ezetimibe; Atherosclerosis; Hypercholesterolemia

1. Ezetimibe in pre-clinical models of hyperlipidemia and atherosclerosis

Ezetimibe potently and selectively inhibits biliary and dietary cholesterol absorption in the intestine. Ezetimibe dose-dependently inhibited diet-induced hypercholesterolemia in hamsters with an ED_{50} of 0.04 mg/kg. In an acute model of intestinal absorption using radiolabeled cholesterol in rats, ezetimibe inhibited the appearance of radiolabeled cholesterol in plasma with an ED_{50} of 0.0015 mg/kg 90 min after dosing, indicating that the onset of activity is rapid. Ezetimibe also dose-dependently reduced intestinal cholesterol absorption in mice [1].

* Tel.: +1-908-740-3242; fax: +1-908-740-3294.
E-mail address: harry.davis@spcorp.com (H.R. Davis).

0531-5131/ © 2003 Published by Elsevier B.V.
doi:10.1016/j.ics.2003.11.026

Pre-clinically, ezetimibe has proven to be most potent in cholesterol-fed rhesus monkeys with an $ED_{50} = 0.0005$ mg/kg/day. A single dose of the ezetimibe analog, SCH 48461, administered to cynomolgus monkeys fed a single cholesterol-containing meal caused a significant reduction of cholesterol in chylomicrons and chylomicron remnants during the postprandial phase without affecting triglyceride content [1].

The effect of ezetimibe on plasma cholesterol levels and atherogenesis was determined in apo E knockout (apo E − / −) mice treated for 6 months. Ezetimibe reduced plasma cholesterol, primarily in the VLDL/chylomicron remnant and LDL lipoprotein fractions. Ezetimibe inhibited the progression of atherosclerosis by greater than 90% under western, low fat, and cholesterol-free dietary conditions in apo E − / − mice [1].

2. Selectivity

Ezetimibe selectively inhibits the transport of cholesteryl across the intestinal wall. Ezetimibe did not affect intestinal cholesterol, ester hydrolysis and the absorption of fatty acid thus generated. The free cholesterol from this hydrolysis, however, was not absorbed in the presence of ezetimibe. Ezetimibe did not affect the absorption of triglyceride, ethinyl estradiol, progesterone, vitamins A and D, and taurocholic acid in rats [1]. Ezetimibe does not affect pancreatic lipase, and therefore shares no properties with orlistat (Xenical). Ezetimibe also does not sequester bile acids and thus differs from cholestyramine (resins). Studies in humans have indicated that ezetimibe does not affect serum fat-soluble vitamin status [2].

A study in patients with sitosterolemia demonstrated that ezetimibe effectively reduced serum plant sterols [3], indicating that ezetimibe also inhibits the absorption of these molecules that are structurally related to cholesterol. This indicates that ezetimibe blocks an intestinal transporter for cholesterol and structurally related plant sterols, and the activity and induction of the ATP binding cassette transporter G5/G8 is not involved in the activity of ezetimibe [3].

3. Metabolism

Ezetimibe is rapidly metabolized in the intestine to its phenolic glucuronide; once glucuronidated, it is excreted in the bile, thereby delivering the drug back to the site of action [1]. Cholesterol absorption studies indicated that the glucuronide appeared more potent than ezetimibe itself, because glucuronidated ezetimibe localizes more avidly to the intestine. Autoradiographic analysis demonstrated that drug-related material was located in the small intestinal villi, and concentrated at the enterocyte brush border (Fig. 1).

In humans, ezetimibe is rapidly absorbed and primarily metabolized in the small intestine and liver to its glucuronide, with little oxidative cytochrome P450-mediated metabolism [4]. Ezetimibe and its glucuronide undergo enterohepatic recycling and have a half-life of approximately 22 h in humans. Ezetimibe and/or the glucuronide metabolite are excreted in the feces (90%) and urine (10%). Since ezetimibe does not influence the activities of cytochrome P450 enzymes, significant pharmacokinetic interactions with many medications have not been noted. Pharmacokinetic interaction ezetimibe studies in humans have found no significant changes in the plasma levels of the other medications, including statins (atorvastatin, simvastatin, pravastatin, lovastatin, and fluvastatin), fibrates

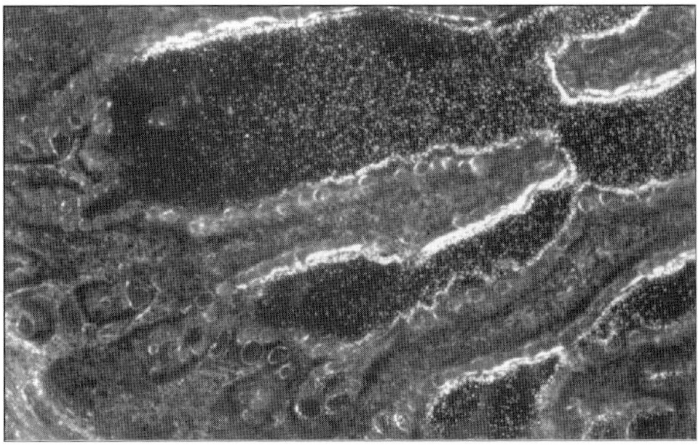

Fig. 1. Localization of radiolabeled ezetimibe glucuronide at the brush border of the small intestinal enterocytes. [I125]-glucuronide-ezetimibe was administered to rats intravenously and localization by autoradiography was determined 3 h post-dose (dark field microscopy; white grains indicate radio-labeled ezetimibe glucuronide).

(gemfibrozil and fenofibrate), digoxin, glipizide, warfarin, and oral contraceptives (ethinyl estradiol and levonorgestrel) [2].

4. Efficacy of ezetimibe in humans

The effect of ezetimibe (10 mg/day) on human cholesterol absorption was investigated in mildly hypercholesterolemic individuals [5]. Fractional cholesterol absorption rate was measured by the continuous dual-isotope feeding method using deuterium-labeled cholesterol and sitostanol. Fractional cholesterol absorption rates averaged 49.8 ± 13.8% on placebo and 22.7 ± 25.8% on ezetimibe, indicating a reduction of 54% ($p<0.001$). LDL and total cholesterol levels following ezetimibe treatment were reduced 20.4% and 15.1%, respectively, whereas campesterol and sitosterol were decreased by 48% and 41%, respectively. The reduction of plasma concentrations of the non-cholesterol sterols, sitosterol and campesterol, which are not endogenously synthesized, suggests a direct effect on the absorption of these sterols by ezetimibe.

In a pooled analysis from two controlled Phase III ezetimibe monotherapy studies in patients with primary hypercholesterolemia, 10 mg/day for 12 weeks reduced LDL-cholesterol levels 18.2%, and significantly decreased triglyceride and apo B levels and increased HDL-cholesterol levels [2]

Ezetimibe inhibits the absorption of biliary and dietary cholesterol and statins inhibit cholesterol synthesis. These mechanisms of action should be complementary in reducing plasma LDL-cholesterol levels. The effect of adding ezetimibe (10 mg/day) to ongoing statin monotherapy was determined in patients with primary hypercholesterolemia. Patients on a stable dose of statin, who had not achieved National Cholesterol Education Program (NCEP) Adult Treatment Panel II goals, were given ezetimibe or placebo for 8 weeks. Ezetimibe caused a 25.1% reduction in LDL-cholesterol and favorable changes in HDL and triglycerides [2]. Of the individuals not at LDL-cholesterol NCEP goal at baseline, 71.5% reach their goal on statin plus ezetimibe compared with 18.9% on statin plus placebo ($p<0.001$) [2].

The addition of ezetimibe to 40 mg of atorvastatin or simvastatin was evaluated in patients with homozygous familial hypercholesterolemia (HoFH) [2]. Patients with HoFH on 40 mg of statin had their statin dose doubled, were given ezetimibe (10 mg) or both for 12 weeks. Compared with increasing the statin dose to 80 mg, the addition of ezetimibe to 40 or 80 mg of statin resulted in an additional 14% LDL-cholesterol reduction (− 20.7% vs. − 6.7%), and adding ezetimibe to 80 mg statin an additional 21% LDL reduction occurred (27.5 vs. 7%). LDL-cholesterol lowering through the inhibition of cholesterol absorption by ezetimibe does not require the expression of LDL receptors, and offers an addition treatment option for patients with HoFH.

The effect of co-administration of ezetimibe (10 mg/day) with statins was evaluated in four 12-week phase III studies, with atorvastatin and simvastatin at 10–80 mg/day, and pravastatin and lovastatin at 10–40 mg/day. LDL-cholesterol reductions with the combination of ezetimibe with statins ranged from − 44% to − 57% for simvastatin (10–80 mg), − 50% to − 60% for atorvastatin (10–80 mg), − 34% to − 41% for pravastatin (10–40 mg), and − 33% to − 45% for lovastatin (10–40 mg). With all statins, the combination of ezetimibe with the lowest statin dose (10 mg) resulted in similar reductions in LDL-cholesterol as for the highest statin alone dose (80 mg for atorvastatin and simvasatin, 40 mg for pravastatin and lovastatin) [2]. C-reactive protein (CRP), an inflammatory marker, which may be a risk factor for atherosclerosis, was evaluated in the simvastatin co-administration study. The reductions in CRP levels were found to be nearly two-fold greater in the ezetimibe plus simvastatin pooled groups (− 34.8%) compared with the simvastatin alone pooled groups (− 18.2%) [6]. For patients with hyperlipidemia, the addition of ezetimibe with statin therapy offers a new treatment option to reach LDL-cholesterol goals and improve CRP and lipid profiles.

References

[1] M. van Heek, H.R. Davis, Pharmacology of ezetimibe, Eur. Heart J. 4 (Suppl. J) (2002) J5–J8.

[2] C.M. Ballantyne, Ezetimibe: efficacy and safety in clinical trials, Eur. Heart J. 4 (Suppl. J) (2002) J9–J18.

[3] K. von Bergmann, G. Salen, D. Lutjohann, T. Musliner, B. Musser, Ezetimibe effectively reduces serum plant sterols in patients with sitosterolemia, Atherosclerosis 3 (2) (2002) 232.

[4] J.E. Patrick, T. Kosoglou, K.L. Stauber, K.B. Alton, S.E. Maxwell, Y. Zhu, et al, Disposition of the selective cholesterol absorption inhibitor ezetimibe in healthy male subjects, Drug Metab. Dispos. 30 (4) (2002) 430–437.

[5] T. Sudhop, D. Lutjohann, A. Kodal, D. Tribble, S. Shah, I. Perevozskaya, K. von Bergmann, Inhibition of intestinal cholesterol absorption by ezetimibe in humans, Circulation 106 (2002) 1943–1948.

[6] P. Sager, L. Melani, L.J. Lipka, J. Strony, R. Suresh, E.P. Veltri, C-reactive protein is reduced during ezetimibe coadministration with simvastatin in patients with primary hypercholesterolemia, J. Am. Coll. Cardiol. 41 (6) (Suppl. A) (2003) 316A–317A.

International Congress Series 1262 (2004) 247–250

www.ics-elsevier.com

Biological therapies for dyslipidemia

Michael H. Davidson*

Rush University Medical Center, Preventive Cardiology, 1725 West Harrison Street, Suite 1159, Chicago, IL 60612, USA

Abstract. Biological therapies involve the utilization of proteins, DNA, antibodies, or other substances derived or synthesized from living tissue for therapeutic effects. There are several biological therapies in clinical development for the prevention and treatment of atherosclerosis. The most advanced in human trials are apolipoprotein mimetics, which include apolipoprotein A-1Milano and phospholipid complexes. Infusions of these apolipoprotein mimetics have been demonstrated to reduce atherosclerotic development in both animal models and humans over a relatively short period of time. Autoimmunization to create neutralizing antibodies to CETP is also in human trials.

Keywords: Dyslipidemia; High-density lipoprotein; Autoimmunization

1. Introduction

Biological therapies are a class of treatments that involve the clinical utilization of substances, either derived or synthesized from biological material. This class of therapies generally includes antibodies, genes, recombinant proteins, structural mimetics, and autoimmunization. There has recently been an explosion of basic studies involving gene transfer and knockout techniques in animals that have been very valuable in elucidating mechanisms for the development of atherosclerosis. Although expectations for human use are high, the number of clinical trials published to date has been relatively limited. This review will focus on the present data available for biological therapies for dyslipidemia and discuss both the potential benefits and challenges that face these emerging treatments.

1.1. Apolipoprotein complexes and mimetics

One of the most promising areas for the utilization of biopharmaceuticals for the treatment of atherosclerosis is a complex that combines recombinant apoA1 with a phospholipid to mimic the structure of newly formed HDL (Fig. 1) [1]. A mutant form of apoA1, known as apolipoprotein A-1Milano (apoA-1M), named after a village in Italy where the variant was discovered because of a low CHD rate, appears to be more effective

* Tel.: +1-312-563-2011; fax: +1-312-563-4417.
E-mail address: michaeldavidson@radiantresearch.com (M.H. Davidson).

doi:10.1016/j.ics.2003.12.028

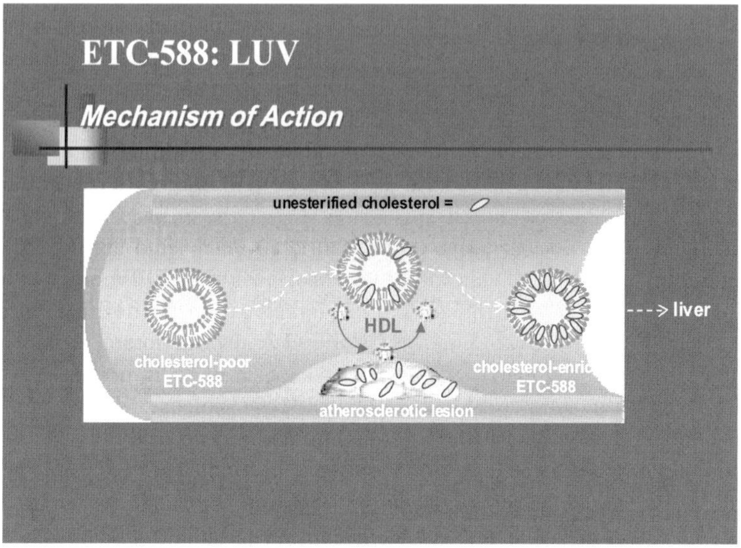

Fig. 1. The function of apoA1 mimetics for reverse cholesterol transport.

in the reverse cholesterol transfer process [2]. Preclinical studies have shown that injections of recombinant apoA-1M/phospholipid can rapidly remove cholesterol and alter the composition and atherosclerotic lesions in rabbits [3,4]. Infusions of pro apoA1 liposomes in humans were shown to promote the net cholesterol excretion from the body by stimulating reverse cholesterol transport [1]. Since HDL facilitates the transfer of cholesterol from peripheral cells to the liver via SRB1 for subsequent elimination as bile acids and neutral steroids, enhanced fecal cholesterol excretion may be used as a measurement of improved reverse cholesterol transport. In four subjects with heterozygous FH, infusion of the recombinant human pro apoA1 liposome complex resulted in approximately a 30–40% increase in the fecal excretion of neutral sterols and bile acids which corresponded to the removal of about 500 mg/day of excess cholesterol after infusion [5,6].

The apoA-1M phospholipid complex infusions are presently undergoing human trials to evaluate clinical outcomes [7]. Recently reported was a study in 47 patients with acute coronary syndromes who received infusions of either 15 or 45 mg/kg of apoA-1M phospholipid complex (ETC-216 Esperion) [8] or placebo weekly for a maximum of five doses. The primary endpoint was the change in percent atheroma volume as measured by coronary intravascular ultrasound (IVUS) at baseline and at the end of the treatments. The study sponsor (Esperion) announced that the preliminary results of the trial demonstrated a significant reduction in plaque volume in the coronary arteries. Although preliminary, these results suggest that apoA1 mimetics have acute effects on plaque regression and potentially preventing vulnerable plaque rupture. The clearance of these apoA1 mimetics from the plasma is relatively rapid (within a few days) and, therefore, repeated infusions may be necessary to demonstrate a clinical benefit. Nevertheless, these early clinical findings are encouraging that short-term benefits may be realized with these infusions that can be extended into longer term clinical outcomes with either multiple treatments or conversion to small molecules (oral apoA1 mimetics) that can be used for chronic therapy.

1.1.1. Autoimmunization

Autoimmunization involves the utilization of a vaccine to stimulate the production of neutralizing antibodies to a specific protein. One potential target for autoimmunization is cholesterol ester transfer protein (CETP). CETP is a 74 kDa plasma glycoprotein that modulates the concentrative gradient transfer of cholesterol ester from HDL to apoB containing lipoproteins [9]. CETP inhibition, as a therapeutic target to raise HDL, remains controversial because HDL levels are increased by delayed catabolism rather than by enhanced production or reverse cholesterol transport. Nevertheless, other anti-atherosclerotic benefits of elevated HDL, such as the increased production of prostacyclin or the inhibition of LDL oxidation, may reduce CHD risk even if reverse cholesterol transport is not upregulated [10]. A vaccine to stimulate anti-CETP antibodies was developed by attaching a B-cell epitope of human CETP to a T-cell epitope of tetanus toxins. This epitope of CETP was previously found to be an important region for CETP activity, and the tetanus toxins help to provide the potent antibody response. In cholesterol-fed rabbit models, CETP inhibition either with oral medication (JTT-7O5) or a vaccine (CET-i) has been demonstrated to reduce atherosclerosis compared with controls [11]. Clinical data regarding the clinical efficacy of CETP inhibition are, however, fairly limited. In a Phase I trial, the CETP vaccine was able to induce anti-CETP antibodies at the highest dose as a single injection in humans, but repeated injections are necessary to induce a significant immune response to markedly inhibit CETP to boost HDL levels [12].

2. Conclusion

Biological therapies are presently under clinical development for the management of dyslipidemia. For patients with atherosclerosis, the biological therapies that are the most advanced in human trials are the apoA1 mimetics. Multiple infusions of an apoA-1M/phospholipid complex have been demonstrated to decrease plaque volume in a relatively short period of time. Autoimmunization to develop anti-CETP antibodies is feasible in humans and a vaccine to create neutralizing antibodies to CETP is in early human trials. These biological therapies, if proven successful in ongoing clinical trials, may significantly expand the armamentarium for the treatment of dyslipidemia.

References

[1] P.K. Shah, J. Yano, O. Reyes, et al., High-dose recombinant apolipoprotein A-I_{milano} mobilizes tissue cholesterol and rapidly reduces plaque lipid and macrophage content in apolipoprotein E-deficient mice: potential implications for acute plaque stabilization, Circulation 103 (2001) 3047–3050.

[2] G. Chiesa, C.R. Sirtori, Apolipoprotein A-IMilano: current perspectives, Curr. Opin. Lipidol. 14 (2003) 159–163.

[3] G. Chiesa, C.R. Sirtori, Recombinant apolipoprotein A-I(Milano): a novel agent for the induction of regression of atherosclerotic plaques, Ann. Med. 35 (2003) 267–273.

[4] G. Chiesa, E. Monteggia, M. Marchesi, et al., Recombinant apolipoprotein A-I(Milano) infusion into rabbit carotid artery rapidly removes lipid from fatty streaks, Circ. Res. 90 (2002) 974–980.

[5] M. Eriksson, L.A. Carlson, T.A. Miettinen, B. Angelin, Stimulation of fecal steroid excretion after infusion of recombinant proapolipoprotein A-I. Potential reverse cholesterol transport in humans, Circulation 100 (1999) 594–598.

[6] B. Angelin, P. Parini, M. Eriksson, Reverse cholesterol transport in man: promotion of fecal steroid excretion by infusion of reconstituted HDL, Atherosclerosis 3 (2002) 23–30.

[7] R.S. Newton, B.R. Krause, HDL therapy for the acute treatment of atherosclerosis, Atherosclerosis 3 (2002) 31–38.

[8] Regression of atherosclerosis seen with ETC-216 (AIM). Esperion Therapeutics, Inc., News Release 6/26/2003.

[9] A.R. Tall, An overview of reverse cholesterol transport, Eur. Heart J. 19 (Suppl. A) (1998) A31–A35.

[10] O. Stein, Y. Stein, Atheroprotective mechanisms of HDL, Atherosclerosis 144 (1999) 285–301 (Review).

[11] C.W. Rittershaus, D.P. Miller, L.J. Thomas, et al., Vaccine-induced antibodies inhibit CETP activity in vivo and reduce aortic lesions in a rabbit model of atherosclerosis, Arterioscler. Thromb. Vasc. Biol. 20 (2000) 2106–2112.

[12] M.H. Davidson, K. Maki, D. Umporowicz, et al., The safety and immunogenicity of a CETP vaccine in healthy adults, Atherosclerosis 169 (2003) 113–120.

State of the art symposium

ELSEVIER

International Congress Series 1262 (2004) 253–256

www.ics-elsevier.com

What happens inside an atherosclerotic plaque?

Peter Libby*

Cardiovascular Medicine, Brigham and Women's Hospital, Mallinckrodt Professor of Medicine, Harvard Medical School, Eugene Braunwald Research Center 307, 77 Avenue Louis Pasteur, NRB 7, 221 Longwood Avenue, Boston, MA 02115, USA

Abstract. Atherogenesis probably begins with endothelial dysfunction, whose triggers include dyslipidemia, smoking, hypertension, and insulin resistance. Endothelial dysfunction may encompass impaired barrier function; induction of endothelial adhesion molecules including VCAM-1; and migration of leukocytes and monocytes into the subendothelial space in response to chemoattractant cytokines such as monocyte chemoattractant protein-1 (MCP-1). Subsequent steps include formation of foam cells, smooth muscle cell migration, T cell activation, and, at sites of plaque disruption, platelet activation and aggregation. The smooth muscle cells form a fibrous cap. Stable plaques have a thick fibrous cap, a small lipid core, and few inflammatory cells. In contrast, lesions with higher risk of rupture have high lipid content, numerous inflammatory cells, and a thin fibrous cap with reduced collagen and vascular smooth muscle cells. Diseased coronary arteries contain multiple such vulnerable plaques, hence the need for systematic therapy to prevent acute coronary events.

Keywords: Endothelial dysfunction; Atherosclerosis; Hypercholesterolemia; Hypertension; Acute coronary syndromes

1. Introduction

We now recognize that thrombus formation causes most acute coronary syndromes, including unstable angina and myocardial infarction. Further, the atherosclerotic plaques most likely to produce these events do not necessarily cause a severe stenosis, but rather undergo physical disruption triggering thrombus formation. We now appreciate that plaque stability is a problem of applied vascular biology. The artery vessel wall is made up of living cells that have important functions in hypertension as well as atherogenesis. Evidence has snowballed that atherosclerosis is fundamentally an inflammatory disease.

2. The role of inflammation in atherosclerosis

Atherosclerotic plaque development involves a complex interaction between the endothelium, inflammatory cytokines, and numerous blood elements [1]. Many factors

* Tel.: +1-617-525-4350, +1-617-525-4383; fax: +1-617-525-4400, +1-617-525-4999.
E-mail address: plibby@rics.bwh.harvard.edu (P. Libby).

0531-5131/
doi:10.1016/j.ics.2003.12.048

associated with heightened risk of atherosclerosis may instigate inflammation. For example, a current concept that links hyperlipidemia with atherogenesis invokes oxidized phospholipids derived from modified lipoproteins as pro-inflammatory stimuli [2].

In an early step in the inflammatory response of atherosclerosis, leukocytes from blood adhere to the endothelium. One candidate for mediating this adhesion is vascular cell adhesion molecule-1 (VCAM-1), expressed at negligible levels on the healthy endothelium. VCAM-1 has garnered a great deal of interest because it binds the monocyte, and the T lymphocyte, precisely the types of leukocytes found in the early atherosclerotic plaque [3]. VCAM-1 expression increases on endothelial cells stimulated with proinflammatory cytokines and over nascent atherosclerotic lesions in a variety of different animal species fed an atherogenic diet [4,5].

Once bound by the endothelial cell, the leukocyte requires a chemoattractant gradient to pull it into the intima. A likely candidate for this role is monocyte chemoattractant protein-1 (MCP-1), a product of various cells including endothelium and smooth muscle [6,7]. We demonstrated reduced lipid deposition in MCP-1 deficient atherosclerotic mice as well as marked reduction in lesion formation [8]. Others showed that inactivation of the MCP-1 receptor CCR2 likewise diminished lesion formation [21].

Once bound in the intima, the leukocyte participates in the inflammatory response in atherosclerosis by maturing from a blood monocyte to a macrophage. In atherosclerosis, macrophages express scavenger receptors for modified lipoproteins, allowing them to ingest lipid and become foam cells. In addition to MCP-1, macrophage colony-stimulating factor (M-CSF) contributes to the shift from blood monocytes into the macrophage foam cells [9].

3. Inflammatory cytokines and the atherosclerotic plaque

Intrinsic vascular wall cells are not mere passive responders to inflammatory stimuli. Atheromata overexpress tumor necrosis factor-alpha (TNF-alpha), interleukin (IL)-beta and IL-6. In the subendothelium, the mononuclear cells produce inflammatory cytokines (IL-1, IL-6, and TNF-alpha) that further augment the expression of adhesion molecules. Various growth factors promote plaque growth by stimulating smooth-muscle cell migration and proliferation. The muscle cells in turn secrete collagen, which forms a stable fibrous cap [10,11].

In contrast, other inflammatory cytokines, such as interferon gamma, IL-1 and TNF-alpha, cause weakening of the fibrous cap [12]. The thinning fibrous cap becomes vulnerable to fissure or rupture, thus exposing the procoagulant atheromatous core to circulating blood elements, which leads to unleashing platelets and the coagulation cascade. Thrombosis can further accentuate inflammation by inducing expression of P-selectin and CD40 ligand on the platelet surface [13]. These molecules fuel the inflammatory process by further leukocyte recruitment.

4. Proinflammatory mediators in atherosclerosis

Nuclear factor κB (NFκB), one of the most important mediators of inflammation in atherogenesis, is ordinarily sequestered in the cytoplasm of the cell in an inactive form. When activated, NFκB translocates to the nucleus, where it regulates the expression of a cassette of genes central to the vascular inflammatory response, including VCAM-1, MCP-1, and IL-6 [14].

Some mediators of hypertension exert proinflammatory actions as well. Preclinical data in hypertensive rats show peri-arteriolar cuffing and arterial infiltration with inflammatory leukocytes [15]. Recent data suggest that angiotensin II and aldosterone may act as proinflammatory stimuli beyond their classically recognized actions on vasomotor tone and salt and water balance. For example, angiotensin II and oxidative stress activate the transcriptional pathways regulated by NFκB in smooth muscle cells and monocytes [16]. Infusion of angiotensin II in rats induces aortic VCAM-1 mRNA accumulation, one of the NFκB-regulated genes [17].

Recent evidence suggests that aldosterone may be an inflammatory mediator as well. Induction of hypertension in rats by administration of aldosterone and salt causes myocardial fibrosis and perivascular cuffing. An aldosterone antagonist abrogated the response [18]. Infusion of aldosterone and consumption of salt in the experimental animal also increased two inflammatory markers, VCAM-1 and the inflammatory isoform of cyclooxygenase (COX-2) [18].

5. Mechanism of plaque rupture

Ruptured plaques characteristically have abundant inflammatory cells, including T cells and macrophages, but a paucity of smooth muscle cells, surmounted by a very thin protective fibrous cap [19]. To investigate whether immune cells inside the plaque might weaken the cap by interfering with the synthesis of collagen by smooth muscle cells, we treated smooth muscle cells with gamma interferon, an inflammatory molecule secreted by T cells in plaques. Exposure to this proinflammatory mediator decreased interstitial collagen production. Not only that, when exposed to other proinflammatory cytokines, macrophages inside the plaque began to overexpress collagen-degrading enzymes, suggesting that the T cells were issuing a double command—one to the smooth muscle cells to stop producing new collagen (gamma interferon); the other to the macrophages to degrade existing collagen (including CD40L) [20]. These alterations produce a net thinning and weakening of the fibrous cap, rendering it friable and susceptible to rupture and hence thrombosis.

6. Conclusion

Atherosclerosis and its clinical sequelae result from longstanding, smouldering inflammatory responses involving intimate interplay between the cells of the immune system, blood, and those of the vessel wall. Appreciation of the role of inflammation in atherogenesis has yielded new insight into the mechanisms by which risk factors promote atherogenesis, and a rational basis for understanding the clinical benefits of lifestyle and pharmacologic interventions that target dyslipidemia, hypertension, and the other components of the metabolic syndrome.

References

[1] P. Libby, et al., Inflammation and atherosclerosis, Circulation 105 (2002) 1135–1143.

[2] U. Schonbeck, et al., Oxidized low-density lipoprotein augments and 3-hydroxy-3-methylglutaryl coenzyme A reductase inhibitors limit CD40 and CD40L expression in human vascular cells, Circulation 106 (2002) 2888–2893.

[3] M.I. Cybulsky, M.A. Gimbrone Jr., Endothelial expression of a mononuclear leukocyte adhesion molecule during atherogenesis, Science 251 (1991) 788–791.
[4] H. Li, et al., An atherogenic diet rapidly induces VCAM-1, a cytokine regulatable mononuclear leukocyte adhesion molecule, in rabbit endothelium, Arterioscler. Thromb. 13 (1993) 197–204.
[5] Y. Nakashima, et al., Upregulation of VCAM-1 and ICAM-1 at atherosclerosis-prone sites on the endothelium in the ApoE-deficient mouse, Arterioscler. Thromb. Vasc. Biol. 18 (1998) 842–851.
[6] B.J. Rollins, et al., Cytokine-activated human endothelial cells synthesize and secrete a monocyte chemoattractant, MCP-1/JE, Am. J. Pathol. 136 (1990) 1229–1233.
[7] J.M. Wang, et al., Expression of monocyte chemotactic protein and interleukin-8 by cytokine-activated human vascular smooth muscle cells, Arterioscler. Thromb. 11 (1991) 1166–1174.
[8] L. Gu, et al., Absence of monocyte chemoattractant protein-1 reduces atherosclerosis in low-density lipoprotein-deficient mice, Mol. Cell 2 (1998) 275–281.
[9] J.H. Qiao, et al., Role of macrophage colony stimulating factor in atherosclerosis: studies of osteopetrotic mice, Am. J. Pathol. 150 (1997) 1687–1699.
[10] C. Betsholtz, E.W. Raines, Platelet-derived growth factor: a key regulator of connective tissue cells in embryogenesis and pathogenesis, Kidney Int. 51 (1997) 1361–1369.
[11] M. Klagsbrun, E.R. Edelman, Biological and biochemical properties of fibroblast growth factors. Implications for the pathogenesis of atherosclerosis, Arteriosclerosis 9 (1989) 269–278.
[12] P. Libby, Molecular bases of the acute coronary syndromes, Circulation 91 (1995) 2844–2850.
[13] U. Schonbeck, P. Libby, CD40 signaling and plaque instability, Circ. Res. 89 (2001) 1092–1103.
[14] T. Collins, M.I. Cybulsky, NF-kappaB: pivotal mediator or innocent bystander in atherogenesis? J. Clin. Invest. 107 (2001) 255–264.
[15] A. Nicoletti, et al., Mediators of perivascular inflammation in the left ventricle of renovascular hypertensive rats, Cardiovasc. Res. 31 (1996) 585–595.
[16] R. Kranzhofer, et al., Angiotensin induces inflammatory activation of human vascular smooth muscle cells, Arterioscler. Thromb. Vasc. Biol. 19 (1999) 1623–1629.
[17] P.E. Tummala, et al., Angiotensin II induces vascular cell adhesion molecule-1 expression in rat vasculature: a potential link between the renin–angiotensin system and atherosclerosis, Circulation 100 (1999) 1223–1229.
[18] R. Rocha, et al., Aldosterone induces a vascular inflammatory phenotype in the rat heart, Am. J. Physiol., Heart Circ. Physiol. 283 (2002) H1802–H1810.
[19] A.C. van der Wal, et al., Site of intimal rupture or erosion of thrombosed coronary atherosclerotic plaques is characterized by an inflammatory process irrespective of the dominant plaque morphology, Circulation 89 (1994) 36–44.
[20] P. Libby, et al., Macrophages and atherosclerotic plaque stability, Curr. Opin. Lipidol. 7 (1996) 330–335.
[21] L. Boring, et al., Decreased lesion formation in CCR-/- mice reveals a role for chemokines in the initiation of atherosclerosis, Nature 394 (1998) 894–897.

International Congress Series 1262 (2004) 257–260

www.ics-elsevier.com

Seeing is believing: imaging techniques to measure atherosclerosis progression

Steven E. Nissen*

Cleveland Clinic Cardiovascular Coordinating Center, The Cleveland Clinic Foundation, 9500 Euclid Avenue, Cleveland, OH 44195, USA

Abstract. Techniques that enable the accurate and reproducible detection and measurement of the pathophysiological changes occurring in atherosclerosis, particularly early on in the disease process, will help to identify those subjects who are at highest cardiovascular risk. It is well established that the extent and composition of atheromatous plaque, rather than the degree of stenosis, determines the risk of plaque disruption and, therefore, has most impact on patient outcome. Traditional techniques that only provide information about lumen size, such as angiography, are therefore of limited value in predicting clinical events. Intravascular ultrasound (IVUS), developed over the past decade, provides unique advantages that have already impacted on the assessment and understanding of coronary atherosclerosis. Several ongoing trials are evaluating the application of IVUS to the study of atherosclerosis progression or regression. These studies, using IVUS, will further increase our understanding of the impact of hyperlipidemia and hypertension on the progression of atherosclerosis, and may help to establish the optimal means of reducing atherosclerotic burden.

Keywords: Intravascular ultrasound; Atherosclerosis; Coronary artery disease; Hyperlipidemia; Statin

1. Introduction

Clinicians have traditionally used angiography and the size of the lumen to predict coronary events. However, coronary artery disease (CAD) is not a disease of the lumen but a disease of the vessel wall.

In its early stages, atherosclerosis outwardly remodels the external elastic membrane [1]. This adventitial enlargement opposes luminal encroachment, thereby concealing the presence of atheroma when assessed angiographically, until the lesion occupies a substantial proportion of the area within the elastic external membrane [2]. Studies have shown that the minimal, or even unseen, angiographic lesion represents the most important source of acute coronary syndromes, including myocardial infarction (MI) [3]. This has

* Tel.: +1-216-445-6852; fax: +1-216-445-6855.
E-mail address: nissens@ccf.org (S.E. Nissen).

doi:10.1016/S0531-5131(03)01864-8

profound implications for drug therapy because approximately 60% of patients present with acute MI or sudden death, and not angina, as the first symptom of coronary disease.

Intravascular ultrasound (IVUS) uses high frequency ultrasound to image not only the coronary lumen, but also the structure of the vessel wall including the atherosclerotic plaque. This review will discuss the impact of IVUS in understanding coronary atherosclerosis and its future management.

2. Limitations of angiography

Although angiography is still the most predominant imaging method used to assess coronary disease, many studies have challenged the accuracy and reproducibility of this technique [4,5]. Angiography only depicts a two-dimensional silhouette of the lumen. In order to assess lesion severity, comparative measurements of luminal diameter within the lesion and a "normal" reference segment are required. However, coronary atherosclerosis is usually diffuse, with no truly normal segment. Angiography is also confounded by outward remodelling of the vessel wall that may conceal early atherosclerosis.

3. Advantages of IVUS

IVUS was developed over the past decade and has many potential advantages in characterizing the atherosclerotic disease process. The tomographical orientation of IVUS enables visualization of the full 360° circumference of the vessel wall, allowing measurement of luminal dimensions by direct planimetering of the cross-sectional image [6]. IVUS is the only technique currently available that enables physicians to routinely visualize coronary plaques and allows the precise assessment of vessels that are often difficult to assess angiographically. Finally, the frequency range of modern ultrasound systems (30–45 MHz) also allows excellent resolution of structures within the artery wall [6]. Due to this sensitivity in measuring plaque volume and content changes over a relatively short period of time, IVUS may be a useful surrogate marker to evaluate the atherosclerotic process, allowing successful clinical trials with fewer patients than required for conventional clinical endpoint trials.

4. Limitations of IVUS

IVUS does have some limitations. Firstly, the ultrasound operator and core laboratory technician must have a thorough knowledge and understanding of potential ultrasonic artifacts, which may adversely affect image quality, increase the difficulty of image interpretation, or reduce the accuracy of quantitative measurements [7]. Secondly, ultrasound catheters currently have a low specificity for the diagnosis of thrombus, although research is underway to overcome this drawback [8,9]. Finally, the physical size of ultrasound catheters (approximately 1.0 mm in diameter) limits the size of vessel that can be imaged.

5. IVUS and the prevalence of atherosclerosis in young adults

IVUS imaging has provided unequivocal in vivo evidence that the atherosclerotic disease process starts at a much younger age than previously realized. A study was conducted in 262 young people (mean age 33.4 ± 13.2 years) from the United States, who died in motor vehicle accidents and who were heart transplant donors. Atherosclerotic lesions (defined as the presence of ≥ 1 site with intimal thickness >0.5 mm) were observed in more than 50% of the cases [10]. Among individuals aged < 20 years, the prevalence of atherosclerosis was an astonishing 17% and at all age ranges, women had nearly as high levels of disease as men. Despite this high prevalence of coronary atherosclerosis in young people, 97% of subjects in the study had completely normal angiograms [10].

6. IVUS and cardiac transplantation

Studies using IVUS have shown regression of donor lesions and the potential for lipid-lowering therapy to regress atherosclerosis. In a case report, a heart was transplanted from a 41-year-old donor with evidence of coronary atherosclerosis to a 42-year-old recipient with normal cholesterol levels (and little or no atherosclerosis) [11]. IVUS imaging was performed 5 years after transplantation and demonstrated that the cholesterol-low environment caused a spontaneous regression of plaques in the coronary vessels of the donor organ [11].

7. IVUS and regression of atherosclerosis

New and emerging applications for IVUS are continuing to evolve. The REVERSal of Atherosclerosis with aggressive Lipid lowering (REVERSAL) trial is a prospective, randomized, double-blind, multicenter study, investigating whether more aggressive lipid-lowering therapy will lead to long-term stabilization or regression of diffuse coronary atherosclerosis [12]. The REVERSAL study randomized 654 patients to treatment with atorvastatin (80 mg) or pravastatin (40 mg) for 18 months. All patients underwent IVUS and quantitative coronary angiography at baseline and at 18 months to assess the primary endpoint of percent change in atheroma volume [12]. The results of the REVERSAL trial will be presented during the American Heart Association Annual Meeting in November 2003.

The Norvasc for Reversal of Manifest Atheroscleroic Lesions by Intravascular Sonographic Evaluation (NORMALISE) study is also ongoing and will assess the effects of blood pressure treatment on onset or progression/regression of coronary artery plaque using IVUS. NORMALISE is a randomized, double-blind, multicenter trial comparing enalapril (10–20 mg), amlodipine (5–10 mg), and placebo treatment in 450 patients over 24 months. The results are due early in 2004.

8. Conclusion

During the next 12 months, pivotal new data from IVUS imaging will further increase our understanding of the impact of hyperlipidemia and hypertension on the progression of atherosclerosis. Adding the information gained from IVUS to conventional risk factors for atherosclerosis may help to establish the optimal means of reducing atherosclerotic burden.

References

[1] V. Fuster, L. Badimon, J.J. Badimon, J.H. Chesebro, The pathogenesis of coronary artery disease and the acute coronary syndromes (1), N. Engl. J. Med. 326 (1992) 242–250.

[2] S. Glagov, E. Weisenberg, C.K. Zarins, R. Stankunavicius, G.J. Kolettis, Compensatory enlargement of human atherosclerotic coronary arteries, N. Engl. J. Med. 316 (1987) 1371–1375.
[3] E.J. Topol, S.E. Nissen, Our preoccupation with coronary luminology: the dissociation between clinical and angiographic findings in ischemic heart disease, Circulation 92 (1995) 2333–2342.
[4] E.N. Arnett, J.M. Isner, D.R. Redwood, K.M. Kent, W.P. Baker, H. Ackerstein, W.C. Roberts, Coronary artery narrowing in coronary heart disease: comparison of cineangiographic and necropsy findings, Ann. Intern. Med. 91 (1979) 350–356.
[5] C.M. Grondin, I. Dyrda, A. Pasternac, L. Campeau, M.G. Bourassa, J. Lesperance, Discrepancies between cineangiographic and postmortem findings in patients with coronary artery disease and recent myocardial revascularization, Circulation 49 (1974) 703–708.
[6] S.E. Nissen, P. Yock, Intravascular ultrasound: novel pathophysiological insights and current clinical applications, Circulation 103 (2001) 604–616.
[7] H. ten Hoff, A. Korbijn, T.H. Smith, J.F. Klinkhamer, N. Bom, Imaging artifacts in mechanically driven ultrasound catheters, Int. J. Card. Imaging 4 (1989) 195–199.
[8] S.L. Bridal, P. Fornes, P. Bruneval, G. Berger, Parametric (integrated backscatter and attenuation) images constructed using backscattered radio frequency signals (25–56 MHz) from human aortae in vitro, Ultrasound Med. Biol. 23 (1997) 215–229.
[9] T. Hiro, C.Y. Leung, H. Karimi, A.R. Farvid, J.M. Tobis, Angle dependence of intravascular ultrasound imaging and its feasibility in tissue characterization of human atherosclerotic tissue, Am. Heart J. 137 (1999) 476–481.
[10] E.M. Tuzcu, S.R. Kapadia, E. Tutar, K.M. Ziada, R.E. Hobbs, P.M. McCarthy, J.B. Young, S.E. Nissen, High prevalence of coronary atherosclerosis in asymptomatic teenagers and young adults: evidence from intravascular ultrasound, Circulation 103 (2001) 2705–2710.
[11] H. Tsutsui, P. Schoenhagen, J.D. Klingensmith, D.G. Vince, S.E. Nissen, E.M. Tuzcu, Regression of a donor atheroma after cardiac transplantation: serial observations with intravascular ultrasound, Circulation 104 (2001) 2874.
[12] S.E. Nissen, for the REVERSAL investigators, Assessing the effects of statins on atherosclerosis progression using intravascular ultrasound: rationale and design of the reversal study, Atherosclerosis 2 (2002) 51–52 (Suppl.).

International Congress Series 1262 (2004) 261–264

www.ics-elsevier.com

Past, present, and future clinical trials of cardiovascular risk reduction—the hypertension perspective

Toshiro Fujita*

Department of Internal Medicine, Chief, Division of Nephrology and Endocrinology, University of Tokyo School of Medicine, 7-3-1, Hongo, Bunkyo, Tokyo 113-8655, Japan

Abstract. The relationship between blood pressure (BP) and risk of cardiovascular (CV) events is continuous, consistent, and independent of other risk factors—the higher the BP, the greater the CV risk. Over the past few decades, numerous clinical trials have shown that reducing BP can reduce the risk of CV events. A wide variety of different antihypertensive drugs were examined in these trials, including "older" BP-lowering agents such as diuretics and β-blockers, and "newer" agents, including ACE inhibitors and calcium channel blockers. The recent ALLHAT trial compared the effects of older with newer antihypertensive agents on CV events in hypertensive patients. Although it remains uncertain whether one antihypertensive drug has superiority over another for CV protection, it is clear that monotherapy is not sufficient to attain currently recommended BP targets in the majority of patients with hypertension; in ALLHAT, for example, a combination of at least two antihypertensive agents was necessary to produce the largest reductions in CV risk. The question of which combination of antihypertensive drugs is most effective will be addressed by the next generation of randomized controlled trials, including the ASCOT trial.

Keywords: Hypertension; Cardiovascular disease; Antihypertensive therapy; Calcium channel blockers; ACE inhibitors

1. Introduction

Over the past few decades, numerous clinical trials have shown that reducing blood pressure (BP) can reduce the mean incidence of stroke by 35–40%, myocardial infarction (MI) by 20–25%, and heart failure by more than 50% [1]. A wide variety of different antihypertensive drug regimens were examined in these trials. It is currently unclear, however, whether any one class of antihypertensive agent, or combination of classes, is superior in efficacy to another. This review will discuss recent and upcoming trials of antihypertensive agents that may influence our future management of hypertension.

* Tel.: +81-3-5800-9735; fax: +81-3-5800-9736.
E-mail address: fujita-dis@h.u-tokyo.ac.jp (T. Fujita).

doi:10.1016/j.ics.2003.11.041

2. Blood pressure and the risk of CVD

In patients between the ages of 40–70 years old, the risk of cardiovascular disease (CVD) doubles with every 20/10 mm Hg increase in BP [2]. The Seventh Report of the Joint National Committee on Prevention, Detection, Evaluation, and Treatment of High Blood Pressure states that BP should be treated to < 140/90 mm Hg, unless an individual has diabetes or chronic renal disease, in which case the target is < 130/85 mm Hg [3].

With increasing age, there is a gradual shift from diastolic BP (DBP) to systolic BP (SBP) as the best predictor of CVD risk. In particular, the greatest burden of CV events occurs in elderly subjects with isolated systolic hypertension (ISH) (SBP>160 mm Hg and DBP < 90 mm Hg).

The Systolic Hypertension in the Elderly Program (SHEP) trial was a landmark, double-blind placebo-controlled outcome trial ($n = 4736$) examining the effects of lowering SBP using a diuretic–based treatment in patients over the age of 60 with ISH [4]. After an average of 4.6 years follow-up, the mean BP in the treatment group was 11/4 mm Hg lower than placebo. This was associated with significant reductions in all CV events (32%), stroke (36%) and left ventricular failure (54%).

The Systolic Hypertension in Europe trial (Syst-Eur) was the first trial to examine the effects of a calcium channel blocker (CCB), nitrendipine, on the risk of stroke in elderly patients with ISH [5]. In this 2-year study, almost 4700 patients were randomly assigned to a CCB, with the possible addition of an angiotensin-converting enzyme (ACE) inhibitor and a diuretic, or matching placebos. Mean BP was reduced by 10.1/4.5 mm Hg and this was associated with a 42% reduction in total stroke rate ($P = 0.003$) and a 44% reduction in non-fatal stroke rate ($P = 0.007$).

Despite the clinical benefits associated with treating high SBP, fewer than 70% of patients < 60 years old, 48% of patients aged 61–75 years, and 34% of patients aged over 75 years are currently treated to target SBP [6].

3. 'Old' versus 'new' antihypertensive therapies

Both "newer" drugs (ACE inhibitors, angiotensin-receptor blockers (ARBs), CCBs) and "older" drugs (diuretics, β-blockers) are available for the treatment of elevated BP. Recent meta-analyses of BP-lowering trials have provided little evidence that any antihypertensive agent is more or less effective than another in reducing the incidence of CVD [7].

The Antihypertensive and Lipid-Lowering treatment to prevent Heart Attack Trial (ALLHAT) was the largest randomised, controlled trial ($n = 33{,}357$) to compare newer drugs with old. ALLHAT examined the effects of a CCB (amlodipine), a diuretic (chlorthalidone), and an ACE inhibitor (lisinopril) on the risk of fatal coronary events and nonfatal MI in patients with hypertension and a high risk of coronary heart disease [8]. After an average of 4.9 years follow-up, no significant difference was observed between amlodipine and chlorthalidone for the primary outcome, or for the secondary outcomes of all-cause mortality, stroke, angina, coronary revascularization, peripheral arterial disease, cancer, or end-stage renal disease. For lisinopril versus chlorthalidone, however, the lisinopril group had a 15% higher risk of stroke ($P = 0.02$), although no significant difference was observed between lisinopril and chlorthalidone for the primary outcome.

This difference in stroke outcome may be partially accounted for by the 2 mm Hg difference in SBP between the lisinopril and chlorthalidone groups.

The Losartan Intervention for Endpoint reduction in hypertension (LIFE) study reported that the ARB, losartan, significantly reduced the incidence of CV mortality, stroke, or MI, compared with the β-blocker, atenolol, in patients aged 55–60 years with essential hypertension (sitting BP 160–200/95–115 mm Hg) and left ventricular hypertrophy [9]. Follow-up was for a minimum of 4 years, until 1040 patients had a primary CV event (death, MI, or stroke). Despite similar reductions in BP in each treatment group (30.2/16.6 mm Hg for losartan vs. 29.1/16.8 mm Hg for atenolol), the ARB was associated with a 25% reduction in the risk of fatal and non-fatal stroke, compared with the β-blocker ($P=0.001$).

4. Combining therapies for the treatment of hypertension

While the evidence for the superiority of one antihypertensive drug over another for CV protection is not compelling, it is clear that monotherapy is not sufficient to attain BP targets in the majority of patients with hypertension. For example, in the ALLHAT and Syst-Eur trials, a combination of at least two antihypertensive agents was often necessary to produce the largest reductions in stroke risk [5,8].

The question of which combination of antihypertensive drugs is most effective will be addressed in part by the Anglo-Scandinavian Cardiac Outcomes Trial (ASCOT). Having enrolled 19,342 patients with untreated SBP ≥ 160 mm Hg or DBP ≥ 100 mm Hg, or treated SBP ≥ 140 mm Hg or DBP ≥ 90 mm Hg, and at least three other pre-specified CV risk factors, ASCOT will compare a newer antihypertensive regimen consisting of the CCB amlodipine (with or without the ACE inhibitor, perindopril) to an older antihypertensive regimen consisting of the β-blocker, atenolol (with or without the diuretic bendrofluazide) for the primary prevention of CVD [10]. ASCOT is expected to be completed in 2005.

5. Conclusions

Several classes of drug are available for the treatment of hypertension but it is not clear whether any one class, or combination of classes, is superior to another. However, since most patients do not reach target BP with a single drug, combinations of drugs from different classes should be used to reduce CV risk. The optimal combination will be examined in the ASCOT trial, which is due to be completed in 2005.

References

[1] B. Neal, et al., Effects of ACE inhibitors, calcium antagonists, and other blood-pressure-lowering drugs: results of prospectively designed overviews of randomised trials. Blood pressure lowering treatment trialists' collaboration, Lancet 356 (2000) 1955–1964.

[2] J.L. Izzo Jr., et al., Clinical advisory statement. Importance of systolic blood pressure in older Americans, Hypertension 35 (2000) 1021–1024.

[3] A.V. Chobanian, et al., National Heart, Lung, and Blood Institute Joint National Committee on Prevention, Detection, Evaluation, and Treatment of High Blood Pressure, National High Blood Pressure Education

Program Coordinating Committee, The seventh report of the Joint National Committee (JNC) on prevention, detection, evaluation, and treatment of high blood pressure: the JNC 7 report, JAMA 289 (2003) 2560–2572.

[4] SHEP Cooperative Research Group, Prevention of stroke by antihypertensive drug treatment in older persons with isolated systolic hypertension. Final results of the Systolic Hypertension in the Elderly Program (SHEP), J. Am. Med. Assoc. 265 (1991) 3255–3264.

[5] R.H. Fagard, et al., Treatment of isolated systolic hypertension in the elderly: the Syst-Eur trial. Systolic Hypertension in Europe (Syst-Eur) trial investigators, Clin. Exp. Hypertens. 21 (1999) 491–497.

[6] D.M. Lloyd-Jones, et al., Differential control of systolic and diastolic blood pressure: factors associated with lack of blood pressure control in the community, Hypertension 36 (2000) 594–599.

[7] J.A. Staessen, et al., Cardiovascular prevention and blood pressure reduction: a quantitative overview updated until 1 March 2003, J. Hypertens. 21 (2003) 1055–1076.

[8] ALLHAT Officers and Coordinators for the ALLHAT Collaborative Research Group, Major outcomes in high-risk hypertensive patients randomized to angiotensin-converting enzyme inhibitor or calcium channel blocker vs. diuretic: the Antihypertensive and Lipid-Lowering Treatment to Prevent Heart Attack Trial (ALLHAT), JAMA 288 (2002) 2981–2997.

[9] B. Dahlöf, et al., LIFE Study Group, Cardiovascular morbidity and mortality in the Losartan Intervention For Endpoint reduction in hypertension study (LIFE): a randomised trial against atenolol, Lancet 359 (2002) 995–1003.

[10] P.S. Sever, et al., Rationale, design, methods and baseline demography of participants of the Anglo-Scandinavian Cardiac Outcomes Trial. ASCOT investigators, J. Hypertens. 19 (2001) 1139–1147.

ELSEVIER

International Congress Series 1262 (2004) 265–268

www.ics-elsevier.com

Past, present, and future clinical trials of cardiovascular risk reduction—the hyperlipidemia perspective

Neil R. Poulter*

Cardiovascular Studies Unit Department of Clinical Pharmacology Imperial College London, NHLI, Faculty of Medicine, St. Mary's Campus, London W2 1PG UK

Abstract. In the 1990s, several randomized trials showed that long-term intervention with statin therapy reduces mortality and recurrent ischemic cardiovascular events both in individuals at increased risk of coronary heart disease (CHD) and in patients with established CHD. Since then, additional trials have illustrated the benefits of statin therapy in a variety of other high-risk patient populations. The HPS and ASCOT-LLA trials showed beneficial effects of statins in individuals with below average, average, or moderately elevated LDL cholesterol levels. The results of the ASCOT-LLA appear to conflict with those of the ALLHAT-LLT study, both of which were carried out among patients with hypertension. In the ALLHAT-LLT trial, significant cardiovascular benefits associated with statin use were not apparent. However, this appears to relate to the inadequate relative reduction in LDL and total cholesterol achieved. The cardiovascular benefits of statins also extend to the elderly and patients with diabetes. This review presents the latest data.

Keywords: Coronary heart disease; Statins; Cholesterol; Diabetes; Hypertension

1. Introduction

During the 1990s, a number of large long-term randomized endpoint trials demonstrated conclusively that lowering serum cholesterol with a statin is associated with significant reductions in cardiovascular morbidity and mortality, both in subjects with, and at high risk of, coronary heart disease (CHD).

This review will discuss recent statin trial data in a variety of high-risk patient populations, as well as identifying remaining uncertainties within the management of hyperlipidemia.

* Tel.: +44-207-594-3445; fax: +44-207-594-3411.
E-mail address: n.poulter@imperial.ac.uk (N.R. Poulter).

0531-5131/
doi:10.1016/j.ics.2003.11.043

2. Statin therapy in patients with normal cholesterol levels

The Heart Protection Study (HPS) enrolled a wide range of patients, aged 40–80 years, who were considered to be at substantial 5-year risk of death from CHD. Patients with total cholesterol levels of ≥ 135 mg/dl (≥ 3.5 mmol/l) were randomized to 40 mg simvastatin daily or placebo. HPS demonstrated that, regardless of baseline LDL cholesterol, 40 mg/day simvastatin significantly decreased the relative risk of major vascular events by 24% ($P \leq 0.0001$) among the 20,536 men and women recruited into the trial. Moreover, there was no apparent cholesterol level below which benefits of statin therapy were not observed [1].

The Lipid-Lowering Arm of the Anglo-Scandinavian Cardiac Outcomes Trial (ASCOT-LLA) compared the effects of 10 mg atorvastatin and placebo on the primary endpoint of nonfatal myocardial infarction (MI) (including silent MI) or fatal CHD in 10,305 hypertensive patients with total cholesterol levels ≤ 250 mg/dl (6.5 mmol/l). In September 2002, the ASCOT Data Safety Monitoring Board recommended that this arm of the trial be prematurely stopped after a median follow-up of 3.3 years. The primary endpoint (nonfatal MI and fatal CHD) was significantly reduced by 36% ($P = 0.0005$) in the atorvastatin group (100 primary events) compared with the placebo group (154 primary events). Reductions were also seen in the rate of fatal or nonfatal stroke in the atorvastatin group (27%, $P = 0.0236$) [2].

A previously reported study, the Antihypertensive and Lipid-Lowering treatment to prevent Heart Attack Trial (ALLHAT-LLT), had also assessed the efficacy of statin therapy in patients with hypertension and moderate hypercholesterolemia. Treatment with 40 mg pravastatin produced nonsignificant reductions in coronary (9%) and stroke (9%) events compared with usual care, and no impact on the primary endpoint of all-cause mortality [3].

The likely explanation for the apparently conflicting results obtained in ASCOT-LLA and ALLHAT-LLT is that, in the latter trial, 28.5% in the usual care group were receiving lipid-lowering drugs and 26.1% took a statin. As a result, the differences in total cholesterol (9.6%) and LDL cholesterol (16.7%) between the pravastatin and usual care groups in ALLHAT-LLT were less than half the equivalent figures in ASCOT-LLA (24% and 35%, respectively) [3,4]. Hence, the apparently disappointing clinical benefits noted in ALLHAT-LLT seem to merely reflect the dose response effect on cardiovascular events associated with achieved LDL cholesterol reduction.

3. Statin therapy in the elderly

Until recently, there was little evidence that lipid-lowering may reduce the risk of CHD in individuals older than 70 years of age. The PROspective Study of Pravastatin in the Elderly at Risk (PROSPER) trial was the first study to examine the effects of statin therapy in an entirely elderly population (70–82 years at trial onset). The trial was of relatively short duration and included 5804 adults, of which the majority ($n = 3000$) were women. Pravastatin (40 mg) produced a 15% reduction in the primary endpoint of fatal and nonfatal coronary and stroke events ($P = 0.014$) compared with placebo. Interestingly, all the benefit was achieved through reduction in coronary events [5].

4. Is there an optimal target for lipid-lowering therapy?

While the HPS and ASCOT-LLA data support the adoption of lower lipid-lowering treatment thresholds and target levels, the optimal cholesterol target for lipid-lowering therapy remains undefined. The Treating to New Targets (TNT), Incremental Decrease in Endpoints through Aggressive Lipid lowering (IDEAL), and the Study of the Effectiveness of Additional Reductions in Cholesterol and Homocysteine (SEARCH) trials will help to establish whether more aggressive lipid-lowering is associated with greater cardiovascular benefit.

5. Treating the patient with diabetes and dyslipidemia

The best agent for diabetic patients with dyslipidemia remains unclear. The key atherogenic features of diabetic dyslipidemia are elevated levels of serum triglycerides, low levels of high-density lipoprotein (HDL) cholesterol, and the preponderance of small, dense LDL. Given fibrates raise HDL cholesterol and lower triglycerides more effectively than statins, it might be expected that they form a central part of any lipid-lowering strategy in this group of patients. However, data comparing statins and fibrates in this context are currently unavailable so on the basis of best evidence to date, statins should be the treatment of choice in patients with diabetic dyslipidemia. Subgroup analyses of the statin trials have reported that statins produce equivalent reductions in CHD risk in diabetic compared with non-diabetic patients [6,7].

More recently, the effects of statins have been evaluated in much larger cohorts of patients with diabetes. For example, the HPS Group reported that allocation to 40 mg simvastatin daily for several years reduced the rate of first major vascular events by about a quarter in 5963 patients with diabetes (90% Type II diabetes), irrespective of their baseline cholesterol levels and whether or not they had existing arterial disease [8].

The relatively small number of patients with diabetes in the ASCOT-LLA was reflected by the non-significant effect of statins on the primary endpoint of fatal CHD and non-fatal MI among diabetics. However, total cardiovascular events and procedures were significantly reduced and to the same extent as among non-diabetic subjects [9]. More recently still, the Collaborative AtoRvastatin Diabetes Study (CARDS) Steering Committee recently stopped this 4-year study 2 years earlier than planned (June 2003) because of a significant benefit associated with atorvastatin therapy for the primary prevention of CHD in patients with Type II diabetes. CARDS recruited nearly 3000 patients aged 40–75 years, without symptomatic CHD but with at least one other CHD risk factor and no previous history of heart disease or stroke [10]. Final results of the trial will be made public when available.

6. Conclusion

Emerging data illustrate the benefits of statin therapy in a variety of patient populations. Furthermore, evidence is accumulating to support the idea that increasing benefits are likely to accrue from more aggressive cholesterol reduction, with no apparent LDL cholesterol threshold for initiating therapy. Looking to the future and the results of further studies, it seems inevitable that this drug class will eventually go "over the counter".

References

[1] Heart Protection Study Collaborative Group, MRC/BHF Heart Protection Study of cholesterol lowering with simvastatin in 20,536 high-risk individuals: a randomized placebo-controlled trial, Lancet 360 (2002) 7–22.
[2] P.S. Sever, et alfor the ASCOT Investigators, Prevention of coronary and stroke events with atorvastatin in hypertensive patients who have average or lower-than-average cholesterol concentrations, in the Anglo-Scandinavian Cardiac Outcomes Trial-Lipid Lowering Arm (ASCOT-LLA): a multicentre randomized controlled trial, Lancet 361 (2003) 1149–1158.
[3] The ALLHAT officers and co-ordinators for the ALLHAT collaborative research group, Major outcomes in moderately hypercholesterolemic, hypertensive patients randomized to pravastatin vs usual care. The anti-hypertensive and lipid-lowering treatment to prevent heart attack trial (ALLHAT-LLT), JAMA 288 (2002) 2998–3007.
[4] R.C. Pasternak, The ALLHAT lipid lowering trial—less is less, JAMA 288 (2002) 3042–3044.
[5] J. Shepherd, et alPROSPER study group, PROspective Study of Pravastatin in the Elderly at Risk. Pravastatin in elderly individuals at risk of vascular disease (PROSPER): a randomized controlled trial, Lancet 360 (2002) 1623–1630.
[6] K. Pyörälä, et alfor the Scandinavian Simvastatin Survival Study (4S) Group, Cholesterol lowering with simvastatin improves prognosis of diabetic patients with coronary heart disease. A subgroup analysis of the Scandinavian Simvastatin Survival Study (4S), Diabetes Care 20 (1997) 614–620.
[7] F.M. Sacks, et alFor the cholesterol and recurrent events Trial Investigators, The effect of pravastatin on coronary events after myocardial infarction in patients with average cholesterol levels, N. Engl. J. Med. 335 (1996) 1001–1009.
[8] Heart Protection Study Collaborative Group, MRC/BHF heart protection study of cholesterol-lowering with simvastatin in 5963 people with diabetes: a randomized placebo-controlled trial, Lancet 361 (2003) 2005–2016.
[9] P.S. Sever, et alon behalf of the ASCOT investigators, Prevention of coronary and stroke events with atorvastatin in hypertensive patients who have average or lower-than-average cholesterol concentrations, in the Anglo-Scandinavian Cardiac Outcomes Trial-Lipid Lowering Arm (ASCOT-LLA): a multicentre randomized controlled trial. Author's response, Lancet 361 (2003) 1986–1987.
[10] H.M. Colhoun, et alCollaborative AtoRvastatin Diabetes Study (CARDS), Design of the Collaborative AtoRvastatin Diabetes Study (CARDS) in patients with type 2 diabetes, Diabet. Med. 19 (2002) 201–211.

ELSEVIER

International Congress Series 1262 (2004) 269–272

www.ics-elsevier.com

A targeted dual therapy approach to cardiovascular risk reduction

R. Preston Mason*

Cardiovascular Division, Brigham and Women's Hospital, Harvard Medical School, USA

Abstract. Endothelial dysfunction is an early feature of the atherosclerotic disease process. Damage to the endothelium leads to reduced nitric oxide (NO) bioavailability and facilitates vessel wall permeability to lipids and inflammatory cells. Endothelial dysfunction is causally related to a variety of risk factors for coronary artery disease (CAD) including hyperlipidemia and hypertension; the strongest predictor of endothelial dysfunction is the total number of risk factors a person has. Elevations in oxidized low-density lipoprotein cholesterol lead to endothelial dysfunction and multiple inflammatory processes such as foam cell formation and increased cytokine production. Hypertension and associated metabolic disorders increase endothelial cell synthesis of collagen IV and fibronectin while reducing NO-dependent renal and cardiovascular relaxation. Several agents known to restore endothelial function and NO bioavailability have been shown to have beneficial antiatherogenic activities and improve cardiovascular outcomes. These observations justify the need for global risk assessment and an integrated therapeutic approach to the treatment of atherosclerosis. Future studies will determine whether combining agents that target different risk factors will have synergistic vascular benefits. © 2003 Elsevier B.V. All rights reserved.

Keywords: Endothelial dysfunction; Hyperlipidemia; Hypertension; Statins; Calcium channel blockers

1. Introduction

Endothelial dysfunction is believed to be the common precursor in the development and progression of atherosclerosis. Damage to the endothelium can lead to reduced nitric oxide (NO) bioavailability and augments vessel wall permeability to lipids and inflammatory cells.

A number of risk factors for atherosclerosis are known to contribute to endothelial dysfunction including hyperlipidemia and hypertension. Evidence shows that both risk factors independently affect NO-mediated vasodilation [1]. NO is associated with many hemodynamic and antiinflammatory benefits including the scavenging of superoxide, inhibition of platelet aggregation, reduced adhesiveness of leukocytes, and enhanced vasodilation. Therefore, any deficiency in the availability of NO has the potential to promote atherogenesis in the vasculature.

* Elucida Research LLC, P.O. Box 7100, Beverly, MA 01915, USA. Tel.: +1-978-921-4194x11; fax: +1-978-921-4195.

E-mail address: rpmason@elucidaresearch.com (R.P. Mason).

doi:10.1016/j.ics.2003.12.022

This review will discuss antihypertensive and lipid-lowering agents that have been shown to have beneficial antiatherogenic effects.

2. Atherogenic protection with calcium channel blockers (CCBs)

Evidence from several clinical trials, including the Prospective Randomized Evaluation of the Vascular Effects of Norvasc Trial (PREVENT) [2], the Coronary Angio-Plasty Amlodipine REStenosis (CAPARES) trial [3], and the European Lacidipine Study on Atherosclerosis (ELSA) [4], suggests that the long-acting calcium channel blockers (CCBs) are capable of atherosclerotic plaque stabilization in patients with coronary artery disease (CAD), independently of their effect on vasodilation.

PREVENT investigated the effects of the CCB, amlodipine, on the development and progression of atherosclerotic lesions in the coronary and carotid arteries of 825 normotensive or controlled hypertensive patients with CAD. Treatment with amlodipine for 3 years was associated with significant slowing ($P=0.007$) of the progression of carotid atherosclerosis in terms of a reduction in carotid intima–media thickness (IMT) compared with placebo. PREVENT also showed significant clinical benefits with amlodipine therapy including a 31% reduction ($P=0.01$) in the composite endpoint of any major vascular event or procedure (nonfatal vascular events, hospitalisation for chronic heart failure, unstable angina, coronary artery bypass grafting/percutaneous transluminal coronary angioplasty, fatal or nonfatal myocardial infarction or stroke, and other fatal vascular events) [2].

These clinical benefits of amlodipine in atherosclerosis appear to be related to its physicochemical properties, including its positive charge, rather than just its ability to effectively lower blood pressure [5].

3. Atherogenic protection with statins

Endothelial dysfunction is reversed by statins, in part, due to direct action on the endothelial vasoactive factors, NO and endothelin [6–9]. Statins have also been shown to inhibit production of proinflammatory cytokines that regulate key functions of the vascular wall such as monocyte adhesion and chemotaxis [10]. Furthermore, several statins have been shown to dose-dependently decrease vascular smooth muscle cell migration and proliferation [11]. These observations suggest a direct antiatherosclerotic effect in the arterial wall that is independent of their effects on plasma lipids.

The results of the Atorvastatin vs. Simvastatin on Atherosclerosis Progression study (ASAP) support a nonlipid-lowering benefit with atorvastatin on atherosclerosis. Atorvastatin 80 mg/day treatment was accompanied by a significant regression in carotid IMT in patients with familial hypercholesterolemia which was not observed with simvastatin 40 mg/day [12]. Post hoc analysis revealed that the reduction of IMT in the atorvastatin treatment group was associated with a significant reduction in the inflammatory marker, C-reactive protein ($r=0.13$, $P=0.03$), but not with changes in plasma lipids [13].

4. Combining antihypertensive and lipid-lowering therapy

The two largest cardiovascular trials to date, the Anglo–Scandinavian Cardiac Outcomes Trial (ASCOT) [14] and the Antihypertensive Lipid-Lowering Heart Attack Trial

(ALLHAT) [15,16], both evaluated the separate and combined effects of antihypertensive and lipid-lowering regimens in patients at risk of CAD.

The ALLHAT lipid-lowering arm compared the effectiveness of statin therapy (pravastatin).vs. "usual care" in 10,355 high-risk hypertensive patients with moderate hypercholesterolemia [15,16]. There was no difference between groups in the primary endpoint of all-cause mortality (relative risk: 0.99, $P=0.88$), but the modest differential in lipid levels limits the interpretation of these data [17].

The ASCOT lipid-lowering arm compared the effects of atorvastatin and placebo in 10,305 hypertensive patients with average or lower-than-average cholesterol levels. This trial was terminated almost 2 years early due to a significant reduction in primary events (hazard ratio: 0.64, $P=0.0005$) in the atorvastatin group, above and beyond antihypertensive therapy. The combined effects of atorvastatin and antihypertensive therapy will be reported during the next 2 years [14].

Future studies will also examine the effect on CAD risk when antihypertensive and lipid-lowering treatments are combined. The forthcoming AVALON trial is a 28-week study to evaluate the efficacy and safety of the combination of atorvastatin 10 mg and amlodipine 5 mg compared with either therapy alone in over 800 patients with hyperlipidemia and hypertension. The RESPOND trial will assess the dose-ranging efficacy and safety of dual therapy with atorvastatin 10 to 80 mg and amlodipine 5 to 10 mg in over 1500 patients with hyperlipidemia and hypertension. The primary objective of this study is to understand the effect of the dual therapy combination on systolic blood pressure and LDL cholesterol reduction compared with amlodipine and atorvastatin alone.

5. Conclusion

Considering that the pathogenesis of atherosclerosis is strongly related to hypertension and dyslipidemia, it is clear that a therapeutic approach aimed at addressing both of these components may not only help to control blood pressure and cholesterol levels but may also optimise any improvement in endothelial function and slow the progression of atherosclerosis. Future studies should be directed towards investigating the possibility of a synergistic antiatherogenic effect when antihypertensive and lipid-lowering treatments are combined. Implementation of global risk assessment and an integrated treatment approach should be advocated if we are to optimise the management of atherosclerosis and its associated cardiovascular morbidity and mortality.

References

[1] O.A. Paniagua, et al., Role of endothelial nitric oxide in shear stress-induced vasodilation in human microvasculature. Diminished activity in hypertensive and hypercholesterolemic patients, Circulation 103 (2001) 1752–1758.

[2] B. Pitt, et al., Effect of amlodipine on the progression of atherosclerosis and the occurrence of clinical events, Circulation 102 (2000) 1503–1510.

[3] B. Jorgensen, et al., Restenosis and clinical outcomes in patients treated with amlodipine after angioplasty: results from the Coronary AngioPlasty Amlodipine REStenosis Study (CAPARES), J. Am. Coll. Cardiol. 35 (2000) 592–599.

[4] A. Zanchetti, et al., On behalf of the ELSA investigators, Calcium antagonist lacidipine slows down progression of asymptomatic carotid atherosclerosis, Circulation 106 (2002) 2422–2427.

[5] R.P. Mason, Membrane interaction of calcium channel antagonists modulated by cholesterol. Implications for drug activity, Biochem. Pharmacol. 45 (1993) 2173–2183.
[6] C.B. Treasure, et al., Beneficial effects of cholesterol-lowering therapy on the coronary endothelium in patients with coronary artery disease, N. Engl. J. Med. 332 (1995) 481–487.
[7] K.C.B. Tan, et al., Atorvastatin lowers C-reactive protein and improves endothelium-dependent vasodilation in type 2 diabetes mellitus, J. Clin. Endocrinol. Metab. 87 (2002) 563–568.
[8] K. Egashira, et al., Reduction in serum cholesterol with pravastatin improves endothelium-dependent coronary vasomotion in patients with hypercholesterolemia, Circulation 89 (1994) 2519–2524.
[9] T.J. Anderson, et al., The effect of cholesterol-lowering therapy on the coronary endothelium in patients with coronary artery disease, N. Engl. J. Med. 332 (1995) 488–493.
[10] R.S. Rosenson, Non-lipid-lowering effects of statins on atherosclerosis, Curr. Cardiol. Rep. 1 (1999) 225–232.
[11] S. Bellosta, et al., Pleiotropic effects of statins in atherosclerosis and diabetes, Diabetes Care 23 (2000) B72–B78 (Suppl.).
[12] T.J. Smilde, et al., Effect of aggressive versus conventional lipid lowering on atherosclerosis progression in familial hypercholesterolaemia (ASAP): a prospective, randomised, double-blind trial, Lancet 357 (2001) 577–581.
[13] S. van Wissen, et al., Differential hs-CRP reduction in patients with familial hypercholesterolemia treated with aggressive or conventional statin therapy, Atherosclerosis 165 (2002) 361–366.
[14] P.S. Sever, et al., For the ASCOT Investigators, Prevention of coronary and stroke events with atorvastatin in hypertensive patients who have average or lower-than-average cholesterol concentrations, in the Anglo–Scandinavian Cardiac Outcomes Trial–Lipid Lowering Arm (ASCOT-LLA): a multicentre randomised controlled trial, Lancet 361 (2003) 1149–1158.
[15] The ALLHAT officers and coordinators for the ALLHAT Collaborative Research Group, Major outcomes in high-risk hypertensive patients randomised to angiotensin-converting enzyme inhibitor or calcium channel blocker vs. diuretic. The Antihypertensive and Lipid Lowering Treatment to Prevent Heart Attack Trial (ALLHAT), JAMA 288 (2002) 2981–2997.
[16] The ALLHAT officers and coordinators for the ALLHAT Collaborative Research Group, Major outcomes in moderately hypercholesterolemic, hypertensive patients randomized to pravastatin vs. usual care. The Antihypertensive and Lipid-Lowering Treatment to Prevent Heart Attack Trial (ALLHAT-LLT), JAMA 288 (2002) 2998–3007.
[17] R.C. Pasternak, The ALLHAT lipid lowering trial—less is less, JAMA 288 (2002) 3042–3044.

International Congress Series 1262 (2004) 273–276

ELSEVIER

www.ics-elsevier.com

Prevalence of low HDL-cholesterol and the metabolic syndrome

Shizuya Yamashita*, Naohiko Sakai, Ken-ichi Tsujii, Tadashi Nakamura, Yuji Matsuzawa

Department of Internal Medicine and Molecular Science, Osaka University Graduate School of Medicine, 2-2 Yamadaoka, Suita, Osaka, Japan

Abstract. The metabolic syndrome (MS), in which glucose intolerance, dyslipidemia, and hypertension are clustered in the individual, is characterized by atherogenic lipoprotein profiles including reduced HDL-cholesterol levels, leading to increased susceptibility to cardiovascular diseases (CVD). The prevalence of MS increases with age and among individuals with "abdominal obesity", which is epidemic in both developed and developing countries. The frequency of subjects with multiple risk factors (MRF) is higher in coronary heart disease (CHD) cases than controls, suggesting that clustering of MRF as seen in MS patients may be important for developing CVD. Accumulation of visceral fat is strongly related to the presence of MRF in both obese and nonobese individuals. Since the prevalence of low HDL-cholesterolemia and MS is high in patients with CHD, treatment of MS by reducing visceral fat is the most important challenge for preventing atherosclerotic CVD.

Keywords: Metabolic syndrome; High-density lipoprotein; Insulin resistance; Visceral fat; Atherosclerosis

1. Introduction

The metabolic syndrome (MS) is characterized by a clustering of multiple risk factors (MRF) such as insulin resistance (IR) and/or impaired glucose metabolism, hypertension, and hyperlipidemia in the individual leading to enhanced susceptibility to atherosclerotic cardiovascular diseases (CVD). Patients with MS display increased plasma triglycerides (TG), apo B-100, and IDL-cholesterol (IDL-C), presence of small dense LDL, and decreased HDL-cholesterol (HDL-C) levels. Low HDL-C levels play a crucial role in the development of CVD. The prevalence of MS increases with age and is rapidly increasing in many countries, largely due to an epidemic of "abdominal obesity".

* Corresponding author. Tel.: +81-6-6879-3732; fax: +81-6-6879-3739.
E-mail address: shizu@imed2.med.osaka-u.ac.jp (S. Yamashita).

0531-5131/ © 2004 Published by Elsevier B.V.
doi:10.1016/j.ics.2004.01.015

2. Importance of MRF in CVD

According to WHO, CVD is the leading cause of death in many populations. Over-nutrition and physical inactivity are causing the number of obese individuals to increase all over the world. In Japan, mean BMI is increasing across the adult population except in young women. In a study of coronary heart disease (CHD) in 122,051 Japanese employees, 10-year retrospective annual comparison of risk factors between cases and controls showed that BMI, serum total cholesterol (TC) and TG, fasting plasma glucose (FPG), and blood pressure were significantly higher and HDL-C levels lower in the case group than in the control group from 10 years prior to onset of disease [1]. The frequency of subjects with MRF was also higher in cases than controls. The study suggested that long duration of MRF is involved in the onset of CHD and clustering of MRF as seen in MS patients may be important for developing CVD.

3. Visceral fat accumulation

Many CHD patients have MRF; they are usually mild to moderate but clustered in the individual. Such patients often have increased mean visceral fat area (VFA). We divided subjects attending annual health examinations into four groups by the presence or absence of obesity and visceral fat accumulation and showed that high VFA is related to having MRF in both obese and nonobese individuals. Accumulation of visceral fat contributes to IR, increases in apo B-containing lipoproteins and small dense LDL, and progression of CHD [2] as well as MRF clustering in Japanese men with IGT [3]. Subjects with high VFA also tend to show ECG abnormalities, further suggesting that clustering of MRF based on visceral fat accumulation enhances risk of CHD. In 1987, we proposed the term “visceral fat syndrome” in which the accumulation of visceral fat is in the upstream of clustering of MRF and CHD. Similar concepts have been proposed since, and recently, MS is the term often used.

4. High VFA and age

We investigated the prevalence of subjects with VFA$\geq$100 cm^2 in relation to age in Japanese volunteers, and found that it was higher in men than women and increased with age in both sexes. In women, VFA dramatically increased after menopause. Furthermore, the prevalence of subjects with MRF increased with age in both genders, corresponding with the increment of subjects with high VFA.

5. Definition of MS and its prevalence

WHO defined MS as having IR and/or impaired glucose regulation in addition to $\geq$2 of central obesity (waist/hip ratio >0.90 in men, >0.85 in women, and/or BMI >30), hypertension, and microalbuminuria [4]. NCEP-ATP III proposed the definition of MS as having $\geq$3 of these criteria [5]. The prevalence of MS varies according to the definition used [6–10]. Most major epidemiological studies put the prevalence at around 20–30% of the US adult population with some variation by race or ethnicity and gender.

The prevalence of MS in Japan may be determined by measuring the total population having $\geq$3 of the following criteria: (1) waist circumference$\geq$85 cm (men)/$\geq$90 cm

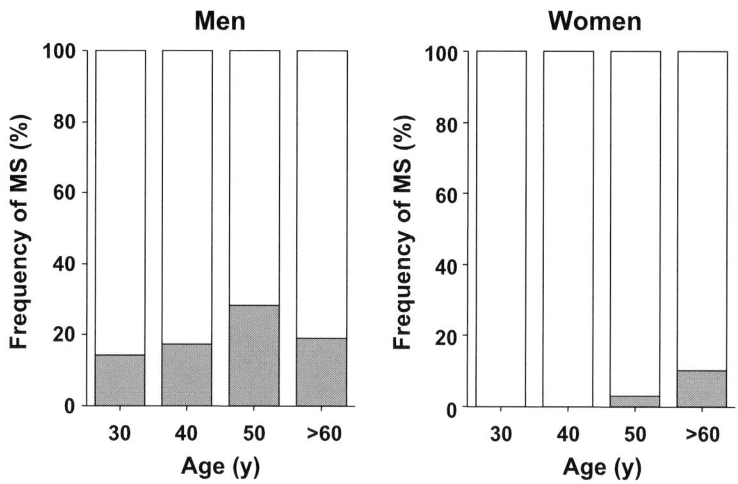

Fig. 1. Frequency of the metabolic syndrome by age in Japanese men and women.

(women); (2) TG≥150 mg/dl; (3) HDL-C<40 mg/dl; (4) sBP≥130 mm Hg and/or dBP≥85 mm Hg; (5) FPG≥110 mg/dl. The prevalence of MS was thus estimated at about 15–30% in men and increasing with age, whereas in women it was much lower but increased after menopause (Fig. 1).

6. Dyslipidemia in MS

The presence of small dense LDL and decreased serum HDL-C are characteristic features of MS. In subjects in the Framingham Offspring and San Antonio Studies, low HDL-C levels were observed in approximately one-third to half of all men and women with MS [8]. Low HDL-C level is a crucial component of dyslipidemia in MS.

7. Contribution of MS to CHD-, CVD-, and all-cause mortality

In a prospective study of 1200 Finnish men who were initially without CVD, cancer, or diabetes, CHD-, CVD-, and all-cause mortality were increased in those with MS [11]. The prevalence of acute coronary events was compared between subjects with and without MS in the PROCAM Heart Study, [12] and proved 2.3-fold higher in those with MS.

8. Molecular mechanism of MS

Visceral fat is a very active tissue in terms of lipogenesis and lipolysis. Free fatty acids released from visceral adipose tissues enter the portal vein, leading to enhanced lipoprotein synthesis and hyperlipidemia. Adipose tissues secrete a variety of bioreactive substances called adipocytokines. TNF-alpha released from visceral fat may cause IR and impaired glucose metabolism. PAI-1 synthesized from visceral fat gives rise to prothrombotic state. Visceral fat accumulation reduces serum adiponectin, an adipocyte-derived protein with antiatherosclerotic effects that can improve IR [13]. Dysregulation of adipocytokines causes IR; clustering of MRF leads to atherosclerotic CVD. Since low HDL-cholesterolemia and MS are common in patients with CHD, treatment of MS by reducing visceral fat is the most important challenge for preventing atherosclerotic CVD.

References

[1] T. Nakamura, et al., Magnitude of sustained multiple risk factors for ischemic heart disease in Japanese employees: a case-control study, Jpn. Circ. J. 65 (2001) 11–17.

[2] H. Kobayashi, et al., Visceral fat accumulation contributes to insulin resistance, small-sized low-density lipoprotein, and progression of coronary artery disease in middle-aged non-obese Japanese men, Jpn. Circ. J. 65 (2001) 193–199.

[3] H. Nagaretani, et al., Visceral fat is a major contributor for risk factor clustering in Japanese men with impaired glucose tolerance, Diabetes Care 24 (2001) 2127–2133.

[4] K.G. Alberti, et al., Definition, diagnosis and classification of diabetes mellitus and its complications: Part 1. Diagnosis and classification of diabetes mellitus. Provisional report of a WHO consultation, Diabet. Med. 15 (1998) 539–553.

[5] Third Report of the National Cholesterol Education Program (NCEP) expert panel on detection, evaluation, and treatment of high blood cholesterol in adults (Adult Treatment Panel III). Final Report, Circulation 106 (2002) 3143–3421.

[6] E.S. Ford, et al., A comparison of the prevalence of the metabolic syndrome using two proposed definitions, Diabetes Care 26 (2003) 575–581.

[7] Y.-W. Park, et al., The metabolic syndrome. Prevalence and associated risk factor findings in the US population from the Third National Health and Nutrition Examination Survey, 1988–1994, Arch. Intern. Med. 163 (2003) 427–436.

[8] J.B. Meigs, et al., Prevalence and characteristics of the metabolic syndrome in the San Antonio Heart and Framingham Offspring studies, Diabetes 52 (2003) 2160–2167.

[9] E.S. Ford, et al., Prevalence of the metabolic syndrome among US adults. Findings from the third national health and nutrition survey, JAMA 287 (2002) 356–359.

[10] The European Group for the Study of Insulin Resistance (EGIR), Frequency of the WHO metabolic syndrome in European cohorts, and an alternative definition of an insulin resistance syndrome, Diabetes Metab. 28 (2002) 364–376.

[11] H.-M. Lakka, et al., The metabolic syndrome and total and cardiovascular disease mortality in middle-aged men, JAMA 288 (2002) 2709–2716.

[12] International Task Force for Prevention of Coronary Heart Disease in cooperation with the International Atherosclerosis Society, Pocket Guide to Prevention of Coronary Heart Disease, 2003, p. 66.

[13] N. Maeda, et al., Diet-induced insulin resistance in mice lacking adiponectin/ACRP30, Nat. Med. 8 (2002) 731–737.

Workshop

International Congress Series 1262 (2004) 279–282

www.ics-elsevier.com

Positive and negative regulation of endothelial cell function

Lena Claesson-Welsh *

Department of Genetics and Pathology, Uppsala University, Sweden, Rudbeck Laboratory, Dag Hammarskjöldsv. 20, 751-85 Uppsala, Sweden

Abstract. Formation of new vessels involves endothelial cell proliferation, migration and differentiation. Vascular endothelial growth factor (VEGF) is known to regulate all aspects of endothelial cell function. We are investigating VEGF-induced signal transduction, with particular emphasis on regulation of cytoskeletal organization and migration, with the aim to identify targets for regulation of excess blood vessel formation in various diseases. © 2003 Published by Elsevier B.V.

Keywords: Angiogenesis; VEGF; Signal transduction; Proteomics; Anti-angiogenesis

1. Introduction

Deregulated, excess blood vessel formation in a number of diseases has received increased attention as a basis for novel therapies. The vascular endothelial growth factor (VEGF) family of ligands and receptors has been the focus of this attention. The VEGFs are crucial for vascular development and neovascularization in physiological and pathological processes in the embryo and adult. This overview presents the current knowledge on the VEGF mechanism of action. Moreover, the therapeutic potential of a group of angiogenesis regulators, denoted endogenous angiogenesis inhibitors, is discussed.

1.1. VEGF-induced signal transduction

Formation of new vessels during embryogenesis and in the adult, in physiological and pathological conditions, is stimulated by growth factors. By virtue of their critical role in the vasculogenic process during development, members of the VEGF family of vascular factors have been of primary interest. The classical VEGF (i.e. VEGF-A165, see Ref. [1] for a review) exerts its effects by binding to two different receptor tyrosine kinases, VEGFR-1 and -2. VEGFR-1 (also denoted Flt-1) occurs in a soluble form as well as a

Abbreviations: HRGP, histidine-rich glycoprotein; VEGF, vascular endothelial growth factor; VEGFR, VEGF receptor.

* Tel.: +46-18-471-43-63; fax: +46-18-55-89-31.

E-mail address: Lena.Welsh@genpat.uu.se (L. Claesson-Welsh).

0531-5131/ © 2003 Published by Elsevier B.V.
doi:10.1016/j.ics.2003.11.045

transmembrane form. The soluble form of VEGFR-1 appears to play a negative regulatory role during embryonal development. Targeted inactivation of the VEGFR-1 gene leads to embryonal death due to obstructed vessels overgrown with endothelial cells. The full length VEGFR-1 is critical in monocyte migration and blocking VEGFR-1 function leads to reduced monocyte infiltration in certain tumor models and increased tumor growth [2]. The signal transduction properties of VEGFR-1 remain essentially unclear due to the poor activity of this kinase.

VEGFR-2, on the other hand, is critical in all aspects of vascular function. Targeted inactivation of the VEGFR-2 gene leads to embryonal death due to arrest in vascular development (see Ref. [1] for a review). Moreover, neutralization of VEGFR-2 function leads to a halt in tumor growth. VEGFR-1 and -2 may form heterodimers, which are functional, at least, in vitro. In response to VEGF-C, VEGFR-2 forms heterodimers also with the third VEGF receptor, VEGFR-3 [3], which is expressed mainly on lymphatic endothelial cells, but also on proliferating endothelial cells. VEGFR-2 is phosphorylated on a number of tyrosine residues in the intracellular domain. Phosphorylation at Y1175 (1173 in the mouse) appears to regulate the proliferative response to VEGF by binding phospholipase Cγ. Phosphorylation at 1214 (1212) mediates binding of the adaptor "growth factor receptor-bound 2". The C-terminal tail of VEGFR-2 is required for activation of focal adhesion kinase (FAK), which is involved in regulating cell-matrix interactions. One of the tyrosine residues in the kinase insert part of VEGFR-2 at position 951 (949), which has not yet been formally shown to be a phosphorylation site, has been implicated in endothelial cell migration (Fig. 1).

1.2. Angiogenesis inhibitors

There is ample evidence that the endothelial cell cytoskeleton and cell–cell, as well as cell–matrix interactions, are potential targets in inhibition of, e.g., tumor vasculari-

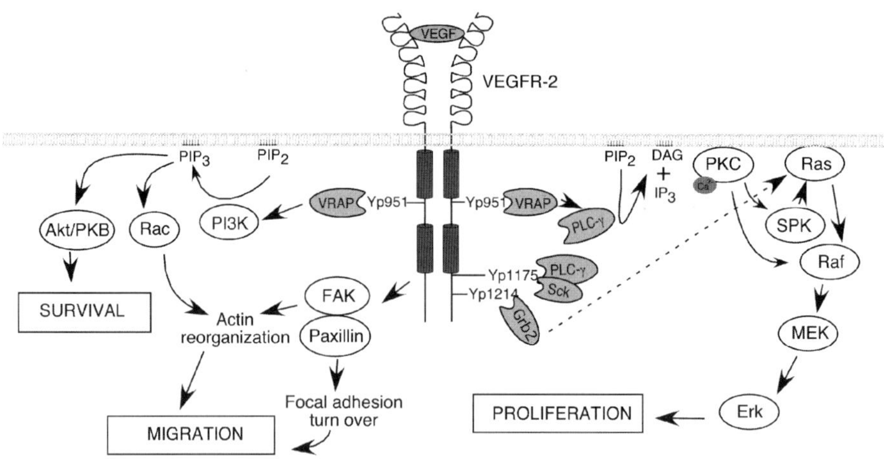

Fig. 1. Signal transduction through VEGFR-2. Receptor-binding signal transduction components (VRAP, VEGF receptor-associating protein; PLCγ, phospholipase Cγ; Sck, Shc-like protein; Grb2, growth factor receptor-bound 2). For further details and references, see Ref. [1].

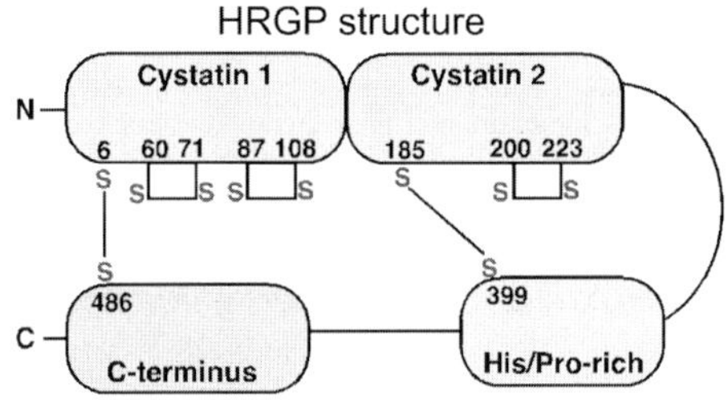

Fig. 2. Structure of histidine-rich glycoprotein. A fragment of HRGP exerts anti-angiogenic effects in vivo.

zation. Thus, several endogenous angiogenesis inhibitors, i.e., inhibitors of endothelial cell function, which are fragments of naturally occurring proteins, appear to exert their action by interfering with endothelial cell attachment and migration [4]. These include endostatin, a fragment of collagen XVIII and tumstatin, a fragment of the collagen αIV chain. Endostatin, as well as tumstatin, bind to endothelial cell integrins, which may obstruct cellular interactions with the matrix. Thrombospondin, another endogenous inhibitor, is a normal constituent of the vascular basement membrane. We have recently identified a fragment of histidine-rich glycoprotein (HRGP), as an inhibitor of tumor vascularization. HRGP is a multi-domain, heparin-binding plasma protein, which carries a central region rich in histidine and proline residues (Fig. 2). We have expressed HRGP recombinantly in mammalian cells. Treatment of T241 fibrosarcoma, a very aggressive tumor form, by subcutaneous injection of recombinant protein (5 mg/kg/day) at a distance from the tumor, led to a 65% reduction in tumor growth. By deletion mapping and screening synthetic peptides, a small region of HRGP has been identified as the minimal active domain. Purified HRGP undergoes limited proteolysis spontaneously, which leads to the release of this domain. Current studies are aimed at identifying a physiological role for this peptide in the regulation of angiogenesis, both during development and in disease.

1.3. Future perspectives

Proof of the principle that angiogenesis inhibition is beneficial in the treatment of tumor diseases also in humans has recently been provided by clinical studies on colorectal cancer (see www.gene.com) and renal cancer [5] patients treated with neutralizing monoclonal antibodies against VEGF. Although we still do not know of potential side effects of long-term treatment, this is a very promising development. Endogenous angiogenesis inhibitors still have not proven useful in clinical studies in humans.

References

[1] M.J. Cross, J. Dixelius, T. Matsumoto, L. Claesson-Welsh, VEGF-receptor signal transduction, Trends Biochem. Sci. 28 (2003) 488–494.

[2] S. Rafii, D. Lyden, R. Benezra, K. Hattori, B. Heissig, Vascular and haematopoietic stem cells: novel targets for anti-angiogenesis therapy? Nat. Rev., Cancer 2 (2002) 826–835.

[3] J. Dixelius, T. Makinen, M. Wirzenius, M. Karkkainen, C. Wernstedt, K. Alitalo, L. Claesson-Welsh, Ligand-induced vascular endothelial growth factor receptor-3 (VEGFR-3) heterodimerization with VEGFR-2 in

primary lymphatic endothelial cells regulates tyrosine phosphorylation sites, J. Biol. Chem., (electronic publication ahead of print).

[4] Y. Cao, Endogenous angiogenesis inhibitors and their therapeutic implications, J. Biol. Chem. 278 (2003) 40973–40979.

[5] J.C. Yang, L. Haworth, R.M. Sherry, P. Hwu, D.J. Schwartzentruber, S.L. Topalian, S.M. Steinberg, H.X. Chen, S.A. Rosenberg, A randomized trial of bevacizumab, an anti-vascular endothelial growth factor antibody, for metastatic renal cancer, N. Engl. J. Med. 349 (2003) 427–434.

International Congress Series 1262 (2004) 283–286

www.ics-elsevier.com

VEGF and its receptors

Napoleone Ferrara*

Department of Molecular Oncology, Genentech, Inc., 1 DNA Way, South San Francisco, CA 94080, USA

Abstract. Vascular endothelial growth factor (VEGF) is a key regulator of physiological angiogenesis. The biological effects of VEGF are mediated by two tyrosine kinase receptors, VEGFR-1 and VEGFR-2. T here is now compelling evidence that VEGF is implicated in pathological angiogenesis such as that occurring in cancer and intraocular neovascular syndromes. It has been also suggested that VEGF may be implicated in angiogenesis in atheromatous plaques. Several VEGF inhibitors are undergoing clinical testing. Very recent data demonstrate that an anti-VEGF antibody has clinical efficacy and prolongs survival in patients with metastatic colorectal cancer.

Keywords: Vascular endothelial growth factor; Endothelium; Apoptosis; Angiogenesis; Tyrosine kinases; Tumor growth; Retinopathy

1. Introduction

For over a decade, the role of vascular endothelial growth factor (VEGF) in the regulation of angiogenesis has been the object of intense investigation. For a historic overview of the VEGF field, see Ref. [1]. While recent evidence indicates that new vessel growth and maturation are highly complex and coordinated processes (for reviews, see Refs. [2,3]), VEGF signaling often represents a critical rate-limiting step in physiological angiogenesis. VEGF appears to be also important in pathological angiogenesis, such as that associated with tumor growth [4]. VEGF (referred to also as VEGF-A) belongs to a gene family that includes placenta growth factor (PlGF), VEGF-B, VEGF-C and VEGF-D. Additionally, homologues of VEGF have been identified in the genome of the parapoxvirus Orf virus and shown to have VEGF-like activities [4]. The main focus of this brief review is the physiology of the prototype member, VEGF-A, a key regulator of blood vessel growth.

2. Activities of VEGF

VEGF promotes growth of vascular endothelial cells derived from arteries, veins and lymphatics (for review, see Ref. [4]). VEGF induces a potent angiogenic response in a variety of in vivo models [5].

* Tel.: +1-650-225-2968; fax: +1-650-225-6443.
E-mail address: nf@gene.com (N. Ferrara).

0531-5131/ © 2003 Published by Elsevier B.V.
doi:10.1016/j.ics.2003.11.003

VEGF is a survival factor for endothelial cells, both in vitro and in vivo [6,7]. In vitro, VEGF prevents apoptosis induced by serum-starvation. Gerber et al. [7] have shown that such activity is mediated by the PI 3′ kinase/Akt pathway. Also, VEGF induces expression of the anti-apoptotic proteins Bcl-2 and A1 in endothelial cells [6].

VEGF also has effects on bone marrow-derived cells. It promotes monocyte chemotaxis [8] and induces colony formation by mature subsets of granulocyte-macrophage progenitor cells [9]. VEGF delivery to adult mice inhibited dendritic cell development [10].

3. Role of VEGF in physiological angiogenesis

3.1. Embryonic and early postnatal development

VEGF plays an essential role in embryonic vasculogenesis and angiogenesis [11]. Inactivation of a single VEGF allele in mice resulted in embryonic lethality between days 11 and 12. The $VEGF^{+/-}$ embryos exhibited a number of developmental anomalies, defective vascularization in several organs and a markedly reduced number of nucleated red blood cells within the blood islands in the yolk sac.

VEGF also plays an important role in early postnatal life [12]. Administration of a soluble, VEGF receptor resulted in nearly complete growth arrest, when the treatment was initiated at day 1 or day 8, postnatally. Such treatment was also accompanied by rapid lethality, primarily due to kidney failure [12]. Defective glomerular development in neonates was also observed in studies using anti-VEGF antibodies [13]. However, VEGF inhibition in adult animals does not result in lethality or any significant adverse effects, indicating that maturation occurs in endothelial cells such that they lose their dependence on VEGF as a survival factor [12].

3.2. Skeletal growth and endochondral bone formation

VEGF mRNA is expressed by hypertrophic chondrocytes in the epiphyseal growth plate, suggesting that a VEGF gradient is needed for directional growth and cartilage invasion by metaphyseal blood vessels [14]. Following VEGF blockade, blood vessel invasion is almost completely suppressed, concomitant with impaired trabecular bone formation, in mice and primates [14]. Although proliferation, differentiation and maturation of chondrocytes were apparently normal, resorption of hypertrophic chondrocytes was inhibited, resulting in expansion of the hypertrophic chondrocyte zone. Importantly, these inhibitory effects are promptly reversible upon interruption of the anti-VEGF treatment [14].

4. Therapeutic implications and perspectives

There is now little doubt that the VEGF family plays an essential role in the regulation of embryonic and postnatal physiologic angiogenesis processes, such as normal growth processes [12,14] and cyclical angiogenesis in the female reproductive tract [15]. Furthermore, VEGF inhibition has been shown to suppress angiogenesis in a wide variety of tumor models, and other modes of pathological angiogenesis leading to the clinical development of a variety of VEGF inhibitors. Clearly, a major question is what impact VEGF inhibition will have in human patients, especially those with highly advanced malignancies. This question will be answered by the several phase III clinical trials that are currently underway, targeting colorectal, lung and renal cell carcinomas. Results of a large phase III in metastatic colorectal cancer patients indicate that there is reason for optimism. Addition of an anti-VEGF antibody to standard chemotherapy resulted in a highly significant increase in survival relative to chemotherapy alone. Furthermore, anti-VEGF therapy has shown efficacy in renal cell carcinoma.

The potential clinical utility of VEGF inhibition is not limited to cancer. Trials inAMD patients are already in phase III. Furthermore, as already noted, gynecologic conditions such as endometriosis or the polycystic ovary syndrome might benefit from this treatment.

The ability of VEGF and other angiogenic factors to promote collateral vessel growth in various animal models of ischemia generated much enthusiasm and led to several clinical trials in patients with coronary or limb ischemia. So far, the clinical results with VEGF (or bFGF) have been somewhat disappointing because the treatment did not significantly increase exercise treadmill time, although some improvement in angina class was measured, in a placebo-controlled trial with recombinant $VEGF_{165}$ in coronary ischemia patients [16]. Currently, the possibility is being explored that a more persistent exposure than that achieved in an early trial [16] may achieve better results. In this context, recent studies using a conditional VEGF switch have shown that early cessation of the VEGF stimulus results in regression of newly formed vessels. However, after a critical duration of exposure, the vessels persisted for months after VEGF withdrawal and resulted in improved organ perfusion [17]. Also, a greater understanding of the differential role of the VEGF receptors may open additional avenues. The recent report that a receptor VEGFR-1-selective mutant may protect the liver from toxic damage extends the potential clinical applications of VEGFR-1 agonists [18]. Other activities of VEGF may have interesting clinical implications. A recent study has shown that VEGF administration leads to enhanced blood vessel formation and ossification in models of bone damage [19].

References

[1] N. Ferrara, VEGF and the quest for tumour angiogenesis factors, Nat. Rev., Cancer 2 (2002) 795–803.

[2] N. Ferrara, K. Alitalo, Clinical applications of angiogenic growth factors and their inhibitors, Nat. Med. 5 (1999) 1359–1364.

[3] G.D. Yancopoulos, et al., Vascular-specific growth factors and blood vessel formation, Nature 407 (2000) 242–248.

[4] N. Ferrara, T. Davis-Smyth, The biology of vascular endothelial growth factor, Endocr. Rev. 18 (1997) 4–25.

[5] D.W. Leung, et al., Vascular endothelial growth factor is a secreted angiogenic mitogen, Science 246 (1989) 1306–1309.

[6] H.P. Gerber, et al., Vascular endothelial growth factor induces expression of the antiapoptotic proteins Bcl-2 and A1 in vascular endothelial cells, J. Biol. Chem. 273 (1998) 13313–13316.

[7] H.P. Gerber, et al., VEGF regulates endothelial cell survival by the PI3-kinase/Akt signal transduction pathway. Requirement for Flk-1/KDR activation, J. Biol. Chem. 273 (1998) 30343–30366.

[8] M. Clauss, et al., Vascular permeability factor: a tumor-derived polypeptide that induces endothelial cell and monocyte procoagulant activity, and promotes monocyte migration, J. Exp. Med. 172 (1990) 1535–1545.

[9] H.E. Broxmeyer, et al., Myeloid progenitor cell regulatory effects of vascular endothelial cell growth factor, Int. J. Hematol. 62 (1995) 203–215.

[10] D.I. Gabrilovich, et al., Production of vascular endothelial growth factor by human tumors inhibits the functional maturation of dendritic cells, Nat. Med. 2 (1996) 1096–1103.
[11] N. Ferrara, et al., Heterozygous embryonic lethality induced by targeted inactivation of the VEGF gene, Nature 380 (1996) 439–442.
[12] H.P. Gerber, et al., VEGF is required for growth and survival in neonatal mice, Development 126 (1999) 1149–1159.
[13] Y. Kitamoto, et al., Vascular endothelial growth factor is an essential molecule for mouse kidney development: glomerulogenesis and nephrogenesis, J. Clin. Invest. 99 (1997) 2351–2357.
[14] H.P. Gerber, et al., VEGF couples hypertrophic cartilage remodeling, ossification and angiogenesis during endochondral bone formation, Nat. Med. 5 (1999) 623–628.
[15] N. Ferrara, et al., Vascular endothelial growth factor is essential for corpus luteum angiogenesis, Nat. Med. 4 (1998) 336–340.
[16] T.D. Henry, et al., The VIVA trial: vascular endothelial growth factor in ischemia for vascular angiogenesis, Circulation 107 (2003) 1359–1365.
[17] Y. Dor, et al., Conditional switching of VEGF provides new insights into adult neovascularization and pro-angiogenic therapy, EMBO J. 21 (2002) 1939–1947.
[18] J. LeCouter, et al., Angiogenesis-independent endothelial protection of liver: role of VEGFR-1, Science 299 (2003) 890–893.
[19] J. Street, et al., Vascular endothelial growth factor stimulates bone repair by promoting angiogenesis and bone turnover, Proc. Natl. Acad. Sci. U. S. A. 99 (2002) 9656–9661.

International Congress Series 1262 (2004) 287–291

www.ics-elsevier.com

Oxygen regulates brain angiogenesis and tight junction formation in blood–brain barrier

Sae-Won Lee[a], Woo Jean Kim[a,b], Yoon Kyung Choi[a], Kyu-Won Kim[a,*]

[a] *Division of Pharmaceutical Bioscience, College of Pharmacy and Research Institute of Pharmaceutical Sciences, Seoul National University, Seoul 151-742, South Korea*

[b] *Department of Molecular Biology, Pusan National University, Pusan 609-735, South Korea*

Abstract. The maintenance of the blood–brain barrier (BBB) is important in the central nervous system because disruption of the BBB may contribute to many brain disorders, including Alzheimer's disease and stroke. However, the molecular mechanism of brain vessel development and BBB formation remains ill-defined. We found that the immunoreactivities of pimonidazol, hypoxic marker and vascular endothelial growth factor (VEGF) were detected in developing brain, and then disappeared after birth. However, the expression of occludin was gradually increased during BBB maturation. Moreover, we found *src*-suppressed C-kinase substrate (SSeCKS)-overexpressed in astrocytes during reoxygenation. Overexpressed SSeCKS strongly reduced the VEGF expression and angiogenesis. Furthermore, SSeCKS overexpression increased the expression of both angiopoietin-1 (Ang-1), an antipermeability factor, and tight junction proteins, consequently decreased [^{3}H]sucrose permeability. We therefore conclude that reoxygenation of astrocytes may act as a significant driving force for the BBB maturation, and SSeCKS is a novel regulator of BBB differentiation by modulating both brain angiogenesis and tight junction formation. © 2004 Published by Elsevier B.V.

Keywords: Blood–brain barrier; Angiogenesis; Oxygen tension; SSeCKS

1. Introduction

During brain vessel formation, permeable capillaries gradually become blood–brain barrier (BBB) capillaries characterized by low vascular permeability and an increase in tight junction protein [1,2]. The BBB is an essential barrier for brain homeostasis [3]; however, it has not been clearly identified as the cellular and molecular mechanism of the BBB development.

We previously reported that hypoxia exists widely in the developing embryonic tissues and regulates the new vessel formation [4]. Here, we identified a strongly upregulated

* Corresponding author. Tel.: +82-2-880-6988; fax: +82-2-872-1795.
E-mail address: qwonkim@plaza.snu.ac.kr (K.-W. Kim).

0531-5131/ © 2004 Published by Elsevier B.V.
doi:10.1016/j.ics.2003.11.044

gene, SSeCKS, in astrocytes under reoxygenation. SSeCKS and its human ortholog, gravin, belong to a family of scaffolding proteins that are also potential tumor suppressors. SSeCKS acts as both an anchoring protein and a substrate for PKC [5].

We found that SSeCKS-overexpressing astrocytes promotes not only the cessation of angiogenesis, but also the differentiation of endothelial cells into a BBB-like state. Therefore, we propose that SSeCKS regulates BBB maturation by controlling brain angiogenesis and vessel differentiation.

2. Results

2.1. Oxygen tension controls developmental vessel formation

To observe the hypoxic states and brain angiogenesis, we detected the immunoreactivities of pimonidazol and vascular endothelial growth factor (VEGF) [4]. These immunoreactivities were slightly detected in embryonic day 13 (E13) rat brain, spread in the whole cerebral cortex at postnatal day 3 (P3), and then gradually disappeared [6].

Next, we examined occludin expression to identify tight junction formation during BBB development. Occludin immunoreactivity was not detected in E13 brain, and then gradually increased and highly detected in adult brain. These results indicate that oxygen gradient from hypoxia to normoxia may regulate brain angiogenesis and BBB maturation during brain development [6].

2.2. SSeCKS-overexpressing astrocytes suppress angiogenesis

We therefore searched in astrocytes for factors upregulated by reoxygenation using cDNA representational difference analysis, and identified a strongly upregulated gene, SSeCKS (Fig. 1A). SSeCKS markedly reduced the expression of VEGF, an endothelial cell mitogen and vascular permeability factor [7] (Fig. 1B). Moreover, the conditioned medium from SSeCKS-transfected astrocytes (SSeCKS-CM) strongly reduced new vessel formation *in vivo* chick chorioallantoic membrane (CAM) assay (Fig. 1C), suggesting that SSeCKS-overexpressing astrocytes potently repress angiogenesis [8].

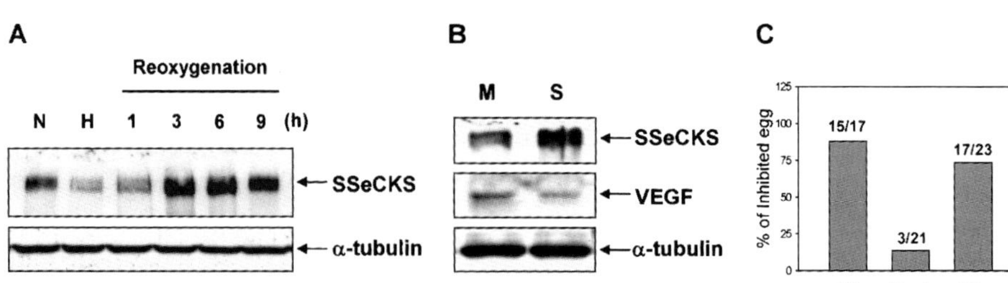

Fig. 1. Antiangiogenic activity of SSeCKS. (A) SSeCKS expression in astrocytes by Western blot analysis. N, normoxia; H, hypoxia. (B) VEGF expression in mock-transfected (M) or SSeCKS-overexpressing astrocytes (S). (C) CAM assay. RA, retinoic acid; Mock, Mock-CM; SSe, SSeCKS-CM.

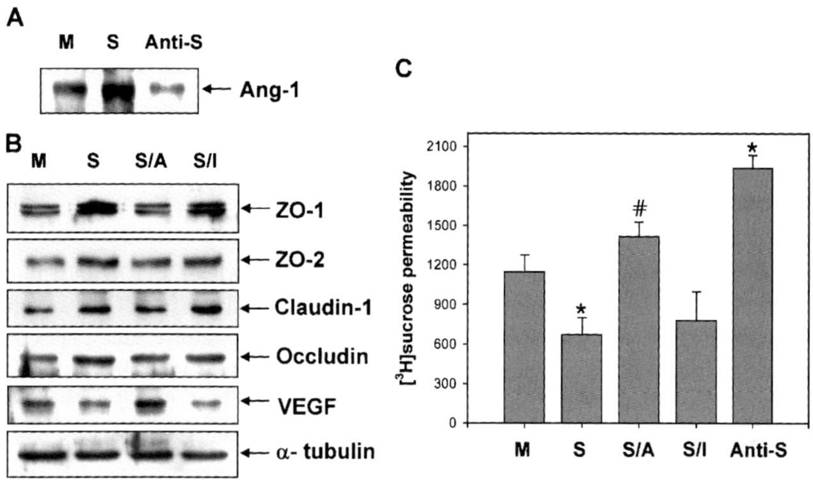

Fig. 2. SSeCKS-overexpressing astrocytes regulates the expression of BBB marker genes and vascular permeability. (A) Expression of Ang-1 in CM. (B) Expression of tight junction proteins and VEGF in HBMECs. (C) [^{3}H]Sucrose permeability of HBMECs. M, Mock-CM; S, sense SSeCKS-CM; Anti-S, antisense SSeCKS-CM; S/A, Ang-1-neutralized SSeCKS-CM; S/I, IgG-neutralized SSeCKS-CM. *$P<0.01$ compared with HBMECs cultured with Mock-CM. #$P<0.05$ compared with HBMECs cultured with SSeCKS-CM.

2.3. SSeCKS-overexpressing astrocytes enhances barriergenesis through Ang-1

We found that the expression of Ang-1 to tighten pre-existing vessels [9] was strongly increased in SSeCKS-CM (Fig. 2A). Moreover, SSeCKS-CM increased the expression of tight junction proteins, zonula occludens-1 (ZO-1), ZO-2, claudin-1 and occludin in human brain microvascular endothelial cells (HBMECs) (Fig. 2B).

We then investigated whether Ang-1 mediates SSeCKS-stimulated BBB formation. The Ang-1-neutralized SSeCKS-CM markedly reduced the expression of tight junction proteins, however, strongly increased the VEGF expression (Fig. 2B). Moreover, we confirmed that the Ang-1-neutralized SSeCKS-CM did not reduce the [^{3}H]sucrose permeability (Fig. 2C). These results indicate that SSeCKS-overexpressing astrocytes may enhance the barrier function of endothelial cells through Ang-1 mediated upregulation of tight junction proteins [8].

3. Discussion

Most studies on the BBB development have mainly examined the effect of the astrocytes without considering oxygen tension. We previously found that astrocytes under reoxygenation might act as a physiological trigger for brain vessel maturation [6]. Here, we identified a potential BBB-inducing protein, SSeCKS (Fig. 1A). Interestingly, SSeCKS overexpression led to a marked reduction of VEGF and an increased expression of Ang-1. In addition, SSeCKS-CM clearly suppressed *in vivo* angiogenesis and vascular permeability (Figs. 1 and 2).

These findings suggest that SSeCKS-expressing astrocytes trigger vessel maturation and stabilization during BBB development by inhibiting brain angiogenesis and by enhancing the expression of tight junction proteins.

4. Materials and methods

4.1. Cells

Brain astrocytes were purified from neonatal Sprague–Dawley rat [10], and cultured in DMEM containing 10% FBS (Life Technologies) and antibiotics. HBMECs (passage 5–8) were purchased from Cell Systems and grown on Attachment Factor-coated plates in CS-C complete SFM media (Cell Systems) or in M199 supplemented with 20% FBS, 3 ng/ml bFGF and 5 U/ml heparin. Culture for hypoxia and reoxygenation was done as described [8]. Transient transfection was performed using Lipofectamine Reagent (Life Technologies) and CM preparation was done as described [8].

4.2. Immunohistochemistry and Western blot analysis

Immunohistochemistry was performed using InnoGenex™ IHC kit (Innogenex). Total proteins (10–25 μg) were purified and immunoblotted as described [8].

4.3. CAM assay

CAM assay was done using a 4.5-day-old chick embryo as described [11].

4.4. [^{3}H]Sucrose permeability assay

HBMECs and astrocytes were cocultured as described [12]. A total of 50 μl (0.8 μCi/ml) of [^{3}H]sucrose (1 μCi/μl, Amersham Pharmacia) was added to the upper compartment. The amount of radioactivity that diffused into the lower compartment was determined after 30 min by liquid scintillation counter (Wallac, PerkinElmer).

Acknowledgements

Financial support was from the Vascular System Research Center grant from the Korea Science and Engineering Foundation, the National Research Laboratory Fund (2002-N-NL-01-C-015) and the Brain Research Center of the 21st Century Frontier Research Program grant (M103KV010005 03K2201 00520) from the Ministry of Science and Technology, Korea (to K-W.K).

References

[1] R.C. Janzer, M.C. Raff, Astrocytes induce blood–brain barrier properties in endothelial cells, Nature 325 (1987) 253–257.

[2] U. Kniesel, H. Wolburg, Tight junctions of the blood–brain barrier, Cell. Mol. Neurobiol. 20 (2000) 57–76.

[3] S. Nag, The blood–brain barrier and cerebral angiogenesis: lessons from the cold-injury model, Trends Mol. Med. 8 (2002) 38–44.

[4] Y.M. Lee, et al., Determination of hypoxic region by hypoxia marker in developing mouse embryos in vivo: a possible signal for vessel development, Dev. Dyn. 220 (2001) 175–186.
[5] I.H. Gelman, The role of SSeCKS/gravin/ AKAP12 scaffolding proteins in the spaciotemporal control of signaling pathways in oncogenesis and development, Front. Biosci. 7 (2002) 11782–11797.
[6] H.S. Song, et al., Oxygen tension regulates the maturation of the blood–brain barrier, Biochem. Biophys. Res. Commun. 290 (2002) 325–331.
[7] C. Ruhrberg, et al., Spatially restricted patterning cues provided by heparin-binding VEGF-A control blood vessel branching morphogenesis, Genes Dev. 16 (2002) 2684–2698.
[8] S.W. Lee, et al., SSeCKS regulates angiogenesis and tight junction formation in blood–brain barrier, Nat. Med. 9 (2003) 900–906.
[9] G. Thurston, et al., Angiopoietin-1 protects the adult vasculature against plasma leakage, Nat. Med. 6 (2000) 460–463.
[10] K.D. McCarthy, J. de Vellis, Preparation of separate astroglial and oligodendroglial cell cultures from rat cerebral tissue, J. Cell Biol. 85 (1980) 890–902.
[11] M.S. Lee, et al., Angiogenic activity of pyruvic acid in in vivo and in vitro angiogenesis models, Cancer Res. 61 (2001) 3290–3293.
[12] L.L. Rubin, et al., A cell culture model of the blood–brain barrier, J. Cell Biol. 115 (1991) 1725–1735.

International Congress Series 1262 (2004) 292–295

www.ics-elsevier.com

Non-genomic activation of protein kinase Akt by steroid hormones

James K. Liao*

Vascular Medicine Research, Cardiovascular Division, Brigham and Women's Hospital, Boston, MA, USA
Vascular Medicine Research, Cardiovascular Division, Harvard Medical School, Boston, MA, USA

Abstract. Many cellular responses to steroid hormones involve the transcriptional modulation of target genes by the prototypical nuclear hormone receptor. In the classic model of steroid hormone action, the glucocorticoid receptor (GR) acts as ligand-dependent transcription factor by either activating or repressing gene expression through direct interactions with DNA or other transcription factors. Recent evidence suggests an important role for non-transcriptional effects of GR in the vascular system. The non-transcriptional actions of GR involve the rapid activation of protein kinases, such as phosphatidylinositol-3 kinase and Akt, leading to the activation of endothelial nitric oxide synthase (eNOS). This novel pathway of steroid hormone action protects against ischemic injury augmenting blood flow and decreasing vascular inflammation. © 2004 Published by Elsevier B.V.

Keywords: Glucocorticoid receptor; Non-transcriptional; Nitric oxide; Ischemia; Protein kinase Akt

Corticosteroids have been used in the treatment of cardiovascular disease, such as acute myocardial infarction and stroke, with conflicting results [1]. Several features make steroids attractive candidates for the treatment of acute ischemia. The degree of ischemic tissue damage is related to the extent of the inflammatory response, which is coordinated through the interaction of leukocytes with activated vascular endothelium. Corticosteroids inhibit endothelial cell activation and leukocyte–endothelial interaction, thereby exerting prominent and very rapid, anti-inflammatory effects on the vasculature [2]. Steroid treatment improves survival of patients with acute myocardial infarction and protects the myocardium from experimental ischemic injury [3–5]. In ischemic stroke, steroids can improve clinical outcome in a subset of patients with severe stroke and administration of high doses of corticosteroids substantially reduces tissue damage in experimental focal cerebral ischemia [6–9]. In addition, we have recently shown that high-dose steroid treatment decreases vascular inflammation and ischemic tissue damage after myocardial infarction and stroke through direct vascular effects involving the non-transcriptional activation of eNOS [10,11].

* Vascular Medicine Research Unit, Brigham and Women's Hospital, 65 Landsdowne Street, Room 275, Cambridge, MA 02139, USA. Tel.: +1-617-768-8424; fax: +1-617-768-8425.
E-mail address: jliao@rics.bwh.harvard.edu (J.K. Liao).

0531-5131/
doi:10.1016/j.ics.2003.12.059

The prolonged use of steroids, however, is often limited by their adverse effects. In most cases, these adverse effects are often attributed to a delayed genomic response initiated by glucocorticoid receptor (GR). This is exemplified by the clinical syndrome of hyperglycemia, dyslipidemia, hypertension, osteoporosis and impaired wound healing in patients with chronic corticosteroid excess (i.e., Cushing syndrome) [12]. Furthermore, downregulation of eNOS and elevated systemic blood pressure are thought to contribute to steroid-induced hypertension [13]. Indeed, continued low-dose steroid administration increases ischemic injury after global ischemia of the brain [14]. In myocardial infarction, impaired wound healing and cardiac remodeling can lead to cardiac rupture within two weeks of myocardial infarction [15,16], and this has lead to discontinuation of steroid treatment for acute ischemia. Therefore, defining the precise molecular mechanisms involved in the beneficial and detrimental effects of GR could have important therapeutic implications, especially if a strategy could be devised to separate these pathways.

1. Non-transcriptional activation of eNOS by corticosteroids

Many beneficial actions of corticosteroids in vivo involve the vascular endothelium. An important endogenous mediator of vascular integrity is endothelium-derived nitric oxide (NO) [17]. NO produced by endothelial NO synthase (eNOS) possesses anti-inflammatory, anti-atherogenic and anti-ischemic properties [18,19]. Enhanced NO production by administration of the eNOS substrate, L-arginine or upregulation of eNOS by statins, confers stroke protection [19–21], and transgenic mice overexpressing eNOS show decreased leukocyte accumulation and reduced vascular lesion formation following vascular injury [22]. Conversely, mice with targeted disruption of eNOS (eNOS$^{-/-}$) exhibit increased vascular inflammation and larger cerebral infarctions following experimental ischemia [23,24], while inhibition of NOS activity decreases cerebral blood flow (CBF) and increases infarct size after ischemia [25].

In two different mouse models of ischemic injury, transient myocardial ischemia and transient focal cerebral ischemia, the protective effects of steroids were mediated by the non-transcriptional activation of eNOS by GR [10,11]. High-dose corticosteroids significantly reduced ischemic tissue damage to the heart and the brain, while low doses were ineffective. Co-treatment with the GR antagonist, RU486, completely reversed the effects of Dex, suggesting that GR-mediated tissue protection. Furthermore, ischemia protection was mediated by NO, since the beneficial actions of steroids were absent in eNOS$^{-/-}$ mice or blocked by co-treatment with the NOS inhibitor N^{ω}-nitro-L-arginine methyl ester (L-NAME). Steroid treatment acutely increased eNOS activity in vitro and in vivo, which led to decreased vascular inflammation and increased vasorelaxation and regional cerebral blood flow in a NO-dependent manner.

2. Activation of PI3K/Akt by corticosteroids

Corticosteroids have recently been reported to activate protein kinase Akt [10,11,26,27], which is an important regulator of cell cycle progression and mediator of cellular survival downstream of PI3K [28]. Phosphorylation of eNOS by Akt leads to increased endothelial NO release [29,30]. In a ligand-dependent manner, corticosteroids activate PI3K and Akt, which is blocked by co-treatment with RU486 or the PI3K inhibitor, LY294002, but not by transcriptional inhibitors [10,11]. Although induction of non-transcriptional actions requires high doses of steroids, these effects are nevertheless specifically mediated by GR. This was demonstrated in transfection studies in COS7 cells, which lack endogenous GR. Whereas Dex did not activate PI3K or Akt in the absence of GR, it readily induced Akt kinase activation after transfection with GR, or the dimerization defective GR mutant (A458T), which is unable to transactivate target genes [10]. This suggests a DNA binding independent mechanism of activation. The fact that PI3K activation can be suppressed by the GR antagonist RU486 further argues against the involvement of transrepression in this process, since the RU486 compound still induces transrepression of AP-1-dependent gene expression in reporter assays [31].

The mechanism of PI3K activation by GR is currently unknown but seems to involve association of GR with the regulatory p85α subunit of PI3K. Also, activation does not require dimerization of the receptor, since the dimerization defective mutant is equally active [10]. Analogies might be drawn to PI3K activation by another steroid receptor, ERα, although there is only modest sequence homology between the two receptors. Activation of PI3K by ERα involves activation of Src and formation of a ternary complex of p85 and Src with the activated receptor, which was mediated by the C-terminus of ERα including the LBD [32]. Since positive cross talk between Src and PI3K has already been described, it might be speculated that this mechanism is also involved in activation of PI3K by GR [33].

Acknowledgements

The work presented in this manuscript was supported, in part, by grants from the National Institutes of Health (HL52233, HL70274 and DK62729), the American Heart Association Bugher Foundation Award and the Deutsche Forschungsgemeinschaft.

References

[1] C. Thiemermann, Corticosteroids and cardioprotection, Nat. Med. 8 (5) (2002) 453–455.

[2] B.N. Cronstein, et al., A mechanism for the antiinflammatory effects of corticosteroids: the glucocorticoid receptor regulates leukocyte adhesion to endothelial cells and expression of endothelial-leukocyte adhesion molecule 1 and intercellular adhesion molecule 1, Proc. Natl. Acad. Sci. U. S. A. 89 (21) (1992) 9991–9995.

[3] D. Barzilai, et al., Use of hydrocortisone in the treatment of acute myocardial infarction. Summary of a clinical trial in 446 patients, Chest 61 (5) (1972) 488–491.

[4] P. Libby, et al., Reduction of experimental myocardial infarct size by corticosteroid administration, J. Clin. Invest. 52 (3) (1973) 599–607.

[5] J.A. Spath Jr., et al., Protective action of methylprednisolone on the myocardium during experimental myocardial ischemia in the cat, Circ. Res. 35 (1) (1974) 44–51.

[6] B.M. Patten, et al., Double-blind study of the effects of dexamethasone on acute stroke, Neurology 22 (4) (1972) 377–383.

[7] A.P. Slivka, et al., High-dose methylprednisolone treatment in experimental focal cerebral ischemia, Exp. Neurol. 167 (1) (2001) 166–172.

[8] G.M. de Courten-Myers, et al., Efficacious experimental stroke treatment with high-dose methylprednisolone, Stroke 25 (2) (1994) 487–492.

[9] R. Bertorelli, et al., MK 801 and dexamethasone reduce both tumor necrosis factor levels and infarct volume after focal cerebral ischemia in the rat brain, Neurosci. Lett. 246 (1) (1998) 41–44.

[10] F. Limbourg, et al., Rapid non-transcriptional activation of endothelial nitric oxide synthase mediates increase in cerebral blood flow and stroke protection by corticosteroids, J. Clin. Invest. 110 (2002) 1729–1738.

[11] A. Hafezi-Moghadam, et al., Acute cardiovascular protective effects of corticosteroids are mediated by non-transcriptional activation of endothelial nitric oxide synthase, Nat. Med. 8 (5) (2002) 473–479.
[12] E. Braunwald, et al., Heart Disease, 6th ed., Saunders, Philadelphia, 2001.
[13] T. Wallerath, et al., Down-regulation of the expression of endothelial NO synthase is likely to contribute to glucocorticoid-mediated hypertension, Proc. Natl. Acad. Sci. U. S. A. 96 (23) (1999) 13357–13362.
[14] R.M. Sapolsky, et al., Glucocorticoids potentiate ischemic injury to neurons: therapeutic implications, Science 229 (4720) (1985) 1397–1400.
[15] B.H. Bulkley, et al., Steroid therapy during acute myocardial infarction. A cause of delayed healing and of ventricular aneurysm, Am. J. Med. 56 (2) (1974) 244–250.
[16] R. Roberts, et al., Deleterious effects of methylprednisolone in patients with myocardial infarction, Circulation 53 (Suppl. 3) (1976) I204–I206.
[17] J. Loscalzo, Nitric oxide and vascular disease, N. Engl. J. Med. 333 (4) (1995) 251–253.
[18] R. De Caterina, et al., Nitric oxide decreases cytokine-induced endothelial activation. Nitric oxide selectively reduces endothelial expression of adhesion molecules and proinflammatory cytokines, J. Clin. Invest. 96 (1) (1995) 60–68.
[19] M. Endres, et al., Stroke protection by 3-hydroxy-3-methylglutaryl (HMG)-CoA reductase inhibitors mediated by endothelial nitric oxide synthase, Proc. Natl. Acad. Sci. U. S. A. 95 (15) (1998) 8880–8885.
[20] T. Dalkara, et al., Blood flow-dependent functional recovery in a rat model of focal cerebral ischemia, Am. J. Physiol. 267 (2 Pt 2) (1994) H678–H683.
[21] E. Morikawa, et al., L-Arginine infusion promotes nitric oxide-dependent vasodilation, increases regional cerebral blood flow, and reduces infarction volume in the rat, Stroke 25 (2) (1994) 429–435.
[22] S. Kawashima, et al., Endothelial NO synthase overexpression inhibits lesion formation in mouse model of vascular remodeling, Arterioscler. Thromb. Vasc. Biol. 21 (2) (2001) 201–207.
[23] Z. Huang, et al., Enlarged infarcts in endothelial nitric oxide synthase knockout mice are attenuated by nitro-L-arginine, J. Cereb. Blood Flow Metab. 16 (5) (1996) 981–987.
[24] M. Moroi, et al., Interaction of genetic deficiency of endothelial nitric oxide, gender, and pregnancy in vascular response to injury in mice, J. Clin. Invest. 101 (6) (1998) 1225–1232.
[25] Z. Huang, et al., Effects of cerebral ischemia in mice deficient in neuronal nitric oxide synthase, Science 265 (5180) (1994) 1883–1885.
[26] M.L. Langdown, et al., Early growth retardation induced by excessive exposure to glucocorticoids in utero selectively increases cardiac GLUT1 protein expression and Akt/protein kinase B activity in adulthood, J. Endocrinol. 169 (1) (2001) 11–22.
[27] T. Simoncini, et al., Interaction of oestrogen receptor with the regulatory subunit of phosphatidylinositol-3-OH kinase, Nature 407 (2000) 538–541.
[28] S.R. Datta, et al., Cellular survival: a play in three Akts, Genes Dev. 13 (22) (1999) 2905–2927.
[29] S. Dimmeler, et al., Activation of nitric oxide synthase in endothelial cells by Akt-dependent phosphorylation, Nature 399 (6736) (1999) 601–605.
[30] D. Fulton, et al., Regulation of endothelium-derived nitric oxide production by the protein kinase Akt, Nature 399 (6736) (1999) 597–601.
[31] S. Heck, et al., A distinct modulating domain in glucocorticoid receptor monomers in the repression of activity of the transcription factor AP-1, EMBO J. 13 (17) (1994) 4087–4095.
[32] G. Castoria, et al., PI3-kinase in concert with Src promotes the S-phase entry of oestradiol-stimulated MCF-7 cells, EMBO J. 20 (21) (2001) 6050–6059.
[33] B.R. Wong, et al., TRANCE, a TNF family member, activates Akt/PKB through a signaling complex involving TRAF6 and c-Src, Mol. Cell 4 (6) (1999) 1041–1049.

ELSEVIER

International Congress Series 1262 (2004) 296–299

www.ics-elsevier.com

Regulation of vascular remodeling and cardiovascular protection: NFκB and vascular remodeling

Bernd R. Binder*, Johannes M. Breuss

Department of Vascular Biology and Thrombosis Research, University of Vienna, Austria, Schwarzspanierstr. 17 A-1090, Vienna, Austria

Abstract. Percutaneous transluminal balloon angioplasty is currently the treatment of choice for obstructive atherosclerotic vascular disease. Still, more than 40% of initially successfully treated patients develop 'restenosis' within 6 months after the intervention, severely hampering the overall success of this therapeutic measure. The proposed mechanisms underlying the process of restenosis have led to respective therapeutic strategies ranging from the use of antiplatelet drugs and antioxidants to radiotherapy. None of the several strategies, however, could decrease the number of patients suffering from restenosis significantly. Inflammation has been implicated as an early step in the development of atherosclerosis and postangioplasty restenosis. The contribution of NFκB to restenosis could be demonstrated in animal experiments using adenoviral-based gene therapy overexpressing the inhibitor of NFκB, I-kB. This treatment resulted in significantly reduced inflammatory response, increased apoptosis, positive remodeling and significantly less lumen loss but no significant change in neointima formation. There is also a crosstalk between the NFκB pathway and the EGR-1/NAK-1 pathways. Modulation of the NAK-1/EGR-1 pathway resulted in reduced neointima formation but no lumen gain because of lack of positive remodeling.

Keywords: Restenosis; Neointima; Vascular remodeling; NFκB; EGR-1; NAB-2; Gene therapy

It is now clear that atherosclerosis is a chronic inflammatory disease [1–5] but much less clear to which extent inflammation also contributes to vascular remodeling. Vascular remodeling occurs whenever a vessel is injured, e.g., by stenting or during balloon angioplasty. Remodeling is a repair process and results either in reconstitution of the vessel wall with no impaired blood flow or in a more or less dramatic narrowing of the vessel

Abbreviations: NFκB, nuclear factor kappa B; EGR-1, early growth response factor 1; NAB-2, corepressor of EGR-1.

* Corresponding author. Tel.: +43-1-4277-62501; fax: +43-1-4277-9625.
E-mail address: bernd.binder@univie.ac.at (B.R. Binder).

doi:10.1016/j.ics.2003.12.038

lumen. The proposed mechanisms underlying the process of restenosis include growth factor-dependent activation of smooth muscle cell proliferation [6], protease-dependent migration of smooth muscle cells into the wounded area [7], cytokine-initiated matrix deposition [6,8] and progression of the atherosclerotic disease itself. These proposed mechanisms have led to respective therapeutic strategies ranging from the use of antiplatelet drugs [9] and antioxidants [10] to radiotherapy [11,12]. None of the several strategies, however, with perhaps the exception of drug releasing stents introduced recently [13], could decrease the number of patients suffering from restenosis significantly and on a permanent basis implying that the mechanisms underlying vascular remodeling are not completely understood.

Activation of the proinflammatory nuclear factor kappa B (NFκB) [14,15] and upregulation of NFκB dependent genes [14,16] by balloon injury has been shown in animal experiments [17]. The contribution of NFκB and its dependent pathways to restenosis are, however, not known. We have chosen an approach to analyze the contribution of the NFκB system at a local level using adenoviral mediated transfer of the inhibitor of NFκB, IκB into the wounded vessel area.

The transcription factor NFκB is a common factor driving the inflammatory response of cells. In resting cells, NFκB is retained in the cytosol by complex formation with its natural inhibitor IκB [18,19]. Upon stimulation by inflammatory cytokines, IκB is phosphorylated, ubiquitinilated and degraded by the proteasome. In turn, NFκB is liberated and enters the nucleus to initiate transcription of certain adhesion molecules, cytokines and other inflammatory mediators [20]. The NFκB signaling process is complex and several negative (e.g., upregulation of the NFκB inhibitor IκB [21]) and positive (e.g., upregulation of XIAP that activates NFκB [22]) feedback loops participate. Among the genes regulated by NFκB are also the family of inhibitors of apoptosis proteins (IAPs) [23] that are responsible for survival of cells especially endothelial cells under inflammatory conditions.

Correspondingly, we could show that local inhibition of the NFκB pathway during the first weeks after balloon angioplasty [24,25] or after stenting [25] significantly inhibits restenosis formation by not only inhibiting the inflammatory response but also by inducing apoptosis. This is reflected by the significantly greater vessel diameter due to positive remodeling seen in IκB-treated dilated vessels, which results in a larger lumen in spite of the unaffected proliferation and neointima formation.

During the inflammatory process, however, not only NFκB becomes activated but also other signal transduction pathways are affected. These pathways include activation of the MAP kinase ERK1/2 and the downstream transcription factor, early growth response factor 1 (EGR-1) [26]. In addition, inflammation upregulates also the orphan nuclear receptor nur77 (NAK-1) [27]. Therefore, whenever the NFκB pathway is inhibited, only part of the inflammatory response is affected. The partially NFκB independent pathways, however, might also participate in feedback loops. In addition to leaving some inflammatory pathways unaffected, shutting off the NFκB system might sometimes result in at first unexpected effects (Fig. 1).

From this scheme, it can be predicted that inhibition of the second major inflammator pathway, the EGR-1 pathway, would result in less apoptosis because the proapoptotic NAK-1 would not be activated and the NFκB dependent antiapoptotic proteins would still be present. It is expected that neointima formation might be reduced because of shutting

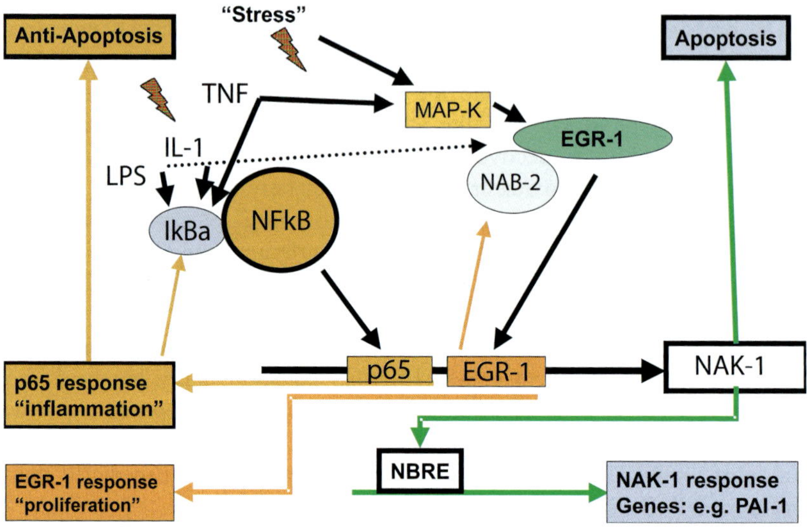

Fig. 1. Pathways operative during vascular remodeling.

off the proliferative activity of EGR-1. However, positive remodeling would also be absent because of a failure to induce apoptosis via NAK-1 and because of the still existing antiapoptotic activity of NFκB. In fact, preliminary data indicate that by use of respective adenovirus constructs, inhibition of the EGR-1 by an adenovirus construct coding for the inhibitor of EGR-1, NAB-2 [28] system results in less neointima formation but no lumen gain because of less positive remodeling (Fig. 2). The adenovirus EGR-1 on the other hand had no significant effect.

In conclusion, inflammation and specifically the NFκB pathway, participate at several steps in vascular remodeling. NFκB directly contributes to an inflammatory loop via

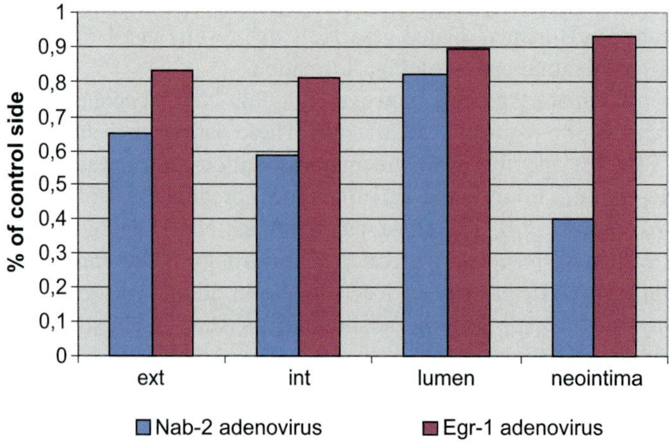

Fig. 2. Adenoviral gene transfer of EGR-1 or NAB-2 in a rabbit balloon restenosis model.

recruitment of monocytes that in turn release growth factors and other cytokines that augment smooth muscle cell proliferation via—at least in part—the EGR-1 pathway. This proliferative effect is counterbalanced to some extent by EGR-1 induced upregulation of proapoptotic Nur77/NAK-1. On the other hand, NFκB induces antiapoptotic proteins that act synergistically with the proliferative EGR-1 pathway and antagonistic to the proapoptotic Nur77/NAK-1. The overall effect is neointima formation and negative remodeling. When NFκB is inhibited, neointima formation is almost unaffected, but the apoptotic/antiapoptotic balance is shifted towards apoptosis and therefore negative remodeling is counterbalanced by positive remodeling. When only the EGR-1 part is inhibited, neointima formation is significantly reduced, but antiapoptotic factors prevail, still resulting in negative remodeling. It can be expected that a combination of inhibitors of NFκB and inhibitors of the EGR-1 pathway might be most efficient in preventing restenosis.

References

[1] A.J. Lusis, Nature 407 (2000) 233–241.
[2] R. Ross, Am. Heart J. 138 (1999) S419–S420.
[3] P. Libby, et al., Circulation 105 (2002) 1135–1143.
[4] P. Libby, Nature 420 (2002) 868–874.
[5] R.N. Ross, Engl. J. Med. 340 (1999) 115–126.
[6] A.C. Newby, et al., Cardiovasc. Res. 41 (1999) 345–360.
[7] E.W. Raines, Int. J. Exp. Pathol. 81 (2000) 173–182.
[8] A.C. Newby, et al., J. Pathol. 190 (2000) 300–309.
[9] L. Schwartz, et al., N. Engl. J. Med. 318 (1988) 1714–1719.
[10] H. Daida, et al., Am. J. Cardiol. 86 (A9) (2000) 550–552.
[11] M. Hoher, et al., Circulation 101 (2000) 2355–2360.
[12] M. Hoher, et al., Circulation 107 (2003) 3022–3027.
[13] R. Waksman, et al., Circulation 108 (2003) 386–388.
[14] D.B. Landry, et al., Am. J. Pathol. 151 (1997) 1085–1095.
[15] B. Cercek, et al., Atherosclerosis 131 (1997) 59–66.
[16] H. Qian, et al., Circulation 99 (1999) 2979–2982.
[17] L.A. Guzman, et al., Arterioscler. Thromb. Vasc. Biol. 16 (1996) 479–487.
[18] P.A. Baeuerle, Cell 95 (1998) 729–731.
[19] P.A. Baeuerle, et al., Science 242 (1988) 540–546.
[20] R. de Martin, et al., Arterioscler. Thromb. Vasc. Biol. 20 (2000) E83–E88.
[21] C.J. Wrighton, et al., J. Exp. Med. 183 (1996) 1013–1022.
[22] R. Hofer-Warbinek, et al., J. Biol. Chem. 275 (2000) 22064–22068.
[23] C. Stehlik, et al., J. Exp. Med. 188 (1998) 211–216.
[24] J.M. Breuss, et al., Circulation 105 (2002) 633–638.
[25] M. Cejna, et al., Radiology 223 (2002) 702–708.
[26] D. Mechtcheriakova, et al., FASEB J. 15 (2001) 230–242.
[27] F. Gruber, et al., Blood 101 (2003) 3042–3048.
[28] M. Lucerna, et al., J. Biol. Chem. 278 (2003) 11433–11440.

International Congress Series 1262 (2004) 300–304

www.ics-elsevier.com

Sitosterolemia; of mice and man

Shailesh B. Patel[a,*], Eric L. Klett[a], Gwang-Sook Anh[a,1], Hongwei Yu[a], Jianling Chen[a], Bhaswati Pandit[a], Mi-Hye Lee[a], Gerald Salen[b]

[a] *Division of Endocrinology, Diabetes and Medical Genetics, Medical University of South Carolina, STR 541, 114 Doughty Street, Charleston, SC 29403, USA*

[b] *Division of Gasteroenterology, University Medical and Dental School New Jersey, NJ, USA*

Abstract. Investigation and study of rare genetic disorders can lead to considerable and rapid advancements into understanding common and basic physiological processes. One such case is the study of the rare human disorder of sitosterolemia. This autosomal recessive disorder is characterized by the accumulation of plant sterols in the blood and tissues. The identification of the molecular defect(s) responsible for causing sitosterolemia has not only advanced our understanding of how we normally regulate dietary sterol entry, but may have also led to the identification of the long sought after transporters responsible for secretion of cholesterol (and other sterols) into bile. This review will summarize the history and current knowledge of how the genetic defects identified have improved our understanding of these important processes.

Keywords: Plant sterols; Biliary sterol excretion; Dietary cholesterol absorption; Genetics; ABC proteins

1. Historical

The structural and biological differences between animal sterols (primarily cholesterol) and plant sterols (primarily sitosterol) have been recognized for more than 80 years. Schoenheimer [1] was the first to demonstrate that herbivores, despite having a diet consisting exclusively of plant sterols, did not absorb any of these sterols, but instead synthesized all of their cholesterol endogenously. The lack of absorption of plant sterols in man, led to the use of these sterols as an internal marker and control for estimating sterol balance and cholesterol absorption in humans [2–4]. Thus, while it was known that mammals did not absorb plant sterols, but could absorb cholesterol from their diets, the reason why these chemically very similar molecules had such different biological pathways was not fully appreciated until very recently. The breakthrough was initiated by a

* Corresponding author. Tel.: +1-843-876-5227; fax: +1-843-876-5133.

E-mail address: patelsb@musc.edu (S.B. Patel).

[1] Present address: Department of Biology, Daejeon University, South Korea.

0531-5131/
doi:10.1016/j.ics.2003.12.044

seminal publication that reported a new disease, β-sitosterolemia[2] by two very astute clinical scientists in 1974 [5].

2. Clinical

Bhattacharyya and Connor [5] described two sisters who presented with tendon xanthomas and arthralgias, but who had normal levels of plasma cholesterol and no family history of cardiovascular or hyperlipidemia. Investigations revealed very elevated non-cholesterol sterols in their blood, the most abundant of which was sitosterol, thus the name of this new disease. Sitosterolemia is an extremely rare autosomal recessive disease, and can present early in childhood, with extremely elevated plasma cholesterol levels and tendon xanthomas, mimicking homozygous familial hypercholesterolemia (FH) [6–8]. Unlike FH, this hyperlipidemia is very sensitive to dietary and drug therapy, a feature that allows its distinction from FH. Other clinical features include hemolytic anemia during childhood and adolescence, arthralgias, tendon as well as tuberous xanthomas and premature atherosclerotic disease. The diagnostic test is the detection of plasma or serum plant sterol levels (almost always >20-fold elevation compared with controls in untreated cases) by the use of GC, or HPLC.

3. Physiology and pathophysiology

The absorption of cholesterol from our diets and many of the mechanisms involved in this process have been studied now for almost a century. Our diets contain as much cholesterol as non-cholesterol sterols (primarily plant sterols, such as sitosterol, campesterol, stigmasterol, avenosterol, etc.). As stated above, our net retention of non-cholesterol sterols, on a daily basis is $<1\%$, whereas our average dietary cholesterol retention is $\sim 55\%$. Schoenheimer [1] had acknowledged that these results could be accounted for not only by a failure to absorb plant sterols, but also by a rapid excretion and breakdown of these sterols. A small amount of plant sterols do enter the circulation and in normal individuals between 0 and 0.5 mg/dl of plants sterols can be detected in plasma. However, while cholesterol enters the metabolic pool, non-cholesterol sterols are rapidly taken up by the liver, and excreted into bile (Fig. 1).

In sitosterolemia, these normal pathways are specifically disrupted [5]. Not only is the absorption of plant sterols in the intestine increased, as originally demonstrated, but any species of non-cholesterol sterol is also absorbed. Additionally, biliary secretion of these sterols, including cholesterol, is disrupted. Thus, sitosterolemia is caused by unregulated sterol entry and failure to excrete sterols into bile. That these highly regulated physiological processes were specifically disrupted by a single locus (based upon the autosomal recessive inheritance) prompted us to initiate a proposal to identify the defective locus.

4. Genetics

Sitosterolemia is an autosomal recessive disease and was mapped to the sitosterolemia locus, STSL, on human chromosome 2p21[9]. This led to the identification of two genes

[2] The term β is no longer necessary, since this is the only naturally occurring form of plant sterol.

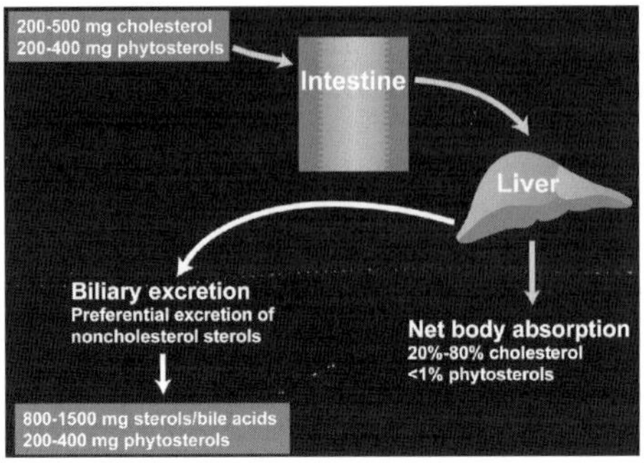

Fig. 1. Dietary sterol balance in humans. Our normal diets contain as much cholesterol (~ 400 mg) as plant sterols (~ 400 mg), but our net output of sterols on a daily basis is ~ 1500 mg. Of this, almost all of the plant sterols are present in the feces (~ 400 mg), the remaining 1100 mg representing bile acids and cholesterol. Studies of normal individuals suggest that our average dietary cholesterol absorption is ~ 55%, thus the net daily output of sterols represents an excess of synthesis and breakdown of cholesterol that needs to be disposed of. Note that the liver is a key organ in this pathway and is responsible for the disposal of not only all of this excess cholesterol, but also any small amounts of non-cholesterol sterols that may enter our bodies, thus ensuring a very low net retention of these species.

that comprise the STSL locus; complete mutations in either ABCG5 or ABCG8 cause sitosterolemia [10–12]. To date, all known cases of sitosterolemia are caused by defects at this locus and no other loci have been implicated [12]. It is important to stress that since complete mutations in either gene causes sitosterolemia, this provides the strongest genetic evidence that their protein products may function as obligate heterodimers [12].

5. Molecular biology

Both ABCG5 and ABCG8 are members of the ATP binding cassette family, sub-group G, which consists of 'half-transporters' [13]. Both of these transporters have ATP binding domains, based upon peptide sequence analyses, though formal demonstration of ATP binding and hydrolysis has not been demonstrated. Based upon mRNA expression analyses, as well as Western blotting analyses, these proteins are expressed only in the liver and the intestine [10,12,14–16]. To date, no in vitro functional assay has been reported, though considerable evidence has accumulated that these proteins are the long sought after biliary cholesterol exporters, as well as functioning to keep non-cholesterol sterols out of the body (see below).

6. Animal models

Clinical studies in sitosterolemia patients had indicated that not only was dietary sterol absorption increased and unregulated, but also there was a severe impairment of biliary excretion of both cholesterol and non-cholesterol sterols [17]. There are now four animal models of sitosterolemia in which these defects can be further tested and delineated. In addition, it over-expresses these proteins and is available for study [18,19].

The Hobbs groups created a mouse model of sitosterolemia by disrupting the STSL locus, such that expression of both Abcg5/sterolin-1 and Abcg8/sterolin-2 was knocked out simultaneously [19]. Biochemical characterization of these animals showed that they had elevated plasma plant sterol levels and had bile that was sterol poor, confirming aspects of human sitosterolemia [19]. In addition, a transgenic mouse for the human STSL has also been created that over-expressed human ABCG5 and ABCG8 that demonstrates that not only is the fractional absorption of dietary cholesterol reduced, but there is also a considerable increase in biliary sterol output [18]. These experiments therefore support the hypothesis that ABCG5 and ABCG8 are key molecules involved in biliary sterol transport.

In collaboration with Tularik, the Kuipers group studied a mouse that had a selective deficiency for Abcg5. Homozygous Abcg5-deficient mice are sitosterolemic and also have a bile that is sterol poor. Interestingly, upon challenge with LXR agonists, their plasma sitosterol levels are also increased. However, biliary sterol levels were also increased, despite the absence of Abcg5 (Kuipers personal communication, Plosch et al., 2004, Gastroenterology, in press).

The Patel group created a mouse that has a selective deficiency of Abcg8/sterolin-2 that is sitosterolemic and also produces a sterol-poor bile. A more detailed characterization of biliary secretion rates, using TUDC infusion showed that Abcg8/sterolin-2 deficient mice could not increase secretion of cholesterol into bile, even in the face of increased bile salt and phospholipid secretion. Remarkably, analyses of the bile sterols showed that while the cholesterol levels were severely reduced, sitosterol secretion into bile was comparable to that of wild-type mice. Nevertheless, all of these data taken together indicate that both Abcg5 and Abcg8 can work independent of each other as well as heterodimers, or that there are as yet unidentified transport mechanisms that can secrete sterols into bile. Further studies, now that a number of these models are available, should help clarify these issues.

7. Conclusions

The identification of the molecular basis for a rare genetic disorder has led to the elucidation two highly conserved and important proteins; the identification of ABCG5 and ABCG8 has allowed us to finally identify the long sought after sterol transporters responsible for biliary sterol export and for selective dietary sterol absorption. Additionally, rapid progress has been made in identifying animal models that will lead to further elucidation of the biological roles of these proteins and whether they play a role beyond regulating cholesterol trafficking in the body.

Acknowledgements

We gratefully acknowledge all of our colleagues and friends Drs. Bert Groen, Astrid Kosters, Ronald Oude-Elferink, Folkert Kuipers, Ikuo Ikeda, Nami Egashira, Masao Sato, and Richard Klein for scientific help, discussion and/or communicating to us pre-publication data. We are particularly grateful to all the medical community and all of the families with sitosterolemia who have allowed us to study them and to the National Institutes of Health, NHLBI for Grant HL060613 for providing funding for this work.

References

[1] R. Schoenheimer, Uber die Bedeutung der Pflanzensterine fur den tierischen Organismus, Hoppe-Seyler Z. Physiol. Chem. 180 (1929) 1–5.

[2] C.R. Treadwell, G.V. Vahouny, Cholesterol absorption, in: C.F. Code, W. Heidel (Eds.), Handbook of Physiology, American Physiological Society, Washington, DC, 1968, pp. 1407–1438.

[3] R.G. Gould, et al., Absorbability of beta-sitosterol in humans, Metabolism 18 (8) (1969) 652–662.

[4] G. Salen, E. Ahrens Jr., S.M. Grundy, Metabolism of beta-sitosterol in man, J. Clin. Invest. 49 (5) (1970) 952–967.

[5] A.K. Bhattacharyya, W.E. Connor, Beta-sitosterolemia and xanthomatosis. A newly described lipid storage disease in two sisters, J. Clin. Invest. 53 (4) (1974) 1033–1043.

[6] G. Salen, et al., Sitosterolemia, J. Lipid Res. 33 (7) (1992) 945–955.

[7] I. Bjorkhem, K.M. Boberg, Inborn errors in bile acid biosynthesis and storage of sterols other than cholesterol, in: C.R. Scriver, et al. (Eds.), The Metabolic Basis of Inherited Disease, McGraw-Hill, New York, 1995, pp. 2073–2102.

[8] G. Salen, S.B. Patel, A.K. Batta, Sitosterolemia, Cardiovasc. Drug Rev. 20 (4) (2002) 255–270.

[9] S.B. Patel, et al., Mapping a gene involved in regulating dietary cholesterol absorption. The sitosterolemia locus is found at chromosome 2p21, J. Clin. Invest. 102 (5) (1998) 1041–1044.

[10] K.E. Berge, et al., Accumulation of dietary cholesterol in sitosterolemia caused by mutations in adjacent ABC transporters, Science 290 (5497) (2000) 1771–1775.

[11] M.H. Lee, et al., Identification of a gene, ABCG5, important in the regulation of dietary cholesterol absorption, Nat. Genet. 27 (2001) 79–83.

[12] K. Lu, et al., Two genes that map to the STSL locus cause sitosterolemia: genomic structure and spectrum of mutations involving sterolin-1 and sterolin-2, encoded by ABCG5 and ABCG8 respectively, Am. J. Hum. Gen. 69 (2001) 278–290.

[13] M. Dean, A. Rzhetsky, R. Allikmets, The human ATP-binding cassette (ABC) transporter superfamily, Genome Res. 11 (7) (2001) 1156–1166.

[14] S. Shulenin, et al., A liver-specific ATP-binding cassette gene (ABCG5) from the ABCG (White) gene subfamily maps to human chromosome 2p21 in the region of the sitosterolemia locus, Cytogenet. Cell Genet. 92 (3–4) (2001) 204–208.

[15] K. Lu, et al., Molecular cloning, genomic organization, genetic variations, and characterization of murine sterolin genes ABCG5 and ABCG8, J. Lipid Res. 43 (4) (2002) 565–578.

[16] H. Yu, et al., The rat STSL locus: characterization, chromosomal assignment, and genetic variations in sitosterolemic hypertensive rats, BMC Cardiovasc. Disord. 3 (1) (2003) 4.

[17] G. Salen, et al., Hyperabsorption and retention of campestanol in a sitosterolemic homozygote: comparison with her mother and three control subjects, J. Lipid Res. 41 (11) (2000) 1883–1889.

[18] L. Yu, et al., Overexpression of ABCG5 and ABCG8 promotes biliary cholesterol secretion and reduces fractional absorption of dietary cholesterol, J. Clin. Invest. 110 (5) (2002) 671–680.

[19] L. Yu, et al., Disruption of ABCG5 and ABCG8 in mice reveals their crucial role in biliary cholesterol secretion. Proc. Natl. Acad. Sci. U. S. A. 99 (25) (2002) 16237-16242.

International Congress Series 1262 (2004) 305–308

www.ics-elsevier.com

Molecular defects in the ABCA1 pathway affect HDL metabolism and function of macrophages

Gerd Schmitz*

Institute for Clinical Chemistry and Laboratory Medicine, University Hospital of Regensburg, Franz-Josef-Strauss-Allee 11, 93053 Regensburg, Germany

Abstract. The ATP-binding cassette transporter 1 (ABCA1) facilitates the cellular release of cholesterol and choline-phospholipids and the formation of apoA-I-rich preβ-HDL. ABCA1 itself is probably not an active transporter, but may act as a regulator protein for the secretion of cholesterol and phospholipid containing vesicles, similar to the role of the sulfonylurea receptor in the vesicular release mechanism that mediates insulin secretion. ABCA1 contains a PDZ binding domain at its C-terminus and associates with β2-syntrophin and utrophin. This protein complex associates within endosomal vesicles but does not co-localize with ABCA1 in Lubrol insoluble membrane rafts, indicating that β2-syntrophin retains ABCA1 in cytoplasmic vesicles and releases ABCA1 to plasma membrane microdomains. Syntaxins play a major role in the fusion of vesicles and have also been demonstrated to interact with members of the ABC-transporter family such as the cystic fibrosis transmembrane conductance regulator. Syntaxin 13 was found to co-localize with ABCA1 in Lubrol rafts and to co-purify with ABCA1 in the phagosome compartment, suggesting a role for syntaxin 13 in ABCA1 processing through the early secretory pathway, the raft compartment and maturing phagosomes. © 2004 Published by Elsevier B.V.

Keywords: ABCA1; HDL; Macrophage

1. Introduction

The ATP-binding cassette transporter 1 (ABCA1) was recently identified as a major regulator of plasma HDL, mediating cellular cholesterol and choline-phospholipid efflux, and mutations in ABCA1 cause genetic HDL deficiency syndromes [1]. ABC-transporters may be classified either as active transporters (high intrinsic ATPase activity) or as regulatory channel-forming proteins like the cystic fibrosis transmembrane conductance regulator (CFTR) and the sulfonylurea receptor 1 (SUR1). ABCA1 binds ATP without measurable ATPase activity, indicating that ABCA1 is probably not an active transporter but a regulator protein, similar to CFTR and SUR1 [2]. CFTR functions as a chloride channel essential for epithelial electrolyte transport and also regulates other ion channels

* Tel.: +49-941-944-6200; fax: +49-941-944-6202.
E-mail address: gerd.schmitz@klinik.uni-regensburg.de (G. Schmitz).

0531-5131/
doi:10.1016/j.ics.2003.12.020

like the inwardly rectifying potassium channel ROMK2. CFTR abundance in the plasma membrane negatively correlates with syntaxin 1A expression and the CFTR N-terminus directly interacts with a peptide-binding site on syntaxin 1A critical for membrane fusion reactions. This bifunctional interaction determines the appearance of CFTR in the plasma membrane and the availability of syntaxin 1A for membrane fusion reactions with a consequence for secretion and trafficking in these cells. SUR1 and the potassium-inward rectifier Kir6.2 together form an ATP-sensitive potassium channel, critical for all of the properties associated with native ATP-sensitive K^+-channels such as surface expression, channel kinetics and response to channel blockers. Furthermore, SUR1 regulates β2-syntrophin dependent exocytosis of insulin containing secretory granules. β2-Syntrophin-utrophin complexes were shown to anchor insulin containing secretory granules to F-actin by interaction with the islet cell autoantigen ICA512. Hyperglycemia associated Ca^+-influx and subsequent release of intracellular Ca^+ leads to dephosphorylation of β2-syntrophin, thereby weakening the interaction with ICA512 and stimulating the exocytosis of secretory granules, suggesting that interactions involving PDZ domains play a role in regulating vesicular trafficking. The hypothesis regarding a functional analogy of ABCA1 to SUR1 may, therefore, be supported by the identification of N-terminal and C-terminal interacting proteins.

2. Association of the ABCA1 C-terminus with PDZ domains

Four amino acids of the ABCA1 C-terminus (ESYV) resemble a PDZ binding motif and direct interaction of ABCA1 with β2-syntrophin was demonstrated in our group using the Yeast-Two-Hybrid System and immunoprecipitation techniques (Fig. 1) [3].

ABCA1 can be detected in the cytosol and Golgi compartment of fibroblasts and monocytes and, while ABCA1 and utrophin are present in Lubrol-rafts and absent in Triton-rafts, β2-syntrophin is absent from both types of rafts, implying a role of β2-syntrophin in vesicular trafficking of ABCA1 rather than acting at the plasma membrane

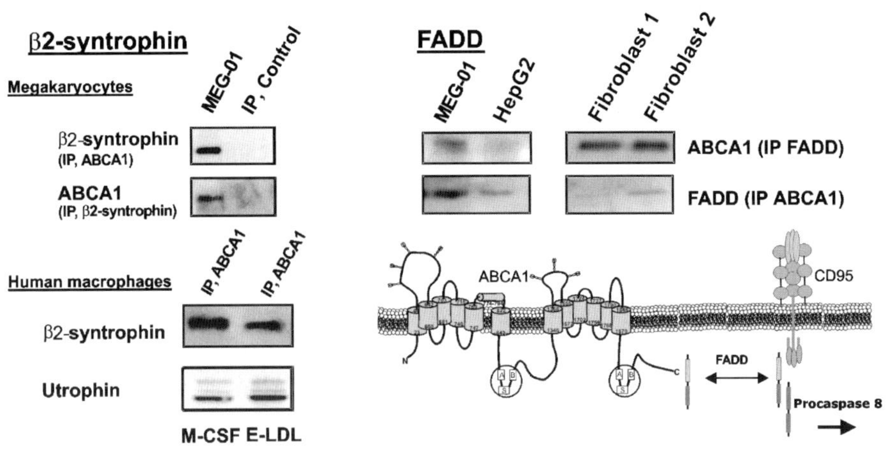

Fig. 1. ABCA1 interacting proteins as detected by immunoprecipitation experiments.

level [4]. β2-Syntrophin may participate in retaining ABCA1 in cytoplasmic vesicles and the targeting of ABCA1 to plasma membrane microdomains when ABCA1 is released from β2-syntrophin (Fig. 2).

ABCA1 was also co-immunoprecipitated with Cdc42, which may explain the altered actin cytoskeleton in cells overexpressing ABCA1 and suggests that ABCA1 regulates actin organization through Cdc42. Moreover, overexpression of Cdc42 increases apoA-I-dependent cholesterol efflux, whereas expression of the dominant-negative form decreases lipid efflux [5].

SNAREs are membrane-associated proteins that act as membrane fusogens or, at the least, as elements that bring membranes into close contact and thereby support fusion events. Syntaxins, which are members of the t-SNARE family and play a major role in vesicle targeting, have been demonstrated to interact with CFTR. The suggested functional analogy of ABCA1 and CFTR and the observation of ABCA1 shuttling in endocytic vesicles prompted us to investigate whether syntaxins may be important in ABCA1 secretory pathways. In a first step, we investigated mRNA and protein expression of all 15 members of the syntaxin family in human monocytes, macrophages, foam cells (E-LDL loaded macrophages) and in cholesterol-loaded macrophages treated with HDL to allow cholesterol efflux. Incubation with E-LDL induced syntaxins 3, 6 and 13 and subsequent addition of HDL reversed this upregulation for syntaxins 3 and 13. Immunoprecipitation revealed that only syntaxin 13 directly interacts with ABCA1. Finally, ABCA1 and syntaxin 13 co-purified with phagosomes and an increased uptake of microspheres could

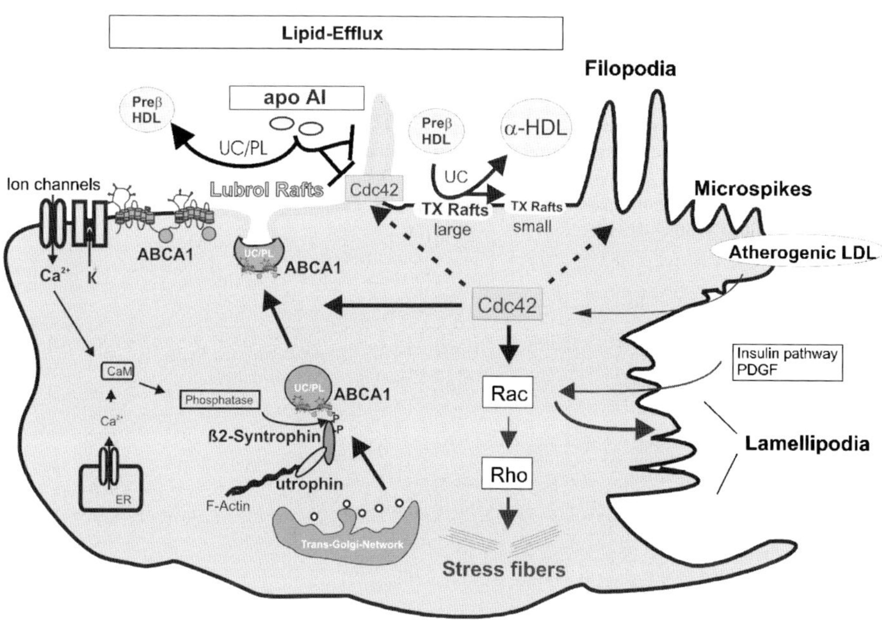

Fig. 2. Proposed role of ABCA1 in vesicular transport and cholesterol release via Lubrol insoluble membrane rafts.

be detected in Tangier disease fibroblasts, indicating that the phagosome compartment may be involved in ABCA1-dependent cholesterol and phospholipid efflux.

3. Interaction of the ABCA1 C-terminus with Fas-associated death domain protein

Interaction of ABCA1 and Fas-associated death domain protein (FADD) was identified by the Yeast-Two-Hybrid System and immunoprecipitation [6]. Recombinant expression of a dominant negative form of FADD markedly reduced the transfer of phospholipids to apoA-I indicating that full-length FADD is required for ABCA1 function. FADD represents an unexpected ABCA1-interacting constituent and links a protein mainly described in the context of death receptor induced apoptosis to reverse lipid efflux. This underlines the importance of proteins associated with the C-terminus of ABCA1 for ABCA1 function and indicates that full-length FADD is one of these accessory proteins. Additional studies evaluating the function of ABCA1/FADD complexes are necessary to further solve the molecular details of ABCA1 and FADD association.

References

[1] M. Bodzioch, E. Orso, J. Klucken, et al., The gene encoding ATP-binding cassette transporter 1 is mutated in Tangier disease, Nat. Genet. 22 (1999) 347–351.

[2] G. Szakacs, T. Langmann, C. Ozvegy, et al., Characterization of the ATPase cycle of human ABCA1: implications for its function as a regulator rather than an active transporter, Biochem. Biophys. Res. Commun. 288 (2001) 1258–1264.

[3] C. Buechler, A. Boettcher, S.M. Bared, M.C. Probst, G. Schmitz, The carboxyterminus of the ATP-binding cassette transporter A1 interacts with a beta2-syntrophin/utrophin complex, Biochem. Biophys. Res. Commun. 293 (2002) 759–765.

[4] W. Diederich, E. Orso, W. Drobnik, G. Schmitz, Apolipoprotein AI and HDL(3) inhibit spreading of primary human monocytes through a mechanism that involves cholesterol depletion and regulation of CDC42, Atherosclerosis 159 (2001) 313–324.

[5] W. Drobnik, H. Borsukova, A. Bottcher, et al., Apo AI/ABCA1-dependent and HDL3-mediated lipid efflux from compositionally distinct cholesterol-based microdomains, Traffic 3 (2002) 268–278.

[6] C. Buechler, S.M. Bared, C. Aslanidis, M. Ritter, W. Drobnik, G. Schmitz, Molecular and functional interaction of the ATP-binding cassette transporter A1 with Fas-associated death domain protein, J. Biol. Chem. 277 (2002) 41307–41310.

International Congress Series 1262 (2004) 309–312

www.ics-elsevier.com

Novel genetic markers for structural coronary artery disease, myocardial infarction, and familial combined hyperlipidemia: candidate and genome scans of functional SNPs

John P. Kane[a,*], Bradley E. Aouizerat[a], May M. Luke[b], Dov Shiffman[b], Olga Iakoubova[b], Dongming Liu[b], Charlie M. Rowland[b], Joseph J. Catanese[b], Diane U. Leong[b], Kit F. Lau[b], Judy Z. Louie[b], Carmen H. Tong[b], Linda B. McAllister[b], Lisa F. Dabby[a], Thomas A. Ports[a], Andrew D. Michaels[a], Christian Zellner[a], Clive R. Pullinger[a], Mary J. Malloy[a], James J. Devlin[b]

[a] *Cardiovascular Research Institute, University of California, 1337 L., 505 Parnassus Ave., San Francisco, CA 94143-0130, USA*

[b] *Celera Diagnostics, Inc., Alameda, CA, USA*

Abstract. Association studies were conducted on a large number of single nucleotide polymorphisms (SNPs) in pooled screening for association with angiographically determined coronary artery disease (CAD) and myocardial infarction (MI), followed by individual genotyping of those showing association. Forty-seven SNPs showed association with severity of CAD in a replication study applying individual genotyping in 1250 patients. Case control analysis of 340 patients with MI and 300 controls revealed significant associations of three novel genes: an immune cell receptor on chromosome 20p ($p=0.02$), a zinc finger protein on chromosome 3 ($p=0.04$), and an unknown gene on chromosome 3 ($p=0.01$). Associations of polymorphisms in three genes with the phenotype of familial combined hyperlipidemia (FCH), Apo A-V, PPAR alpha and microsomal triglyceride transfer protein (MTP) were established, supporting a metabolic model for the disorder based on misdirection of fatty acid metabolism. Congruence of SNP associations in non-alcoholic steatohepatitis suggests overlap of this syndrome with FCH. © 2003 Published by Elsevier B.V.

Keywords: Coronary artery; Atherosclerosis; Genetics; Combined hyperlipidemia

* Corresponding author. Tel.: +1-415-476-1517; fax: +1-415-502-5658.
E-mail address: kane@itsa.ucsf.edu (J.P. Kane).

0531-5131/ © 2003 Published by Elsevier B.V.
doi:10.1016/j.ics.2003.11.002

1. Angiographically determined coronary artery disease and myocardial infarction

1.1. Introduction

Common diseases, such as coronary artery disease (CAD) or myocardial infarction (MI), are mechanistically and phenotypically heterogeneous. A number of interrelated processes are involved, including dyslipidemia, oxidative stress, impaired sterol recovery, inflammation, thrombosis, impaired thrombolysis, and pathological calcification. Thematic complementarity of genomic determinants within these processes would be expected to underlie significant multiple and combinatorial gene–gene and gene–environment interactions. We used high throughput genotyping to discover and replicate single nucleotide polymorphisms (SNPs) associated with CAD and MI by both candidate gene and gene-centric "functional" SNP genome scan strategies.

1.2. Methods

To discover markers for severe CAD, 280 SNPs were genotyped in 1250 individual DNA samples, deeply annotated with angiographic and clinical data. Cases and controls were selected from the UCSF Genomic Resource in Arteriosclerosis, a collection of over 14,000 individual specimens of DNA and plasma from extensively documented cases of CAD, MI, stroke, hypertension, and disorders of lipoprotein and carbohydrate metabolism. Controls included an unselected population and a cohort of healthy individuals in the eighth decade of life and beyond.

For genetic markers for MI, allele frequencies of 16,000 SNPs (predicted to alter the amount, activity, or stability of encoded proteins: 80% mis-sense, non-sense, or splice donor/acceptor, and 15% promoters) were determined in pooled DNA samples from 843 males (340 MI, 503 controls) stratified by age and smoking history. SNPs were drawn from public databases and a compendium of 294,000 SNPs determined by resequencing of the coding and regulatory regions of 24,000 genes in the genomes of 39 individuals. Seventy-five percent of these were novel compared with public databases. Forty-five thousand exhibited altered amino acid sequence of the gene product. SNPs were determined by allele-specific PCR analysis and analyzed in dominant, recessive, additive, and allelic modes. Reproducibility was verified on 96 SNPs in 250 samples, replicated after a 5-month interval. Only 0.02% of the assignments were discordant.

1.3. Results

1.3.1. Structural coronary disease

Forty-seven SNPs, representing 10 selected mechanisms were associated with CAD (p-values <0.05 and odds ratios >1.3) among CAD candidate genes. Two endothelial nitric oxide synthase (NOS 3, Glu298Asp) and ApoE4 confirmed reported associations. Comparing the highest and lowest quartiles of the Gensini score of angiographic severity, the p-value for NOS 3 was 0.027 (odds ratio 1.3). Among hypertensives, the p-value was 0.017 (OR 1.5). Similar analysis for Apo E4 yielded a p-value of 0.021 for homozygotes compared with other genotypes (OR 5.4), and $p=0.0074$ E4 versus all other alleles (OR 1.5). Other SNPs showing association are being retested in a large independent cohort.

1.3.2. Myocardial infarction

Eighty of the 1000 SNPs showed association with MI in sets of 50 pooled samples. These were retested in an independent cohort by individual genotyping. Three SNPs in genes encoding an immune cell receptor on chromosome 20p ($p=0.02$ in the recessive mode, OR 1.4), a zinc finger protein on 3q ($p=0.04$ in the recessive mode, OR 1.7), and an unknown gene on chromosome 3 ($p=0.01$ in the allelic mode, OR 1.4) showed significant association with MI in both cohorts. The risk allele frequency for the zinc finger protein increased with disease severity and with early (< 60 years) MI. At-risk allele frequencies were 41–95%. Thus, these are common variants that could potentially account for significant fractions of the population-attributable risk.

2. Familial combined hyperlipidemia

2.1. Introduction

Familial combined hyperlipidemia (FCH), the most prevalent lipoprotein disorder, significantly contributes to the risk of CAD and MI. We propose an alternative locus model, in which increased mobilization of fatty acids from adipose tissue or misdirection of fatty acids from degradative pathways into hepatic triglyceride synthesis and export into plasma underlie the hyperlipidemia, comporting with the increased secretion of apoB-100 observed in FCH. To test this model, we studied the association of three candidate genes with the FCH phenotype.

2.2. Methods

Sequence anomalies were sought in the coding regions and regulatory sequences of candidate genes by differential DNA melting analysis. Anomalies were identified by sequencing, and SNPs were chosen on the basis of putative function and allele frequencies. SNP analysis was performed using allele-specific techniques. The Apo AV gene was studied because of association with hypertriglyceridemia in the population. PPAR alpha was selected because it transcriptionally regulates genes that function in the oxidation of fatty acids, directing fatty acids into degradative pathways. It also upregulates lipoprotein lipase. Microsomal triglyceride transfer protein (MTP) was selected because it is rate limiting in the lipidation of Apo B-100 in the hepatic export of triglycerides in very low-density lipoproteins.

2.3. Results

2.3.1. Apo A-V

Significant association of the − 1131 C allele of the Apo A-V gene was found in a case control study of FCH. Gender dimorphism was evidenced by resistance of women to the effect of the − 1131C allele.

2.3.2. PPAR alpha

Forty-four L162 V heterozygotes and 3 homozygotes were identified among 260 FCH patients (variant allele frequency of 9.62%). The allele frequency was 2.03% among a control cohort of 344 patients without the FCH phenotype ($p<0.001$).

2.3.3. MTP

The promoter polymorphism (G493T) at the initiation site alters MTP expression in carriers of the T allele. In a case, control study of 182 patients with the FCH phenotype and 300 controls strikingly decreased representation of the T allele in FCH was found: 16.8% vs. 24.5% ($p = 0.03$). Whereas the T allele is associated with decreased HDL cholesterol among normolipidemic subjects, it was found to correlate with higher levels in FCH ($p = 0.004$).

3. Discussion

High throughput genomic analysis is essential for establishing the relationship of individual gene loci and functional polymorphisms to multifactorial disorders, such as atherosclerosis. It is probable that many significant risk factors will have modest odds ratios but relatively high allele frequencies, and thus confer quantitatively significant impact in the population. The replicability of reported risk factors in additional cohorts has been very low until now, reflecting the small size of cohorts employed in initial screens and stratification of patient populations. Thus, it is critical that large samples be studied and that positive associations be verified in additional cohorts, avoiding stratification of study populations. Likewise, clinical annotation of the samples is crucial to informative analyses. The selection of candidate genes using paradigms of experimental atherosclerosis and cell biology can provide a high yield of associations and important mechanistic insights into the processes of atherogenesis and infarction. However, application of a wide screen for disease-associated polymorphisms will yield novel genes, such as those discovered in this project that can lead to previously unsuspected mechanisms of disease. Whereas the aggregate of associations will provide information for predicting both risk and mechanism, sophisticated analysis of gene–gene and gene–environment interactions will provide much greater insights, due to the importance of thematic complementarity among gene products within a single mechanistic process. For example, simultaneous, functional polymorphisms in several genes involved in inflammatory signaling might be expected to have an amplified effect on inflammation in the vessel wall.

Association of functional polymorphisms in three genes involved in fatty acid metabolism with the FCH phenotype in this study comports with the proposed metabolic model that posits misdirection of fatty acids from degradative pathways toward export from the liver in VLDL. Increased secretion of ApoB-100 in several kinetic studies, probably reflecting rescue by increased lipidation, provides strong inferential support for this model. Modifying factors, such as increased mobilization of fatty acids from adipose tissue, reflecting either insulin resistance or primary genetic determinants could aggravate the metabolic defect. The association of insulin resistance with many FCH cases is consistent with this interaction. Likewise, defects in intravascular hydrolysis of triglycerides could amplify the hyperlipidemia. Defects in lipoprotein lipase in some cases also consistent with this model and may reflect in part the impact of genomic variation in the PPAR alpha gene.

Identification of genomic determinants that participate in different mechanistic elements active in multifactorial diseases may provide the basis, ultimately, for accurate clinical analysis of risk, but more importantly, may lead to individualization of treatment based on the patient's predominant disease mechanisms.

International Congress Series 1262 (2004) 313–316

ELSEVIER

www.ics-elsevier.com

Nutrition and inflammation: role of dietary cholesterol

Alan Chait*, Katherine Lewis, Lisa Tannock, Kevin O'Brien, Barbara Retzlaff, Steven Kahn, Robert Knopp, Thomas Wight

Department of Medicine, Division of Metabolism, Endocrinology and Nutrition, 1959 NE Pacific Street, Box 356426 University of Washington, Seattle, WA 98195-6426, USA

Abstract. Most HDL particles are anti-atherogenic by virtue of their role in reverse cholesterol transport. However, the presence of apolipoproteins such as apo E and serum amyloid A (SAA) on a subset of HDL particles allows these particles to bind to vascular proteoglycans. This can lead to the retention of these HDL subspecies in the artery wall, their subsequent modification by oxidation and enzyme digestion, and thus their ability to be pro-atherogenic. Because dietary cholesterol can increase circulating SAA levels, it may play a role in atherogenesis by facilitating the retention of SAA-containing HDL by vascular proteoglycans. © 2003 Published by Elsevier B.V.

Keywords: Diet; Inflammation; Atherosclerosis; Serum amyloid A; Proteoglycans

1. Introduction

The retention of atherogenic lipoproteins by extracellular vascular proteoglycans is believed to play an important role in atherogenesis [1]. Retained lipoproteins can undergo modifications that render them potentially atherogenic. It is widely believed that the apo B- and E-containing lipoproteins, VLDL remnants and LDL are atherogenic, whereas HDL is anti-atherogenic by way of its role in reverse cholesterol transport. Apo B and apo E contain positively charged amino acids that are binding domains for the negatively charged sulfate and carboxylic acid groups on proteoglycans. Apo A–I, the major apolipoprotein of HDL is present extensively in both human and mouse atherosclerotic lesions [2–4], but does not posses proteoglycan binding domains. This raises the question of whether other apolipoproteins that may be present on a small subset of HDL might lead to its retention by the vascular matrix, thereby rendering these HDL subsets atherogenic, rather than anti-atherogenic, as is the case for most HDL particles.

Abbreviations: VLDL, very low density lipoproteins; LDL, low density lipoproteins; HDL; high density lipoproteins, SAA; serum amyloid A.

* Corresponding author. Tel.: +1-206-543-3158; fax: +1-206-685-8346.
E-mail address: achait@u.washington.edu (A. Chait).

0531-5131/ © 2003 Published by Elsevier B.V.
doi:10.1016/j.ics.2003.11.019

2. Methods and results

Using an in vitro gel mobility shift assay to assess the binding of lipoproteins to purified proteoglycans [5,6], we showed that HDL that did not contain apo E failed to bind to purified proteoglycans in vitro, whereas apo E-containing HDL bound in proportion to its content of apo E [6]. Although apo E is present on a small subset of HDL particles, somewhere around 5%, these apo E-containing HDL particles could be retained by vascular proteoglycans, and thereby be pro-atherogenic.

The presence of serum amyloid A (SAA) on HDL also facilitates proteoglycan binding. SAA is an acute phase reactant that has stretches of positively charged residues, and is modestly increased by chronic inflammatory stimuli such as occur with obesity, the metabolic syndrome and diabetes [7,8]. Increased SAA levels also predict an increased risk of cardiovascular disease [7]. The addition of a small amount of dietary cholesterol to high fat diets fed to LDL receptor-deficient mice resulted in a doubling of their circulating SAA levels without additional adverse effects on their plasma lipids and lipoproteins. This was associated with a doubling in size of aortic lesions. The extent of the lesions correlated with circulating SAA levels, but not with plasma lipids and lipoproteins. HDL from these animals bound isolated proteoglycans in vitro in proportion to their SAA content, and apo A–I, SAA and proteoglycans were co-localized in atherosclerotic lesions. Thus, SAA-containing HDL also may be pro-atherogenic.

To test whether dietary cholesterol also affected the levels of inflammatory markers in human subjects, plasma from approximately 200 subjects who had been categorized by their degree of insulin sensitivity and obesity were analyzed for SAA and C-reactive protein (CRP), a molecule that is an acute phase reactant in humans but not in mice. Baseline levels of both CRP and SAA increased progressively from lean insulin sensitive through lean insulin resistant individuals (with similar BMI values) and were highest in obese insulin resistant individuals (with similar S_i levels to the lean insulin resistant group). However, when comparing the effect of 0 versus 4 eggs per day in these groups, SAA and CRP levels increased in response to egg feeding only in lean insulin sensitive individuals. The presence of insulin resistance or obesity appeared to preclude an increase in the levels of these inflammatory markers.

3. Discussion

There has been a recent resurgence of interest in the role of inflammation in atherosclerosis. Inflammatory markers such as CRP and SAA have been used to predict cardiovascular disease risk, and are increased in conditions such as the metabolic syndrome [9,10]. What is less clear, however, is whether these molecules are just markers of atherosclerosis, or whether they actually mediate the atherosclerotic process. Several potential mechanisms have been postulated whereby CRP might play a role in the pathogenesis of atherosclerosis. However, there are less data about mechanisms by which SAA may mediate atherosclerosis. Mice, which clearly develop atherosclerosis in response to inflammatory stimuli, do not increase CRP levels in response to inflammation [11]. The inflammatory marker, SAA, is present in all vertebrate species [12] and has positively charged residues that would predict proteoglycan binding. Retention of SAA-containing lipoproteins by the vascular matrix is one mechanism by which this marker of inflammation actually might mediate atherosclerosis.

Our findings in mice are consistent with this notion. Dietary cholesterol (against a background of a high fat diet) resulted in an increase in both SAA levels and atherosclerosis, without an adverse effect on plasma lipids and lipoproteins. These findings suggest that dietary cholesterol is an inflammatory stimulus. The observation in human subjects that the inflammatory markers SAA and CRP increased in response to egg feeding is consistent with this notion, although it is surprising that this only occurred in insulin sensitive individuals.

These findings also suggest that HDL can actually be pro-atherogenic under certain circumstances, rather than anti-atherogenic, as is the case for most HDL particles. The presence on HDL of apolipoproteins such as apo E and SAA, which can bind to vascular proteoglycans, could lead to their retention in the extracellular matrix of the vascular wall, where they could undergo the various forms of modifications that could render them atherogenic. In conclusion, not all HDL particles are necessarily beneficial. Mild degrees of chronic inflammation due to a variety of stimuli can render HDL potentially atherogenic, e.g. by the presence of SAA.

Acknowledgements

This work is supported in part by National Institutes of Health Grants HL030086, DK035816, an Atorvastatin Research Award and a Medical School Grant from Merck and Co.

References

[1] K.J. Williams, I. Tabas, The response-to-retention hypothesis of early atherogenesis, Arterioscler. Thromb. Vasc. Biol. 15 (1995) 551–561.

[2] H.F. Hoff, R.L. Jackson, A.M. Gotto Jr., Apo-lipoprotein localization in human atherosclerotic arteries, Adv. Exp. Med. Biol. 67 (1976) 109–120.

[3] K.D. O'Brien, K.L. Olin, C.E. Alpers, W. Chiu, M. Ferguson, K. Hudkins, T.N. Wight, A. Chait, Comparison of apolipoprotein and proteoglycan deposits in human coronary atherosclerotic plaques: colocalization of biglycan with apolipoproteins, Circulation 98 (1998) 519–527.

[4] V.V. Kunjathoor, K.D. O'Brien, R.C. LeBoeuf, Presence and relationships of proteoglycan and apolipoprotein deposits in lesions of atherosclerosis-prone mice, Circulation 96 (1997) 1–39.

[5] E. Hurt-Camejo, G. Camejo, P. Sartipy, Measurements of proteoglycan–lipoprotein interaction by gel mobility shift assay, Methods Mol. Biol. 110 (1998) 79–267.

[6] K.L. Olin, S. Potter-Perigo, P.H. Barrett, T.N. Wight, A. Chait, Biglycan, a vascular proteoglycan, binds differently to HDL(2) and HDL(3): role of apoE, Arterioscler. Thromb. Vasc. Biol. 21 (2001) 35–129.

[7] P. Jousilahti, V. Salomaa, V. Rasi, E. Vahtera, T. Palosuo, The association of c-reactive protein, serum amyloid A and fibrinogen with prevalent coronary heart disease-baseline findings of the PAIS project, Atherosclerosis 156 (2001) 6–451.

[8] Y. Kumon, T. Suehiro, T. Itahara, Y. Ikeda, K. Hashimoto, Serum amyloid A protein in patients with non-insulin-dependent diabetes mellitus, Clin. Biochem. 27 (1994) 469–473.

[9] E. Leinonen, E. Hurt-Camejo, O. Wiklund, L.M. Hulten, A. Hiukka, M.R. Taskinen, Insulin resistance and adiposity correlate with acute-phase reaction and soluble cell adhesion molecules in type 2 diabetes, Atherosclerosis 166 (2003) 94–387.

[10] A. Festa, R. D'Agostino, G. Howard, L. Mykkanen, R. Tracy, S. Haffner, Chronic subclinical inflammation

as part of the insulin resistance syndrome: the insulin resistance atherosclerosis study (IRAS), Circulation 102 (2000) 42–47.
[11] A.J. Szalai, M.A. McCrory, Varied biologic functions of C-reactive protein: lessons learned from transgenic mice, Immunol. Res. 26 (2002) 87–279.
[12] C.M. Uhlar, A.S. Whitehead, Serum amyloid A, the major vertebrate acute-phase reactant, Eur. J. Biochem. 265 (1999) 501–523.

International Congress Series 1262 (2004) 317–319

ELSEVIER

www.ics-elsevier.com

Isoflavones: effects on cardiovascular risk and functions

Paul Nestel*

Baker Heart Research Institute, P.O. Box 6492 St. Kilda Rd., Central, Melbourne 8008, Australia

Abstract. Isoflavones, plant polyphenols with estrogenic activity, are becoming widely distributed in foods and sold as supplements. Their similarity to estrogens suggests potential cardiovascular benefits. Two major areas, those of lipid lowering and of improved vascular function, will be reviewed. The novel properties of isoflavone metabolites formed in vivo that may confer specific cardiovascular protection are documented. Although lipid lowering is at best modest, effects on vasculature have been more consistent. Arterial compliance, a parameter of the elasticity or distensibility of large arteries is improved by as much as reported for estrogens. Vasodilatory effects of isoflavones or their metabolites on the microcirculation, suppression of adhesion molecules, antioxidant properties and inhibition of experimental atherosclerosis may provide opportunities for pharmacological intervention. © 2003 Published by Elsevier B.V.

Keywords: Isoflavones; Lipoproteins; Vascular function; Antioxidants

1. Isoflavones and plasma lipids

The authorization in 1999 by the Food and Drug Administration for a health claim relating to modest intakes of soy protein has been controversial. The evidence was based largely on a meta-analysis published in 1995 [1], although about half of the quoted studies showed minor or no cholesterol lowering effect. However, there have been sufficient, well-executed studies to indicate a likely though modest effect on plasma lipids. Soy protein, containing defined amounts of isoflavones or protein that had been depleted of isoflavones by ethanolic extraction, has been compared with another source of protein, mostly casein or whole milk. Purified isoflavones, from soy or red clover have also been trialed. The isoflavones in soy have been the postulated active constituent but may require cofactors in the whole food for optimal activity.

A study by Crouse et al. [2] showed an LDL-C lowering effect among those with elevated LDL-C concentration but not in those with normal LDL-C levels, and among the hypercholesterolemic subjects a dose effect was noted across two levels of isoflavone intake. Lichtenstein et al. [3], in a comparison of soy protein with animal protein each with

* Tel.: +61-3-8532-1383; fax: +61-3-8532-1100.
E-mail address: paul.nestel@baker.edu.au (P. Nestel).

doi:10.1016/S0531-5131(03)01737-0

either trace amounts of isoflavones or delivering 50 mg isoflavones daily, showed an LDL lowering of 5% with soy protein but only in subjects whose LDL-C concentrations exceeded 4.14 mmol/l. Other trials have been either negative or delivered small changes in LDL-C.

Trials of purified isoflavones have been disappointing to date. Nestel et al. [4,5] found no effects with isoflavones derived from either soy or red clover. Similar negative findings were published also by other researchers. The suggestion that equol producers, about a quarter of the population, may respond better to isoflavone consumption has not been tested adequately. That not all isoflavones might be effective has been suggested by the finding that biochanin, but not formononetin-enriched isoflavones, lowered LDL-C [6].

2. Isoflavone effects on vascular function

Several reports on the effects of isoflavones from soy and red clover on a variety of arterial circulations have been tested, including large arteries that test the distensibility or elasticity of the aorta, predominantly those in muscular, medium-sized arteries and in the microcirculation of the forearm.

The effects on endothelial function have been tested directly in the human microcirculation by infusing isoflavones into the brachial artery and with the demonstration of a powerful vasodilatory response with genistein, but not with daidzein [7]. Similar effects have been reported with several metabolites of isoflavones on preparations of rat aortic rings. Equol, dehydroequol, dihydrodaidzein, *cis*- and *trans*-terahydrodiadzein were at least as potent as 17β-estradiol in vasorelaxation and opposing constriction induced by norepinephrine and oxidized LDL [8]. Squadrito et al. [9] reported improved flow-mediated dilatation in 30 subjects taking genistein supplements for 6 months.

The distensibility or compliance in the large arterial system is the converse of arterial stiffness and declines with age, menopause, raised blood pressure and hyperlipidemia.

Teede et al. [10] and Nestel et al. [4,5] have reported a significant reduction in arterial stiffness with purified isoflavones from soy [4], red clover [5] and formononetin extracted and purified from red clover [10].

The effect on blood pressure has been inconsistent. No effect was observed in a large trial with isolated isoflavones based on 24-h ambulatory blood pressure testing [10].

3. Antioxidant and anti-inflammatory effects

Isoflavones are likely to exert potential benefits via the reduction of cardiovascular risk through multiple, other mechanisms. The antioxidant effects of several isoflavones (genistein, daidzein and equol) have been documented in vitro. Tikkanen et al. [11] reported diminished oxidizability of LDL studied ex vivo despite the fact that the LDL contained very little isoflavone. Wiseman et al. [12] observed a reduction in plasma F_2-isoprostane, a biomarker of in vivo lipid peroxidation, in subjects eating a high isoflavone, soy-based diet.

Expression of adhesion molecules and of inflammatory cytokines has also been found to be suppressed in vitro when endothelial and other cells have been incubated with isoflavones or metabolites. One in vivo study showed that supplementing with formononetin reduced circulating concentrations of VCAM-1, an adhesion molecule associated with atherosclerosis [10].

4. Experimental atherosclerosis

In a recent unpublished study by Kanellakis, Nestel and Bobik, the carotid arteries of rabbits were damaged by balloon angioplasty and the animals fed a supplement of the daidzein metabolite, *trans*-tetrahydrodiadzein. Control rabbits showed early neointimal hyperplasia and superoxide production in the damaged artery. By contrast, isoflavone-treated rabbits showed substantially less superoxide production and neointimal proliferation throughout the 28 days of the investigation.

Yamakoshi et al. [13] also demonstrated that an isoflavone extract from soybean without the protein reduced the extent of atherosclerosis in cholesterol-fed rabbits.

References

[1] J.W. Anderson, B.M. Johnstone, M.B. Cooke-Newell, Meta-analysis of the effects of soy protein on serum lipids, New Engl. J. Med. 332 (1995) 276–282.

[2] J.R. Crouse, T. Morgan, J.G. Terry, J. Ellis, M. Vitollins, G.L. Burke, A randomized trial comparing the effect of casein with soy protein containing varying amounts of isoflavones on plasma concentrations of lipids and lipoproteins, Arch. Intern. Med. 159 (1999) 2070–2076.

[3] A.H. Lichtenstein, S.M. Jalbert, H. Adlercreutz, B.R. Goldin, H. Rasmussen, E.J. Shaefer, L.A. Ausman, Lipoprotein response to diets high in soy or animal protein with and without isoflavones in moderately hypercholesterolemic subjects, Arterioscler. Thromb. Vasc. Biol. 22 (2002) 1852–1858.

[4] P.J. Nestel, T. Yamashita, T. Sasahara, S. Pomeroy, A. Dart, P. Komesaroff, A. Owen, M. Abbey, Soy isoflavones improve arterial compliance but not plasma lipids in menopausal and perimenopausal women, Arterioscler. Thromb. Vasc. Biol. 17 (1997) 3392–3398.

[5] P.J. Nestel, S. Pomeroy, S. Kay, P. Komesaroff, J. Behrsing, J.D. Cameron, L. West, Isoflavones from red clover improve systemic arterial compliance but not plasma lipids in menopausal women, J. Clin. Endocrinol. Metab. 84 (1999) 895–898.

[6] P. Nestel, M. Cehun, A. Chronopoulos, L. De Silva, H. Teede, B. McGrath, A biochanin-enriched isoflavone from red clover lowers LDL-cholesterol in men, Eur. J. Clin. Nutr., (in press).

[7] H.A. Walker, T.S. Dean, T.A.B. Sanders, The phytoestrogen genistein produces acute nitric oxide-dependent dilation of human forearm vasculature with similar potency to 17β-estradiol, Circulation 103 (2001) 258–262.

[8] J.P.F. Chin-Dusting, L. Fisher, T.V. Lewis, A. Piekarska, P. Nestel, A. Husband, The vascular activity of some isoflavone metabolites: implications for a cardioprotective role, Br. J. Pharmacol. 133 (2001) 595–605.

[9] F. Squadrito, D. Altavilla, N. Morabito, The effect of the phytoestrogen genistein on plasma nitric oxide concentrations, endothelin-1 levels and endothelium dependent vasodilation in postmenopausal women, Atherosclerosis 163 (2002) 339–347.

[10] H.J. Teede, B. McGrath, L. DeSilva, M. Cehun, A. Fassoulakis, P.J. Nestel, Isoflavones reduce arterial stiffness, Arteroscler. Thromb. Vasc. Biol. 23 (2003) 1066–1071.

[11] M.J. Tikkanen, K. Wahala, S. Ojala, V. Vihma, H. Adlercreutz, Effect of soybean phytoestrogen intake on low density lipoprotein oxidation resistance, Proc. Natl. Acad. Sci. U. S. A. 95 (1998) 3106–3110.

[12] H. Wiseman, J.D. O'Reilly, H. Adlercreutz, A.J. Mallet, E.A. Bowery, I.R. Rowland, T.A.B. Sanders, Isoflavone phytoestrogens consumed in soy decrease F_2-isoprostane concentrations and increase resistance of low-density lipoprotein to oxidation in humans, Am. J. Clin. Nutr. 72 (2000) 395–400.

[13] J. Yamakoshi, M.K. Piskula, T. Izumi, M. Saito, S. Kataoka, A. Obata, H. Kikechi, Isoflavone aglycone-rich extract without soy protein attenuates atherosclerosis development in cholesterol-fed rabbits, J. Nutr. 130 (2000) 1887–1893.

International Congress Series 1262 (2004) 320–327

www.ics-elsevier.com

Flavonoids-rich nutrients with potent antioxidant activity prevent atherosclerosis development: the licorice example

Michael Aviram*

The Lipid Research Laboratory, Technion Faculty of Medicine, The Rappaport Family Institute for Research in the Medical Sciences and Rambam Medical Center, Bat-Galim 31096, Haifa, Israel

Received 18 August 2003; received in revised form 26 August 2003; accepted 1 September 2003

Abstract. *Background*: Macrophage-mediated oxidation of low-density lipoprotein (LDL) has a major role in early atherogenesis, and, thus, intervention means to inhibit this process by flavonoids-rich nutrients (pomegranate, red wine, licorice) are being extensively studied. In the present study, we questioned the ability of the isoflavan glabridin from licorice root to accumulate in macrophages and to affect cell-mediated oxidation of LDL and atherogenesis. *Results*: Macrophages accumulated glabridin, and this process was time and glabridin dose dependent. In parallel, macrophage-mediated oxidation of LDL was inhibited by up to 80%. Glabridin inhibited superoxides release from MPM by up to 60%, and in glabridin-enriched macrophages, reduced protein kinase C activity by 70% was noted, in comparison to control cells. Translocation of P-47phox, the cytosolic component of NADPH oxidase, to the plasma membrane was substantially inhibited by glabridin. Macrophages (MPM) isolated from the atherosclerotic apolipoprotein E-deficient (E^o) mice that consumed glabridin (20 μg/mouse/day) for 6 weeks demonstrated reduced capability to oxidize LDL by 80%, in comparison to placebo-treated mice. This latter phenomenon was associated with a substantial 50% reduction in the mice aortic lesion size. *Conclusions*: Glabridin accumulation in macrophages affects cell-signaling processes, which are associated with activation of the cellular NADPH oxidase system. These phenomena are responsible for the inhibition of cell-mediated oxidation of LDL and the attenuation of atherosclerosis developments by dietary glabridin. © 2003 Elsevier B.V. All rights reserved.

Keywords: Antioxidants; Flavonoids; Licorice; Glabridin; Lipid peroxidation; LDL; Oxidized-LDL; Aggregated-LDL; Paraoxonase; Atherosclerosis

* Tel.: +972-4-8542970; fax: +972-4-8542130.
E-mail address: aviram@tx.technion.ac.il (M. Aviram).

doi:10.1016/S0531-5131(03)01453-5

1. Atherogenic modifications of low-density lipoprotein (LDL) and atherosclerosis

Most of the accumulated cholesterol in foam cells originates from plasma LDL, which is internalized into the cells via the LDL receptor. Native LDL, however, does not induce cellular cholesterol accumulation because the LDL receptor activity is downregulated by the cellular cholesterol content [1]. LDL has to undergo some modifications, such as oxidation, in order to be taken up by macrophages at enhanced rate via the macrophage scavenger receptors pathway, which, unlike the LDL receptor, are not subjected to downregulation by cellular cholesterol content [1–3]. The underlying mechanisms leading to the formation of atherosclerotic lesion under oxidative stress are complicated and represent the outcome of multiple interactive processes.

The "oxidative modification of lipoproteins" hypothesis of atherosclerosis proposes that LDL oxidation plays a pivotal role in early atherogenesis, and this hypothesis is supported by evidence that LDL oxidation occurs in vivo and contributes to the clinical manifestation of atherosclerosis.

2. Macrophage-mediated oxidation of LDL

The identity of the cells responsible for the oxidation of LDL along atherogenesis in the arterial wall is uncertain. Monocyte-derived macrophages are likely candidates to induce the oxidation of LDL during early atherogenesis, as they are prominent in arterial lesions, and because they generate reactive oxygen and nitrogen species. LDL oxidation by arterial wall cells was suggested to involve the activation of macrophage 15-lipoxygenase and of nicotinamide adenine dinucleotide phosphate (NADPH) oxidase [4]. Macrophage-mediated oxidation of LDL can also result from an initial cellular lipids peroxidation. When cultured macrophages were exposed to ferrous ions, cellular lipid peroxidation took place [5]. These "oxidized macrophages" could easily oxidize LDL even in the absence of any added transition metal ions.

3. Paraoxonase and LDL oxidation

Human serum paraoxonase 1 (PON1) is an esterase, which is physically associated with HDL and is also distributed in tissues such as liver, kidney and intestine [6].

Human serum paraoxonase activity was shown to be inversely related to the risk of cardiovascular disease, as shown in atherosclerotic, hypercholesterolemic and diabetic patients [7]. HDL-associated PON1 has recently been shown to protect LDL, as well as the HDL particle itself, against oxidation induced by either copper ions or by free radicals generators, and this effect could be related to the hydrolysis of the specific lipoprotein's oxidized lipids such as cholesteryl linoleate hydroperoxides and some specific oxidized phospholipids. Protection of HDL from oxidation by PON1 was shown to preserve the antiatherogenic effect of HDL in reverse cholesterol transport, as shown by its beneficial effect on HDL-mediated macrophage cholesterol efflux. These effects of PON1 may be relevant to its beneficial properties against cardiovascular disease. Antioxidants were shown to preserve PON1's activity as they decrease the formation of lipid peroxides, which can, in turn, inactivates PON1.

4. Flavonoids and cardiovascular disease

Dietary consumption of flavonoids was shown to be inversely related to morbidity and mortality from coronary heart diseases. Flavonoids compose the largest and most studied group of plant phenols. Over 4000 different flavonoids have been identified to date.

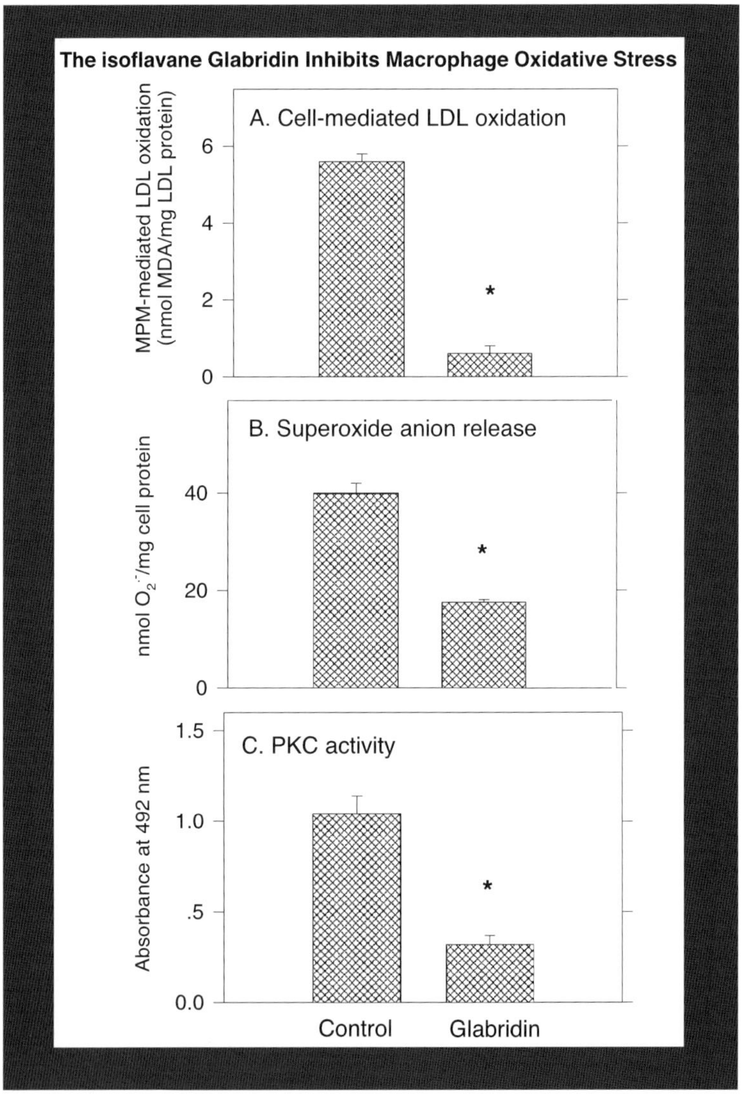

Fig. 1. Licorice-derived glabridin inhibits superoxide-induced macrophage-mediated oxidation of LDL: a role for protein kinase C.

Flavonoids are powerful antioxidants, and their activity is related to their chemical structures [8]. Plant flavonoids can act as potent inhibitors of LDL oxidation via several mechanisms including scavenging of free radicals, chelation of transition metal ions, or preservation of serum paraoxonase (PON1) activity (and as a result, hydrolysis of LDL-associated lipid peroxides).

5. Licorice, LDL oxidation and atherosclerosis: characterization of antioxidant constituents from the licorice roots

Glycyrrhiza glabra, the licorice plant, has been known as a healthy nutrient for more than 3000 years. The licorice roots have long been used as flavoring and sweetening agents.

Among licorice flavonoids, glabridin constituted the major flavonoid in the licorice root extract (500 mg/kg of root ethanolic extract). Upon LDL incubation with glabridin, the latter was shown to bind to the LDL and subsequently protect it from oxidation [9–11].

Glabridin inhibited AAPH-induced LDL oxidation in a dose-dependent manner.

Addition of glabridin (30 μM) to LDL that was incubated with AAPH or with copper ions inhibited the formation of oxidized lipids and oxysterols (7-hydroxycholesterol, 7-ketocholesterol and epoxycholesterol) by 65%, 70% and 45%, respectively. Glabridin inhibited the consumption of β-carotene and that of lycopene by 41% and 50%, respectively, after 1 h of LDL oxidation in the presence of AAPH, but failed to protect vitamin E, the major LDL-associated antioxidant, from oxidation [11]. Glabridin was also found to preserve the arylesterase activity of human serum PON1, including its ability to hydrolyze oxidized LDL cholesteryl linoleate hydroperoxides, since PON1 was found to be more potent in reducing the amount of cholesteryl linoleate hydroperoxides when added to Ox-LDL in the presence of glabridin, in comparison to its effects in the absence of glabridin. Glabridin was also shown to accumulate in macrophages in a dose- and time-dependent manner and in parallel, in glabridin-enriched cells, macrophage-mediated oxidation of LDL was inhibited by up to 80%, in comparison to control cells (Fig. 1A). These effects could be related to glabridin-mediated inhibition of superoxide anion release from macrophages in response to phorbol 12-myristate 13-acetate (PMA) (Fig. 1B), to inhibition of the translocation of P-47 (a cytosolic component of NADPH oxidase) to the plasma membrane and to a reduction in cellular protein kinase C activity [12] (Fig. 1C), which is required for P-47 phosphorylation and activation. Thus, glabridin-induced inhibition of P-47 phosphorylation may be the primary event responsible for its inhibitory effect on NADPH oxidase-induced macrophage-mediated oxidation of LDL. All of the above inhibitory effects of glabridin on the events related to cell-mediated oxidation of LDL required the hydroxyl groups on the isoflavan B ring [10].

6. The antioxidative properties of licorice consumption in humans

Evaluation of the protective effect of licorice root extract on the resistance of LDL to ex vivo oxidation was studied in normolipidemic human subjects [13], as well as in hypercholestero-lemic patients [14]. LDL, which was isolated from the plasma of ten

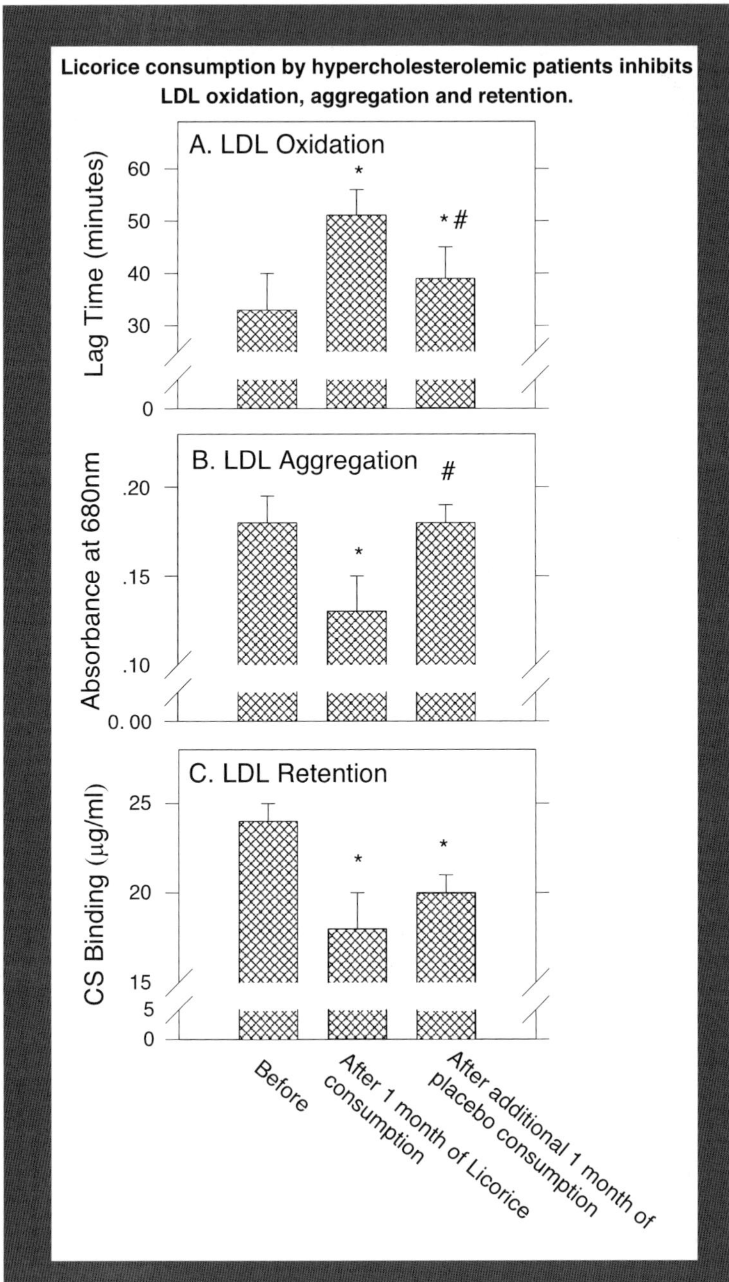

Fig. 2. Licorice consumption by hypercholesterolemic patients inhibits LDL modifications.

healthy volunteers after consumption of 100 mg of licorice root ethanolic extract per day, for a period of 2 weeks, was more resistant to copper ion-induced oxidation, as well as to AAPH-induced oxidation, by 44% and 36%, respectively, in comparison to LDL isolated prior to licorice supplementation. Supplementation of licorice root extract (0.1 g/day) to hypercholesterolemic patients for a period of 1 month was followed by an additional 1 month of placebo consumption [14]. Licorice consumption resulted in a moderate reduction in the patients' plasma susceptibility to lipid peroxidation (by 19%), and in a marked reduction in the susceptibility of the patients' plasma LDL to oxidation, as shown by a prolongation of the lag time required for the initiation of LDL oxidation by 55%, in comparison to the lag time of LDL isolated from plasma derived before licorice extract consumption (Fig. 2A). This effect was even partially sustained after an additional 1 month of placebo supplementation, since LDL derived after this period was still less susceptible to copper ion-induced lipid peroxidation, as demonstrated by an 18% increment in the lag time, in comparison to the baseline lag time (before licorice administration).

Atherogenicity of LDL is attributed not only to its oxidative modification but also to its aggregation. Upon analyzing the susceptibility to aggregation of LDL isolated from hypercholesterolemic patients that consumed licorice extract for 1 month, a significant reduction of 28% in LDL aggregation was observed (Fig. 2B). After an additional 1 month of placebo consumption, LDL aggregation rates returned towards baseline values.

Retention of LDL, which is an early step in atherogenesis, was measured by analysis of LDL binding to the proteoglycan chondroitin sulfate (CS). Following licorice consumption, LDL CS binding ability was significantly reduced by 25%, and this effect was partially sustained for the additional 1 month of placebo consumption (Fig. 2C).

Licorice extract supplementation resulted also in a 10% reduction in the patients' systolic blood pressure, which sustained for an additional month (during the placebo consumption). Thus, dietary consumption of licorice root extract by hypercholesterolemic patients may act as a moderate hypotensive nutrient and as a potent antioxidant agent, which confer its health benefit against cardiovascular disease.

7. The effect of licorice consumption by mice on LDL oxidation, macrophage foam cell formation and atherosclerosis development

Dietary supplementation of licorice (200 μg/day/mouse) to the apolipoprotein E-deficient (E^o) mice for a period of 6 weeks resulted in 80% reduction in the susceptibility of their LDL to copper ion-induced oxidation, in comparison to LDL isolated from placebo-treated mice [13]. Administration of purified glabridin to E^o mice in their drinking water was followed by analysis of its antioxidative effect against ex vivo LDL oxidation [13]. GC–MS analysis of the LDL, derived from E^o mice after consumption of glabridin, revealed that glabridin was absorbed and bound to the LDL particle. Whereas no glabridin could be detected in LDL from control mice, LDL from mice that consumed glabridin (20 μg/day/mouse) contained about 2 nmol of glabridin/mg LDL protein. LDL derived from E^o mice after consumption of 20 μg glabridin/day/mouse for a period of 6 weeks was significantly more resistant to copper ion-induced oxidation by 22% than LDL derived from placebo-treated mice. Administration of glabridin (25 μg/day/mouse) to E^o mice for a

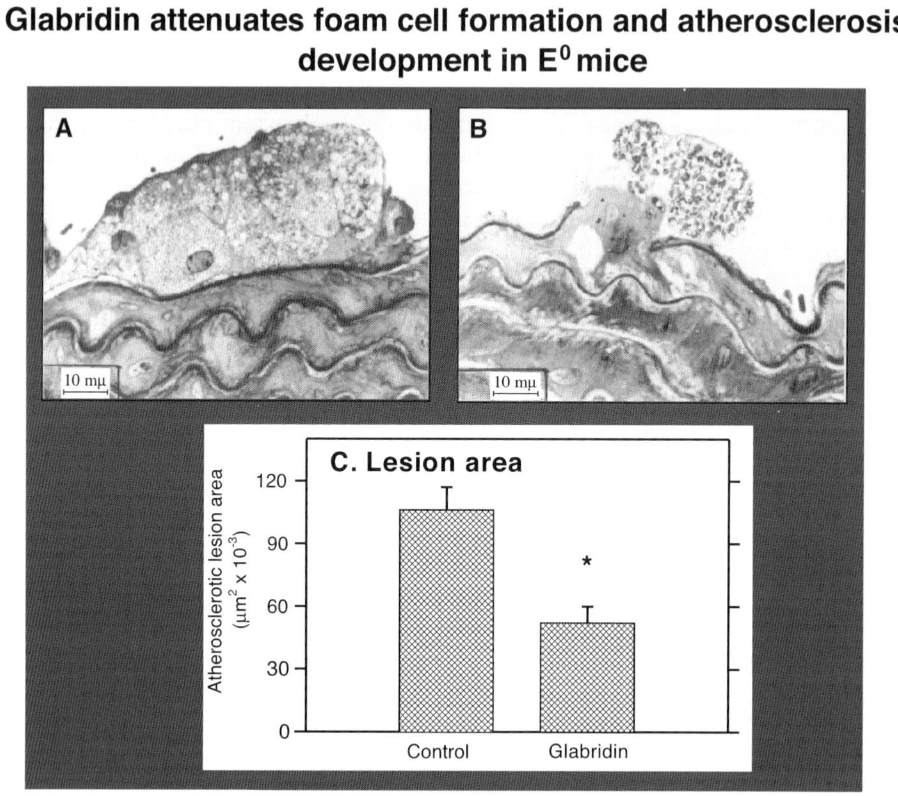

Fig. 3. Licorice-derived glabridin consumption decreased macrophage foam cell formation and attenuated atherosclerosis progression in the atherosclerotic E^0 mice.

period of 3 months also reduced (by 50%) an additional atherogenic modification of LDL, i.e., its susceptibility to aggregation induced by vortexing. Most important, inhibition of atherogenic modifications of LDL (oxidation and aggregation) in E^0 mice following glabridin consumption was associated with a substantial reduction in macrophage foam cell formation (Fig. 3B vs. A) and in the development of the atherosclerotic lesion area (Fig. 3C).

We thus conclude that licorice-derived glabridin can protect LDL against cell-mediated oxidation via two major pathways, including a direct interaction with the lipoprotein and/ an indirect effect through accumulation in arterial macrophages. Licorice thus represents a most potent nutrient, which can attenuate the development of atherosclerosis, secondary to its antioxidation properties against lipids peroxidation in arterial cells and in lipoproteins.

References

[1] J.L. Goldstein, M.S. Brown, Regulation of the mevalonate pathway, Nature 343 (1990) 425–430.

[2] D. Steinberg, S. Parthasarathy, T.E. Carew, J.C. Khoo, J.L. Witztum, Beyond cholesterol: modifications of low-density lipoprotein that increase its atherogenicity, N. Engl. J. Med. 320 (1989) 915–924.

[3] M. Aviram, Review of human studies on oxidative damage and antioxidant protection related to cardiovascular disease, Free Radic. Res. 33 (2000) S85–S97.
[4] M. Aviram, M. Rosenblat, A. Etzioni, R. Levy, Activation of NADPH oxidase is required for macrophage-mediated oxidation of low density lipoprotein, Metabolism 45 (1996) 1069–1079.
[5] B. Fuhrman, J. Oiknine, S. Keidar, M. Kaplan, M. Aviram, Increased uptake of low density lipoprotein (LDL) by oxidized macrophages is the result of enhanced LDL receptor activity and of progressive LDL oxidation, Free Radic. Biol. Med. 23 (1997) 34–46.
[6] B.N. La Du, S. Adkins, C.L. Kuo, D. Lipsig, Studies on human serum paraoxonase/arylesterase, Chem. Biol. Interact. 87 (1993) 25–34.
[7] M. Aviram, Does paraoxonase play a role in susceptibility to cardiovascular disease? Mol. Med. 5 (1999) 381–386.
[8] C.A. Rice-Evans, N.J. Miller, G. Paganga, Structure–antioxidant activity relationships of flavonoids and phenolic acids, Free Radic. Biol. Med. 20 (1996) 933–956.
[9] J. Vaya, P.A. Belinky, M. Aviram, Antioxidant constituents from licorice roots: a. Isolation, structure elucidation and antioxidative capacity toward LDL; b. Oxidation, Free Radic. Biol. Med. 23 (1997) 302–313.
[10] P.A. Belinky, M. Aviram, S. Mahmood, J. Vaya, Structural aspects of the inhibitory effect of glabridin on LDL oxidation, Free Radic. Biol. Med. 24 (1998) 1419–1429.
[11] P.A. Belinky, M. Aviram, B. Fuhrman, M. Rosenblat, J. Vaya, The antioxidative effects of the isoflavan glabridin on endogenous constituents of LDL during its oxidation, Atherosclerosis 137 (1998) 49–61.
[12] M. Rosenblat, P. Belinky, J. Vaya, R. Levy, T. Hayek, R. Coleman, S. Merchav, M. Aviram, Macrophage enrichment with the isoflavan glabridin inhibits NADPH oxidase-induced cell mediated oxidation of low density lipoprotein, J. Biol. Chem. 274 (1999) 13790–13799.
[13] B. Fuhrman, S. Buch, J. Vaya, P.A. Belinky, R. Coleman, T. Hayek, M. Aviram, Licorice extract and its major polyphenol glabridin protect low-density lipoprotein against lipid peroxidation: in vitro and ex vivo studies in humans and in atherosclerotic apolipoprotein E-deficient mice, Am. J. Clin. Nutr. 66 (1997) 267–275.
[14] B. Fuhrman, N. Volkova, M. Kaplan, D. Presser, J. Attias, T. Hayek, M. Aviram, Anti-atherosclerotic effects of licorice extract supplementation to hypercholesterolemic patients: increased resistance of their LDL to atherogenic modifications, reduced plasma lipids levels, and decreased systolic blood pressure, Nutrition 18 (2002) 268–273.

International Congress Series 1262 (2004) 328–331

www.ics-elsevier.com

Recent lifestyle trials in the prevention of type 2 diabetes

Jaakko Tuomilehto[a,b,*], Jaana Lindström[b]

[a] *Department of Public Health, University of Helsinki, Helsinki, Finland*
[b] *Diabetes and Genetic Epidemiology Unit, Department of Epidemiology and Health Promotion, National Public Health Institute, Helsinki, Finland*

Abstract. Knowledge about the natural history of type 2 diabetes (T2D) with a preclinical phase, modifiable risk factors, an effective and simple screening tool to identify high-risk subjects and effective intervention that is affordable and acceptable are necessary. In addition, the efficacy of the intervention has to be proven in a clinical trial setting. Such proof for lifestyle prevention of T2D from randomised clinical trials has accumulated as several major lifestyle intervention trials have been successfully carried out. The results are consistent: the risk of T2D in high-risk subjects can be halved; the effect of lifestyle changes is rapid; the magnitude of lifestyle changes required to achieve a significant risk reduction does not have to be drastic, and benefits are similar in different ethnic groups.

Keywords: Type 2 diabetes; Primary prevention; Lifestyle

1. Introduction

Primary prevention of type 2 diabetes (T2D) was first proposed 80 years ago [1] and more recently stressed by the World Health Organization (WHO) [2]. Until recently, the two main questions related to the potential for prevention of T2D have remained unanswered: (1) Is lifestyle intervention really efficacious to prevent T2D and a solution to the prevention of the global epidemic of T2D?; (2) Does lifestyle intervention work in different countries, ethnic groups and cultural settings?

2. Lifestyle intervention studies

The main lifestyle issues in the prevention of T2D are body weight, diet and physical activity. One of the largest early intervention studies was the Malmöhus study in Sweden [3] which comprised 267 men. A significant difference in the rates of development of T2D

* Corresponding author. Diabetes and Genetic Epidemiology Unit, Department of Epidemiology and Health Promotion, National Public Health Institute, Mannerheimintie 166, 00300 Helsinki, Finland. Tel.: +358-9-47448316; fax: +358-9-47448338.

doi:10.1016/j.ics.2003.12.025

was found between IGT subjects randomised to treatment and those randomised to no therapy. It is unclear what kind of dietary and physical changes occurred. Nevertheless, this trial suggested that the worsening from IGT to diabetes might be prevented or delayed. More recently, a few trials have tested this hypothesis; we may call them the "major lifestyle trials in prevention of T2D".

2.1. The Malmö feasibility study

The feasibility of diet and exercise intervention in 217 men with IGT was assessed in the Malmö feasibility study [4]. The effect of exercise and diet was compared with a reference group with no intervention. The reference group consisted of men who themselves decided not to join the intervention programme. By the end of the 5-year study period, 10.6% of the intervention group (IG) and 28.6% of the reference group had developed diabetes. Thus, the relative risk reduction in the incidence in the intervention group was 63%, and the absolute risk reduction was 18%.

2.2. The Da Qing study

The Da Qing study [5] included 577 people with IGT. The participating clinics were randomised to carry out the intervention according to one of the four specified intervention protocols (diet alone, exercise alone, diet–exercise combined or none). The 6-year incidence of type 2 diabetes was lower in the three intervention groups (41–46%) compared with the control group (CG; 68%). The study subjects were relatively lean, (mean BMI: 25.8 kg/m^2) making inferences for other ethnic groups, where IGT subjects are usually obese, difficult. In this study, the relative risk reduction was approximately 40%, while the absolute risk reduction was 22–26% during the 6-year period.

2.3. The Finnish diabetes prevention study (DPS)

The Finnish Diabetes Prevention Study (DPS) is the first properly randomised controlled trial aiming at preventing T2D with lifestyle modification alone [6–8]. A total of 522 middle-aged, overweight (BMI>25 kg/m^2) individuals with IGT were randomised into the control group (CG) or the intervention group (IG). The intervention comprised dietary and exercise advice [9]. The goals of the intervention were a reduction in weight of 5% or more, total intake of fat less than 30 E%, intake of saturated fat less than 10 E%, intake of dietary fiber 15 g/1000 kcal or more, and moderate- or high-intensity physical activity 30 min/day or more.

The first analysis of diabetes incidence was carried out after a median follow-up duration of 3.2 years. There were 27 diabetes cases in the IG and 59 in the CG. Based on life-table analysis, the risk of diabetes was reduced by 58% ($p < 0.001$) during the trial in the IG compared with the CG. The absolute risk of diabetes was *32/1000* person-years in the IG and *78/1000* person-years in the CG. This indicates that 22 subjects with IGT need to be treated for 1 year or five people for 5 years with such a lifestyle intervention to prevent one case of diabetes.

2.4. The diabetes prevention program (DPP)

The Diabetes Prevention Program (DPP) [10,11] was a multicenter randomised clinical trial carried out in the United States. It compared the efficacy and safety of three interventions—an extremely intensive lifestyle intervention [12] or standard lifestyle recommendations combined with metformin or placebo. The study focused on high-risk individuals ($n = 3234$) with IGT who also had slightly elevated fasting plasma glucose (>5.5 mmol/l). Weight loss goal for all participants was a 7% weight reduction and to maintain it throughout the trial. The physical activity goal was approximately 700 kcal/week expenditure from physical activities. In DPP, intensive lifestyle intervention resulted in a 58% reduction in T2D diabetes risk compared with the placebo group. In the metformin group, T2D risk was reduced by 31% compared with placebo.

3. Discussion

The results from the recent major T2D prevention trials have now provided unequivocal evidence that T2D can be prevented, at least in high-risk individuals. The risk reductions yielded by the trials are strikingly similar. The data from the Chinese Da Qing study [5] were slightly different; while the relative risk reduction was somewhat less, about 40%, the absolute risk reduction was higher, 27%, due to the fact that the overall incidence in the Chinese was higher.

The public health implications of these results are very wide. The primary prevention of type 2 diabetes is possible by a nonpharmacological intervention that can be implemented in the primary health care setting. We can now assume that whenever and wherever unhealthy lifestyles are corrected, the individual disease risk should be reduced regardless of the demographic background.

It is, however, important to note that, in the DPP, people aged over 60 years at baseline benefited more from lifestyle intervention than younger ones [11]. Similar results have been observed from the DPS (Tuomilehto, unpublished data). Thus, the immediate benefits are likely to be even greater because the absolute risk of T2D in a short term is higher in older than in younger people.

The evidence to initiate intensive action to prevent type 2 diabetes is clearly sufficient. According to the estimates derived from the US Third National Health and Nutrition Examination Survey, 11% of US adults aged 40–74 years meet the DPP eligibility criteria [13]. This illustrates the magnitude of the problem; the number of subjects at high risk of T2D who would benefit from lifestyle intervention is large. It will be a major challenge for the health care systems to implement the necessary action to prevent or postpone T2D in these people.

References

[1] E. Joslin, The prevention of diabetes mellitus, JAMA 76 (1921) 79–84.

[2] WHO Study Group, Primary prevention of diabetes mellitus—Technical Report Series No. 844, Geneva (1994), Report No.: 844.

[3] G. Sartor, B. Schersten, S. Carlstrom, A. Melander, A. Norden, G. Persson, Ten-year follow-up of subjects with impaired glucose tolerance. Prevention of diabetes by tolbutamide and diet regulation, Diabetes 29 (1980) 41–49.

[4] K.F. Eriksson, F. Lindgarde, Prevention of type 2 (non-insulin-dependent) diabetes mellitus by diet and physical exercise. The 6-year Malmo feasibility study, Diabetologia 34 (1991) 891–898.
[5] X.R. Pan, G.W. Li, Y.H. Hu, J.X. Wang, W.Y. Yang, Z.X. An, et al., Effects of diet and exercise in preventing NIDDM in people with impaired glucose tolerance. The Da Qing IGT and diabetes study, Diabetes Care 20 (1997) 537–544.
[6] J. Eriksson, J. Lindström, T. Valle, S. Aunola, H. Hämäläinen, P. Ilanne-Parikka, et al., Prevention of type 2 diabetes in subjects with impaired glucose tolerance: the Diabetes Prevention Study (DPS) in Finland-study design and 1-year interim report on the feasibility of the lifestyle intervention programme, Diabetologia 42 (1999) 793–801.
[7] M. Uusitupa, A. Louheranta, J. Lindström, T. Valle, J. Sundvall, J. Eriksson, et al., The Finnish diabetes prevention study, Br. J. Nutr. 83 (Suppl. 1) (2000) S137–S142.
[8] J. Tuomilehto, J. Lindström, J. Eriksson, T. Valle, H. Hämäläinen, P. Ilanne-Parikka, et al., Prevention of type 2 diabetes mellitus by changes in lifestyle among subjects with impaired glucose tolerance, N. Engl. J. Med. 344 (2001) 1343–1350.
[9] J. Lindström, A. Louheranta, M. Mannelin, M. Rastas, V. Salminen, J. Eriksson, et al., The Finnish Diabetes Prevention Study (DPS): lifestyle intervention and 3-year results on diet and physical activity, Diabetes Care 26 (2003) 3230–3236.
[10] The Diabetes Prevention Program Research Group, The Diabetes Prevention Program: baseline characteristics of the randomized cohort, Diabetes Care 23 (2000) 1619–1629.
[11] The Diabetes Prevention Program Research Group, Reduction in the incidence of type 2 diabetes with lifestyle intervention or metformin, N. Engl. J. Med. 346 (2002) 393–403.
[12] The Diabetes Prevention Program Research Group, The Diabetes Prevention Program (DPP): description of lifestyle intervention, Diabetes Care 25 (2002) 2165–2171.
[13] S.H. Saydah, D. Byrd-Holt, M.I. Harris, Projected impact of implementing the results of the Diabetes Prevention Program in the U.S. population, Diabetes Care 25 (2002) 1940–1945.

International Congress Series 1262 (2004) 332–338

www.ics-elsevier.com

Therapeutic angiogenesis: cellular approach from bone marrow, cord blood and peripheral blood ☆

Toyoaki Murohara *

Department of Cardiology, Nagoya University Graduate School of Medicine, 65 Tsurumai, Showa-ku, Nagoya, 466-8559, Japan

Abstract. Adult peripheral blood, umbilical cord (placental) blood and bone marrow contain endothelial progenitor cells (EPCs) that participate in neovascularization, consistent with postnatal vasculogenesis. Cultured EPCs participated in endothelial network formation (capillary formation) with HUVEC, and transplanted EPCs were incorporated into sites of neovascularization in vivo. For example, transplanted human EPCs formed capillaries among preserved skeletal myocytes in the ischemic hindlimb of athymic nude rats. Furthermore, transplantation of EPCs functionally augmented neovascularization in response to hindlimb ischemia. Thus, transplantation of EPCs may become a useful strategy to modulate postnatal neovascularization.

Keywords: Angiogenesis; Vasculogenesis; Ischemia; Progenitor/stem cell therapeutic neovascularization

1. Therapeutic angiogenesis

The therapeutic effficacies of several angiogenic growth factors on severe ischemic diseases were first identified by Folkman [1], who demonstrated that tumor growth was dependent on nutritional neovascularization which is mediated by neoplasm-specific angiogenic growth factors. Subsequently, the feasibility of using recombinant angiogenic growth factor protein to augment collateral artery development was established in animal models of myocardial and/or hindlimb ischemia [2]. This novel strategy for the treatment of vascular insufficiency was later termed "therapeutic angiogenesis" [3].

Therapeutic angiogenesis is an important means of preserving the integrity of tissues subjected to severe ischemia [4,5]. Supplemental administration of angiogenic cytokines, including vascular endothelial growth factor (VEGF), basic fibroblast growth factor (bFGF) and hepatocyte growth factor (HGF) in the form of either genes with expression vectors or recombinant proteins, has been shown to augment collateral vessel development when endogenous neovascularization is insufficient.

☆ A part of this review was presented at the 13th International Symposium on Atherosclerosis, Kyoto, Japan, September 28–October 2, 2003.

* Tel.: +81-52-744-2149; fax: +81-52-744-2157.

E-mail address: murohara@med.nagoya-u.ac.jp (T. Murohara).

0531-5131/ © 2004 Published by Elsevier B.V.
doi:10.1016/j.ics.2004.01.099

Recent advances in vascular and developmental biology have led us to a new paradigm of therapeutic angiogenesis, namely, cell-mediated vascular regeneration. This concept has gained special impetus since the discovery of endothelial progenitor cells (EPCs) or angioblasts in circulating adult human peripheral blood [6]. Transplantation of either culture-expanded EPCs or adult stem cells isolated from bone marrow or umbilical cord blood have recently been shown to augment neovascularization in ischemic tissues [7–9]. This review summarizes the recent progress in therapeutic angiogenesis by means of cell transplantation strategy and presents possible future clinical application of EPCs.

2. Vasculogenesis and angiogenesis

The development of vascular tissues may be considered in several different contexts. Vasculogenesis and angiogenesis are the two major processes responsible for the development of new blood vessels (i.e., neovascularization). Vasculogenesis is referred to as the formation of blood vessels from EPCs or angioblasts [10]. It begins with the formation of cell clusters or blood islands in the embryonic process. Growth and fusion of multiple blood islands in the embryo ultimately give rise to the capillary network structure [11]. After the onset of blood circulation, this network differentiates into an arteriovenous vascular system. EPCs are located at the periphery of the blood islands, while hematopoietic stem cells (HSCs) are located in the center of the blood islands during the early embryonic stages. EPCs give rise to endothelial cells, whereas HSCs develop into mature blood cells after blood island fusion. In addition to this spatial association, HSCs and EPCs share several angiogenic determinants, including Flk-1/KDR/VEGF-receptor 2, Tie-2/TEK, VE-cadherin and CD34. These progenitor cells have consequently been considered to derive from a common precursor, termed a hemangioblast [12,13].

On the other hand, angiogenesis is a process mediated through the sprouting of new capillaries from preexisting mature small vessels. Angiogenesis has been suggested to begin with the "activation" of endothelial cells within a parent vessel, followed by a disruption of the extracellular matrices and the subsequent migration and outgrowth of endothelium into the interstitial space, possibly in response to an ischemic stimulus [14,15]. Subsequent EC proliferation, pericyte recruitment and production of a new basement membrane matrix complete the angiogenesis process. Thus, the proliferative and migratory activities of endothelial cells constitute the basal mechanism of angiogenesis.

3. Postnatal vasculogenesis

Until recently, vasculogenesis has been considered to be restricted to the embryo [16], while neovascular formation in adults was thought to be the consequence of angiogenesis alone. We, however, recently discovered that the peripheral blood of adult species contains EPCs that are predominantly derived from CD34-positive mononuclear blood cells (MNC^{CD34+}) located in the bone marrow [6]. In vitro, these cells differentiate into mature endothelial cells. In animal models of tissue ischemia, transplanted heterologous, homologous and/or autologous EPCs were incorporated into sites of active angiogenesis [6]. These findings suggest that not only naturally circulating EPCs, but also exogenously transplanted EPCs contribute to neovascular formation in adults, consistent with "postnatal vasculogenesis."

This paradigm may have implications regarding the enhancement of collateral vessel growth and angiogenesis in ischemic tissues, therapeutic angiogenesis as well as the delivery of anti- or pro-angiogenic agents to sites of pathologic or utilitarian angiogenesis, respectively. In fact, transplantation of culture-expanded EPCs has been shown to effectively augment angiogenesis and collateral vessel formation in ischemic tissues in several animal models [7,8,17]. EPCs identified in peripheral blood have been shown to derive from bone marrow in response to ischemic stimuli [18,19].

4. Human umbilical cord blood is an additional source of endothelial progenitor cells

We recently identified EPCs in human umbilical cord blood, a previously unknown source for HSCs. Human umbilical cord blood has been shown to contain a large number of hematopoietic colony-forming cells [20,21]. In fact, the transfusion of human cord blood in severe combined immunodeficiency (SCID) mice demonstrated repopulation of the bone marrow with colonogenic progenitors which support the development of erythroid, myeloid and B- and T-lymphocyte lineages. In contrast to HSCs isolated from adult bone marrow, cord blood progenitors have distinctive proliferative characteristics, including the capacity to form a greater number of colonies, a higher cell-cycle rate and self-renewal potential and longer telomeres [22,23]. When used for stem cell transplantation to reconstitute hematopoiesis (HSC transplantation), all of these properties should favor the growth of the cord blood progenitors compared with adult bone marrow-derived progenitors.

Because HSCs and EPCs are considered to derive from a common precursor cell (i.e., hemangioblast) and because cord blood contains a great number of HSCs, cord blood would be a novel source for isolating EPCs. Cell surface molecules such as CD34, KDR, Tie-2 and VE-cadherin are expressed by ECs at an early stage of differentiation [24–27]. Similarly, HSCs express CD34, KDR and Tie-2 on their surface [28,29]. However, as they differentiate into mature blood cells, HSCs lose CD34 [30]. Importantly, Rafii et al. [31] showed the colonization of the flow surface of left ventricular assist devices with CD34-positive ECs, and Shi et al. [32] demonstrated that transplanted bone marrow-derived CD34-positive cells participated in the endothelialization of impervious Dacron grafts in vivo. Therefore, we consider that CD34 antigen is an appropriate marker for isolation of EPCs from human umbilical cord blood [8].

Flow cytometric analysis revealed that cord blood contained a 10-fold excess of MNC^{CD34+} compared with adult peripheral blood. When cord blood MNCs were isolated and cultured on fibronectin-coated plates, numerous cell clusters appeared within 48 h, and spindle-shaped and attached (AT) cells sprouted from the edge of those clusters. Cell clusters and AT cells formed linear cordlike structures. Mature ECs differentiated and sprouted from these structures and eventually formed cobblestone-like EC monolayers. The morphological structure of AT cells resembled that of EPCs derived from adult peripheral blood. AT cells express multiple endothelial-lineage markers and functions [6].

5. Therapeutic vasculogenesis using human endothelial progenitor cells

We examined whether transplanted cord blood-derived EPCs participated in postnatal neovascularization in vivo in immunodeficient animals. EPCs were isolated on day 7 of culture and then fluorescence-labeled. Unilateral hindlimb ischemia was surgically induced in nude rats, and 3 days after surgery, the animals were injected with fluorescence-labeled cord blood-derived EPCs (3×10^5 cells/animal) in the ischemic thigh skeletal muscles. On day 14 after limb ischemia, frozen tissue sections were prepared from the ischemic tissues. Fluorescence microscopy revealed that numerous labeled EPCs had been incorporated and had arranged themselves into EC capillary-like structures among the preserved skeletal myocytes in the ischemic limbs. Moreover, transplanted EPCs often formed tubular structures with a round lumen. When adjacent sections were stained for alkaline phosphatase to identify ECs, capillary ECs were detected at exactly the same locations where fluorescence-positive implanted EPCs had been identified. Thus, transplanted EPCs had survived and had been incorporated into capillary-like network structures in the ischemic hindlimb in vivo.

Finally, we examined whether in vivo transplantation of EPCs would quantitatively augment neovascularization in the ischemic limb in nude rats. Unilateral limb ischemia was surgically induced, and human umbilical cord blood-derived EPCs isolated on day 7 of culture were directly transplanted into the ischemic thigh muscles (3×10^5 EPCs/rat). Serial laser Doppler blood flow analyses revealed significantly augmented ratios of the ischemic/normal hindlimb blood flow in the EPC-transplanted group compared with saline-treated control animals on days 7, 14 and 21. Moreover, on day 14, immunohistochemical analysis of vWF expression and histochemical staining for alkaline phosphatase in the ischemic tissues revealed a significant increase in capillary density after transplantation of EPCs compared with the controls. No significant difference in capillary density was observed between the two groups in the contralateral nonischemic limb. Thus, transplantation of human cord blood-derived EPCs is a novel strategy for enhancing tissue neovascularization in adult animals [6], a notion consistent with "therapeutic vasculogenesis" [5].

6. Utilization of bone marrow stem cells for therapeutic neovascularization

Because at present it is still difficult to use autologous cord blood-derived EPCs clinically in adults, other source(s) of EPCs should be explored. Currently, autologous EPCs can be isolated and expanded from adult human peripheral blood for therapeutic angiogenesis [7]; however, the number of EPCs obtained from peripheral blood may be limited. To overcome this problem, the use of genetically modified EPCs transfected with adenovirus vector encoding VEGF gene is being considered [33]. This strategy seems to show promise in animal experiments, but its clinical application may need further careful evaluation since a recent study showed that a powerful expression of VEGF transgene has been shown to induce angioma formation in experimental animal models [34,35]. Instead, a combined administration of culture expanded EPCs together with naked plasmid vectors containing VEGF gene would be a safer and more feasible strategy in clinics.

Autologous bone marrow cells are receiving great attention as an alternative source [9,36,37]. Bone marrow contains a large number of HSCs and other stem cells for stroma tissues [38], including EPCs [18,32]. In fact, the implantation of autologous bone marrow cells has been shown to effectively augment angiogenesis in ischemic tissues [9,37,39]. The greatest advantage of using bone marrow-derived EPCs is that one can use the patient's own EPCs (autologous cell implantation), thus eliminating any immunological adverse reactions. Secondly, one can obtain a significant number of CD34-positive MNCs from bone marrow. Taken together, these advantages appear to confirm the utilization of autologous BM-MNCs as an efficient and safe strategy for therapeutic neovascularization in humans.

We recently reported on the safety and efficacy of the autologous implantation of bone marrow-derived MNCs (i.e., stem cell-rich fraction) for therapeutic angiogenesis in patients with critical limb ischemia in a multicenter clinical trial in Japan [Therapeutic Angiogenesis by Cell Transplantation Study (TACT study)] [40]. The long-term efficacy and potential side effects of this procedure should be carefully followed in the future.

7. Perspectives on the clinical utility of EPCs

Previous studies, including those from our laboratory, clearly showed the usefulness of implanting EPCs for therapeutic neovascularization in ischemic tissues. Currently, the utilization of EPCs for other forms of vascular insufficiency is being considered. Shin'oka et al. [41] created a low-thrombogenic arterial biograft, successfully combining a culture of a biodegradable scaffold together with autologous bone marrow cells. In their study, EPCs contained in the bone marrow could repopulate mature endothelial cells after being seeded onto the arterial scaffold.

Because EPCs are avidly incorporated into an active angiogenic site, the inhibition of EPC mobilization and/or incorporation could be a novel strategy for the treatment of angiogenic disorders such as malignant neoplasms. In fact, Rafii et al. recently demonstrated that genetically modified mice, with reduced HSC/EPC mobilization from BM, revealed significantly retarded tumor growth and suppressed tumor-related angiogenesis as compared with wild-type animals [42].

Future studies will clarify the mechanisms and circumstances that may be responsible for modulating the contribution of vasculogenesis to postnatal neovascularization. Specifically in this regard, it is intriguing to consider the possibility that certain angiogenic growth factors acknowledged to promote both angiogenesis and vasculogenesis in the embryo, but that have been assumed to promote neovascularization exclusively by angiogenesis in the adult, may in fact promote the migration, proliferation and mobilization of EPCs from BM. Finally, the possibility that the modulation of vasculogenesis can be used therapeutically to augment as well as inhibit neovascularization deserves further investigation.

References

[1] J. Folkman, Tumor angiogenesis: therapeutic implications, N. Engl. J. Med. 285 (1971) 1182–1186.
[2] A. Yanagisawa-Miwa, et al., Salvage of infarcted myocardium by angiogenic action of basic fibroblast growth factor, Science 257 (1992) 1401–1403.
[3] S. Takeshita, et al., Therapeutic angiogenesis: a single intra-arterial bolus of vascular endothelial growth factor augments revascularization in a rabbit ischemic hindlimb model, J. Clin. Invest. 93 (1994) 662–670.
[4] J.M. Isner, et al., Clinical evidence of angiogenesis following arterial gene transfer of $phVEGF_{165}$, Lancet 348 (1996) 370–374.
[5] J.M. Isner, T. Asahara, Angiogenesis and vasculogenesis as therapeutic strategies for postnatal neovascularization, J. Clin. Invest. 103 (1999) 1231–1236.
[6] T. Asahara, et al., Isolation of putative progenitor endothelial cells for angiogenesis, Science 275 (1997) 965–967.
[7] C. Kalka, et al., Transplantation of ex vivo expanded endothelial progenitor cells for therapeutic neovascularization, Proc. Natl. Acad. Sci. U. S. A. 97 (2000) 3422–3427.

[8] T. Murohara, et al., Transplanted cord blood-derived endothelial precursor cells augment postnatal neovascularization, J. Clin. Invest. 105 (2000) 1527–1536.
[9] S. Shintani, et al., Augmentation of postnatal neovascularization with autologous bone marrow transplantation, Circulation 103 (2001) 897–903.
[10] W. Risau, Differentiation of endothelium, FASEB J. 9 (1995) 926–933.
[11] W. Risau, I. Flamme, Vasculogenesis, Annu. Rev. Cell Dev. Biol. 11 (1995) 73–91.
[12] I. Flamme, W. Risau, Induction of vasculogenesis and hematopoiesis in vitro, Development 116 (1992) 435–439.
[13] M. Weiss, S.H. Orkin, In vitro differentiation of murine embryonic stem cells: new approaches to old problems, J. Clin. Invest. 97 (1996) 591–595.
[14] P.A. D'Amore, R.W. Thompson, Mechanisms of angiogenesis, Annu. Rev. Physiol. 49 (1987) 453–464.
[15] J. Folkman, Angiogenesis in cancer, vascular, rheumatoid and other disease, Nat. Med. 1 (1995) 27–31.
[16] W. Risau, et al., Vasculogenesis and angiogenesis in embryonic stem cell-derived embryoid bodies, Development 102 (1988) 471–478.
[17] A. Kawamoto, et al., Therapeutic potential of ex vivo expanded endothelial progenitor cells for myocardial ischemia, Circulation 103 (2001) 634–637.
[18] T. Asahara, et al., Bone marrow origin of endothelial progenitor cells responsible for postnatal vasculogenesis in physiological and pathological neovascularization, Circ. Res. 85 (1999) 221–228.
[19] T. Takahashi, et al., Ischemia- and cytokine-induced mobilization of bone marrow-derived endothelial progenitor cells for neovascularization, Nat. Med. 5 (1999) 434–438.
[20] T. Nakahata, M. Ogawa, Hemopoietic colony-forming cells in umbilical cord blood with extensive capability to generate mono- and multipotential hemopoietic progenitors, J. Clin. Invest. 70 (1982) 1324–1328.
[21] E. Gluckman, et al., Hematopoietic reconstitution in a patient with Fanconi's anemia by means of umbilical-cord blood from an HLA-identical sibling, N. Engl. J. Med. 321 (1989) 1174–1178.
[22] H. Mayani, P.M. Lansdorp, Thy-1 expression is linked to functional properties of primitive hematopoietic progenitor cells from human umbilical cord blood, Blood 83 (1994) 2410–2417.
[23] H. Vaziri, et al., Evidence for a mitotic clock in human hematopoietic stem cells: loss of telomeric DNA with age, Proc. Natl. Acad. Sci. U. S. A. 91 (1994) 9857–9860.
[24] T.P. Yamaguchi, et al., flk-1, and flt-related receptor tyrosine kinase is an early marker for endothelial cell precursors, Development 118 (1993) 489–498.
[25] B. Millauer, et al., High affinity VEGF binding and developmental expression suggest Flk-1 as a major regulator of vasculogenesis and angiogenesis, Cell 72 (1993) 835–846.
[26] T.N. Sato, et al., Distinct roles of the receptor tyrosine kinases Tie-1 and Tie-2 in blood vessel formation, Nature 376 (1995) 70–74.
[27] S. Nishikawa, Progressive lineage analysis by cell sorting and culture identifies FLK1+VE-cadherin+cells at a diverging point of endothelial and hemopoietic lineages, Development 125 (1998) 1747–1757.
[28] O. Katoh, et al., Expression of the vascular endothelial growth factor (VEGF) receptor gene, KDR, in hematopoietic cells and inhibitory effect of VEGF on apoptotic cell death caused by ionizing radiation, Cancer Res. 55 (1995) 5687–5692.
[29] M. Yano, et al., Expression and function of murine receptor tyrosine kinases, TIE and TEK, in hematopoietic stem cells, Blood 89 (1997) 4317–4326.
[30] C.I. Civin, et al., Antigenic analysis of hematopoiesis: III. A hematopoietic progenitor cell surface antigen defined by a monoclonal antibody raised against KG-1a, J. Immunol. 133 (1984) 157–165.
[31] S. Rafii, et al., Characterization of hematopoietic cells arising on the textured surface of left ventricular assist devices, Ann. Thorac. Surg. 60 (1995) 1627–1632.
[32] Q. Shi, et al., Evidence for circulating bone marrow-derived endothelial cells, Blood 92 (1998) 362–367.
[33] H. Iwaguro, et al., Endothelial progenitor cell vascular endothelial growth factor gene transfer for vascular regeneration, Circulation 105 (2002) 732–738.
[34] R.J. Lee, et al., VEGF gene delivery to myocardium. Deleterious effects of unregulated expression, Circulation 102 (2000) 898–901.
[35] P. Carmeliet, VEGF gene therapy: stimulating angiogenesis or angioma-genesis?, Nat. Med. 6 (2000) 1102–1103.

[36] S. Tomita, R.K. Li, R.D. Weisel, Autologous transplantation of bone marrow cells improves damaged heart function, Circulation 100 (1999) II247–II256.
[37] K. Kamihata, et al., Implantation of autologous bone marrow cells into ischemic myocardium enhances collateral perfusion and regional function via side-supply of angioblasts, angiogenic ligands and cytokines, Circulation 104 (2001) 1046–1052.
[38] D.J. Prockop, Marrow stromal cells as stem cells for non-hematopoietic tissues, Science 276 (1997) 71–74.
[39] T. Ueno, et al., Therapeutic angiogenesis by bone marrow-derived cell transplantation in pigs with coronary constrictor-induced chronic myocardial ischemia, J. Am. Coll. Cardiol. 37 (Suppl. A) (2001) 48A.
[40] E. Tateishi-Yuyama, et al., for the Therapeutic Angiogenesis using Cell Transplantation (TACT) Study Investigators, Therapeutic angiogenesis for patients with limb ischaemia by autologous transplantation of bone-marrow cells: a pilot study and a randomised controlled trial, Lancet 360 (2002) 427–435.
[41] T. Shin'oka, Y. Imai, Y. Ikada, Transplantation of a tissue-engineered pulmonary artery, N. Engl. J. Med. 344 (2001) 532–533.
[42] D. Lyden, K. Hattori, S. Dias, Impaired recruitment of bone-marrow-derived endothelial and hematopoietic precursor cells blocks tumor angiogenesis and growth, Nat. Med. 7 (2001) 1194–1201.

ELSEVIER

International Congress Series 1262 (2004) 339–343

www.ics-elsevier.com

Cardiomyocyte regeneration following angioblast-dependent neovascularization of ischemic myocardium

M.D. Schuster, A.A. Kocher, T. Seki, G. Xiang, S. Homma, S. Itescu*

Departments of Surgery and Medicine, Columbia University, New York NY, USA

Abstract. In the adult, new blood vessel formation can occur either through angiogenesis from preexisting mature endothelium or vasculogenesis mediated by bone marrow-derived endothelial precursors. We recently isolated endothelial progenitor cells, or angioblasts, in human adult bone marrow, which have selective migratory properties for ischemic tissues, including myocardium, to where they home and induce vasculogenesis. Angioblast trafficking to the infarct zone enables development of progressively larger-sized capillaries. Here, we show that this results in sustained improvement in cardiac function by mechanisms involving induction of proliferation/regeneration of endogenous cardiomyocytes. © 2004 Published by Elsevier B.V.

Keywords: Regeneration; Stem cells; Myocardial infarction

1. Introduction

An integral component of the healing process following a myocardial infarct is compensatory hypertrophy of viable cardiomyocytes at the peri-infarct rim in order to increase pump function in response to the loss of infarcted tissue [1]. However, cardiomyocyte hypertrophy initiates a genetic program that culminates in apoptotic loss of the cardiomyocytes, expansion of the initial infarct area, progressive collagen replacement and heart failure [2], a process termed cardiac remodelling.

We have recently put forward the hypothesis that hypertrophied cardiac myocytes undergo apoptosis because the endogenous capillary network cannot provide the compensatory increase in perfusion required for cell survival [3]. Intravenous administration of bone marrow derived angioblasts resulted in induction of neovascularization at the peri-infarct region, salvage of hypertrophied cardiomyocytes and significant improvement in myocardial function [3].

* Corresponding author. Transplantation Immunology, Columbia-Presbyterian Medical Center, 630 West 168th Street, PH 14W, Room 1485, New York, NY 10032, USA. Tel.: +1-212-305-7176; fax: +1-212-305-8304.
E-mail address: si5@columbia.edu (S. Itescu).

0531-5131/ © 2004 Published by Elsevier B.V.
doi:10.1016/j.ics.2003.12.064

Recent observations have suggested that a second compensatory response of viable cardiomyocytes at the peri-infarct region is to proliferate and regenerate following injury [4]. While cardiomyocyte regeneration can be accomplished by providing exogenous precursors, for example from the bone marrow [5], no approaches are known to effectively induce endogenous cardiomyocytes to enter the cell cycle. Here, we investigated whether inductive cues from human bone marrow-derived angioblasts might result in cycling and regeneration of endogenous cardiomyocytes.

2. Methods

2.1. Animals, surgical procedures and injection of human cells

Rowett (rnu/rnu) athymic nude rats (Harlan Sprague–Dawley, Indianapolis, IN, USA) were used in studies approved by the "Columbia University Institute for Animal Care and Use Committee". After anesthesia, a left thoracotomy was performed, and the left anterior descending (LAD) coronary artery was ligated. 2.0×10^6 $CD34^+$ $CD117^+$ cells obtained from a single donor after G-CSF mobilization were injected into the tail vein 48 h after LAD ligation. Controls received saline after LAD ligation [3]. Each group consisted of 6–10 rats. Histologic and functional studies were performed at 2 and 15 weeks.

2.2. Quantitation of capillary density

In order to quantitate capillary density and species origin of the capillaries, sections were stained freshly with mAbs directed against factor VIII (Dako, CA, USA), and confirmed with anti-CD31 (Research Diagnostics, NJ, USA) and rat or human MHC class I (Accurate Chemicals, CT, USA). Staining was performed by immunoperoxidase technique using an Avidin/Biotin Blocking Kit, a rat-absorbed biotinylated anti-mouse IgG and a peroxidase-conjugate (all Vector Laboratories Burlingame, CA, USA). Capillary density was determined at 2 weeks post-infarction and expressed per HPF (400 ×).

2.3. Quantitation of cardiomyocyte proliferation

Cardiomyocyte DNA synthesis and cell cycling was determined by dual staining for cardiomyocyte-specific troponin I and rat-specific Ki-67. Briefly, paraffin embedded sections were microwaved in a 0.1 M EDTA buffer, and stained with a polyclonal rabbit antibody with specificity against rat Ki-67 at 1:3000 dilution (gift of Giorgio Cattoretti, Columbia University) incubated overnight at 4 °C. For confocal microscopy, fluorescein isothiocyanate (FITC)-conjugated rabbit anti-mouse IgG was used as secondary antibody to detect Ki-67 in nuclei. A Texas Red-conjugated anti-mouse mAb (Vector Laboratories) against troponin I was used to detect cardiomyocytes, and slides were coverslipped with 4′,6-diamidine-2-phenylindole dihydrochloride (DAPI) vectashield to visualize all nuclei. Images were viewed at 100x magnification, acquired and analyzed using a Zeiss LSM 510 Multiphoton Confocal Microscope and LSM software.

2.4. Analyses of myocardial function

Echocardiographic studies were performed using a high frequency liner array transducer (SONOS 5500, Hewlett Packard, Andover, MA, USA). 2D images were obtained at mid-papillary and apical levels. Percent left ventricular ejection fraction (LVEF) was calculated as [(EDV − ESV)/EDV] × 100.

3. Results

3.1. Angioblast migration to the ischemic myocardium results in generation of capillaries with large lumen size

At 2 weeks after intravenously injecting either 2×10^5 angioblasts or control medium following myocardial infarction the number of small-sized, medium-sized and large-sized capillaries at the peri-infarct zone were quantified. Capillaries were considered to be small-sized if they had < 3 nuclei (mean lumen diameter 0.056 mm ± 0.006) medium-sized if they

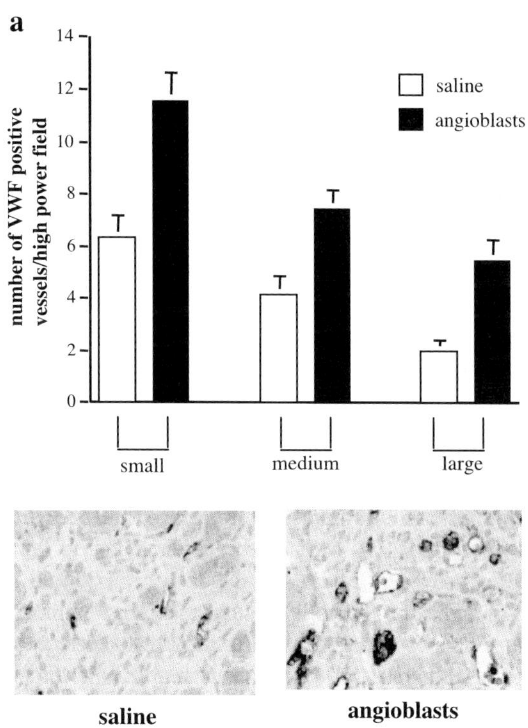

Fig. 1. Redirected trafficking of human angioblasts to ischemic myocardium induces neovascularization and protects cardiomyocytes against apoptosis. (a) Myocardial infarct bed 2 weeks post-LAD ligation from representative animals in each group stained with immunoperoxidase after binding of VWF and confirmed with anti-CD31 staining. The infarct zones of rats injected with 2×10^5 angioblasts show an increase in small diameter capillaries (< 3 nuclei with diameters < 7 μm), medium-sized capillaries (3–6 nuclei with diameters 7–25 μm) and an additional increase in large-sized vessels of human origin (>6 nuclei with diameters >20 μm). Results are expressed as the mean ± S.E.M. of at least 15 hpf in three separate experiments.

had 3–6 nuclei (mean lumen diameter 0.020 mm ± 0.002), and large-sized if they had >6 contiguous endothelial lining cells (mean lumen diameter of 0.053 mm ± 0.004). As shown in Fig. 1a, the group receiving 2×10^5 angioblast demonstrated 1.8-fold higher number of small-sized capillaries, 1.7-fold higher number of medium-sized capillaries compared with saline controls ($p < 0.01$). The group receiving 2×10^5 angioblasts additionally demonstrated 2.75-fold higher number of large-lumen capillaries compared with the group receiving saline controls ($p < 0.01$).

3.2. Development of capillaries with large lumen size correlates with sustained regeneration of endogenous cardiomyocytes

Recent observations have suggested that human cardiomyocytes have the capacity to proliferate and regenerate in response to injury [4]. Therefore, we investigated whether the additive improvement in cardiac function observed after injection of 2×10^5 human angioblasts and development of the islands of cardiomyocytes at the peri-infarct rim in animals receiving 2×10^5 human angioblasts contained a high frequency of rat myocytes with DNA activity, as determined by dual staining with a mAb reactive against but not human, Ki-67 (Fig. 2a). Triple immunofluorescence using confocal microscopy confirmed the presence of cycling rat cardiomyocytes, and demonstrated a speckled pattern of Ki-67 reactivity within cycling nuclei, Fig. 2a. In contrast, in animals receiving saline, there was a high frequency of cells with fibroblast morphology and reactivity with rat Ki-67, but not troponin I, within the infarct zone.

The number of cardiomyocytes progressing through cell cycle at the peri-infarct region of rats receiving 2×10^5 human angioblasts was 40-fold higher than that at sites distal to the

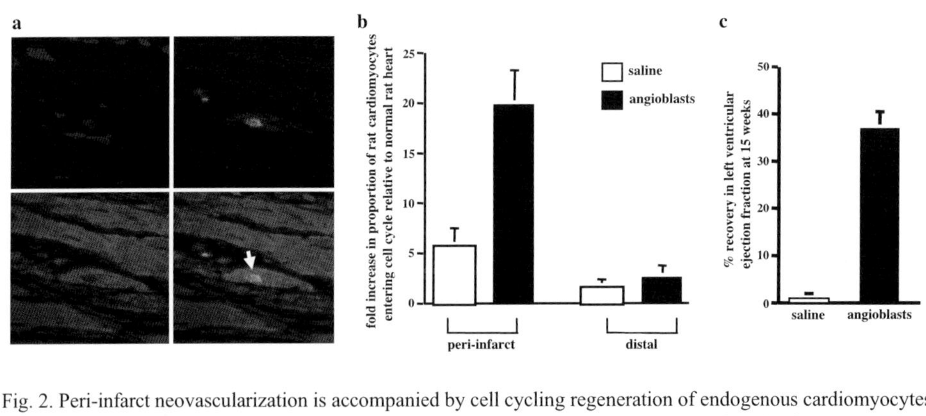

Fig. 2. Peri-infarct neovascularization is accompanied by cell cycling regeneration of endogenous cardiomyocytes and improvement in cardiac function. (a) Shows confocal microscopy of section of peri-infarct tissue from representative animal receiving human angioblasts demonstrates cardiomyocytes whose nuclei (labeled blue by DAPI) concomitantly expressed Ki-67 antigen (labeled green by FITC-conjugated secondary antibody) and whose cytoplasm concomitantly stained for troponin I (labeled red by Texas Red). (b) Bar graph showing that the group of animals receiving 2×10^5 human angioblasts has a significantly higher index of cell cycling cardiomyocytes at the peri-infarct region than saline controls or sham operated animals (both $p < 0.01$). No difference between the groups is seen at sites distal to the infarct. (c) Shows the improvement in myocardial function at 15 weeks in the group receiving angioblasts, defined as mean improvement in LVEF. No significant improvement in these parameters was observed in the groups receiving saline.

infarct, where myocyte DNA activity was no different than in sham-operated rats. As shown in Fig. 2b, animals receiving 2×10^5 human angioblasts had a 20-fold higher number of cycling cardiomyocytes at the peri-infarct rim than that found in non-infarcted hearts ($1.19 \pm 0.2\%$ vs. $0.06 \pm 0.03\%$, $p < 0.01$) and 3.5-fold higher than in the same region in LAD-ligated controls receiving saline ($1.19 \pm 0.2\%$ vs. $0.34 \pm 0.1\%$, $p < 0.01$).

We next examined whether there was a direct relationship between the number of human angioblasts trafficking to ischemic myocardium, the size of capillaries generated, protection against cardiomyocyte apoptosis and long-term myocardial function. As shown in Fig. 2c, animals receiving only saline did not demonstrate any functional cardiac recovery defined as the degree of improvement in LVEF and reduction in left ventricular end-systolic area (LVAs) at 15 weeks after intravenous injection. Strikingly, the group receiving 2×10^5 angioblasts had a mean recovery in LVEF of $34 \pm 4\%$ ($p < 0.001$).

4. Discussion

Perhaps the most striking finding in this study is that in parallel with growth of larger-sized capillaries accompanying injection of high concentrations of human angioblasts, ischemic rat hearts developed prominent islands of regenerating myocytes at the peri-infarct region. This regenerative response bears striking similarity to the spontaneous myocardial regeneration seen in MRL mice which accompanies prominent spontaneous neovascularization and wound repair following myocardial or other injury [6]. Together, our results indicate that angioblast-dependent neovascularization gives rise to two complementary mechanisms by which heart function is improved: (i) protection of at-risk, but otherwise viable, myocytes against apoptosis after injection of low angioblast concentrations and development of capillaries of small lumen size, and (ii) proliferation/regeneration of endogenous cardiomyocytes after injection of high angioblast concentrations and development of capillaries of large lumen size.

References

[1] M.H. Soonpaa, L.J. Field, Assessment of cardiomyocyte DNA synthesis in normal and injured adult mouse hearts, Am. J. Physiol. 272 (1997) H220–H226.

[2] J.M. Pfeffer, M.A. Pfeffer, P.J. Fletcher, E. Braunwald, Progressive ventricular remodeling in rat with myocardial infarction, Am. J. Physiol. 260 (1991) H1406–H1414.

[3] A.A. Kocher, et al., Neovascularization of ischemic myocardium by human bone-marrow-derived angioblasts prevents cardiomyocyte apoptosis, reduces remodeling and improves cardiac function, Nat. Med. 7 (2001) 430–436.

[4] A.P. Beltrami, et al., Evidence that human cardiac myocytes divide after myocardial infarction, N. Engl. J. Med. 344 (2001) 1750–1757.

[5] D. Orlic, et al., Bone marrow cells regenerate infarcted myocardium, Nature 410 (2001) 701–705.

[6] J.M. Leferovich, et al., Heart regeneration in adult MRL mice, Proc. Natl. Acad. Sci. U. S. A. 98 (2001) 9830–9835.

International Congress Series 1262 (2004) 344–347

www.ics-elsevier.com

Changes in incidence and mortality of stroke and risk factors in a Japanese general population: the Hisayama study

M. Fujishima*, Y. Kiyohara

Department of Medicine and Clinical Science, Graduate School of Medical Sciences, Kyushu University, Maidashi 3-1-1, Higashiku, Fukuoka 812-8582 Japan

Abstract. Stroke is the third leading cause of death in Japan, but it is more common than coronary heart disease in Japanese. Our autopsy-based, long-term prospective cohort study, the Hisayama study, demonstrated that stroke incidence and mortality markedly decreased from the 1960s to 1970s mainly due to treatment of hypertension. Thereafter, the reduction of stroke incidence became smaller and almost ceased in 1980 to 1990s in Japan. Stroke risk factors other than hypertension, such as obesity, hypercholesterolemia and diabetes, have been increasing in recent years probably due to the westernization of lifestyle. They become more important risk factors for ischemic stroke and seem to be responsible for the recent decline in the reduction of stroke incidence. © 2003 Published by Elsevier B.V.

Keywords: Stroke; Epidemiology; Japanese; Hisayama study

1. Introduction

The Japanese population is characterized by a higher susceptibility to stroke rather than coronary heart disease compared with Western populations; however, stroke mortality has been consistently decreasing since the early 1970s [1]. Whether this change reflects decreased stroke and ischemic heart disease, case-fatality rates could not be determined from vital statistics. For the last 2–3 decades, Japan has experienced a great change in dietary and living patterns [2] which may have an effect on stroke morbidity and mortality. Thus, to determine the basis of the change in stroke death, secular trends in incidence and risk factors for stroke were examined in a general population of Hisayama Town where a prospective population survey of cerebrovascular disease was initiated in 1961 [3].

* Corresponding author. Nishinippon Medical Institute, Tanaka 275, Sasagurimachi, Kasuyagun, Fukuoka 811-2416 Japan. Tel.: +81-92-947-0511; fax: +81-92-947-1552.

E-mail address: m-fujishima@kitakyu-hp.or.jp (M. Fujishima).

0531-5131/ © 2003 Published by Elsevier B.V.
doi:10.1016/j.ics.2003.12.032

2. Subjects and methods

Hisayama Town is located in the neighborhood of Fukuoka City (population: 1.35 million), a metropolitan area on Kyushu Island in Japan. The population of the town was 6500 in 1960 and increased very little to 7600 in 2000. We established three study cohorts of the residents that were free from stroke and ischemic heart disease, aged 40 years or over in 1961 (1618 men and women, the 1st cohort), in 1974 (2074 subjects, the 2nd cohort) and in 1988 (2637 subjects, the 3rd cohort) [4]. The most prominent characteristic of our study is in the detailed protocol for detecting new cardiovascular events during the follow-up period (the follow-up rate>99%).

The cause of death was determined clinically and verified pathologically (the autopsy rate>80%). The clinical diagnoses of stroke were determined on the basis of a detailed history, neurological examination and, recently, by brain imaging.

To assess changes in stroke risk, we compared the risk factors in 1961, 1974 and 1988 including: (1) hypertension (BP $\geq$ 160/95 mmHg), (2) obesity (BMI $\geq$ 25.4 kg/m^2), (3) hypercholesterolemia (serum cholesterol $\geq$ 220 mg/dl) and (4) glucose intolerance including diabetes and impaired glucose tolerance (IGT) [2].

3. Results

3.1. Secular trends in stroke mortality

The age- and sex-adjusted mortality for all stroke, cerebral infarction and cerebral hemorrhage significantly decreased in the 2nd and 3rd cohort (Table 1). Death from subarachnoid hemorrhage did not change at all. In contrast, coronary heart disease mortality remained unchanged among the three cohorts.

Table 1
Changes in the age- and sex-adjusted mortality and incidence of stroke and coronary heart disease among three cohorts of Hisayama residents aged 40 years or over

	1st cohort (1961–1969)	2nd cohort (1974–1982)	3rd cohort (1988–1996)
Mortality (1000 pys)			
Stroke	4.8	1.6*	1.1*
Cerebral infarction	1.8	0.8*	0.5*
Cerebral hemorrhage	2.0	0.5*	0.2*,†
Subarachnoid hemorrhage	0.6	0.2	0.4
Coronary heart disease	0.9	0.7	0.9
Incidence (1000 pys)			
Stroke	10.5	5.0*	4.7*
Cerebral infarction	7.0	3.7*	3.1*
Cerebral hemorrhage	2.3	0.8*	1.0*
Subarachnoid hemorrhage	0.9	0.5	0.7
Coronary heart disease	2.1	1.9	2.3

*$p<0.05$ vs. 1st cohort.
† $p<0.05$ vs. 2nd cohort.

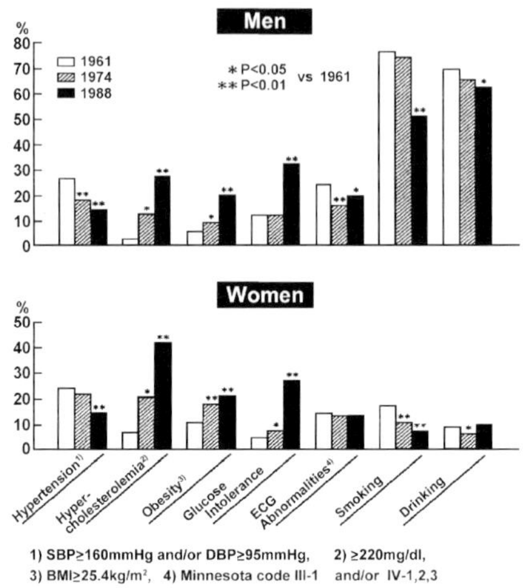

Fig. 1. Comparison of age-adjusted prevalence of cardiovascular risk factors among three cross-sectional examinations of Hisayama residents aged 40 years or over.

3.2. Changes in stroke incidence

Stroke incidence decreased from the 1st cohort to the 2nd cohort but remained unchanged in the 3rd cohort (Table 1). Among stroke subtypes, cerebral infarction and hemorrhage decreased significantly in the 2nd cohort but did not change in the 3rd cohort, while subarachnoid hemorrhage remained unchanged among the cohorts. Likewise, the incidence of coronary heart disease did not change among the three cohorts.

3.3. Changes in risk factors for stroke

The prevalence of hypertension decreased consistently by 50% in 1988 compared with that in 1961 due to increased antihypertensive treatment (Fig. 1). In contrast, the frequency of obesity increased 2–4 times, hypercholesterolemia 6–9 times and glucose intolerance 2–5 times in 1988 compared with those in 1961.

The increased prevalence of such metabolic abnormalities strongly suggests recent changes in dietary habits and westernization of lifestyle in Japanese who take more animal fat and protein but less carbohydrate or eat more meat but less rice. In fact, food intake and nutritional state of Japanese population have been changing since 1975; particularly, both animal fat and protein intakes increased by 15% and currently remain high.

4. Discussion

Mortality rates for stroke have been declining for several decades in developed countries, and this decline accelerated in the late 1960s and 1970s [5–7]. In the Hisayama study, the incidence of stroke, especially cerebral infarction, significantly decreased from the 1st cohort (1960s) to the 2nd cohort (1970s) leading to a decline of stroke mortality. Among cerebral infarction subtypes, the incidence of lacunar infarction decreased significantly in the 2nd cohort, while atherothrombotic infarction and cerebral embolism

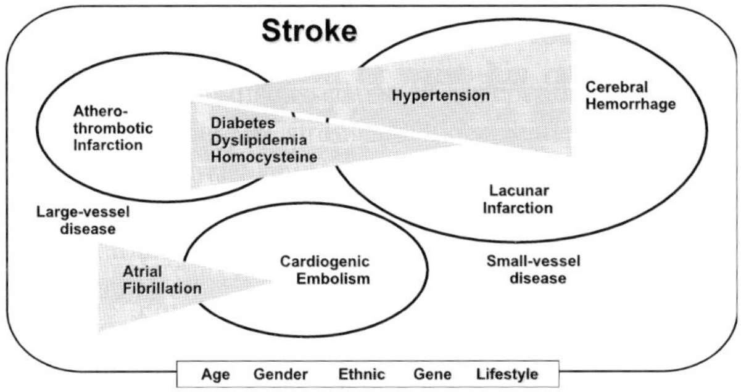

Fig. 2. Frequency of stroke subtypes and risk factors in Japanese.

relatively increased. Our autopsy studies demonstrated that fibrinoid necrosis in small cerebral penetrating arteries of the putamen was found less frequently in the 1970s than in the 1960s [6], indicating that decreased stroke incidence and mortality seemed related to the successful management of hypertension. However, during the 1980–1990s, the decline of stroke incidence slowed down and almost ceased, although the prevalence of hypertension continued to decline due to popularization of hypertension treatment [4]. Meanwhile, metabolic disorders, such as obesity, hypercholesterolemia and glucose intolerance, have increased progressively due to changes in dietary habits. A five-year follow-up of the 3rd cohort revealed that diabetes was 3.2 times risk for cerebral infarction and 2.6 times for ischemic heart disease than normoglycemia [8]. These findings indicate recent changing of the risk factor profile for stroke in Japanese.

From the Hisayama study, frequency of stroke subtypes of Japanese and their association to stroke risk factors could be illustrated in Fig. 2 [4,9,10].

References

[1] Statistics and Information Department, Minister's Secretarist, Ministry of Health and Welfare Vital Statistics, Japan, 1993.

[2] M. Fujishima, Y. Kiyohara, K. Ueda, et al., Smoking as cardiovascular risk factor in low cholesterol population: the Hisayama study, Clin. Exp. Hypertens., Part A Theory Pract. 14 (1992) 99–108.

[3] S. Katsuki, Epidemiological and clinicopathological study on cerebrovascular disease in Japan, Prog. Brain Res. 21B (1966) 64–89.

[4] M. Fujishima, Cardiovascular disease in the elderly: the Hisayama study, Jpn. J. Geriat. 36 (1999) 16–21.

[5] H. Baum, M. Goldstein, Cerebrovascular disease type specific mortality, Stroke 13 (1982) 810–817.

[6] K. Ueda, T. Omae, Y. Hirota, et al., Decreasing trend in incidence and mortality from stroke in Hisayama residents, Japan, Stroke 12 (1981) 154–160.

[7] R.A. Wolf, R.B. D'Agostino, M.A. O'Neal, et al., Secular trends in stroke incidence and mortality: the Framingham study, Stroke 23 (1992) 1551–1555.

[8] M. Fujishima, Y. Kiyohara, I. Kato, et al., Diabetes and cardiovascular disease in a prospective population survey: the Hisayama study, Diabetes 45 (Suppl. 3) (1996) S14–S16.

[9] Y. Tanizaki, Y. Kiyohara, I. Kato, et al., Incidence and risk factors for subtypes of cerebral infarction in a general population: the Hisayama study, Stroke 31 (2000) 2616–2622.

[10] H. Shimizu, Y. Kiyohara, I. Kato, et al., Plasma homocyst(e)ine concentrations and the risk of subtypes of cerebral infarction: the Hisayama study, Cerebrovasc. Dis. 13 (2002) 9–15.

International Congress Series 1262 (2004) 348–351

ELSEVIER

www.ics-elsevier.com

Stroke in Korea

Jong S. Kim*

Department of Neurology, University of Ulsan, Asan Medical Center, Song-pa PO Box 145, 138600 Seoul, South Korea

Abstract. Stroke is the second most important cause of death, followed by cancer, in Korea. There has been no evidence of decrease in stroke mortality until recently. Although intracerebral hemorrhage (ICH) outnumbered cerebral infarction (CI) before 1980, recent large hospital registry studies reported that the proportion of ICH is approximately 20%. As compared with the western population, small arterial disease is relatively common and cardiogenic embolism is uncommon. The middle cerebral artery is the most common site of atherosclerosis in patients with ischemic stroke. Hypertension is present in 60–70%, and diabetes mellitus in 25–30% among admitted stroke patients. Increased intake of fat or animal protein and increased incidence of diabetes mellitus appear to explain the decrease in ICH in our country. The stroke knowledge of the general population is deviated from scientific facts, possibly due to the strong influence of alternative medicine. Moreover, due to an increase in life expectancy and decrease in birth rate, the proportion of aged population increases rapidly. Therefore, stroke will remain as a major social burden in Korea. Nationwide efforts are required for risk factor reduction, stroke education and the proper care of stroke patients. © 2004 Published by Elsevier B.V.

Keywords: Stroke; Risk factors; Stroke knowledge; Herbal medicine; Korea

In Korea, stroke is the second most important cause of death followed by cancer. The stroke mortality rate, 77/100,000 in 2002, has not significantly changed since 1985 [1]. As shown in Table 1, the prevalence of stroke is higher in men than in women in both Seoul and Cheong-Song. Although intracerebral hemorrhage (ICH) outnumbered cerebral infarction (CI) in the past, the latter has outnumbered the former since mid-1980. A multicenter study conducted in the early 1990s showed that ICH occupied approximately 30% of all admitted stroke patients [2]. However, recent hospital-based registries reported that this rate is approximately 20%, suggesting that the proportion of ICH is further decreasing. Aneurysmal rupture occupies approximately 10% of all strokes.

According to several hospital registry studies [3–5], the mean age of stroke patients was 62 or 63 years. Approximately 60% of the admitted patients were male. The 30-day

* Tel.: +82-2-3010-3442; fax: +82-2-474-4691.
E-mail address: jongskim@amc.seoul.kr (J.S. Kim).

doi:10.1016/j.ics.2003.12.081

Table 1
Prevalence of stroke among 1000 subjects

Age	Seoul[a]		Cheong-Song[b]	
	Male	Female	Male	Female
50–59	0.7	0.3	2.6	0.4
60–69	5.4	6.8	5.8	5.7
70–	38.7	15.7	17.4	6.6

[a] 63,603 subjects, year 1980.
[b] 36,609 subjects, year 1998.

mortality rate is 5–8%. The proportion of ischemic stroke subtypes varies among registries (Table 2). However, it seems clear that the proportion of small arterial diseases is relatively high and that of cardiac embolism low, as compared with western societies. The difference in the proportion of large arterial disease probably results from the different rate of angiographic investigation. For instance, small subcortical infarcts may be caused by intracranial atherosclerosis, which would be classified as small arterial diseases unless angiograms are performed. In our AMC registry, we performed MR angiogram in more than 90% of the cases. Table 2 shows our results among the patients who underwent MR angiogram.

In admitted stroke patients, hypertension was present in 60–70%, diabetes mellitus in 25–30%, hypercholesteromia in 15–20%, cigarette smoking in 35%, and emboligenic cardiac disease in 15–20% [3–5]. In our case control study [6], multivariate analyses identified the following independent risk factors: for CI in men, hypertension, diabetes mellitus, high salt intake, low intake of vegetables, abdominal obesity; for ICH in men, hypertension, heavy alcohol drinking and high salt intake; for CI in women, hypertension, high salt intake, abdominal obesity and lack of exercise. Diabetes mellitus was found to be a discriminant risk factor favoring development of CI (vs. ICH) [7]. Among patients with a prior history of hypertension, the mode of hypertension treatment was a significant factor related to subtype differences, such that inadequately treated hypertension favored ICH (vs. CI) [7]. It seems that low fat intake [7] or nutritional deficiency [8] is related to the development of ICH.

According to the national statistics, consumption of animal protein and fat has gradually increased from 1980 to 2000 while rice consumption has decreased. Moreover, there has been evidence that hypertension is now better controlled than before. Considering our results that untreated hypertension and nutritional deficits are related to ICH and that diabetes mellitus is preferentially related to CI, increased compliance of hypertension

Table 2
Stroke subtypes (% among ischemic stroke)

Year	Hospital	Number of patients	Large arterial disease	Small arterial disease	Cardiac embolism	Other etiologies	Undetermined etiologies	Angiogram
2003	AMC	1045	41.5	26.1	12.9	1.7	17.8	100%
2001	Yonsei	1000	16.5	21.5	18.5	3.1	40.6	53.90%
1999	Hallym	1018	35.4	37	15.9	2	15.2	not mentioned

treatment, increased prevalence of diabetes mellitus and increased meat consumption seem to explain the gradually decreased occurrence of ICH in this country.

It has been shown that Orientals more often have intracranial atherosclerosis (vs. extracranial diseases) than Caucasians [9]. In our hospital-based study, the frequency of extracranial and intracranial atherosclerosis was similar [10]. Among patients who underwent angiograms, atherosclerotic diseases were found in the middle cerebral artery (MCA) in 38% and in the internal carotid artery (ICA) in 28% (extracranial carotid artery disease in 15%). Therefore, MCA seems to be the most common site for atherosclerosis in patients with ischemic stroke [5]. Although we were not able to identify risk factors that differentiate extracranial diseases from intracranial atherosclerosis [10], the incidence of extracranial diseases appears to increase gradually, and accordingly, cases of carotid endarterectomy increased recently.

It seems that Koreans have a heavy burden of stroke risk factors. In the general population, the incidence of hypertension is not particularly high as compared with other countries [11]. However, only a small portion of hypertensive patients are treated by doctors, illustrating that hypertension is still not adequately treated. The cigarette smoking rate in adult males is >60%, which is one of the highest in the world. Another important problem we are facing is the rapidly increasing aged population due to prolonged life expectancy and a markedly decreased birth rate. It is expected that by the year 2030, 23% of Koreans will be older than 65 years. Thus, stroke will remain as a major health burden in this country.

Finally, according to our interview with 1000 randomly selected subjects living in Seoul, knowledge of stroke in the general population significantly deviated from scientific facts. For instance, although 65% of the subjects correctly identified paresis as the most important symptom of stroke, tremor was indicated incorrectly as an important symptom of stroke. Considering that a tremor has been regarded as a symptom of stroke by traditional medicine, it seems clear that the general stroke knowledge of our population is heavily influenced by the presence of alternative medicine [12]. Moreover, less than 50% of the respondents answered that they would visit a western-style general hospital immediately if they developed stroke symptoms, while others favored traditional, alternative ways of treating stroke. The preference for alternative medicine was especially high in old subjects (vs. young ones) or less-educated subjects (vs. well-educated ones) [12].

In conclusion, stroke is and will be a major social burden in Korea. Nationwide efforts are required for risk factor reduction, stroke education and the proper care of stroke victims.

References

[1] Korea National Statistical Office, Annual Report on the Cause of Death Statistics (Based on Vital Registration in year 2002), National Statistical Office, 2002.

[2] The Korean Neurological Association, Epidemiology of cerebrovascular disease in Korea: a collaborative study, 1989–1990, J. Korean Med. Sci. 8 (1993) 281–289.

[3] B.C. Lee, S.C. Jeong, S.H. Hwang, H.C. Kim, J.C. Bae, H.I. Ma, K.H. Yu, I.H. Lee, Analysis of 1129 consecutive patients with acute stroke: the Hallym stroke registry, J. Korea Stroke 1 (1999) 21–27.

[4] B.I. Lee, H.S. Nam, J.H. Heo, D.I. Kim, Yonsei stroke registry: analysis of 1000 patients with acute cerebral infarctions, Cerebrovasc. Dis. 12 (2001) 145–151.

[5] J.T. Kim, S.H. Yoo, J.H. Kwon, S.U. Kwon, J.S. Kim, Magnetic resonance angiography (MRA) based

classification of ischemic stroke: analysis of 1045 acute, consecutive patients, J. Kor. Neurol. Ass. 22 (suppl.) (2003) 39.
[6] S. Choi-Kwon, J.S. Kim, Lifestyle factors and risk of stroke in Seoul, Korea, J. Stroke Cerebrovas. Dis. 7 (1998) 414–420.
[7] J.S. Kim, S.S. Yoon, Stroke subtypes and risk factors in patients living in southern Seoul, Korea: the impact of hypertension control on stroke subtypes, J. Stroke Cerebrovasc. Dis. 7 (1998) 205–210.
[8] S. Choi-Kwon, T.H. Yang, E.K. Kim, M.Y. Jeon, J.S. Kim, Nutritional status in acute stroke: undernutrition versus overnutrition in different stroke subtypes, Acta Neurol. Scand. 98 (1998) 187–192.
[9] H.M. Liu, Y.K. Tu, P.K. Yip, C.T. Su, Evaluation of intracranial and extracranial carotid steno-cocclusive diseases in Taiwan Chinese patients with MR angiography: preliminary experience, Stroke 27 (1996) 650–653.
[10] J.S. Kim, S. Choi-Kwon, Risk factors for stroke in different levels of cerebral arterial disease, Eur. Neurol. 42 (1999) 150–156.
[11] J.S. Kim, S.J. Kim, D.W. Jones, Hypertension in Korea: a national survey, Am. J. Prev. Med. 10 (1994) 200–204.
[12] J.S. Kim, S.S. Yoon, Perspectives of stroke in persons living in Seoul, South Korea: a survey of 1000 subjects, Stroke 28 (1997) 1165–1169.

ELSEVIER

International Congress Series 1262 (2004) 352–355

ICS

www.ics-elsevier.com

Stroke therapies in Asian populations

G.A. Donnan*, M. Koga, B.B. Pedreira

Department of Neurology, National Stroke Research Institute, 300 Waterdale Rd., Heidelberg Heights, Victoria, 3081 Australia

Abstract. In spite of concerns about differing risk factor profiles in patients with stroke in Asian populations, there is some evidence that, for acute stroke therapies and secondary prevention, benefits may be at least equal to the benefits seen in Western countries. Some of the earliest evidence of potential benefits for intravenous tissue plasminogen activator (tPA) using surrogate outcome measures and randomised controlled clinical trial design were shown in a Japanese population, and one of the largest trials of acute stroke therapy was conducted on mainland China—Chinese Acute Stroke Trial (CAST) [Lancet 349 (1997) 1641]. For secondary stroke prevention, both the PATS and Perindopril Protection Against Recurrent Stroke Study (PROGRESS) trials suggested that lowering of blood pressure with either indapamide alone or indapamide + perindopril was as effective or even more so in Asian populations. Generalisation to a broad range of racial groups should be considered when conducting large international trials of stroke therapy. © 2003 Published by Elsevier B.V.

Keywords: Stroke; Therapies; Asian

1. Background

Thirty years ago, there were no interventions for patients with acute stroke or secondary prevention which were of proven benefit. Fortunately, that has changed, and there are now three acute stroke interventions for which there exists level 1 evidence of efficacy and five secondary prevention strategies.

It is often suggested that there may be racial differences in response to various forms of therapy in vascular and other diseases. This is an extension of the observation that different patterns of disease occur in different societies. In the article, we briefly discuss the response of therapies in acute stroke and secondary prevention in the context of their level of evidence for efficacy generally and in Asian countries specifically.

2. Acute therapies

There is level 1 evidence that the use of intravenous tissue plasminogen activator (tPA) given within 3 h of acute ischaemic stroke, oral aspirin within 48 h and management

* Corresponding author. Tel.: +613-9496-2699; fax: +613-9496-2650.
E-mail address: amm@austin.unimelb.edu.au (G.A. Donnan).

0531-5131/ © 2003 Published by Elsevier B.V.
doi:10.1016/j.ics.2003.12.027

within a Stroke Care Unit (SCU) improves outcomes. The administration of neuroprotective therapies has been the subject of numerous clinical trials, but none have proven to be effective. For both intravenous tPA and aspirin, there is additional evidence that these approaches may be effective in Asian populations.

2.1. tPA

Yamaguchi et al. [2]were pioneers in the use of intravenous tPA. Using reperfusion seen on angiography as a surrogate outcome measure, they conducted a randomised, double-blind, placebo-controlled trial of the use of intravenous tPA given within 6 h of stroke onset using 20 million international units (MIU) of duteplase vs. placebo in 98 patients. Posttreatment angiography demonstrated complete and > 50% reperfusion in 21.3% of rtPA and 4.3% placebo groups (P= 0.034). Furthermore, clinical outcome at about 4 weeks poststroke was significantly better in the rtPA group, and there were no differences between groups in the frequency of haemorrhagic transformation [1,2]. These findings preceded the later studies of intravenous tPA within 3 h. Improved clinical outcomes with a relative risk reduction of approximately 30%, and absolute risk reduction of around 12–14% were shown [3].

2.2. Aspirin

The Chinese Acute Stroke Trial (CAST) was published in 1997 [4]. In CAST, 21,106 patients with acute ischaemic stroke were enrolled from 413 Chinese hospitals at a mean 25 h after the onset of symptoms to receive either aspirin or placebo. Out of all the subjects, 87% had a CT prior to therapy. The investigators found a significant 14% (SD7) reduction in mortality. For their predefined endpoint of death or nonfatal stroke at 4 weeks, there was a 12% (SD6) risk reduction with aspirin compared with placebo (2P= 0.03). This was equated to an absolute difference of 6.8 fewer cases per 1000 treated. At discharge, there was an absolute reduction of 11.4 per 1000 treated in favour of aspirin (2P= 0.08). When analysed in conjunction with a similar trial, International Stroke Trial (IST), an a priori hypothesis—significant reductions in death and disability—was found [5]. Hence, the evidence that aspirin is equally effective in Asian (Chinese) populations as in Western (20,000 patients were randomised with IST to a largely European-based population) is strong.

2.3. Other therapies

Although there is no level 1 evidence for efficacy, a number are currently being evaluated. For example, fraxipirin was studied by Kay et al. [6] who conducted a randomised double-blind, placebo-controlled trial comparing two doses of low molecular weight heparin (fraxipirin) with placebo in the treatment of ischaemic stroke. There was a significant dose-dependent effect among the three studied groups in favour of low molecular weight heparin (P= 0.005, chi square test for trend). However, when a larger study was conducted using much the same protocol except for a shorter time window (24 h), no significant benefit was observed. Because of the uncertainty generated by the initial finding, a further trial (FIS-TRIS) is currently in progress (Chen, personal communication).

Interestingly, edaravone, the free radical scavenger, was approved in Japan for the treatment of acute brain infarction within 24 h after onset in April 2001. A multicentre, randomised, placebo-controlled, double-blind study on acute ischemic stroke patients commencing within 72 h of onset was conducted [7]. Edaravone was infused at a dose of 30 mg twice daily for 14 days. Patients (252) were initially enrolled. Of these, 125 were allocated to the edaravone group, and 125 were allocated to the placebo group for analysis. A significant improvement in functional outcome at discharge within 3 months or at 3 months after onset was observed in the edaravone group as evaluated by the modified Rankin Scale ($P = 0.0382$).

3. Secondary prevention

Five secondary prevention strategies have now been proven to be of benefit based on level 1 evidence. Because hypertension is the most powerful risk factor for stroke apart from increasing age, it is of particular interest in Asian populations.

3.1. Blood pressure lowering

Based partly on data from collections of large-cohort studies such as the Eastern Collaborative Group [8], there was a well-established linear relationship between increasing systolic and diastolic blood pressure levels and increased relative risk of stroke. It was estimated that about 30% of the relative risk reduction in stroke would result from about a 10-mm reduction of mean arterial blood pressure. These findings led indirectly to the Perindopril Protection Against Recurrent Stroke Study (PROGRESS) [9]. Here, 6105 patients were randomised to receive either perindopril-based therapy (perindopril alone or perindopril + indapamide) or placebo. There were 172 centres from UK, Sweden, Italy, Australia and New Zealand as well as Asian populations which included Japan and the People's Republic of China. A total of 1520 patients were randomised in China, and 815 were randomised in Japan. Overall, there was a 28% relative risk reduction in fatal and nonfatal stroke. For those in Asian regions, the hazard ratio was somewhat lower [0.37 (95%, CI 0.27–0.52)] than non-Asian groups [hazard ratio 0.76 (95%, CI 0.58–0.98)]. The efficacy of blood pressure lowering was similarly shown in the Chinese PATS trial [10] of indapamide vs. placebo. A total of 2824 patients received placebo, and 2841 received indapamide. Hazard ratio was 0.71 (95%, CI 0.58–0.88).

3.2. Antiplatelet agents

For composite vascular endpoints, the overall relative risk reduction is about 25% for antiplatelet agents. There is some evidence that aspirin alone provides about 13% relative risk reduction for the endpoints of recurrent fatal or nonfatal stroke. Furthermore, the phosphodiasterase inhibitor, dipyridamole plus aspirin may be more efficacious than either aspirin or dipyridamole alone (ESPS2) [11]. Clopidogrel is slightly superior to aspirin when composite vascular endpoints are considered (CAPRIE) [12]. The majority of studies have been performed in Western populations. However, there is one exception and that is the use of the phosphodiesterase inhibitor Cilostazol reported by Gotoh et al. [13]. The investigators conducted a randomised, controlled trial of 1200 patients with recent minor ischaemic stroke and followed these for approximately 5 years. Unfortunately, there was about 50% dropout rate, but there was an observed fatal and nonfatal stroke rate per year of 3.37% for the Cilostazol group and 5.78% for the placebo group (relative risk reduction of 41.7%). This is a somewhat more powerful effect for dipyridamole alone than in ESPS2 in which about a 16% relative risk reduction was seen compared with placebo. The study provides evidence that antiplatelet agents may be as effective among Asian populations as elsewhere.

3.3. Use of warfarin in patients with AF

Anticoagulation with warfarin using international normalised ratios (INRs) ranging from 2.0 to 3.0 is recommended for patients with nonvalvular atrial fibrillation (NVAF) who have additional risk factors. Yamaguchi et al. [14] studied the efficacy and safety of conventional- and low-intensity warfarin therapy for secondary prevention of stroke in patients with NVAF in a prospective, randomised, multicentre trial. Fifty-five and 60 patients were allocated into the conventional-intensity group (INR 2.2 to 3.5) and low-intensity group (INR 1.5–2.1), respectively. The trial was stopped when major haemorrhagic complications occurred in 6 patients of the conventional-intensity group (0%/yr, $P = 0.01$). All 6 patients with major bleeding were elderly, and their mean INR was 2.8. The annual rate of ischaemic stroke was low and similar in both groups (1.1%/yr and 1.7%/yr). For secondary prevention of stroke in persons with NVAF in Asian populations, especially in older patients, the low-intensity warfarin treatment seems to be safer than conventional-intensity treatment.

References

[1] Cerebrovasc. Dis. 3 (1993) 269–272.
[2] T. Yamaguchi, et al., in: W. Hacke, et al. (Ed.), Thrombolytic Therapy in Acute Ischemic Stroke, Springer Verlag, Berlin, 1990, pp. 161–167.
[3] Cochrane Database Syst. Rev., 2 (2000) (CD000213).
[4] Lancet 349 (1997) 1641–1649.
[5] Lancet 349 (1997) 1569–1581.
[6] N. Engl. J. Med. 333 (1995) 1588–1593.
[7] Cerebrovasc. Dis. 15 (2003) 222–229.
[8] Lancet 352 (1998) 1801–1807.
[9] Lancet 358 (2001) 1033–1041.
[10] Chin. Med. J. (Engl.) 108 (1995) 710–717.
[11] J. Neurol. Sci. 143 (1–2) (1996) 1–13.
[12] Lancet 348 (9038) (1996) 1329–1339.
[13] J. Stroke Cerebrovasc. Dis. 9 (2000) 147–157.
[14] Stroke 31 (4) (2000) 817–821.

International Congress Series 1262 (2004) 356–359

www.ics-elsevier.com

Administration of control-released basic fibroblast growth factor—Is it a more effective angiogenic therapy than bone marrow cell transplantation for severely ischemic hearts?

K. Tambara[a], Y. Sakakibara[a], G. Sakaguchi[a], Y. Tabata[b], M. Komeda[a,*]

[a] *Department of Cardiovascular Surgery, Graduate School of Medicine, Kyoto University, 54 Kawaharacho, Shogoin, Sakyo, Kyoto 606-8507, Japan*

[b] *Department of Biomaterials, Institute for Frontier Medical Sciences, Kyoto University, Kyoto, Japan*

Abstract. Therapeutic angiogenesis is an important treatment option in patients with severe ischemic heart disease because they have diffusely stenosed coronary arteries that are not suitable targets for conventional revascularization. Among such therapies, we mainly addressed administration of control-released, basic fibroblast growth factor (bFGF) as a safe and effective treatment. We applied this method in various animal models with satisfactory results, and the clinical trial will soon be started. Based on our experiments, we concluded that both control-released bFGF administration and bone marrow cell (BMC) transplantation induce angiogenesis, but only bFGF produces arteriogenesis. Future study is warranted for safe and effective clinical application of the bFGF control-release system. © 2004 Published by Elsevier B.V.

Keywords: Angiogenesis; Basic fibroblast growth factor; Bone marrow cells; Cell transplantation; Ischemic heart disease

1. Introduction

Although coronary angioplasty or coronary artery bypass grafting (CABG) have been widely accepted as standard treatments for ischemic heart disease, the efficacy in hearts with diffuse and severe coronary stenoses is often questionable or insufficient because those conventional revascularization remedies cannot secure enough blood supply to the myocardium at cell levels. From this perspective, therapeutic angiogenesis for severely ischemic hearts has recently drawn the increasing attention of cardiologists and cardiac surgeons. Among such therapies, we attend to administration of control-released basic

* Corresponding author. Tel.: +81-75-751-3780; fax: +81-75-751-3098.
E-mail address: masakom@kuhp.kyoto-u.ac.jp (M. Komeda).

0531-5131/ © 2004 Published by Elsevier B.V.
doi:10.1016/j.ics.2003.11.046

fibroblast growth factor (bFGF) to the ischemic heart [1–4]. We achieved control-release of a number of biological peptides, including growth factors, by incorporation of the peptide into gelatin hydrogel with electrostatic force. Using this method, impregnated bFGF can be gradually released over 4 weeks in situ without any systemic side effect, which is considered to be one of the hurdles for gene therapy to overcome for its safe clinical use. As another key modality for therapeutic angiogenesis, bone marrow cell (BMC) transplantation may be promising [5,6]. This method has a theoretical advantage as treatment for chronic heart failure that BMCs can be transdifferentiated to cardiomyocytes, endothelial cells, or other components.

In this review, we briefly show our results of various animal studies with the administration of control-released bFGF to the ischemic heart. Then we attend to comparisons of control-released bFGF with BMC transplantation as angiogenic agents, which may lead to animportant speculation of the difference in angiogenic properties induced by the two treatments. Finally, we refer to future prospects of therapeutic angiogenesis using the control-release system.

2. Control released bFGF in the ischemic heart

We conducted a number of studies applying the bFGF control-release system to ischemic hearts. In rat and pig myocardial infarction (MI) models, administration of control-released bFGF induced inhibition of left ventricular (LV) enlargement and improvement in LV systolic function [3,4]. Regional myocardial blood flow in the peri-MI area was increased with bFGF administration [3]. We also demonstrated that prevascularization by bFGF administration enhances the efficacy in cell transplantation [1]. When applied with CABG, control-released bFGF enabled revascularization of numerous coronary branches via an arterial graft in a rabbit acute MI model [2].

3. Comparisons with BMC transplantation

3.1. Control-release of bFGF vs. BMC transplantation

We conducted a comparative study to investigate the difference in quantity and quality of angiogenesis between control-release of bFGF and BMC transplantation using a pig MI model [7].

MI was created in 18 swine by transcatheter embolization of the left anterior descending artery [8]. Four weeks later, they were randomized into 3 groups. Group I (n=6) served as control with only saline injection, Group II (n=6) had bone marrow-derived mononuclear cell transplantation (totally $1-2\times10^8$ cells), and Group III (n=6) received injection of bFGF (200 μg)-impregnated gelatin hydrogel microspheres. Each agent was subepicardially or intramuscularly injected at 5 peri-MI areas per animal. Four weeks after the treatment, LV function was estimated by an echocardiograph and cardiac catheterization. Plasma levels of brain natriuretic peptide (BNP) were measured at baseline and at 4 weeks.

Before treatment, there was no significant difference in cardiac function among the 3 groups. Four weeks after the treatment, Groups II and III had smaller LV end-diastolic dimension (LVEDD: I, II, III; 56.7±6.2 vs. 49.2±4.6 vs. 49.1±4.9 mm, respectively, $p<0.05$), better ejection fraction (45.7±9.1% vs. 62.6±12.0% vs. 63.4±10.1%, $p<0.05$)

and better end-systolic elastance (1.34±0.26 vs. 1.52±0.83 vs. 1.72±0.65 mm Hg/ml, $p<0.01$) than Group I. There were no significant differences between Groups II and III in any parameters. The plasma levels of BNP were highest in Group I (1394±383, 1031±91, 934±306 pg/ml, $p<0.05$). Under microscopic examination, neovascularization was found at the peri-MI area in Groups II and III. It should be noted that the number of vessels more than 50 μm in Group III was higher than those in Groups I and II (6.9±3.9, 15.0±5.2, 26.2±7.1/mm^2, $p<0.05$). In an occasional section, we found cartilage formation derived from donor BMCs.

3.2. Combination therapy with skeletal myoblast (SM) transplantation

We investigated the effectiveness of control-released bFGF and transplanted BMCs in SM transplantation using a rat MI model.

In the bFGF study, we administered control-released bFGF via gelatin sheets concomitantly with SM transplantation in a rat MI model [9]. In brief, MI was created by ligating the left coronary artery in Lewis rats. Among the survivors, 30 rats with moderate-sized MI were enrolled in the study. Four weeks after ligation, they were randomized into 3 groups. In Group I (n=10), neonatal SMs (5×10^6) were subepicardially transplanted in the MI area, and then a gelatin sheet (20×20 mm) containing 100 μg bFGF was placed onto the LV surface to cover the MI and peri-MI areas. In Group II (n=10), SM transplantation and a sheet with saline alone were applied in the same manner. Group III (n=10) had culture medium injection with a sheet containing saline alone and served as control. Four weeks after treatment, all rats were sacrificed following echocardiography and cardiac catheterization. Each heart specimen was sliced at 100-μm thickness intervals, and the sections were stained with von Willebrand factor and fast skeletal myosin heavy chain to calculate vascular density and graft volume (using Simpson's method), respectively. Four weeks later, in Group I, LVEDD (I, II, III; 0.92±0.02 vs. 0.96±0.02 vs. 0.99±0.02 cm) and the MI size was smallest ($p<0.05$, respectively). Also, end-systolic elastance was highest and tau was lowest in Group I (both $p<0.01$). The graft volume in Group I was much larger than that in Group II (13.3±2.1 vs. 4.9±1.0 mm^3, $p<0.01$). Vascular density in the MI and peri-MI area was highest in Group I (peri-MI; 109±13 vs. 53±6 vs. 50±7/mm^2, $p<0.01$). Within the graft, the number of vessels with diameters over 50 μm was 1.8±0.6/mm^2 in Group I, while there were no such large vessels seen in Group II.

In the BMC study, we performed cotransplantation of SMs and BMCs using syngeneic Lewis rats. Briefly, MI was induced by ligating the left coronary artery. Four weeks later, animals were randomized into 3 groups. Group I (n=8) received culture medium alone (control), Group II (n=8) had SM transplantation (5×10^6 cells), and Group III (n=6) had cotransplantation of SMs (5×10^6) and BMCs (1×10^6). Each agent was subepicardially injected in the MI area. BMCs were labeled and green fluorescent LV function was assessed by echocardiography for 4 weeks. LVEDD was gradually increased in Group I, while that in Groups II and III was unchanged at 4 weeks (9.99±0.29 vs. 8.31±0.36 vs. 8.18±0.48 mm, $p<0.01$). Fractional area change was unchanged in Groups I and II, while that in Group III was increased at 4 weeks (30±2% vs. 35±4% vs. 46±5%, $p<0.05$). Histologically, the survival extent of the transplanted SM was similar between Groups II and III. In addition, the number of vessels found in the peri-MI area was largest in Group III, followed by Group II.

3.3. Conclusion

We should be careful when summarizing the results because the studies were independently conducted on various experimental models. However, our findings suggested a significant difference in angiogenic properties between bFGF administration and BMC transplantation. Namely, bFGF induces arteriogenesis, but BMC does not. It may be reasonably attributed to arteriogenesis induced by control-released bFGF that SM-derived graft volume was increased in SM transplantation with bFGF administration.

4. Future prospects of control-released bFGF to ischemic hearts

As demonstrated in Sections 2 and 3, administration of control-released bFGF may be a safe and effective angiogenic therapy for patients with severe ischemic heart disease. However, the optimal regimen of control-released angiogenic factors with gelatin hydrogel is still unclear, for instance concerning factors such as dosage and timing. In addition, there remain some biotechnological issues in the bFGF control-release system as the releasing period is limited to 2–3 months and the releasing curve is not linear.

Recent development in robotic surgery is remarkable, and the minimally invasive drug delivery system using such instruments may enable repetitively or serially transthoracic administration of angiogenic factors to the heart in patients with end-stage heart failure. Basic and clinical research on this field is warranted.

References

[1] Y. Sakakibara, et al., Prevascularization with gelatin microspheres containing basic fibroblast growth factor enhances the benefits of cardiomyocyte transplantation, J. Thorac. Cardiovasc. Surg. 124 (2002) 50–60.

[2] K. Ueyama, et al., Developing "bio-CABG": revascularizing numerous coronary branches by the arterial graft, Circulation 106 (Suppl. 2) (2002) 552.

[3] A. Iwakura, et al., Intramyocardial sustained delivery of basic fibroblast growth factor improves angiogenesis and ventricylar function in a rat infarct model, Heart Vessels 18 (2003) 93–99.

[4] Y. Sakakibara, et al., Toward surgical angiogenesis using slow-released basic fibroblast growth factor, Eur. J. Cardio-Thorac. Surg. 24 (2003) 105–111.

[5] H. Kamihata, et al., Implantation of bone marrow mononuclear cells into ischemic myocardium enhances collateral perfusion and regional function via side supply of angioblasts, angiogenic ligands, and cytokines, Circulation 104 (2001) 1046–1052.

[6] K. Hamano, et al., Local implantation of autologous bone marrow cells for therapeutic angiogenesis in patients with ischemic heart disease: clinical trial and preliminary results, Jpn. Circ. J. 65 (2001) 845–847.

[7] Y. Sakakibara, et al., Which is a more effective angiogenic therapy, bone marrow cell transplantation or control-released basic fibroblast growth factor administration? Circulation 106 (Suppl. 2) (2002) II419.

[8] G. Sakaguchi, et al., A pig model of chronic heart failure by intracoronary embolisation with gelatin sponge, Ann. Thorac. Surg. 75 (2003) 1942–1947.

[9] K. Tambara, et al., Simultaneous administration of control-released basic fibroblast growth factor enhances the efficacy of skeletal myoblast transplantation by increasing vascular density and graft volume, Circulation (2003) (in press).

International Congress Series 1262 (2004) 360–363

www.ics-elsevier.com

Will all postinfarction patients receive defibrillators? Recent trials and expanding indications

Paul A. Friedman*

Mayo Clinic, Cardiovascular Diseases Department, 200 First Street SW, Mary Brigh, 4-523, Rochester, MN 55905, USA

Abstract. Implantable defibrillators have been demonstrated to be the most effective therapy for secondary prevention of sudden cardiac death. Unfortunately, however, many patients succumb to their initial episode of cardiac arrest so that primary prevention strategies are warranted. Several studies have demonstrated the mortality benefit of prophylactic, implantable defibrillators in patients with coronary artery disease depressed ventricular function and nonsustained ventricular tachycardia with inducible ventricular tachycardia during electrophysiologic study. However, widespread application of this approach is limited by the need for invasive risk stratification. The results of the MADIT II study, which demonstrate mortality reduction with prophylactic ICD implantation in patients with previous myocardial infarction and severe left ventricular dysfunction in the absence of invasive risk stratification, have dramatic implications for the management of this high-risk population. This article will review these data and their implications. © 2004 Published by Elsevier B.V.

Keywords: Sudden cardiac death; Myocardial infarction; Congestive heart failure; Ventricular tachycardia; Ventricular fibrillation

Michel Mirowski pioneered the implantable defibrillator in the 1960s after the death of a close friend and mentor from recurrent ventricular arrhythmias. His frustration with available therapies led to the idea of an implantable device to continuously monitor the cardiac rhythm and deliver lifesaving shocks immediately when needed. Over the ensuing years, technical advances, including the introduction of biphasic waveforms, the development of transvenous lead systems, and the use of painless antitachycardia pacing, have resulted in diminished, device-related morbidity, greater ease of implantation, and greater acceptance of device therapy by patients and physicians [1]. Given their effectiveness, implantable defibrillators (ICDs) are now nearly universally chosen for those individuals fortunate enough to survive out-of-hospital cardiac arrest. However, because 95% of

* Tel.: +1-507-255-2446; fax: +1-507-255-2550.
E-mail address: pfriedman@mayo.edu (P.A. Friedman).

0531-5131/ © 2004 Published by Elsevier B.V.
doi:10.1016/j.ics.2004.02.010

victims of out-of-hospital cardiac arrest succumb to the initial episode, identification and prophylactic treatment of high-risk individuals (primary prevention) is desirable [2]. The challenge for the clinician has been to identify the high-risk individual.

It has long been known that patients with depressed ventricular function following myocardial infarction are at increased risk for sudden death [3]. However, whether treatment of ventricular arrhythmias would lead to increased heart failure death or improved survival in this population was hotly debated. Two large primary prevention studies, the first Multicenter Automatic Defibrillator Implantation Trial (MADIT) [4] and the Multicenter Unsustained Tachycardia Trial (MUSTT) [5] enrolled patients with coronary artery disease, nonsustained ventricular tachycardia, and depressed ventricular function (ejection fraction 0.35 or less, or 0.40 or less, respectively). Patients underwent an invasive electrophysiologic study, and those with inducible ventricular arrhythmias had improved survival with ICD implantation. Subsequent analysis demonstrated that those patients with the poorest ventricular function derived the greatest benefit [6]. Despite obvious mortality reduction in this high-risk population, the need for invasive screening of asymptomatic individuals prevented widespread adoption of this approach.

The second MADIT study [7] overcame these limitations by eliminating invasive screening. In this prospective, randomized, clinical trial, patients with an ejection fraction 0.30 or less, in the absence of recent myocardial infarction or surgical revascularization, derived significant benefit from prophylactic ICD placement compared with conventional medical therapy. During 20 months of follow-up, there was a 20% relative risk reduction (6% absolute reduction) of death from any cause in the ICD group. Importantly, defibrillator therapy was found beneficial when added to effective drug therapy. Study patients received angiotensin-concerting enzyme inhibitors (68%), beta-blockers (70%), and lipid-lowering statins (67%). Moreover, in the context of other major cardiovascular trials that have significantly impacted practice, the MADIT II study results remain compelling (Fig. 1, courtesy of Dr. Arthur Moss).

How should the clinician apply the findings of these trials? While the MADIT II findings are persuasive, they should be applied judiciously. Patients not on optimal medical therapy for depressed ventricular function and coronary disease should receive those medications proven to improve survival, and then undergo reevaluation of ventricular function at a reasonable interval, such as 3 months. Similarly, patients with an ejection fraction of 0.30 or less and recent surgical revascularization are best treated with optimal medical therapy in the perioperative period. Reassessment of ventricular function at 3 months, with the use of defibrillator therapy in the absence of improvement, is supported by available data. In contrast, prophylactic ICD placement at the time of surgical revascularization has not improved survival, likely due to the potent benefit from coronary bypass [8]. Asymptomatic patients with an ejection fraction greater than 0.30 but less than or equal to 0.40 with nonsustained arrhythmia are at intermediate risk, and are best risk-stratified by an invasive, electrophysiologic study at present [4,5].

Many important questions remain. The observation in MADIT II of a higher rate of new or worsening heart failure is worrisome. The authors speculate that improved survival may have allowed time for heart failure to develop. However, right ventricular pacing may be deleterious in this population; it is conceivable that reprogramming defibrillators to minimize pacing, or use of two ventricular leads to permit cardiac resynchronization, may

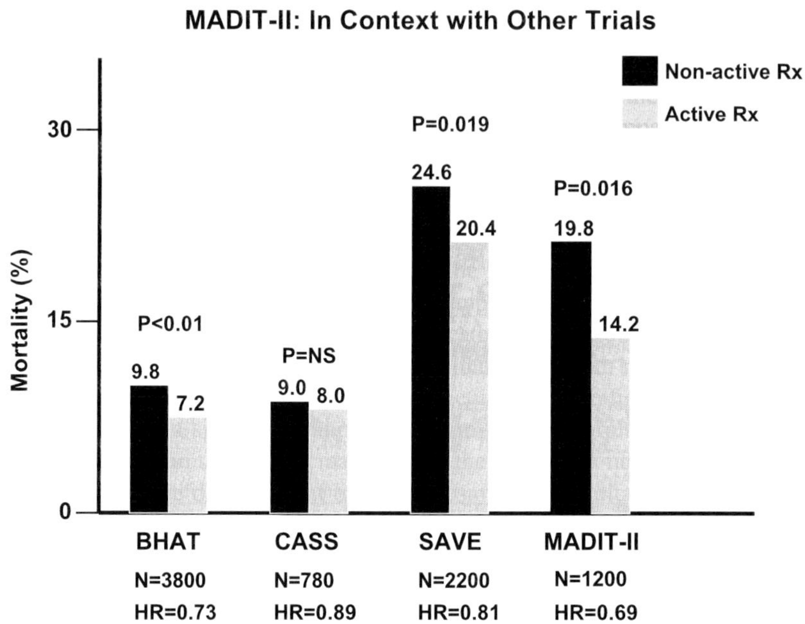

Fig. 1. MADIT II in context with other cardiovascular trials. Hazard ratio (HR). (Courtesy of Dr. A.J. Moss).

mitigate this complication [9]. A pressing need for enhanced, noninvasive risk stratification exists to identify patients with an ejection fraction above 0.30 at high risk of sudden death. Additionally, a method to determine which patients with ejection fractions 0.30 or less are at reduced risk is lacking; these patients might be spared surgical device placement. Identification of high-risk individuals in other disease states, including dilated cardiomyopathy, hypertrophic cardiomypathy, long QT syndrome, Brugada syndrome and other conditions remains challenging. Despite these gaps in our knowledge, the MADIT II study, in conjunction with previous trials, provides an evidence-based approach for selecting coronary disease patients who may benefit from primary, sudden death prevention with implantable defibrillator therapy.

References

[1] M. Glikson, P. Friedman, The implantable cardioverter defibrillator, Lancet 357 (2001) 1107.

[2] J.T. Bigger, Expanding indications for implantable cardiac defibrillators, New England Journal of Medicine 346 (2002) 931–933.

[3] J. Bigger, et al.., Multicenter Post-Infarction Research Group, The relationships among ventricular arrhythmias, left ventricular dysfunction, and mortality in the 2 years after myocardial infarction, Circulation 69 (1984) 250–258.

[4] A.J. Moss, et al., Improved survival with an implanted defibrillator in patients with coronary disease at high risk for ventricular arrhythmia. Multicenter Automatic Defibrillator Implantation Trial Investigators, New England Journal of Medicine 335 (1996) 1933–1940.

[5] A.E. Buxton, et al., A randomized study of the prevention of sudden death in patients with coronary artery disease. Multicenter Unsustained Tachycardia Trial Investigators, New England Journal of Medicine 341 (1999) 1882–1890.

[6] A.J. Moss, Implantable cardioverter defibrillator therapy: the sickest patients benefit the most [editorial; comment], Circulation 101 (2000) 1638–1640.
[7] A.J. Moss, et al., Prophylactic implantation of a defibrillator in patients with myocardial infarction and reduced ejection fraction, New England Journal of Medicine 346 (2002) 877–883.
[8] J.T. Bigger Jr., Prophylactic use of implanted cardiac defibrillators in patients at high risk for ventricular arrhythmias after coronary-artery bypass graft surgery. Coronary Artery Bypass Graft (CABG) Patch Trial Investigators [see comments], New England Journal of Medicine 337 (1997) 1569–1575.
[9] S. Cazeau, et al., Effects of multisite biventricular pacing in patients with heart failure and intraventricular conduction delay, New England Journal of Medicine 344 (2001) 873–880.

International Congress Series 1262 (2004) 364–367

www.ics-elsevier.com

First human randomized trial of G-CSF stem cell mobilization to treat large acute myocardial infarction—preliminary results of a pilot study

Stephen G. Ellis*, Marc Penn, Brian Bolwell, Gerry McConnell, Kelly Brezina, Eric J. Topol

Department of Cardiovascular Medicine, The Cleveland Clinic Foundation, 9500 Euclid Avenue, F-25, Cleveland, OH 44195, USA

Abstract. Based upon substantial preclinical testing, we initiated an FDA-sanctioned, single-site dose escalation study of granulocyte colony stimulation factor (G-CSF) to attempt to enhance myocardial healing for patients with large acute MI via mobilization of stem cells. Principal inclusion criteria were age ≤ 80 yrs, acute ST elevation MI reperfused late (4–48 h), EF 20–39%, and coronary anatomy unlikely to require CABG. Patients were randomized to G-CSF or placebo in a 2:1 fashion and treated for 5 days starting <48 h from MI onset. Initial daily SQ dose was 5 μg/kg day. Primary safety and efficacy endpoints are rupture-free survival and change in EF to 30 days. To date, six patients have been randomized. Final results of this pilot study will provide important information upon which to base further trials of G-CSF in the setting of acute MI.

Keywords: Acute MI; Bone marrow stimulant

1. Introduction

Although reperfusion therapy has revolutionized the management of patients presenting with acute myocardial infarction, approximately 15% of the 1.3 million patients in the United States who initially survive acute infarction to present in the emergency room each year still expire within 30 days of the event [1]. Patient age, early heart muscle function, and infarction location are the primary factors, other than therapy, that determine outcome [1]. Multiple, randomized clinical trials (RCT) have shown that the principal benefit of reperfusion therapy on survival accrues to patients who present within 3 h of symptom onset [1], yet the typical patient presents to hospital beyond this therapeutic window [1].

With the increased understanding of the plasticity of stem cells normally resident in bone marrow, peripheral circulating blood, skeletal muscle, and elsewhere, there has been a

* Corresponding author. Tel.: +1-216-445-6712; fax: +1-216-445-6714.
E-mail address: elliss@ccf.org (S.G. Ellis).

0531-5131/ © 2004 Published by Elsevier B.V.
doi:10.1016/j.ics.2003.11.042

dramatic increase in interest in repopulating damaged myocardium to improve cardiac function. Many types of cells, when injected directly into normal or scarred myocardium, can take up residence there [2], although few have been shown to establish the typical markers of normal myocyte–myocyte interaction such as connexin-43 [2]. Even so, chronic improvement in left ventricular performance has been demonstrated, probably due to decreased wall stress consequent to cell-induced passive wall thickening and possibly from increased systolic contractility [2]. Studies with skeletal muscle satellite cells have progressed to human trials [3].

Alternatively, injection of primitive bone marrow-derived cells (Lin^{-}c-kit^{pos}) into recently infarcted myocardium has yielded newly resident cells in large numbers that express markers of myocytes (e.g. Csx/Nkx 2.5, GATA-4, MEF2, cardiac myosin) or endothelial cells (e.g. F1k-1, VE-cadherin, factor VIII) and appear to augment both systolic left ventricular performance measured by dp/dt and improve regional blood flow [2]. Importantly, G-CSF-mobilized $CD34^{+}$ cells injected intravenously or released directly from stimulated allogenic bone marrow appear both to home to recently infarcted myocardium and improve survival and cardiac function after infarction in a rat model [2]. Transplantation of cytokine-mobilized peripheral blood stem cells was first accomplished in humans in 1989 [4] and is now a common means to repopulate the bone marrow in patients undergoing chemotherapy for cancer. The stage appears set, then, for the treatment of damaged human myocardium using these concepts.

2. Methods

2.1. Inclusion/exclusion criteria

Patients: Acute myocardial infarction 4–48 h after onset treated with successful primary or rescue intervention and

(i) age < 80 years
(ii) left ventricular ejection fraction 20–39%
(iii) new proximal or mid-LAD or dominant RCA/circumflex occlusion
(iv) absence of cardiogenic shock, contradictions to filgrastim, etc.

Rationale: A new therapy that carries with it many unknown risks should be applied only to patients whose risk without therapy is reasonably high, hence the inclusion criteria i–iv. The rationale for the time window for inclusion is that patients treated within 4 h, even with initially poor left ventricular function, have far greater likelihood of left ventricular recovery and survival than those presenting later. The upper end of the window is based upon the typical approximate 3 days required to mobilize large numbers of stem cells using G-CSF and the probable need to speed such cells to the damaged myocardium. Capacity for G-CSF mobilization of marrow stem cells is inversely related to patient age, hence criteria i.

2.2. Allocation to treatment

Randomized, double-blind 2:1 active/placebo, two-step dose escalation study ($n = 6$ per group).

Table 1
Preliminary results ($n=6$)

Age	54 ± 12 years	fold increase baseline to max CD117	16.4 ± 9.2 ×
Time MI to reperfusion	12 ± 6 h	baseline WBC	12.3 ± 4.1
Time MI to G-CSF/placebo	33 ± 22 h	peak WBC	22.6 ± 5.5
Fold increase baseline to max CD34	12.8 ± 7.7 ×	baseline LVEF	31 ± 4
		30-day LVEF	39 ± 4
		30-day survival	100%

The rationale for the need for a placebo group is, primarily, that one needs to establish some benchmark for the typical follow-up wall thickness in the type of patients to be enrolled. Without this, it would be very difficult to establish safety criteria other than the absence of perforation, which hopefully will be an extremely rare event. The rationale for the two-step dosing aspect of the trial configuration is that since there is a concern about possible risk, we should start out with a lower dose than is typically used in oncology and only progress to a higher dose once we are reasonably satisfied of the safety of the lower dose.

2.3. Primary endpoints

(i) Safety—Absence of myocardial rupture or significant thinning
(ii) Efficacy—Measures of global and regional left ventricular performance (change in LVAF, baseline to 30 days) and stem cell mobilization

3. Results

Patient recruitment is ongoing. Initial blinded data are provided in Table 1.

4. Discussion

Chronic congestive heart failure complicating large myocardial infarction continues to be the source of considerable morbidity, mortality, and expenditure for industrialized countries [1]. There is now ample evidence that cells of a number of origins when injected directly into the damaged myocardium may take up residence there and, under certain circumstances, survive for a protracted period of time [2]. Typically, but not always, these cells do not fully integrate into their new milieu and, in fact, electrical mechanical coupling of injected and remaining viable cells is infrequently accomplished. We and others have taken the tact that to recapitulate normal organ development, the body needs to rely on more natural mechanisms of cell "homing" [5]. The presently described study is the first randomized trial attempting to ascertain whether or not there may be safety and clinical efficacy with this approach. The results, whatever they may be, will provide initial guidance for subsequently more definitive studies, which will establish or refute the role of stem cell therapy for treatment of acute myocardial infarction and chronic congestive heart failure.

References

[1] E.J. Topol, et al., Acute myocardial infarction: early diagnosis and management, Textbook of Cardiovascular Medicine, 2nd ed. pp., Lippincott Williams & Wilkins, New York, 2002.
[2] J.S. Forrester, et al., Stem cell repair of infarcted myocardium, Circulation 108 (2003) 1139–1145.

[3] P. Menasché, et al., Myoblast transplantation for heart failure, Lancet 357 (2001) 279–281.
[4] A.M. Gianni, et al., Granulocyte-macrophage colony-stimulating factor to harvest circulating haemopoietic stem cells for autotransplantation, Lancet 2 (1989) 580–585.
[5] A.T. Askari, et al., Effect of stromal- cell-derived factor-1 on stem cell homing and tissue regeneration in ischaemic cardiomyopathy, Lancet 362.

International Congress Series 1262 (2004) 368–371

www.ics-elsevier.com

Adiponectin as a potential key player in metabolic syndrome Insights into atherosclerosis, diabetes and cancer

Tohru Funahashi[a,*], Yuji Matsuzawa[b], Shinji Kihara

[a] *Department of Internal Medicine and Molecular Science, Osaka University Graduate School of Medicine, 2-2 Yamada-oka, Suita, Osaka 565-0871, Japan*

[b] *Sumitomo Hospital, 5-3-20 Nakanoshima, Kita, Osaka 530-0005, Japan*

Abstract. The adipose tissue produces and secretes many bioactive substances, collectively referred to as adipocytokines. Adiponectin is an adipocytokine, which we identified by screening the adipose-specific genes from human fat. Plasma concentration of adiponectin is reduced in visceral obesity. Adiponectin accumulated in injured vascular wall, and exhibited anti-atherogenic moieties. Adiponectin knockout mice exhibit a more severe insulin resistance. The human mutation of adiponectin gene accompanying hypoadiponectinemia is strongly associated with both atherosclerotic vascular diseases and type 2 diabetes. We conclude that hypoadiponectinemia stands upstream of the pathophysiology of metabolic syndrome leading to atherosclerosis. © 2004 Published by Elsevier B.V.

Keywords: Adiponectin; Visceral obesity; Metabolic syndrome

1. Introduction

The World Health Organization has reported that cardiovascular diseases are currently the most common cause of death throughout the world, including Asia and Africa. The metabolic syndrome, a cluster of glucose intolerance, hypertension, dyslipidemia, and visceral obesity is the common basis of atherosclerotic vascular diseases. What is the molecular mechanism that links visceral fat and metabolic syndrome? In this review, we describe the discovery of adipocyte-derived protein, adiponectin, and its role as a potential key player in the metabolic syndrome.

2. Discovery of adiponectin

In the early 1990s, our group investigated the expression profile of adipose tissue in collaboration with the human body map project team. Traditionally, adipose tissue

* Corresponding author. Tel.: +81-6-6879-3732; fax: +81-6-6879-3739.
E-mail address: tohru@imed2.med.osaka-u.ac.jp (T. Funahashi).

0531-5131/ © 2004 Published by Elsevier B.V.
doi:10.1016/j.ics.2004.01.091

has been regarded as a simple energy storage organ. Surprisingly, adipose tissues, particularly visceral fat, expressed a variety of genes for secretory proteins including growth factors, cytokines and vasoactive substances. We collectively named these adipocyte-derived molecules as 'adipocytokines'. Through systemic analysis of adipose-expressed genes, we discovered a novel adipocyte-derived factor, named adiponectin. Adiponectin has two distinguished characteristics. One is that plasma concentration of adiponectin decreases upon accumulation of visceral fat. Another characteristic is that adiponectin accumulates in injured vascular walls; adiponectin bound to collagens I, III, and V present in the subendothelial intima. This is the reason we named this protein 'adiponectin'.

3. Adiponectin and atherosclerosis

Administration of adiponectin suppressed TNF-α-induced expression of adhesion molecules by inhibiting nuclear translocation of NFκB [1]. Adiponectin also suppressed growth factor-induced proliferation of smooth muscle cells by inhibiting classical mitogen activated protein (MAP) kinase pathway. In macrophages, adiponectin suppressed the expression of scavenger receptor and foam cell formation. These data suggest that circulating adiponectin accumulates in the locus, in which the endothelial barrier is damaged, and exhibits protective activities against almost all the process of atherosclerosis. To test this hypothesis, we generated adiponectin knockout mice [2]. Adiponectin knockout mice showed severer neointimal thickening in response to vascular injury compared with the wild-type mice [3]. To elucidate the effect of adiponectin on the fat-rich atheromatous lesions, we overexpressed adiponectin in apoE knockout mice. Overexpression of adiponectin significantly reduced the fatty streak area [4]. Expression of vascular cell adhesion molecule 1 (VCAM-1) and class A scavenger receptor was decreased.

Clinically, plasma adiponectin levels in subjects with coronary artery disease were significantly lower compared with those of body mass index (BMI)-matched controls [1]. The low concentrations of plasma adiponectin were significantly associated with the risk of coronary artery disease in men.

4. Adiponectin and diabetes mellitus

Type 2 diabetes mellitus is a common cause of atherosclerotic vascular disease. Plasma adiponectin level correlated positively with insulin sensitivity determined by glucose clamp test in humans and nonhuman primates. We investigated insulin sensitivity in adiponectin knockout mice [2]. Plasma glucose and insulin levels were normal under normal chow, but once high-fat/high sucrose diet was loaded, plasma glucose and insulin concentrations in the knockout mice increased to levels higher than in wild-type mice. The knockout mice exhibited severer insulin resistance relative to the wild-type mice.

Pima Indians are prone to developing obesity and type 2 diabetes, but not all Pima develop type 2 diabetes. Pima Indians with high plasma adiponectin at baseline had low risk of the development of diabetes. Adiponectin is the first example of adipocytokines to

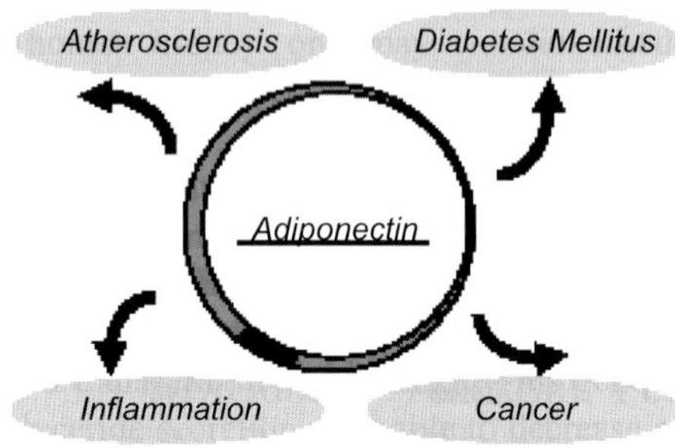

Fig. 1. Adiponectin and obesity-related diseases. Hyposecretion of adiponectin may play an important role in the development of obesity-related diseases.

demonstrate a protective effect against the development of diabetes. Therefore, adiponectin has dual functions; protecting against insulin resistance and atherosclerosis.

We also analyzed the genetic cause of hypoadiponectinemia in humans. For this purpose, we screened patients for mutations in the adiponectin gene, and found several mutations. Among them, we focused on missense mutation with the substitution of isoleucine 164 to threonine in the globular domain. Disturbed secretion of this mutant protein was noted, together with markedly low plasma adiponectin levels. The subjects carrying this mutation were frequently hypertensive, hyperlipidemic, diabetic, and had atherosclerotic vascular diseases (i.e., clinical phenotype of metabolic syndrome). Thus, both environmental and genetic causes of hypoadiponectinemia are associated with the metabolic syndrome. Adiponectin may be a key player in metabolic syndrome.

5. Adiponectin and cancer

The associations of obesity with breast cancer, and endometrial cancer risks have been well established. Aromatizing conversion of the androgens to estrone in the adipose tissue may contribute to the development of these cancers. However, dysregulation of adipocyte-derived hormones may also participate in increasing the risk of carcinogenesis. We have recently reported that low serum adiponectin level is associated with an increased risk of breast cancer [5]. It has been also reported that serum adiponectin level is inversely related to the risk of endometrial cancer independent of BMI in women younger than 65 years of age. The molecular mechanism of adiponectin-induced enhancement of the carcinogenic process of various cancers needs further examination.

Hyposecretion of adiponectin may play an important role in the development of various obesity-related diseases (Fig. 1).

References

[1] N. Ouchi, et al., Novel modulator for endothelial adhesion molecules: adipocyte-derived plasma protein adiponectin, Circulation 100 (1999) 2473–2476.

[2] N. Maeda, et al., Diet-induced insulin resistance in mice lacking adiponectin/ACRP30, Nat. Med. 8 (2002) 731–737.

[3] M. Matsuda, et al., Role of adiponectin in preventing vascular stenosis. The missing link of adipo-vascular axis, J. Biol. Chem. 277 (2002) 37487–37491.

[4] Y. Okamoto, et al., Adiponectin reduces atherosclerosis in apolipoprotein E-deficient mice, Circulation 106 (22) (2002) 2767–2770.

[5] Y. Miyoshi, et al., Association of serum adiponectin levels with breast cancer risk, Clin. Cancer Res., 2003 (in press).

International Congress Series 1262 (2004) 372–375

www.ics-elsevier.com

Obesity and other risk factors for cardiovascular diseases among Africans: results from CARDIAC study in Tanzania

Marina Njelekela[a,*], Katsumi Ikeda[b], Jacob Mtabaji[a], Yukio Yamori[c]
On behalf of the WHO-cardiovascular diseases and alimentary comparison (CARDIAC) study group

[a] *Department of Physiology, School of Medicine, Muhimbili University College of Health Sciences, P.O. Box 65001, Dar es salaam, Tanzania*
[b] *Department of Human and Environmental Science, Mukogawa Women's University, Koshien, Hyogo, Japan*
[c] *WHO Center for Primary Prevention of CVD, Kyoto, Japan*

Abstract. *Objective*: To investigate the prevalence of obesity and central adiposity and to assess if any significant relationship exists between obesity and other risk factors for cardiovascular diseases (CVD) in an African population. *Methods*: A cross-sectional, epidemiological study was conducted in three distinct areas: urban, rural and a pastoralist population in Tanzania. *Results*: The overall prevalence of obesity (body mass index (BMI) ≥ 30 kg/m^2) was 14.2% and that of adiposity was 16.9%. Of the obese participants, 40.5% had reached higher education levels and 59.1% lived in the urban area. Significant hypertension (48.1%), hypercholesterolemia (32.4%), hypertriglyceridemia (20.3%), elevated LDL-C (33.8%), and hyperglycemia (4.6%) were seen among obese participants. Elevated plasma leptin concentration and low REE were observed among obese participants. *Conclusion*: Obesity, associated with significant biochemical derangement, is now a health problem in Tanzania. Effective strategies for primary prevention of obesity need to be introduced, especially in urban areas in Tanzania.

Keywords: Obesity; CVD risk factors; Urban; Education; Occupation; Africans

1. Introduction

Many developing countries, including Tanzania, are still contending with infectious diseases although the prevalence of a number of non-communicable diseases, such as diabetes and hypertension, is increasing rapidly, particularly in urban areas [1]. Obesity is one of the modifiable major risk factors for cardiovascular diseases (CVD) and one of the

* Corresponding author. Tel.: +255-22-2150302; fax: +255-22-2150465.
E-mail address: mnjelekela@muchs.ac.tz (M. Njelekela).

0531-5131/
doi:10.1016/j.ics.2003.11.047

contributing factors in the development of diabetes and hypertension [2]. In some African countries, the prevalence of obesity has been found to be higher in urban areas as compared with rural areas [3]. Factors contributing towards obesity in African countries have also been previously reported [4]. With a higher body mass index (BMI), other CVD risk factors, such as hypertension, hypercholesterolemia, and hyperglycemia, tend to be elevated as well. Thus, this study reports on the prevalence of obesity and central adiposity and assesses if any significant relationship exists between obesity and other risk factors for CVD in Tanzania.

2. Materials and methods

Data for this study were collected as part of the CARDIAC-MONALISA (MONeo ALImentation SAnae) Study, which was conducted in Tanzania in 1998. The study aimed at monitoring past trends in the populations previously included in the original CARDIAC study. The methodology has been described in detail in one of our previous publications [5]. In summary, the survey involved approximately 100 men and 100 women aged 46–58 years from the three areas of Dar es Salaam, Handeni and Monduli, respectively.

Anthropometric measurements and BP were measured. REE was estimated using Hosoya's portable indirect calorimeter (HPIC, METAVINE, VINE Limited, Osaka, Japan). In this analysis, education and occupation were taken as measures of socio-economic status (SES) [6]. Samples of blood and urine were shipped to the central WHO CARDIAC Study laboratory in Kyoto, Japan, for analysis.

3. Statistical analysis

All analyses were done using Stat view statistical software. The difference between the means across groups was tested by analysis of variance. Proportions were compared by contingency table analysis with a chi (χ^2) square test. Statistical significance was defined as $p<0.05$. Separate analyses were conducted for men and women.

4. Results

The analysis included 545 participants from the three distinct areas. The response rate was 90.8%. The overall prevalence of obesity (BMI $\geq$ 30 kg/m^2) was 14.2% and that of central adiposity (WC>102 cm) was 16.9% among men and 49.6% among women (WC > 88 cm). Participants from the urban area showed a significantly higher mean weight, WC, BMI, and blood pressure level, a higher prevalence of obesity and central adiposity compared with those in the rural and pastoralist populations. Resting energy expenditure was highest among the pastoralists and participants from rural areas (results not shown).

Fig. 1 shows the prevalence of CVD risk factors among lean, obese and morbidly obese participants for both men and women. The overall prevalence of hypertension was 48.1%, hypercholesterolemia 32.4%, hypertriglyceridemia 20.3%, elevated LDL-C 33.8%, and hyperglycemia 4.6%, respectively. Of the obese participants, 40.5% had formal education and 59.1% lived in the urban area. Participants who received formal education for 9 years or more showed a significantly higher BMI (men, $p<0.001$, women $p<0.0001$) and a higher prevalence of elevated HBA1c percent ($\geq$ 7%) (women 40.0%, $p<0.05$). Consumption of

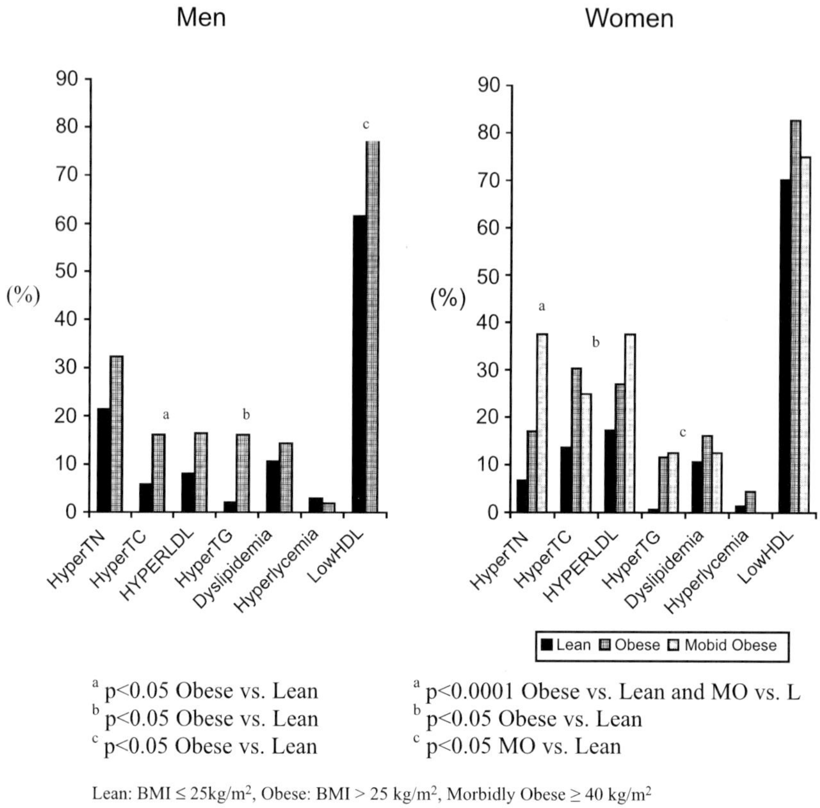

Fig. 1. Prevalence of risk factors for CVD among lean (L), obese (O) and morbidly obese (MO) men and women.

a high calorie diet, such as coconut milk and meat for more than 3 days in a week, was higher in the educated group: meat (men 52.7%, $p<0.001$; women 30.4%, $p<0.0001$) and coconut milk (men 51.9%, $p<0.001$; women 32.3%, $p<0.0001$), respectively.

5. Discussion

The elevated BMI and waist circumference in urban dwellers and among skilled workers indicates that as people become more affluent obesity levels tend to increase [7]. The change in diet structure and acquisition of professional and leisure occupation strongly relate to urbanization [8], which results in a change in CVD risk factor pattern in the urban areas compared with rural areas. In most developing countries, obesity is not yet recognized as a major health problem and resources set for non-communicable disease prevention and treatment are few [1]. The findings of this study attest to an association between obesity with the expected lipid derangements that would constitute part of the predisposition to cardiovascular disease and the metabolic syndrome in urban areas in Africa. Both WC and BMI elevations are commonly associated with dyslipidemia [2,7]. Blood pressure levels and prevalence of hypertension increased with obesity. The association between elevated BMI and hypertension has been reported in another study in Africa [9]. Obesity decreases insulin signal transduction of the insulin receptor leading to insulin resistance [10]. The findings of this study tend to reinforce the fact that diagnosing obesity and identifying an individual and populations at risk requires at most a measuring tape and a weighing scale. The derived BMI and WC allow the identification of "action points" for intervention. The addition of lipid measurements, blood pressure readings and a fasting blood sugar would enable clinical diagnosis of the metabolic syndrome, which should be a target for intensive therapeutic lifestyle changes.

Acknowledgements

We would like to express our sincere appreciation to our participants and to the Center for Primary Prevention of Cardiovascular Diseases Kyoto for funding this project.

References

[1] N. Unwin, et al., Noncommunicable diseases in sub-Saharan Africa: where do they feature in the health research agenda? Bull. World Health Organ., Suppl. 79 (2001) 907.
[2] P. Poirier, et al., Obesity and cardiovascular disease, Curr. Atheroscler. Rep. 4 (2002) 448–453.
[3] M.A. Van der Sande, et al., Blood pressure patterns and cardiovascular risk factors in rural and urban Gambian communities, J. Hum. Hypertens. 14 (2000) 489–496.
[4] P. Bovet, et al., Distribution of blood pressure, body mass index and smoking habits in the urban population of Dar Es Salaam, Tanzania, and associations with economic status, Int. J. Epidemiol. 31 (2002) 240–247.
[5] M. Njelekela, et al., Prevalence of obesity in middle aged men and women in Tanzania Africa: relationship with resting energy expenditure and dietary factors, J. Nutr. Sci. Vitaminol. 48 (2002) 352–358.
[6] G.A. Kaplan, J.E. Keil, Socioeconomic factors and cardiovascular disease: a review of the literature, Circulation 88 (1993) 1973–1998.
[7] R. Martorell, et al., Obesity in women from developing countries, Eur. J. Clin. Nutr. 54 (2000) 247–252.
[8] B.M. Popkin, The nutrition transition in low-income countries: an emerging crisis, Nutr. Rev. 52 (1994) 285–298.
[9] F.A. Ukoli, et al., Body fat distribution and other anthropometric blood pressure correlates in a Nigerian urban elderly population, Cent. Afr. J. Med. 41 (1995) 154–161.
[10] G.L. Dohm, Mechanisms of muscle insulin resistance in obese individuals, Int. J. Sport Nutr. Exerc. Metab. 11 (2001) S64–S70(Suppl.).

International Congress Series 1262 (2004) 376–379

www.ics-elsevier.com

Homocysteine as a risk factor of cardiovascular disease

M. Merkel*

Department of Internal Medicine I, University Hospital Hamburg-Eppendorf, University of Hamburg, Martinistr. 52, 20251 Hamburg, Germany

Abstract. Homocysteine (Hcy) is an amino acid, which is a product of methionine demethylation and a precursor to cysteine biosynthesis. Slight elevations in plasma homocysteine (homocysteinemia) are frequently found in the general population. Possible causes are widespread conditions such as a variant of the enzyme methylene-tetrahydrofolate reductase (MTHFR) or a shortage of folate, vitamin B_6 and B_{12}.

There is evidence that moderate homocysteinemia may increase the risk for coronary artery disease (CAD), venous thrombosis and stroke. In vitro experiments and animal studies showed that homocysteine injures the endothelium and promotes atherosclerosis. In the case of control studies, it was found that a 5-μmol increase of homocysteine is associated with a 20–50% increased risk of vascular disease. However, interventional trials do not unanimously prove that a homocysteine reduction by folate or vitamin supplementation reduces coronary events. Therefore, a supplementation of folate and vitamins cannot be generally recommended for patients with vascular disease.

Keywords: Homocysteine; Homocysteinemia; Atherosclerosis; Coronary heart disease; Review

1. Introduction

Homocysteine (Hcy) is an amino acid which is a byproduct of the transmethylation and transsulfuration pathway. It is not used for protein assembly and is not a significant part of the human diet. Together with its oxidized dimer, the thiolactone homocystine, it is often referred to as homocyst(e)ine. Increased plasma Hcy (homocysteinemia) is usually defined as Hcy>15 μmol/l. Whereas a dramatic increase of plasma Hcy due to enzymatic defects results in an increased risk of vascular disease, the effect of a moderate increase of plasma Hcy on coronary artery disease (CAD), thromboembolism and stroke is a subject of debate.

Abbreviations: Hcy, Homocysteine; MTHFR, Methylene-tetrahydrofolate reductase; CAD, Coronary artery disease.

* Tel.: +49-40-42803-5542; fax: +49-40-42803-8903.

E-mail address: merkel@uke.uni-hamburg.de (M. Merkel).

0531-5131/ © 2003 Published by Elsevier B.V.
doi:10.1016/j.ics.2003.12.014

2. Homocystein metabolism

Hcy is formed by demethylation of methionine (first step of transsulfuration). The enzymes, ATP/L-methionine-*S*-adenosyltransferase, several methyl transferases and *S*-adenosyl-methionine-hydrolase, work independently from vitamins and folate. This important pathway of methylation is present in all tissues.

Hcy degradation can be performed via several pathways. Firstly, Hcy is metabolised to cysteine (second step of transsulfuration). The rate-limiting enzyme, cystathionine-β-synthase (CBS), is vitamin B_6-dependent, as is the second enzyme γ-cystathionase. Secondly, Hcy can be remethylated to methionine. For this pathway, either betaine or 5-methyl-tetrahydrofolate acts as a methyl donor. Betaine-dependent methylation is carried out by two enzymes which are expressed only in the liver. This reaction is independent of vitamins and cofactors. The alternative way is performed by methionine synthase in virtually all cells. This pathway is vitamin B_{12} (cobalamin)-dependent and uses 5-methyl-tetrahydrofolate, from the folate cycle, as a methyl donor. Therefore, deficiencies or defects both in folate metabolism and in vitamin B_{12} metabolism can impair this reaction.

3. Homocysteinemia and homocysteinuria

Both dietary (vitamin B_6, B_{12} or folate deficiency) and genetic (enzyme defects in the transsulfuration, transmethylation, folate and cobalamin pathways) can cause homocysteinemia. Whereas dietary vitamin or folate shortage usually results in a slight increase of Hcy, enzymatic disorders can cause Hcy levels above 100 μmol/l and homocysteinuria, usually combined with other symptoms. These diseases are rare, and severe metabolic disorders for which at least nine distinct enzymatic defects have been described. Homozygous deficiencies of cystathionine-β-synthase (1:200,000–1:1,000,000 persons), methionine synthase, methylene-tetrahydrofolate reductase (MTHFR) and disturbances of the cobalamin (vitamin B_{12}) pathway are the most common defects [1].

4. Methylene-tetrahydrofolate reductase (MTHFR) C677T variant

A moderate increase of Hcy often occurs as a result of the mutation C677T in the MTHFR gene. This variant, also referred to as thermolabile MTHFR, has reduced activity resulting in an elevation of serum Hcy concentrations of about 20–50% due to an impaired methionine synthase reaction. The mutation is surprisingly common, with about 10% of the population being homozygous-affected (TT), 47% homozygous-unaffected (CC), and 43% heterozygotes (CT) [2]. However, because the increase in Hcy is relatively small, and the impact of the mutation varies according to the folate intake, studies comparing the risk of CAD with and without the TT mutation need large numbers to be able to show an effect.

5. Hcy and endothelial integrity

The first evidence that Hcy affects the integrity of endothelium was found in homocysteinuric patients. Besides the clinical observation of frequent vascular thrombosis and embolism, arterial intimal proliferation, elastic lamina disruption, smooth muscle hypertrophy, fibrosis and platelet accumulation were found upon histological investigations [3]. A central pathogenetic mechanism as to how Hcy may cause vascular wall injury and thromboembolism may be the formation of homocystine which causes oxidative stress and production of free radicals. This process alters LDL and directly injures cells. Other possible atherogenic properties of Hcy include leucocyte recruitment, enhancement of collagen and smooth muscle cell production, nitric oxygen (NO) reduction and NF-κB activation. In addition, Hcy has prothrombotic effects, presumably by direct modification of tissue plasminogen activator or clotting factors.

Some animal studies support the hypothesis that Hcy may be directly atherogenic. Apo-E-deficient mice fed with a methionine-rich folate, vitamin B_6 – and vitamin B_{12} – poor diet had increased atherosclerosis [4], and cynomolgus monkeys on a methionine-rich diet had an impaired endothelial function [5].

6. Hcy levels and human vascular disease

Homocysteinuric patients were reported to have a very high risk of thromboembolism affecting half of the patients by the age of 30 [1]. However, to define vascular injury due to slight homocysteinemia in humans is difficult. A cross-sectional study in subjects from the Framingham Heart Study found Hcy levels to be associated with an increased risk of extracranial carotid artery stenosis [6]. A metastudy to assess the relationship between plasma Hcy and vascular disease found that a 25% (3 μmol/l) Hcy decrease results in a risk reduction of CAD (11%) and stroke (19%) [7]. A meta-analysis focussing on the MTHFR C677T polymorphism found for homozygote TT carriers increased odds ratios for CAD (1.21; 1.06–1.39), stroke (1.31; 0.8–2.15) and deep vein thrombosis (1.29; 1.08–1.54) [2]. A stronger association was observed in retrospective studies of Hcy measured after the onset of disease than in prospective studies among individuals with no CAD when blood was collected. However, these data clearly establish an association between Hcy levels and vascular disease.

7. Interventional studies

Although there is undoubtedly an independent association between plasma Hcy and vascular disease, final proof of a causal relationship can only be done by interventional studies. In the Swiss Heart Study, it was shown that supplementation of folate (1 mg/d), vitamin B_6 (10 mg/d) and vitamin B_{12} (400 μg/d) after percutanous coronary intervention resulted in decreased plasma Hcy (11 to 7.2 μmol/l), increased minimum lumen diameter (1.45 to 1.72 mm), decreased restenosis rate (38% to 19.6%) and decreased major coronary event rate (23% to 15%) after 11 months [8]. An open label study investigating the effects of 500 μg/d folate in patients with stable CAD revealed that, although plasma Hcy level was significantly reduced, within two years, there was no reduction in cardiovascular death and major coronary events [9]. The Folate After Coronary Intervention Trial (FACIT) showed after stent implantation that addition of folate (1.2 mg/d), vitamin B_6 (48 mg/d) and vitamin B_{12} (60 μg/d) resulted in a significantly increased rate of restenosis (26% to 34%) and major coronary events (11% to 17%) after 6 months [10]. The reasons for these striking differences in interventional studies are not clear; patient selection and vitamin dosage have been discussed.

8. Conclusion

Plasma Hcy level has been discussed as an independent cardiovascular risk factor. Based on the present data, there is strong evidence that plasma Hcy is correlated with CAD, venous thrombosis and stroke. However, interventional trials do not unanimously prove that a reduction of Hcy by folate and vitamin supplementation reduces coronary events. Some authors found such nutritional additions to improve clinical and angiographic outcome, whereas others fail to show a beneficial effect. Therefore, a supplementation of folate and vitamins cannot be generally recommended for all patients with vascular disease. Further studies need to elucidate the conditions under which an Hcy reduction by medication with folate, vitamin B_6 and/or vitamin B_{12} should be suggested.

References

[1] S.H. Mudd, H.L. Levy, S. Flemmung, Disorders of transsulfuration, in: C.R. Scriver, A.L. Beaudet, W.S. Sly, D. Valle (Eds.), The Metabolic and Molecular Bases of Inherited Disease, McGraw-Hill, New York, 1995, pp. 1279–1327.

[2] D.S. Wald, M. Law, J.K. Morris, Homocysteine and cardiovascular disease: evidence on causality from a meta-analysis, BMJ 325 (7374) (2002) 1202.

[3] K.S. McCully, Vascular pathology of homocysteinemia: implications for the pathogenesis of arteriosclerosis, Am. J. Pathol. 56 (1) (1969) 111–128.

[4] M.A. Hofmann, E. Lalla, Y. Lu, et al., Hyperhomocysteinemia enhances vascular inflammation and accelerates atherosclerosis in a murine model, J. Clin. Invest. 107 (6) (2001) 675–683.

[5] S.R. Lentz, C.G. Sobey, D.J. Piegors, et al., Vascular dysfunction in monkeys with diet-induced hyperhomocyst(e)inemia, J. Clin. Invest. 98 (1) (1996) 24–29.

[6] J. Selhub, P.F. Jacques, A.G. Bostom, et al., Association between plasma homocysteine concentrations and extracranial carotid-artery stenosis, N. Engl. J. Med. 332 (5) (1995) 286–291.

[7] The homocysteine studies collaboration, Homocysteine and risk of ischemic heart disease and stroke: a meta-analysis, JAMA 288 (16) (2002) 2015–2022.

[8] G. Schnyder, M. Roffi, Y. Flammer, et al., Effect of homocysteine-lowering therapy with folic acid, vitamin B12, and vitamin B6 on clinical outcome after percutaneous coronary intervention: the Swiss heart study: a randomized controlled trial, JAMA 288 (8) (2002) 973–979.

[9] A. Liem, G.H. Reynierse-Buitenwerf, A.H. Zwinderman, et al., Secondary prevention with folic acid: effects on clinical outcomes, J. Am. Coll. Cardiol. 41 (12) (2003) 2105–2113.

[10] H.W. Lange, Folate therapy increases in-stent restenosis: results from the folate after coronary intervention trial (FACIT), 52nd Meeting of the American College of Cardiology, 2003, Abstract www.hartziekten.nl/cardio.nl/ACC2003.

ELSEVIER

International Congress Series 1262 (2004) 380–383

www.ics-elsevier.com

Omega-3 fatty acids, thrombosis and vascular disease

William S. Harris*

Lipid and Diabetes Research, Mid America Heart Institute, Saint Luke's Hospital, 4320 Wornall Road, Suite 128, Kansas City, MO 64111, USA

Abstract. The cardioprotective effects of long-chain, marine omega-3 fatty acids (ω3 FA) have been demonstrated in animal and human experimental studies, in epidemiological investigations and in randomized, controlled trials. In Western countries, effective intakes of eicosapentaenoic acid (EPA) and docosahexaenoic acid (DHA) appear to be in the 0.5–1 g/day range. The mechanism behind the ω3 FA effect is not known with certainty, but appears to involve the prevention of fatal arrhythmias associated with myocardial ischemia. The extent to which this may be secondary to ω3 FA-induced reductions in thrombotic tendencies is not known. Although the anti-thrombotic properties of larger quantities (>3 g/day) of ω3 FA have been examined, the impact of < 1 g/day has not. Current evidence suggests that at very low intakes (150 mg/day of EPA) ex vivo platelet function may be inhibited, and individuals with higher blood levels of ω3 FA have lower levels of tissue plasminogen activator. On the other hand, supplementation with 800–1600 mg/day of EPA + DHA had no effect on coagulation factors. Although further research is needed, these data imply that hemostatic processes may be beneficially impacted by low intakes of ω3 FA, and CHD risk may thereby be reduced. © 2003 Published by Elsevier B.V.

Keywords: Eicosapentaenoic acid; Docosahexaenoic acid; Fish oils; Platelet aggregation; Cardiovascular disease; Thrombosis; Hemostasis

1. Introduction

The purpose of this review is to examine some of the evidence for an antithrombotic mechanism behind the cardioprotective effect of omega-3 fatty acids (ω3 FA) derived from fish oils, eicosapentaenoic acid (EPA) and docosahexaenoic acid (DHA). Evidence from several types of studies suggest that, especially in cultures with typically very low intakes of ω3 FA such as the USA, increasing daily intakes by 500–1000 mg of EPA + DHA may reduce risk of death from coronary heart disease (CHD). This evidence includes population studies [1–4] and supplementation trials [5–7].

* Tel.: +1-816-932-8235; fax: +1-816-932-8278.
E-mail address: wharris@saint-lukes.org (W.S. Harris).

0531-5131/ © 2003 Published by Elsevier B.V.
doi:10.1016/j.ics.2003.12.097

2. Clinical trial evidence of efficacy

The best evidence for the cardioprotective effects of ω3 FA comes from the GISSI Prevenzione study [7,8]. Here, supplementation with 850 mg/dayay of EPA + DHA reduced risk of death from any cause by 20% and risk of sudden death by 45% in post-MI patients.

3. Potential cardioprotective mechanisms

The mechanism(s) responsible for this beneficial effect are not known. Almost all the past studies that have explored "mechanistic" questions have used far greater intakes of ω3 oils than were used in the GISSI and DART studies. Intakes of 3 to over 20 g of EPA + DHA have had effects on blood lipids (notably triglycerides), platelet function, blood pressure, blood vessel flexibility, and inflammation (reviewed in Ref. [9]). However, there is very little information on the biological effects of the low intakes (less than 1 g/day) as used in the major clinical trials and as suggested from epidemiological studies.

At present, it appears that ω3 FA feeding decreases risk for sudden cardiac death by reducing the susceptibility of the heart to malignant arrhythmias (see review, by Leaf et al. [10]). Whether there is a thrombotic element in the causal chain leading to this outcome is not presently known.

3.1. Effects of low intakes of ω3 FA on platelet aggregation

A supplementation experiment was conducted in elderly men from Lyon, France (average age 72) in which eleven were given 150 mg of EPA in capsule form and another eight were given placebo for four weeks [11]. Ex vivo platelet aggregation studies were carried out at the beginning and end of the study using several concentrations of three agonists: epinephrine, adenosine diphosphate (ADP), and collagen. Although a very small study, statistically significant reductions in platelet aggregation were found with all three agonists in the EPA group (Fig. 1). Interestingly, no change in platelet membrane FA

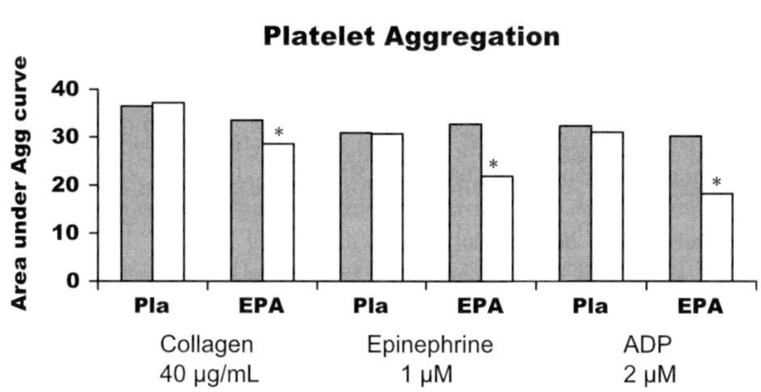

Fig. 1. Platelet aggregation. Effects of the indicated concentrations of three agonists on ex vivo platelet aggregation in 8 elderly subjects treated with placebo (Pla) or 11 treated with 150 mg/d of eicosapentaenoic acid (EPA). The bars represent the areas under the aggregation curves measured at baseline (black) and after four weeks of treatment (white). $^*p<0.02$. Adapted from Dolecek [12].

composition (either arachidonic acid or EPA) was detected suggesting that EPA may be able to operate via a mechanism that does not depend on release of arachidonic acid or EPA from membrane phospholipids with subsequent conversion via cyclooxygenase to thromboxanes and other eicosanoids. This study implies that very small intakes of ω3 FA may have physiological activity. This would be consistent with the reported reductions in risk for CHD death reported in several epidemiological studies in which fish intake, not supplements, were the source of ω3 FA [1,12–17].

3.2. Effects of low intakes of ω3 FA on coagulation and fibrinolytic factors

Reduced thrombotic tendencies can arise not only from altered platelet function but also from changes in hemostatic factors. The effects of either low-dose, supplemental ω3 FA and of background fish intake (assessed by a biomarker of intake, erythrocyte ω3 FA levels) on several factors has been examined.

The PRIME study (Prospective Epidemiological Study of Myocardial Infarction) [18] examined the relationship between erythrocyte FA composition and factor (F) VII coagulant activity (FVIIc) and antigen (FVIIag), von Willibrand's factor, plasminogen activator inhibitor-1 (PAI-1), fibrinogen, D-dimer (fibrin degradation product), and tissue plasminogen activator (tPA). The latter was the only hemostatic marker related to RBC ω3 FA levels in 283 men (average age 55 years with normal lipid profiles and body weights). There was an inverse correlation between these two factors such that a 10% increase in RBC ω3 FA was associated with a 26% reduction in tPA ($p<0.01$). Lower tPA levels would suggest reduced systemic endothelial activation and thus lower risk for vascular disease [19].

These epidemiological findings were not supported, however, by the results of a recent intervention trial in 150 mildly hyperlipidemic but otherwise healthy men and women [20]. In this study, individuals were randomized to one of five treatment groups: placebo, EPA + DHA (800 or 1700 mg), or α-linolenic acid (4.5 or 9.5 g) for 6 months. The latter is an 18-carbon ω3 FA found in certain plant oils. Compared with the changes observed in the placebo group, there was no effect on either coagulation factors (FVIIa, FVIIc, FVIIag, FXIIa, FXIIag, or fibrinogen) or fibrinolytic markers (PAI-1 or tPA). Whether the results would have been different for subjects at higher risk for CHD is not known.

These studies provide too little data to make any firm statement regarding the effects of low intakes of ω3 FA on either platelet function, or on coagulation or fibrinolytic factors. Nevertheless, future studies are clearly warranted in light of the impressive reduction in clinical events associated with these doses of ω3 FA.

4. Conclusion

At nutritionally achievable intakes of ω3 FA, risk of death from cardiovascular is reduced. Because the vast majority of past studies on potential mechanisms have provided 3–10 times more EPA + DHA than has been shown to be effective in reducing risk for clinical events, we cannot know whether the effects seen at those doses are responsible for the observed benefits associated with lower intakes. While some evidence suggests that ω3 FA may have an anti-thrombotic effect at intakes of less than 1 g/day, much more research is needed at this intake level to sort out the relevant mechanisms of action.

References

[1] D.S. Siscovick, et al., Dietary intake and cell membrane levels of long-chain n − 3 polyunsaturated fatty acids and the risk of primary cardiac arrest, J. Am. Med. Assoc. 274 (1995) 1363–1367.

[2] C.M. Albert, et al., Blood levels of long-chain n − 3 fatty acids and the risk of sudden death, N. Engl. J. Med. 346 (2002) 1113–1118.

[3] T. Rissanen, et al., Fish oil-derived fatty acids, docosahexaenoic acid and docosapentaenoic acid, and the risk of acute coronary events. The Kuopio ischaemic heart disease risk factor study, Circulation 102 (2000) 2677–2679.

[4] R.N. Lemaitre, et al., N-3 polyunsaturated fatty acids, fatal ischemic heart disease and non-fatal myocardial infarction in older adults. The cardiovascular health study, Am. J. Clin. Nutr. 76 (2002) 319–325.

[5] M.L. Burr, et al., Effects of changes in fat, fish, and fibre intakes on death and myocardial reinfarction: diet and reinfarction trial (DART), Lancet 2 (1989) 757–761.

[6] C. von Schacky, et al., The effect of dietary ω-3 fatty acids on coronary atherosclerosis. A randomized double-blind placebo-controlled trial, Ann. Intern. Med. 130 (1999) 554–562.

[7] R. Marchioli, et al., Early protection against sudden death by n-3 polyunsaturated fatty acids after myocardial infarction: time-course analysis of the results of the Gruppo Italiano per lo Studio della Sopravvivenza nell'Infarto Miocardico (GISSI)-Prevenzione, Circulation 105 (2002) 1897–1903.

[8] GISSI-Prevenzione Investigators, Dietary supplementation with n-3 polyunsaturated fatty acids and vitamin E in 11,324 patients with myocardial infarction: results of the GISSI-Prevenzione trial, Lancet 354 (1999) 447–455.

[9] P.M. Kris-Etherton, et al., Fish consumption, fish oil omega-3 fatty acids and cardiovascular disease, Circulation 106 (2002) 2747–2757.

[10] A. Leaf, et al., Clinical prevention of sudden cardiac death by n-3 polyunsaturated fatty acids and mechanism of prevention of arrhythmias by n-3 fish oils, Circulation 107 (2003) 2646–2652.

[11] F. Driss, et al., Inhibition of platelet aggregration and thromboxane synthesis after intake of small amounts of icosapentaenoic acid, Thromb. Res. 36 (1984) 389–396.

[12] T.A. Dolecek, Epidemiological evidence of relationships between dietary polyunsaturated fatty acids and mortality in the multiple risk factor intervention trial, Proc. Soc. Exp. Biol. Med. 200 (1992) 177–182.

[13] C.M. Albert, et al., Fish consumption and risk of sudden cardiac death, JAMA 279 (1998) 23–28.

[14] F.B. Hu, et al., Fish and omega-3 fatty acid intake and risk of coronary heart disease in women, JAMA 287 (2002) 1815–1821.

[15] D. Mozaffarian, et al., Cardiac benefits of fish consumption may depend on the type of fish meal consumed: the cardiovascular health study, Circulation 107 (2003) 1372–1377.

[16] F.B. Hu, et al., Fish and long-chain omega-3 fatty acid intake and risk of coronary heart disease and total mortality in diabetic women, Circulation 107 (2003) 1852–1857.

[17] A. Ascherio, et al., Dietary intake of marine n-3 fatty acids, fish intake, and the risk of coronary disease among men, N. Engl. J. Med. 332 (1995) 977–982.

[18] P.Y. Scarabin, et al., Haemostasis in relation to dietary fat as estimated by erythrocyte fatty acid composition: the prime study, Thromb. Res. 102 (2001) 285–293.

[19] I. Juhan-Vague, et al., Fibrinolytic function and coronary risk, Curr. Cardiol. Rep. 1 (1999) 119–124.

[20] Y.E. Finnegan, et al., Plant and marine-derived (n-3) polyunsaturated fatty acids do not affect blood coagulation and fibrinolytic factors in moderately hyperlipidemic humans, J. Nutr. 133 (2003) 2210–2213.

International Congress Series 1262 (2004) 384–387

www.ics-elsevier.com

Genetic manipulation of macrophage—and vascular genes in mouse models of atherosclerosis

Th.J.C. van Berkel*, J.H. von der Thüsen, J. Kuiper, E.A.L. Biessen, M. van Eck

Division of Biopharmaceutics, LACDR, Gorlaeus Laboratories, Leiden University, P.O. Box 9502, 2300 RA Leiden, The Netherlands

Abstract. Macrophage-derived foam cells play an essential role in the development of atherosclerosis. The population of macrophages in the arterial wall highly depends on monocyte infiltration from the blood circulation. Transplantation of the hematopoietic system offers a unique opportunity to replace genes in cells from hematopoietic origin, including macrophages. We have exposed atherosclerosis susceptible mice (LDL-receptor −/−, apoE −/− and apoE3-Leiden mice) to total body irradiation 1 day before the transplantation of donor bone marrow lacking either apoE, LDL-receptor, LRP, ABCA-1, LPL, CCR2, SR-BI or overexpressing SR-A, ApoE3-Leiden or apoE2. This allowed the evaluation of the individual role of these gene products in the development of atherogenesis.The evaluation of new strategies for the prevention of atherosclerotic lesion formation and plaque rupture has thus far been hampered by the lack of a practical animal model. A mouse model of rapid and site-controlled atherogenesis was developed by the placement of silastic collars around the carotid arteries of apoE −/− and LDL-R −/− mice, leading to rapid lesion development (3–6 weeks) proximal to the collar [Circulation 103 (2001) 1164]. Local transfection of the arteries with IL-10, PAF-AH or IL-9 led to inhibition of atherosclerotic lesion development, while administration of adenovirus p53 induced plaque rupture. Being the first example of inducible rupture at a predefined location, this model offers a unique opportunity to delineate the processes that precede rupture, as well as to evaluate plaque-stabilizing therapies.

Keywords: Atherosclerosis; Mouse models; Gene therapy; Bone marrow transplantation; Adenovirus

1. Introduction

Macrophage-derived foam cells play an essential role in the initiation and progression of atherosclerosis. The population of macrophages in the arterial wall depends on monocyte infiltration from the circulation. Transplantation of the hematopoietic system

* Corresponding author. Tel.: +31-71-527-6216; fax: +31-71-527-6032.
E-mail address: t.berkel@lacdr.leidenuniv.nl (Th.J.C. van Berkel).

0531-5131/ © 2004 Published by Elsevier B.V.
doi:10.1016/j.ics.2003.12.047

offers a unique opportunity to replace genes in cells from hematopoietic origin, including macrophages. In irradiated recipients, introduction of donor bone marrow cells leads to total replacement in about 7 days. We applied the bone marrow transplantation system to analyse the relative importance of macrophage genes, which are involved in the regulation of macrophage cholesterol homeostasis.

The use of mouse models in preclinical evaluation of therapeutic strategies has major advantages over other animals with respect to practicality. Mouse models of accelerated atherogenesis and plaque disruption are, however, needed in order to evaluate both systemic and local gene therapeutic protocols. We developed in hypercholesterolemic mice a model for rapid progression of atherosclerosis by placement of a perivascular collar in the common carotid artery. In this model, plaque rupture can be induced by local incubation with an adenovirus carrying a p53 transgene.

2. Results and discussion

2.1. Bone marrow transplantation

In the last couple of years, we have exposed atherosclerosis susceptible mice (LDL-receptor $-/-$, apoE $-/-$ and apoE3-Leiden mice) to total body irradiation 1 day prior to the transplantation of donor bone marrow lacking either apoE, the LDL-receptor, ABCA-1, LPL or overexpressing scavenger-receptor A, apoE3-Leiden or ApoE2 [1–7]. Expression of the LDL-receptor, scavenger-receptor A and LPL in macrophages appears to stimulate atherosclerotic lesion formation [3–6], while ABCA1 [7] and apoE expression [1,2,6] appears to be protective. Apparently, the regulation of cholesterol homeostasis in the macrophages leads directly to consequences for atherosclerotic lesion formation.

Recently, we also determined the role of CC–chemokine receptor 2 (CCR2) in the early development of atherosclerosis [8]. The absence of CCR2 on leukocytes induces an 86% reduction of aortic lesion area as compared with controls ($n = 10$, $P < 0.01$). These results provide direct evidence that CCR2 expressed by leukocytes plays a critical role in the initiation of early atherosclerosis and that pharmacological intervention in CCR2 function represents an attractive target to inhibit atherogenesis.

2.2. Mouse model for rapid and site controlled atherogenesis

The aim of this study was to evaluate the intimal response of the carotid artery to silastic collar placement in apoE $-/-$ and LDLr $-/-$ mice, which are known to spontaneously develop extensive and complex atherosclerotic lesions. One week after bilateral insertion of a 0.3-mm diameter collar, intimal thickening was not detectable in either strain. By 3 weeks, however, a neointima had appeared in the area proximal to the collar in apoE $-/-$ mice. Six weeks after collar insertion, a significant increase in intimal surface area had occurred in both strains, although this was more extensive in the apoE $-/-$ group ($1.46 \pm 0.50 \times 10^5$ μm^2 in apoE $-/-$, $0.59 \pm 0.23 \times 10^5$ μm^2 in LDLr $-/-$; $P < 0.05$ compared with sham-operated in both strains). The increase with time in neointimal surface proximal to the collar was found to be significant in both apoE $-/-$ and LDLr $-/-$ mice ($P < 0.01$, one-way ANOVA).

The intimal area within and distal to the collar remained virtually unaltered at all time points examined; these values were confirmed to differ significantly from the values obtained at the proximal site ($P < 0.0001$, two-way ANOVA). The medial surface area did not rise significantly with time at any site in either strain, and medial SMC loss was not found to have occurred at the time points examined (data not shown). No plaques were found in the corresponding sites of the common carotid arteries of sham-operated animals of either strain. The intima–media ratios of the proximal site are in agreement with the absolute data, being highest in both strains 6 weeks after insertion (apoE −/−, 2.96 ± 1.72; LDLr −/−, 1.42 ± 0.88). The degree of proximal lumen stenosis (as expressed by the intima–lumen ratio) was highest in the apoE −/− mice, being $36 \pm 26\%$ at 3 weeks and approaching occlusion ($85 \pm 5\%$) by 6 weeks. The corresponding values for LDLr −/− mice were $9 \pm 7\%$ and $61 \pm 23\%$. Distal and midsection sites did not display a significant increase in intima–edia or intima–lumen ratio. Our model [9] is characterized by site-controlled and accelerated atherogenesis, which mirrors the differences seen between apoE −/− and LDLr −/− mice in spontaneous atherosclerosis.

2.3. Mouse model for plaque rupture

To study the effect of p53-mediated apoptosis in pre-existing atherosclerosis, we transfected collar-induced carotid lesions in $ApoE^{-/-}$ mice with adenovirus carrying a p53 transgene. One day after transfection, we analyzed these plaques for transgene expression and markers of apoptosis and proliferation. After 2 weeks, we assessed lesion stability by analyzing plaque composition and by inducing plaque stress in vivo through systemic administration of phenylephrine [10].

Whereas the core area in Ad5-CMV.p53-treated animals was increased compared with the Ad5-CMV.lacZ control group ($54.1 \pm 16.6 \times 10^3$ versus $32.0 \pm 5.5 \times 10^3$ μm^2, $P = 0.25$), the cap area was decreased by Ad5-CMV.p53 treatment ($14.7 \pm 5.4 \times 10^3$ versus $25.3 \pm 2.3 \times 10^3$ μm^2, $P = 0.11$). This effect was seen to translate to a highly significant decrease in the cap/intima ratio in Ad5-CMV.p53-treated arteries (0.21 ± 0.04 versus 0.46 ± 0.03, $P < 0.001$), which was mirrored by a decrease in the cap/core ratio (0.28 ± 0.13 versus 0.86 ± 0.24, $P < 0.01$). Histological analysis of the collar-induced plaques revealed evidence of plaque rupture in seven animals and in one additional plaque out of 20 Ad5-CMV.p53-treated vessels. This was accompanied by intracarotid thrombosis in one case and by intraplaque hemorrhage in seven vessels. Because we did not find evidence of plaque rupture or its sequelae in the Ad5-CMV.lacZ-treated control plaques ($n = 20$), the number of events in the Ad5-CMV.p53-treated group was highly significant (Fisher's exact test, $P = 0.003$). In our model [10], rupture occurs frequently and in a control led fashion, allowing the delineation of the molecular pathways involved and the evaluation of therapies aimed at plaque stabilization and the prevention of acute cardiovascular events.

Acknowledgements

This work was supported by The Netherlands Hearts Foundation (Grant 98.192, 93.001 and 2001 D041).

References

[1] M. van Eck, N. Herijgers, J. Yates, N.J. Pearce, P.M. Hoogerbrugge, P.H.E. Groot, Th.J.C. van Berkel, Bone marrow transplantation in apolipoprotein E-deficient mice. Effect ApoE gene dosage on serum lipid concentrations, (beta) VLDL catabolism, and atherosclerosis, Arterioscler. Thromb. Vasc. Biol. 17 (11) (1997) 3117–3126.

[2] M. van Eck, N. Herijgers, M. Vidgeon-Hart, N.J. Pearce, P.M. Hoogerbrugge, P.H.E. Groot, Th.J.C. van Berkel, Accelerated atherosclerosis in C57Bl/6 mice transplanted with ApoE-deficient bone marrow, Atherosclerosis 150 (1) (2000) 71–80.

[3] N. Herijgers, M. van Eck, S.J. Korporaal, P.M. Hoogerbrugge, Th.J.C. van Berkel, Relative importance of the LDL receptor and scavenger receptor class B in the beta-VLDL-induced uptake and accumulation of cholesteryl esters by peritoneal macrophages, J. Lipid Res. 41 (7) (2000) 1163–1171.

[4] N. Herijgers, M. van Eck, P.H.E. Groot, P.M. Hoogerbrugge, Th.J.C. van Berkel, Low density lipoprotein receptor of macrophages facilitates atherosclerotic lesion formation in C57Bl/6 mice, Arterioscler. Thromb. Vasc. Biol. 20 (8) (2000) 1961–1967.

[5] M. van Eck, R. Zimmerman, P.H.E. Groot, R. Zechner, Th.J.C. van Berkel, Role of macrophage-derived lipoprotein lipase in lipoprotein metabolism and atherosclerosis, Arterioscler. Thromb. Vasc. Biol. 20 (9) (2000) E53–E62.

[6] M. van Eck, K.W. van Dijk, N. Herijgers, M.H. Hofker, P.H.E. Groot, Th.J.C. van Berkel, Essential role for the (hepatic) LDL receptor in macrophage apolipoprotein E-induced reduction in serum cholesterol levels and atherosclerosis, Atherosclerosis 154 (1) (2001) 103–112.

[7] M. van Eck, I.S. Bos, W.E. Kaminski, E. Orso, G. Rothe, J. Twisk, A. Bottcher, E.S. van Amersfoort, T.A. Christiansen-Weber, W.P. Fung-Leung, Th.J.C. van Berkel, G. Schmitz, Leukocyte ABCA1 controls susceptibility to atherosclerosis and macrophage recruitment into tissues, Proc. Natl. Acad. Sci. U. S. A. 99 (9) (2002) 6298–6303.

[8] J. Guo, M. van Eck, J. Twisk, N. Maeda, G.M. Benson, P.H.E. Groot, Th.J.C. van Berkel, Transplantation of monocyte CC–chemokine receptor 2-deficient bone marrow into ApoE3-Leiden mice inhibits atherogenesis, Arterioscler. Thromb. Vasc. Biol. 23 (3) (2003) 447–453.

[9] J.H. von der Thüsen, Th.J.C. van Berkel, E.A.L. Biessen, Induction of rapid atherogenesis by perivascular carotid collar placement in apolipoprotein E-deficient and low-density lipoprotein receptor-deficient mice, Circulation 103 (8) (2001) 1164–1170.

[10] J.H. von der Thüsen, B.J. van Vlijmen, R.C. Hoeben, M.M. Kockx, L.M. Havekes, Th.J.C. van Berkel, E.A.L. Biessen, Induction of atherosclerotic plaque rupture in apolipoprotein E −/− mice after adenovirus-mediated transfer of p53, Circulation 105 (17) (2002) 2064–2070.

International Congress Series 1262 (2004) 388–391

www.ics-elsevier.com

ApoE4 trapping by the low density lipoprotein receptor

Michael K. Altenburg[a], Sudi I. Malloy[a], Chris Knouff[a], John S. Parks[b], Nobuyo Maeda[a,*]

[a] *Department of Pathology and Laboratory Medicine, University of North Carolina at Chapel Hill, 703 Brinkhouse Bullitt Bldg., CB 7525, Chapel Hill, NC 27599, USA*

[b] *Department of Pathology, Wake Forest University School of Medicine, Winston-Salem, NC 27157, USA*

Abstract. Low density lipoprotein receptor (LDLr) is critical for plasma lipoprotein clearance and a decreased LDLr expression has been thought to explain the increased plasma cholesterol and atherosclerosis risk in humans with apolipoprotein (apo) E4. However, in mice expressing human apoE4 instead of their mouse counterpart, increased LDLr expression caused accumulation of cholesterol-rich apoE-poor chylomicron remnants, and resulted in significant atherosclerosis. The production rates of chylomicrons and very low density lipoproteins (VLDL) were unchanged, as was the clearance rate of exogenously given apoE-deficient remnants. These data suggest an enhanced conversion of nascent lipoprotein particles to cholesterol-rich remnants that are poorly cleared. We hypothesize that the negative effects from increased LDLr are due to the high binding affinity of apoE4 for the receptor which reduces the availability of apoE4 for transfer to triglyceride-rich lipoproteins (TRL), thereby inhibiting their rapid internalization.

Keywords: ApoE; LDLr; Plasma lipoprotein clearance

1. Introduction

The low density lipoprotein receptor (LDLr) plays a pivotal role in the removal of atherogenic lipoproteins from the circulation by removing lipoproteins containing the LDLr ligands apoB100 and apoE [1]. In humans, apoE is polymorphic with three isoforms, apoE2, apoE3, and apoE4. These isoforms differ at positions 112 and 158, with apoE2 having two cysteines, apoE3 cysteine at 112 and arginine at 158, and apoE4 has two arginines. ApoE2 has a reduced LDLr affinity and apoE4 an increased affinity compared with apoE3 [2–4]. Paradoxically, apoE4 is associated with an elevated plasma cholesterol level and atherosclerosis, while apoE2 is associated with a reduction in cholesterol and risk in humans [5,6]. The increased risk associated with

* Corresponding author. Tel.: +1-919-966-6916; fax: +1-919-966-8800.
E-mail address: Nobuyo@med.unc.edu (N. Maeda).

doi:10.1016/j.ics.2003.11.035

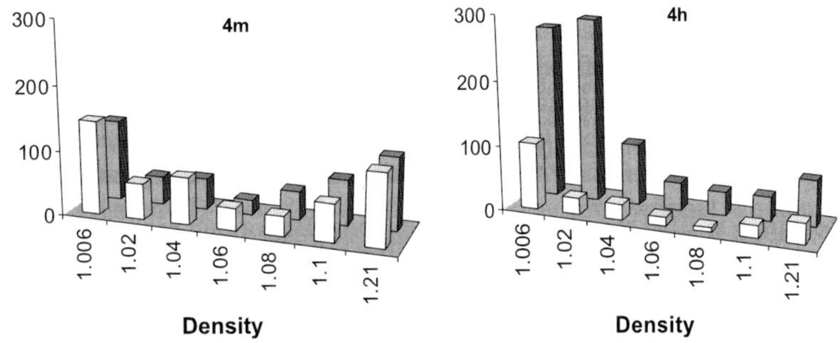

Fig. 1. Cholesterol (mg/dl) in UC fractions before (shaded) and after an 18h fast (white). Plasma was pooled from HFW fed 4m ($n=5$) and 4h ($n=5$) and separated by ultracentrifugation into density fractions.

apoE4 is thought to be due to elevated intracellular cholesterol from increased apoE4-mediated lipid delivery, leading to down-regulation of the LDLr. Here we describe the over-expression of the LDLr in mice with apoE4 and found increased cholesterol and atherosclerosis.

2. Experimental procedures and results

To examine the effects of LDLr expression level on mice with apoE4, mice homozygous for the replacement of APOE*4 allele (4m) were bred to mice heterozygous for targeted replacement of the mouse LDLr gene with a human LDLr minigene (4h) that results in a stabilized LDLr mRNA [4,7]. Total mRNA for LDLr in 4h mice was 2.3 times that of 4m mice. On normal chow (NC), plasma cholesterol in 4h mice was about one-third that of 4m mice, resulting from reduced HDL cholesterol. When fed a high-fat western diet (HFW), 4h mice became markedly hypercholesterolemic with accumulation of apoE-poor, but cholesterol-enriched, particles in their plasma predominantly in their chylomicron/very low density lipoproteins (VLDL) remnant ($1.006<d\leq 1.02$) fractions [7]. Plasma lipoprotein fractions from 4m mice fed HFW diet did not change before and after fasting (Fig. 1). In contrast, fasting 18 h almost

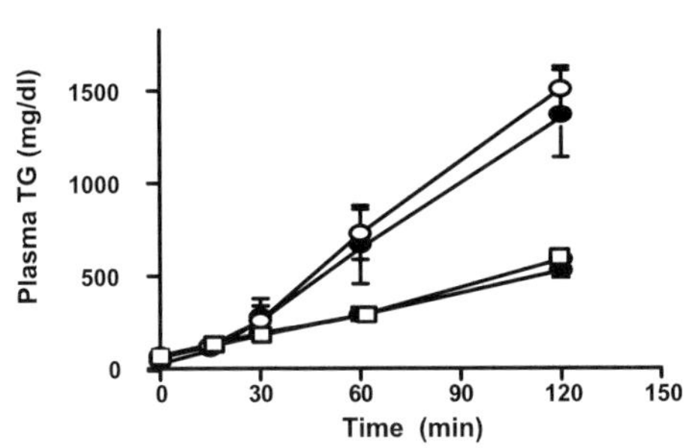

Fig. 2. Triglyceride secretion of 4m (open symbol) and 4h (closed symbol) mice after inhibition of lipolysis and uptake with Triton WR1339. Mice ($n=4$) after olive oil gavage reflects VLDL and chylomicron secretion (circles). VLDL secretion in mice ($n=4$) fasted 4h (squares). The difference between the top and bottom reflects chylomicron production.

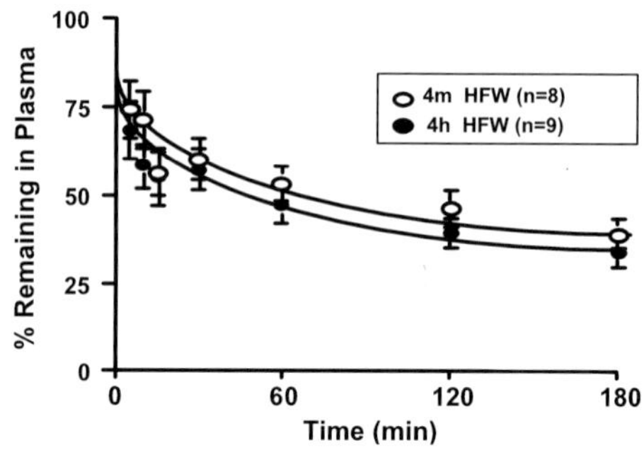

Fig. 3. Clearance of apoE −/− VLDL in 4 m and 4 h mice. Radioactivity remaining in the plasma after injection of I^{125} labeled VLDL into HFW fed 4 m and 4 h mice. There was no significant difference between 4m and 4h mice.

completely eliminated 4h remnants, suggesting that these particles are derived primarily from the diet. Interestingly, similar prolonged postprandial lipemia has also been observed in humans with apoE4 [8].

Triglyceride secretion was indistinguishable in 4m and 4h mice, suggesting that their VLDL production from the liver is the same. When mice were gavaged with a 200 μl olive oil bolus immediately after Triton WR 1339 injection, the rate of TG accumulation after gavage was also the same in both 4m and 4h mice (Fig. 2). These results indicate that chylomicron secretion from the intestine is also the same in 4m and 4h mice [7].

There was no significant difference in clearance of remnant particles between 4m and 4h mice (Fig. 3). Therefore, the elevated cholesterol associated with increased LDLr in the 4h mice is not due to delayed clearance of cholesterol-rich apoE-poor remnants. The inference from these data is that the conversion of nascent triglyceride-rich lipoproteins (TRL) to apoE-poor remnants is increased in 4h mice.

3. Discussion

ApoE is normally associated with various proteins and proteoglycans on the surface of capillaries and the hepatic space of Disse where it can be transferred to circulating lipoproteins. We propose that the increased LDLr can "trap" apoE protein and limit its transfer to circulating nascent lipoproteins, which in turn reduces the apoE-mediated removal of larger particles and forces their remodeling to slowly cleared remnants. The clearance of these cholesterol-rich apoE-poor remnants is equally slow in both 4m and 4h and is seemingly LDLr-independent. The higher affinity of apoE4 for the LDLr may make it more susceptible to trapping than apoE3 and apoE2.

Thus, mice expressing human apoE isoforms have revealed important interactions between apoE genotype, LDLr expression, and diet. Contrary to the currently accepted hypothesis that increased atherosclerosis risk in humans with apoE4 is due to down-regulation of LDLr, we found that increased LDLr has adverse effects on mice expressing apoE4. Our proposed mechanism of apoE4 trapping by LDLr is likely to be contributing to the paradoxical association between apoE4 and increased atherosclerosis risk. We expect

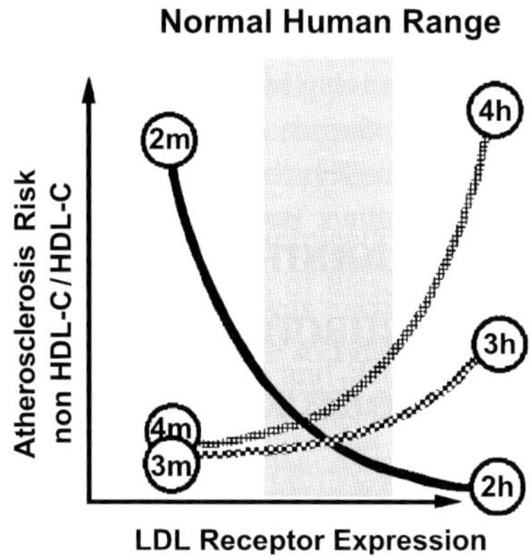

Fig. 4. Interaction between apoE isoforms and LDLr level. On the left-hand side are mice expressing the different apoE isoforms with a relatively low wild-type LDLr level. On the right-hand side are the same mice with an elevated LDLr level. We suggest that the human LDLr level mean is centered between the extremes in our mice.

that humans vary in their basal expression of LDLr, and its levels influence the atherosclerosis risk differently depending on the apoE genotype (Fig. 4). Control of diet would then be more important in individuals with apoE4 than those with apoE2 or apoE3 when the LDLr level is relatively high.

Acknowledgements

This work is supported by grants from NIH (HL42360) to N.M.

References

[1] M.S. Brown, J.L. Goldstein, A receptor-mediated pathway for cholesterol homeostasis, Science 232 (4746) (1986) 34–47.

[2] K. Bohnet, et al., Apolipoprotein (apo) E genotype and apoE concentration determine binding of normal very low density lipoproteins to HepG2 cell surface receptors, J. Lipid Res. 37 (6) (1996) 1316–1324.

[3] C. Knouff, et al., Apo E structure determines VLDL clearance and atherosclerosis risk in mice, J. Clin. Invest. 103 (11) (1999) 1579–1586.

[4] K.H. Weisgraber, Apolipoprotein E: structure-function relationships, Adv. Protein Chem. 45 (1994) 249–302.

[5] E. Boerwinkle, G. Utermann, Simultaneous effects of the apolipoprotein E polymorphism on apolipoprotein E, apolipoprotein B, and cholesterol metabolism, Am. J. Hum. Genet. 42 (1) (1988) 104–112.

[6] J. Davignon, R.E. Gregg, C.F. Sing, Apolipoprotein E polymorphism and atherosclerosis, Arteriosclerosis 8 (1) (1988) 1–21.

[7] S.I. Malloy, et al., Harmful effects of increased LDLR expression in mice with human APOE*4 but not APOE*3, Arterioscler. Thromb. Vasc. Biol. (2003) (available online).

[8] N. Bergeron, R.J. Havel, Prolonged postprandial responses of lipids and apolipoproteins in triglyceride-rich lipoproteins of individuals expressing an apolipoprotein epsilon 4 allele, J. Clin. Invest. 97 (1) (1996) 65–72.

International Congress Series 1262 (2004) 392–395

www.ics-elsevier.com

Signal transduction pathways in free cholesterol-loaded macrophages: cell biological insight into the progression of atherosclerosis

Ira Tabas*

Departments of Medicine and Anatomy and Cell Biology, Columbia University, 630 West 168th Street, New York, NY 10032, USA

Abstract. Macrophage death in advanced atherosclerotic lesions gives rise to lesional necrosis and plaque instability. Late lesional macrophages accumulate large amounts of unesterified, or "free" cholesterol (FC), and FC loading of macrophages is cytotoxic. Therefore, FC-induced macrophage death in advanced atherosclerosis may represent an important turning point in lesion progression. This brief review summarizes recent findings on the cellular and molecular mechanisms of FC-induced macrophage death. These mechanisms suggest novel therapeutic strategies directed at maintaining plaque stability and inhibiting acute vascular events. © 2004 Published by Elsevier B.V.

Keywords: Atherosclerosis; Plaque rupture; Macrophage; Cholesterol; Apoptosis

1. Introduction

The development of the so-called "culprit" lesion during atherogenesis represents a critical series of events, because it is these lesions that are prone to rupture or erosion, leading to acute thrombotic vascular occlusion and tissue infarction [1]. Pathologists have noted that these lesions are often associated with necrosis due to death of macrophages and with the accumulation of unesterified, or "free" cholesterol (FC) [2]. One hypothesis to emerge from these observations is that macrophage death, perhaps induced by FC accumulation, leads to the release of cellular substances, such as inflammation-inducing molecules, proteases, and tissue factor, which promote plaque inflammation and breakdown as well as acute thrombosis [3–8]. Indeed, both cell culture and in vivo atherosclerosis studies have revealed that FC accumulation is a potent inducer of cell death in macrophages [9–13]. In the context of these observations, an important goal in atherosclerosis research is to elucidate the cellular and molecular mechanisms of lesional macrophage death in general and FC-induced macrophage death in particular.

* Tel.: +1-212-305-9430; fax: +1-212-305-4834.
E-mail address: iatl@columbia.edu (I. Tabas).

0531-5131/ © 2004 Published by Elsevier B.V.
doi:10.1016/j.ics.2003.12.095

2. Mechanisms of FC-induced apoptosis in macrophages

The end effect of prolonged FC loading of cultured macrophages is a mixture of apoptotic and necrotic cells [9–12], which is similar to what occurs in advanced atherosclerotic lesions [14,15]. At earlier time points, apoptosis is prominent and characterized by caspase activation, phosphatidylserine externalization, nuclear condensation, and DNA fragmentation. At later time points of FC loading, necrotic changes, such as membrane permeabilization and organelle swelling, occur. While it is possible that some of the necrosis may result from direct FC-induced damage to the plasma membrane [16], it is likely that most results from the progression of apoptosis-related cytotoxicity that occurs in the absence of phagocytosis of the apoptotic macrophages, both in vitro and in atherosclerotic lesions [17–19].

Initial studies on the mechanism of FC-induced apoptosis focused on the pathways leading to caspase activation and revealed that both Fas and mitochondrial pathways were involved [11,12]. The goal of more recent studies was to explore how FC loading initiates these apoptotic pathways. Previous work had suggested that FC trafficking to and loading of the plasma membrane was the key cellular event [16]. However, using a variety of cellular manipulations, our laboratory showed that the key site was the ER [20]. In particular, we showed that specific inhibitors of cholesterol trafficking to the ER, namely, nanomolar doses of the amphipathic amine U18666A and partial deficiency of NPC1 protein, could prevent FC-induced apoptosis, while direct loading of the plasma membrane with FC was an inefficient inducer [20]. Based upon these findings, we then discovered that FC loading is a potent inducer of an ER stress-related signal transduction pathway known as the unfolded protein response, or UPR [20]. The UPR is an integrated stress response that attempts to correct defects in protein folding and, if that fails, trigger apoptosis [21].

In FC-loaded macrophages, induction of the UPR is specifically blocked by the aforementioned inhibitors of cholesterol trafficking to the ER. Moreover, genetic alterations of either the protective or apoptosis-inducing pathways of the UPR in macrophages have dramatic effects on FC-induced apoptosis in these cells, providing molecular genetic evidence that the UPR is causally related to FC-induced apoptosis. In addition, we showed that the UPR effector CHOP is expressed in atherosclerotic lesions, particularly in those areas enriched in macrophages and FC. Finally, we have begun to elucidate how FC loading induces the UPR. The earliest detectable event after FC loading is depletion of ER calcium pools [20], which is a known and potent inducer of the UPR [22]. Preliminary data suggest that FC enrichment of the normally cholesterol-poor ER cause dysfunction of sarco-endoplasmic reticulum calcium ATPase (SERCA), which functions to pump calcium back into the ER.

To test the overall concept of that cholesterol trafficking to the ER is an important cause of macrophage apoptosis in advanced atherosclerotic lesions, we bred the *Npc1+/−* mouse onto the *Apoe −/−* atherosclerosis background. Despite similar plasma lipid levels and similar lesion sizes, the *Apoe −/−;Npc1+/−* lesions had substantially less macrophage apoptosis and lesional necrosis than the *Apoe −/−;Npc1+/+* lesions [23]. These data not only suggest that cholesterol trafficking to the ER is important in lesional macrophage apoptosis, but they also are consistent with the notion that FC accumulation in lesional macrophages is due to ACAT dysfunction rather than blockage of FC trafficking to ACAT. The latter conclusion is based upon the understanding that the Npc1+/− mutation, which is specific for blocking cholesterol trafficking to the ER, would not have an anti-apoptotic effect if FC were accumulating in a pre-ER compartment.

3. Conclusions

Based on these studies, we propose that FC accumulation in advanced lesional macrophages triggers the apoptosis branch of the UPR, leading to macrophage death and lesional necrosis. This working model is simplistic in the sense that other factors undoubtedly contribute to both macrophage death (e.g., oxidized lipids) and plaque instability (e.g., defective collagen production by intimal smooth muscle cells). However, the *Npc1+/−* mouse study suggests that by targeting the specific process of cholesterol trafficking to the ER, a substantial improvement in plaque morphology can result. Thus, the findings disclosed in this review may provide the basis for a novel therapeutic strategy designed to prevent the development of culprit lesions and resultant acute cardiovascular events.

Acknowledgements

These studies were supported in part by grants HL54591 and HL56984 from the National Institutes of Health. The author gratefully acknowledges the contributions of the following scientists: Bo Feng, Pin Mei Yao, David Ron, Yankun Li, Cecilia M. Devlin, Dajun Zhang, Heather P. Harding, Michele Sweeney, James X. Rong, George Kuriakose, Edward A. Fisher, Andrew R. Marks, and Mark Kockx.

References

[1] R. Virmani, A.P. Burke, F.D. Kolodgie, A. Farb, Vulnerable plaque: the pathology of unstable coronary lesions, J. Interv. Cardiol. 15 (2002) 439–446.

[2] A.P. Burke, R. Virmani, Z. Galis, C.C. Haudenschild, J.E. Muller, 34th Bethesda Conference: task force #2—what is the pathologic basis for new atherosclerosis imaging techniques? J. Am. Coll. Cardiol. 41 (2003) 1874–1886.

[3] I. Tabas, Consequences of cellular cholesterol accumulation: basic concepts and physiological implications, J. Clin. Invest. 110 (2002) 905–911.

[4] P.A. Berberian, W. Myers, M. Tytell, V. Challa, M.G. Bond, Immunohistochemical localization of heat shock protein-70 in normal-appearing and atherosclerotic specimens of human arteries, Am. J. Pathol. 136 (1990) 71–80.

[5] R.Y. Ball, E.C. Stowers, J.H. Burton, N.R. Cary, J.N. Skepper, M.J. Mitchinson, Evidence that the death of macrophage foam cells contributes to the lipid core of atheroma, Atherosclerosis 114 (1995) 45–54.

[6] V. Fuster, L. Badimon, J.J. Badimon, J.H. Chesebro, The pathogenesis of coronary artery disease and the acute coronary syndromes, N. Engl. J. Med. 326 (1992) 242–250.

[7] F.D. Kolodgie, J. Narula, A.P. Burke, N. Haider, A. Farb, Y. Hui-Liang, J. Smialek, R. Virmani, Localization of apoptotic macrophages at the site of plaque rupture in sudden coronary death, Am. J. Pathol. 157 (2000) 1259–1268.

[8] P. Libby, S.K. Clinton, The role of macrophages in atherogenesis, Curr. Opin. Lipidol. 4 (1993) 355–363.

[9] G.J. Warner, G. Stoudt, M. Bamberger, W.J. Johnson, G.H. Rothblat, Cell toxicity induced by inhibition of acyl coenzyme A: cholesterol acyltransferase and accumulation of unesterified cholesterol, J. Biol. Chem. 270 (1995) 5772–5778.

[10] I. Tabas, S. Marathe, G.A. Keesler, N. Beatini, Y. Shiratori, Evidence that the initial up-regulation of

phosphatidylcholine biosynthesis in free cholesterol-loaded macrophages is an adaptive response that prevents cholesterol-induced cellular necrosis, J. Biol. Chem. 271 (1996) 22773–22781.

[11] P.M. Yao, I. Tabas, Free cholesterol loading of macrophages induces apoptosis involving the fas pathway, J. Biol. Chem. 275 (2000) 23807–23813.

[12] P.M. Yao, I. Tabas, Free cholesterol loading of macrophages is associated with widespread mitochondrial dysfunction and activation of the mitochondrial apoptosis pathway, J. Biol. Chem. 276 (2001) 42468–42476.

[13] S. Fazio, A.S. Major, L.L. Swift, L.A. Gleaves, M. Accad, M.F. Linton, R.V. Farese Jr., Increased atherosclerosis in LDL receptor-null mice lacking ACAT1 in macrophages, J. Clin. Invest. 107 (2001) 163–171.

[14] M.J. Mitchinson, S.J. Hardwick, M.R. Bennett, Cell death in atherosclerotic plaques, Curr. Opin. Lipidol. 7 (1996) 324–329.

[15] M.M. Kockx, Apoptosis in the atherosclerotic plaque: quantitative and qualitative aspects, Arterioscler. Thromb. Vasc. Biol. 18 (1998) 1519–1522.

[16] G. Kellner-Weibel, Y.J. Geng, G.H. Rothblat, Cytotoxic cholesterol is generated by the hydrolysis of cytoplasmic cholesteryl ester and transported to the plasma membrane, Atherosclerosis 146 (1999) 309–319.

[17] M.-K. Chang, C. Bergmark, A. Laurila, S. Horkko, K.-H. Han, P. Friedman, E.A. Dennis, J.L. Witztum, Monoclonal antibodies against oxidized low-density lipoprotein bind to apoptotic cells and inhibit their phagocytosis by elicited macrophages, Proc. Natl. Acad. Sci. U. S. A. 96 (1999) 6353–6358.

[18] M. Khan, S. Pelengaris, M. Cooper, C. Smith, G. Evan, J. Betteridge, Oxidised lipoproteins may promote inflammation through the selective delay of engulfment but not binding of apoptotic cells by macrophages, Atherosclerosis 171 (2003) 21–29.

[19] J.J. Lemasters, V. Necrapoptosis and the mitochondrial permeability transition: shared pathways to necrosis and apoptosis, Am. J. Physiol. 276 (1999) G1–G6.

[20] B. Feng, P.M. Yao, Y. Li, C.M. Devlin, D. Zhang, H.P. Harding, M. Sweeney, J.X. Rong, G. Kuriakose, E.A. Fisher, A.M. Marks, I. Tabas, The endoplasmic reticulum is the site of cholesterol-induced cytotoxicity in macrophages, Nat. Cell Biol. 5 (2003) 781–792.

[21] K.J. Travers, C.K. Patil, L. Wodicka, D.J. Lockhart, J.S. Weissman, P. Walter, Functional and genomic analyses reveal an essential coordination between the unfolded protein response and ER-associated degradation, Cell 101 (2000) 249–258.

[22] M. Treiman, Regulation of the endoplasmic reticulum calcium storage during the unfolded protein response—significance in tissue ischemia? Trends Cardiovasc. Med. 12 (2002) 57–62.

[23] B. Feng, D. Zhang, G. Kuriakose, C.M. Devlin, M. Kockx, I. Tabas, Niemann-Pick C heterozygosity confers resistance to lesional necrosis and macrophage apoptosis in murine atherosclerosis, Proc. Natl. Acad. Sci. U. S. A. 100 (2003) 10423–10428.

International Congress Series 1262 (2004) 396–399

www.ics-elsevier.com

Caveolin and cholesterol in lipid transport and signaling

Christopher J. Fielding*

Department of Physiology, Cardiovascular Research Institute, University of California , San Francisco, CA 94143, USA

Abstract. Caveolae are free cholesterol-rich invaginated microdomains of the cell surface characterized by the presence of one or more structural proteins (caveolins). The cholesterol-binding capacity of caveolin plays a key role in the organization of signaling complexes within caveolae. Caveolae are particularly rich in multiprotein signaling complexes containing protein growth factor receptors or integrins. Immunoprecipitation of caveolins from cells labeled with ^{3}H free cholesterol (FC) allows proteins and lipids present in caveolae to be identified at intervals following the initiation of signal transduction. Signaling was found to be associated with transient loss of caveolin-associated FC, stimulation of FC efflux, and phosphorylation of caveolin at a sensitive tyrosine residue. FC within caveolae is labile and responsive to changes in the local composition of signaling complexes. In view of the extended residence of caveolae at the cell surface, these data imply that caveolae take part in an FC cycle initiated by the binding of ligand to its transmembrane kinase. Regulated loss of FC from caveolae is followed by a recovery phase when FC content is restored. These changes form an essential part of signal transduction from the cell surface for caveolae-associated signaling complexes.

Keywords: Caveola; Caveolin; Cholesterol; Signaling

1. Introduction

It is now widely accepted that the cell surface is made up of a heterogenous mixture of microdomains differentiated by the presence of different lipids and proteins. Well-recognized examples include coated pits, distinguished by a low free cholesterol (FC) content relative to glycerophospholipid and by the structural protein, clathrin. Other microdomains are enriched in FC and sphingolipids. These were formerly considered to form a single population, described as lipid rafts or caveolae. From the research of several laboratories, it is now clear that this fraction contains at least two distinct structures. Planar FC, sphingolipid-rich domains (lipid rafts), enriched in glycerophosphatidylinositol (GPI)-

* Tel.: +1-415-476-4307; fax: +1-415-476-2283.
E-mail address: cfield@itsa.ucsf.edu (C.J. Fielding).

0531-5131/ © 2003 Published by Elsevier B.V.
doi:10.1016/j.ics.2003.12.023

linked proteins, are labile structures particularly enriched in lymphocytes and involved in cytokine and chemokine signaling. Caveolae are stable invaginations, rich in FC and sphingolipids, containing caveolins as their major structural proteins, and deficient in GPI-anchored proteins [1–4]. Caveolae are present at high levels in endothelial cells, muscle cells, lung cells, adipocytes, and other terminally differentiated peripheral cells that respond to protein growth factors. It is of particular interest that many transformed cell lines and human cancer cells, whose replication has become independent of growth factors, are deficient in or completely lack caveolae. Transfection of these cell lines with caveolin cDNA may restore dependence on growth factors.

There is some crosstalk between caveolae and lipid rafts. Loss of caveolae is associated with an increase in the level of GPI-anchored proteins in rafts, and vice versa [3]. In caveolin $-/-$ mice and cultured cells lacking caveolin, signaling complexes normally organized in caveolae become associated with lipid rafts [5]. However, this adoption is incomplete, since the vascular and pulmonary tissues of these animals show a characteristic hyperplasia, suggestive of imperfect growth control [6].

Both lipid rafts and caveolae contain unusual concentrations of gangliosides [2]. There may be unrecognized subclasses of both microdomains distinguished by different subclasses of sphingolipids and, possibly, different complexes of signaling proteins. However, techniques that could isolate these in a native state are not yet available.

2. Caveolin function and primary sequence

FC binding by caveolin-1 is mediated by a motif (V/L x_{1-4} Y x_{1-4} K^+/R^+, where x is any amino acid) [7], which has also been identified in a number of other documented FC-binding proteins. In caveolin, this site is located at the boundary of the cytoplasm with the cytofacial leaflet of the membrane bilayer. Within the caveolin primary sequence, this site is adjacent to a “scaffold” site ($\varphi x_{2-4} \varphi x_{2-4} \varphi$, where φ is Y, W, or F and x is any amino acid) [8] that interacts with many recognized signaling intermediate proteins. Examples include transmembrane receptor kinases, downstream nonreceptor kinases, and linkers. The presence of a single scaffold site on each molecule and of more than one scaffold-binding protein in a single complex (e.g., EGFR, Src) suggests the cooperative interaction of multiple caveolins during a single signaling event. Several models of caveolin aggregates have been recently suggested. Based on the size distribution of molecular aggregates, the C-terminal domain of caveolin has been implicated in oligomerization, although this is a poorly conserved region compared with other domains in the primary sequence. Finally, caveolin is phosphorylated on Y_{14} in response to the action of several protein growth factors [9–11]. Chronic exposure to tyrosine phosphatase inhibitors leads to both phosphorylation of caveolin, and dissociation of its surface complexes to FC-rich intracellular vesicles [12]. However, the transient phosphorylation of caveolin observed in response to epidermal growth factor (EGF) or vascular epidermal growth factor (VEGF) occurs at the cell surface. The EGF, VEGF, and platelet-derived growth factor (PDGF) receptor proteins and c-Src all show binding sites for the caveolin ‘scaffold’ domain. These data suggest tertiary structure within the N-terminal moiety of the caveolin primary sequence to bring Y_{14} to the scaffold sequence. No details are yet available on the tertiary structure of signaling proteins bound to caveolin.

3. Interaction of FC and protein binding during signal transduction

The FC content of caveolae, modified, for example, by cyclodextrin (a soluble extracellular FC acceptor) or cholesterol loading from low-density lipoprotein (LDL), plays a major role in determining both the composition of signaling complexes and their activity [13,14], but this response appears to be complex. In some cases, FC activates signal transduction; in others, it inhibits it. In different cell lines, loss of FC can have contrary effects on the same kinase activity. Within a branching signaling pathway responding to the same ligand, FC may stimulate one pathway and inhibit another. Finally, within the same pathway, FC may activate some reaction steps and inhibit others [15]. Taken together, these data suggest that FC levels within caveolae can be differentially regulated in terms of both space and time. That is, local events, most probably the phosphorylation of signaling proteins bound to the caveolin scaffold domain, can locally influence FC content while at the same time, the FC content of other signaling complexes remains unchanged.

4. Caveolae and FC homeostasis

Early work focused on the role of caveolae as preferred receptables for newly synthesized and recycling preformed FC. This, no doubt, mainly reflects the concentration of FC in the exofacial leaflet of the cell membrane to lipid rafts and caveolae, and the ability of caveolin to bind FC. Several additional functions for caveolin have been described [16]. Findings in these areas may be sensitive to differences in the cells and conditions used, particularly in the level of FC-rich microdomains in different models. The functions proposed include roles in recycling of FC, either directly, via weakly acidified endosomes, or indirectly, after cholesteryl ester hydrolysis, in postlysosomal vesicles; in the formation or maintenance of intracellular lipid droplets; as part of a chaperone complex with heat shock proteins and cyclophyllins; in maintaining the FC gradient across Golgi stacks; and in FC efflux. It has not been determined unambiguously if caveolin determines the level of FC in membranes, or if increased membrane FC leads to a redistribution of caveolin within the cell. The functional implication of these alternatives is quite different. In either case, contrary to earlier suggestions, caveolin-bound FC seems to be quite labile, possibly because the network of protein molecules to which caveolar FC is directly bound prevents the formation of a classical liquid ordered phase. (This may not be the case with planar lipid rafts, which lack caveolin.) Both the N- and C-termini of caveolin are cytoplasmic, and the protein lacks an extracellular domain. At least part of caveolar FC is within the exofacial domain of the plasma membrane—not directly accessible to the caveolin FC binding site.

5. PDGF-mediated signal transduction and caveolar function

Signaling initiated by the reaction of PDGF with its receptor protein has been the basis for several studies in which levels of FC and protein associated with caveolae have been determined. The effects of FC on sequential kinase activities in these multiprotein signaling complexes were determined. One unexpected feature was the magnitude of transient changes in caveolin-associated FC. Up to 80% of total FC in this fraction was lost

7.5–15 min following PDGF binding, and associated with a stimulation of FC efflux [17]. This FC was subsequently replaced from intracellular pools, probably mainly the *trans*-Golgi network. A second unexpected feature was that the presence of an extracellular FC acceptor (the major protein of plasma high-density lipoprotein, apo A-1) not only increased loss of FC from the caveolar fraction, but also stimulated phosphoprotein levels in response to PDGF. These findings suggest complex interplay between protein kinase activity and FC binding within the caveola that is variable as a function of time. In particular, it suggests that even modest changes in ambient plasma membrane FC could have significant effects on the ability of cells to respond to extracellular signals and attachment mediated by integrins. It is of interest that both are modified during mitosis. At the same time, FC levels in the cell membrane decrease, as does expression of caveolin at the cell surface. Together, these data support the concept that FC is a key regulator of the major functions of caveolae.

References

[1] J.E. Schnitzer, et al., Separation of caveolae from associated microdomains of GPI-anchored proteins, Science 269 (1995) 1398–1399.

[2] K. Iwabuchi, et al., Separation of "glycosphingolipid signaling domain" from caveolin-containing membrane fractions in mouse melanoma B16 cells and its role in cell adhesion coupled with signaling, J. Biol. Chem. 273 (1998) 33766–33773.

[3] L. Abrami, et al., Cross-talk between caveolae and glycosylphosphatidylinositol-rich domains, J. Biol. Chem. 276 (2001) 30729–30736.

[4] G. Sowa, et al., Distinction between signaling mechanisms in lipid rafts vs caveolae, Proc. Natl. Acad. Sci. U. S. A. 98 (2001) 14072–14077.

[5] S. Vainio, et al., Dynamic association of human insulin receptor with lipid rafts in cells lacking caveolae, EMBO Rep. 3 (2002) 95–100.

[6] S.E. Woodman, et al., Caveolin-1 knockout mice show an impaired response to exogenous stimuli, Am. J. Pathol. 162 (2003) 2059–2068.

[7] H. Li, et al., Peripheral-type benzodiazepine receptor function in cholesterol transport. Identification of a putative cholesterol recognition/interaction amino acid sequence and consensus pattern, Endocrinology 139 (1998) 4991–4997.

[8] E.J. Smart, et al., Caveolins, liquid-ordered domains, and signal transduction, Mol. Cell. Biol. 19 (1999) 7289–7304.

[9] C.C. Mastick, et al., Insulin-stimulated tyrosine phosphorylation of caveolin is specific for the differentiated adipocyte phenotype of 3T3-L1 cells, J. Biol. Chem., (1997) 20706–20714.

[10] Y.N. Kim, et al., Epidermal growth factor-stimulated tyrosine phosphorylation of caveolin-1, J. Biol. Chem. 275 (2000) 7481–7491.

[11] L. Labreque, et al., Regulation of vascular endothelial growth factor receptor-2 activity by caveolin-1 and plasma membrane cholesterol, Mol. Cell. Biol. 14 (2003) 334–347.

[12] R.G. Parton, et al., Regulated internalization of caveolae, J. Cell Biol. 127 (1994) 1199–1215.

[13] S.V. Matveev, et al., Heterologous desensitization of EGF receptors and PDGF receptors by sequestration in caveolae, Am. J. Physiol. 282 (2002) C935–C946.

[14] Y. Zhu, et al., Lipoprotein promotes caveolin-1 and Ras translocation to caveolae: role of cholesterol in endothelial signaling, Arterioscler. Thromb. Vasc. Biol. 20 (2000) 2465–2470.

[15] C.J. Fielding, Membrane cholesterol and the regulation of signal transduction. Biochem. Soc. Trans 32 (2004) in press.

[16] C.J. Fielding, et al., Relationship between cholesterol trafficking and signaling in rafts and caveolae. Biochim. Biophys. Acta 1610 (2003) 219–228.

[17] P.E. Fielding, et al., Sterol efflux to apolipoprotein A-1 originates from caveolin-rich microdomains and potentiates PDGF-dependent protein kinase activity, Biochemistry 41 (2002) 4929–4937.

International Congress Series 1262 (2004) 400–403

www.ics-elsevier.com

MTP/apoB mediated lipoprotein assembly: an emerging pathway for lipid secretion and transport

John R. Wetterau*

Department of Metabolic Research, Bristol-Myers Squibb, P.O. Box 5400, Princeton, NJ 08543-5400, USA

Abstract. Phospholipid, free and esterified cholesterol, triglyceride, and apolipoprotein B (apoB) are assembled into lipoprotein particles in hepatocytes and intestinal enterocytes, and then secreted from the cell in the form of very low density lipoproteins or chylomicrons for transport throughout the body. Studies have shown that the formation of the mature lipoprotein particle requires the microsomal triglyceride transfer protein (MTP), a lipid transfer protein found within the endoplasmic reticulum of liver and intestine. Although the MTP/apoB lipid secretion and transport pathway was originally thought to be unique to the liver and intestine, recent reports suggest a similar pathway may have additional roles in other tissues. © 2004 Elsevier B.V. All rights reserved.

Keywords: Microsomal triglyceride transfer protein; Apolipoprotein B; Abetalipoproteinemia; Fatty acids; Triglyceride

1. Introduction

The microsomal triglyceride transfer protein is an intracellular lipid transfer protein found in high concentrations in the lumen of the microsomal fraction of liver and intestinal mucosa. It catalyzes the transport of triglyceride (TG), cholesteryl ester (CE), and phospholipid between membranes in in vitro assays. Following its purification from bovine liver, it was shown to consist of two subunits, a unique 97 kDa subunit and the multifunctional protein, protein disulfide isomerase. The role of MTP in lipid transport and metabolism was revealed by studies demonstrating that a defect in MTP is the proximal cause of abetalipoproteinemia, an autosomal recessive defect in the production of apoB-containing lipoproteins, chylomicrons and very low-density lipoproteins (VLDL) (reviewed in Ref. [1]).

2. Role of MTP in lipoprotein assembly

As newly synthesized apoB is translocated into the lumen of the endoplasmic reticulum (ER), it co-translationally associates with lipid to form a small nascent, lipid poor, lipoprotein particle. MTP helps initiate the transfer of lipid to apoB as the

* Tel.: +1-609-818-4254; fax: +1-609-818-3600.
E-mail address: john.wetterau@bms.com (J.R. Wetterau).

doi:10.1016/j.ics.2003.12.082

polypeptide is translocated into the ER lumen. MTP also binds to the newly synthesized apoB and is thought to play a chaperone like role in directing apoB into the ER lumen. Both roles are believed to be important in promoting lipoprotein production (reviewed in Refs. [2,3]).

Once formed, the nascent particle with a density of high-density lipoprotein (HDL) or low-density lipoprotein (LDL) may be directly secreted in some cases, or it may acquire additional lipid to form a mature VLDL or chylomicron. There are conflicting views on how the nascent particle is further lipidated to form a mature lipoprotein. This uncertainty may in part reflect the different model systems used to study the assembly of apoB-containing lipoproteins. It has been proposed that lipid may be added to the nascent particle through a series of events leading to the mature lipoprotein particle, or alternatively, the nascent particle may fuse with a preformed lipid emulsion to form a lipid rich, mature lipoprotein particle. Whether MTP is required for the maturation of the nascent particle is still the topic of debate.

3. Role of MTP/apoB in fatty acid trafficking

Hepatic fatty acids (fa) can be oxidized directly, incorporated into the cytosolic triglyceride pool, or be secreted as TG in a lipoprotein particle. The majority of fa delivered to the liver appears to first cycle through a cytosolic fat droplet before entering the VLDL synthetic pathway (reviewed in Ref. [4]). Following lipolysis of the TG in the intracellular droplet, a portion of the free fa enters the VLDL secretion pathway, while the majority is recycled back to the cytosolic TG droplet. Hebbachi and Gibbons [5] studied fa recycling following MTP inhibition in rat hepatocytes. They found, as expected, an MTP inhibitor decreased TG secretion. In addition, they found MTP inhibition did not decrease cytosolic TG turnover, while it increased the rate of fa re-esterification into the intracellular TG pool. The influx of fa into the total TG pool (intracellular and secreted) was decreased by MTP inhibition. Blocking the triglyceride secretion pathway with an MTP inhibitor may not shift fa metabolism towards an oxidative pathway, as hepatic fatty acid oxidation activity was not increased in rats treated with an MTP inhibitor for two weeks [6].

4. ApoB-containing lipoproteins in other tissues

Co-expression of MTP and apoB in HeLa cells results in the production and secretion of apoB-containing lipoproteins [7]. This suggests that lipoprotein production does not require a liver or intestinal specific assembly apparatus and that the expression of apoB, MTP, and lipid availability are sufficient for the production of lipoprotein particles. Since apoB and MTP expression have been detected in tissues other than the liver and intestine, the work by Gordon et al. [7] raises the question as to whether MTP/apoB-mediated lipoprotein production may occur in these tissues.

ApoB-containing lipoproteins have been reported to be synthesized and secreted from rat yolk sac [8]. Rodent yolk sac lipoprotein production is thought to play an important role in the transport of nutrients to the embryo. The epithelial cells of the proximal tubules of chickens have also been shown to secrete apoB on VLDL, LDL, and HDL density particles [9,10]. Given the reported expression of MTP [11] and apoB [12] message in human kidney, one may wonder whether mammalian kidneys have the capacity to synthesize and secrete apoB-containing lipoproteins under some circumstances.

Young and colleagues found that both apoB and MTP are expressed in mouse cardiac myocytes [13] and that mouse and human heart tissue secrete apoB-containing lipoproteins [14]. The secretion was abolished in the presence of an MTP inhibitor. A role for lipoprotein secretion in regulating intracellular triglyceride levels was supported by the overexpression of an apoB transgene in mouse heart. This genetic manipulation, which is expected to increase triglyceride secretion, was able to decrease cardiac TG stores under a number of conditions associated with increased TG accumulation [15]. The apoB transgene was also able to attenuate the cardiac dysfunction in a diabetic mouse model. In contrast, genetic manipulation that results in decreased MTP expression resulted in increased TG accumulation in the heart [16]. From these studies, it was concluded that the apoB/MTP lipoprotein secretion pathway has an important role in controlling cardiac lipid homeostasis, and ultimately, cardiac function.

5. Conclusions

The MTP/apoB secretion pathway in the liver and intestine is recognized for its importance in the transport and partitioning of esterified fatty acids (in the form of triglyceride) throughout the body. However, in addition to its role in whole body fuel transport, it appears that MTP/apoB-mediated transport has other roles. These may include a more limited nutrient transport role in specific tissues, for example the yolk sac, or a role in fa trafficking in other tissues. In the liver and intestine, fatty acids enter the cell where they may be temporarily stored as TG or oxidized. A portion of the fatty acid is also secreted as triglyceride in lipoproteins. The magnitude of this depends upon the availability of fatty acids. Thus, there is a balance between utilization, storage, and secretion. A similar balance may occur in other tissues that have a large flux of fatty acids and rely heavily upon fatty acid oxidation as a source of fuel, for example the heart and kidney. When an imbalance between fa input and utilization occurs in these cells, like liver and intestine, storage of fa in cytosolic fat droplets may become excessive. One could speculate that disturbances in the balance may also induce the capacity to secrete TG in the form of a lipoprotein particle. Although the amount of TG secreted may be quantitatively small, this secretion may nevertheless play an important role for the cell.

References

[1] N. Berriot-Varoqueaux, L.P. Aggerbeck, M.-E. Samson-Bouma, J.R. Wetterau, The role of the microsomal triglyceride transfer protein in abetalipoproteinemia, Annu. Rev. Nutr. 20 (2000) 663–697.

[2] E.A. Fisher, H.N. Ginsberg, Complexity in the secretory pathway: the assembly and secretion of apolipoprotein B-containing lipoproteins, J. Biol. Chem. 277 (2002) 17377–17380.

[3] D.A. Gordon, H. Jamil, Progress towards understanding the role of microsomal triglyceride transfer protein in apolipoprotein-B lipoprotein assembly, Biochim. Biophys. Acta 1486 (2000) 72–83.

[4] G.F. Gibbons, K. Isam, R.J. Pease, Mobilisation of triacylglycerol stores, Biochim. Biophys. Acta 1483 (2000) 37–57.

[5] A.-M. Hebbachi, G.F. Gibbons, Inactivation of microsomal triglyceride transfer protein impairs the normal redistribution but not the turnover of newly synthesized glycerolipid in the cytosol, endoplasmic reticulum and Golgi of primary rat hepatocytes, Biochim. Biophys. Acta 1441 (1999) 36–50.

[6] T. Funatsu, H. Kakuta, T. Takasu, K. Miyata, Atorvastatin increases hepatic fatty acid beta-oxidation in sucrose-fed rats: comparison with an MTP inhibitor, Eur. J. Pharm. 455 (2002) 161–167.
[7] D.A. Gordon, et al., Secretion of apolipoprotein B-containing lipoproteins from HeLa cells is dependent on expression of the microsomal triglyceride transfer protein and is regulated by lipid availability, Proc. Natl. Acad. Sci. U. S. A. 91 (1994) 7628–7632.
[8] H. Franke, D. Plonné, L. Winkler, R. Dargel, Synthesis, secretion and immunoelectron microscopic demonstration of apolipoprotein B-containing lipoprotein particles in the visceral rat yolk sac, Histochemistry 97 (1992) 283–292.
[9] P. Tarugi, et al., Secretion of apoB-and apoA-I-containing lipoproteins by chick kidney, J. Lipid Res. 39 (1998) 731–743.
[10] R.L. Walzem, R.J. Hansen, D.L. Williams, R.L. Hamilton, Estrogen induction of VLDLy assembly in egg-laying hens, J. Nutr. 129 (1999) 467S–472S.
[11] C.C. Shoulders, et al., Abetalipoproteinemia is caused by defects of the gene encoding the 97 kDa subunit of a microsomal triglyceride transfer protein, Hum. Mol. Genet. 2 (1993) 2109–2116.
[12] B. Teng, M. Verp, J. Salomon, N. Davidson, Apolipoprotein B messenger RNA editing is developmentally regulated and widely expressed in human tissues, J. Biol. Chem. 265 (1990) 20616–20620.
[13] L.B. Nielsen, et al., Genes for apolipoprotein B and microsomal triglyceride transfer protein are expressed in the heart, Circulation 98 (1998) 13–16.
[14] J. Borén, M.M. Véniant, S.G. Young, Apo B100-containing lipoproteins are secreted by the heart, J. Clin. Invest. 101 (1998) 1197–1202.
[15] L.B. Nielsen, E.D. Bartels, E. Bollano, Overexpression of apolipoprotein B in the heart impedes cardiac triglyceride accumulation and development of cardiac dysfunction in diabetic mice, J. Biol. Chem. 277 (2002) 27014–27020.
[16] J. Björkegren, et al., Lipoprotein secretion and triglyceride stores in the heart, J. Biol. Chem. 276 (2001) 38511–38517.

International Congress Series 1262 (2004) 404–406

www.ics-elsevier.com

The pro-inflammatory nature of the vascular extracellular matrix

Thomas N. Wight[a,*], Stephen Evanko[a], Michael Kinsella[a], Mary Chang[b], Chang Yeop Han[b], Sana Sakr[a], Robert Huang[c], Mervyn Merrilees[c], Michael Rosenfeld[d], Alan Chait[b]

[a] *Department of Vascular Biology, The Hope Heart Institute, 1124 Columbia Street, #783, Seattle, WA 98104-2046, USA*

[b] *Division of Endocrinology and Metabolism, Department of Medicine, University of Washington, School of Medicine, Seattle, WA, USA*

[c] *Department of Anatomy with Radiology, School of Medical Sciences, The University of Auckland, Auckland, New Zealand*

[d] *Department of Pathobiology, University of Washington, Seattle, WA 98195, USA*

Abstract. Chronic inflammation in vascular disease affects the organization of the extracellular matrix (ECM) in such a way as to promote the events associated with atherosclerosis and restenosis. Versican and hyaluronan are two ECM components that are affected by inflammation and, in turn, affect the inflammatory response. Inflammatory growth factors such as TGF-β1 and PDGF stimulate the production of versican and hyaluronan by arterial smooth muscle cells (ASMCs). These ECM components accumulate in vascular disease and promote the proliferation and migration of ASMCs, contributing to intimal hyperplasia. Hyaluronan also serves as attachment ligand for inflammatory cells and may be partly responsible for leukocyte retention as part of the early inflammatory response. Inflammation also leads to destruction of the ECM and failure of the ECM to remodel. Elastic fibers are absent in atherosclerotic and restenotic lesions and controlled expression of a versican variant, V3, in ASMCs restores the ability of these cells to form elastic fibers. ECM assembly is critical to vascular healing and the prevention of vascular disease.

Keywords: Proteoglycans; Hyaluronan; Versican; Elastin; Atherosclerosis; Restenosis

Chronic inflammation is involved in the development of atherosclerosis [1,2], for example, inflammation disrupts the structure and organization of the extracellular matrix (ECM) during disease progression [3]. ECM remodeling can be likened to wound healing [4,5] in which the ECM goes through a series of stages that culminate in the advanced

* Corresponding author. Tel.: +1-206-903-2070; fax: +1-206-903-2088.
E-mail address: twight@hopeheart.org (T.N. Wight).

0531-5131/
doi:10.1016/j.ics.2003.12.061

atherosclerotic plaque. Inflammation plays a role in several of these stages. Different inflammatory stimuli regulate the assembly and disassembly of specific ECM components which, in turn, control many of the events that lead to vascular disease. So, two important questions to consider are: (1) do specific ECM components play a role in retention of inflammatory cells in vascular disease?; (2) is it possible to reverse the destruction of the ECM induced by inflammation in vascular disease?

Two ECM components that are likely to play a role in inflammation in vascular disease are versican and hyaluronan [3]. Versican is a chondroitin sulfate proteoglycan enriched in vascular lesions. Hyaluronan is a glycosaminoglycan that interacts with versican and forms high molecular weight complexes that fill the ECM as vascular lesions develop. These two molecules increase in the early phases of atherosclerosis and are particularly enriched in human restenotic lesions induced by mechanical injury during surgical intervention [6–9]. These early changes are most likely due to inflammatory cytokines and growth factors since both PDGF and TGF β1 increase the synthesis of both versican and hyaluronan in ASMCs [10]. These molecules also form a provisional ECM which supports arterial smooth muscle cell (ASMC) proliferation and migration [11]. In addition, studies with intestinal SMCs induced to synthesize hyaluronan demonstrate that hyaluronan interacts with monocytes through CD44-HA connections [12], suggesting that this ECM component could serve as a partial substrate for leukocytes as part of the inflammatory response. Furthermore, in lipid-induced atherosclerotic lesions in experimental animals, hyaluronan and macrophages tend to co-localize [13]. This is especially prominent in animal models of atherosclerosis in which lipid metabolism is perturbed such as in the LDL receptor negative Watanabe rabbit. Hyaluronan and macrophages co-localize to the more superficial regions of the lesions in this animal model. Enrichment of hyaluronan in these lesions suggests that hyaluronan metabolism may be altered. In fact, cultures of ASMCs derived from Watanabe rabbits synthesize more hyaluronan and have more hyaluronan associated with their cell surface than similar cells from wild type animals. It remains to be determined whether these differences are responsible for the retention of the macrophage in these lesions.

The second question is whether it is possible to reverse the destructive effects of inflammation on the organization of the ECM. Inflammation destroys the architecture of the ECM during atherogenesis. Healing involves rebuilding this structure to limit disease progression. The usual repair response as part of the end stage of inflammation in vascular disease is the formation of fibrous tissue enriched in collagen fibrils and associated proteoglycans and glycoproteins. What do not reform during this phase are the elastic fibers. In fact, atherosclerotic and restenotic lesions are usually devoid of elastic fibers. One factor that appears to inhibit elastic fiber formation is chondroitin sulfate which is a part of the versican molecule [14]. We have found that overexpressing the versican variant that lacks chondroitin sulfate, V3, promotes elastic fiber assembly in ASMC [15]. Furthermore, when these transduced SMCs are seeded into injured blood vessels, elastic fibers develop in response to the injury. If the synthesis of the chondroitin sulfate containing form of versican is blocked by antisense, elastic fibers form as well. Such results indicate that the adverse effect of inflammation on elastic fiber destruction can be repaired by regulating the expression of the proteoglycan versican in ASMC.

In conclusion, the ECM is of considerable importance when considering the role of inflammation in vascular disease. While it is true that inflammation is driven by the immune cells and their products, they must operate in a "soil" that provides the proper signals. It appears that this "soil" is made from specific components of the ECM and regulating how this soil is assembled may provide a key to controlling vascular lesion development.

Acknowledgements

This work was supported by NIH grants HL18645 (TNW), DK02456 (AC) and the Marsden Foundation (MM). The authors thank Ms. Ellen Briggs for the preparation of the manuscript.

References

[1] R. Ross, Atherosclerosis—an inflammatory disease, N. Engl. J. Med. 340 (2) (1999) 115–126.
[2] G.K. Hansson, et al., Innate and adaptive immunity in the pathogenesis of atherosclerosis, Circ. Res. 91 (4) (2002) 281–291.
[3] T. Wight, The vascular extracellular matrix, in: V. Fuster, E. Topol, E. Nabel (Eds.), Atherosclerosis and Coronary Artery Disease, Lippincott, Williams and Wilkins, Philadelphia, 2003, in press.
[4] R.A. Clark, et al., Fibronectin and fibrin provide a provisional matrix for epidermal cell migration during wound reepithelialization, J. Invest. Dermatol. 79 (5) (1982) 264–269.
[5] R.L. Geary, et al., Wound healing: a paradigm for lumen narrowing after arterial reconstruction, J. Vasc. Surg. 27 (1) (1998) 96–106.
[6] R. Riessen, et al., Distribution of hyaluronan during extracellular matrix remodeling in human restenotic arteries and balloon-injured rat carotid arteries, Circulation 93 (1996) 1141–1147.
[7] T.N. Wight, et al., Selective deposits of versican in the extracellular matrix of restenotic lesions from human peripheral arteries, Am. J. Pathol. 151 (1997) 963–973.
[8] A.V. Finn, et al., A novel rat model of carotid artery stenting for the understanding of restenosis in metabolic diseases, J. Vasc. Res. 39 (5) (2002) 414–425.
[9] I.M. Chung, et al., Enhanced extracellular matrix accumulation in restenosis of coronary arteries after stent deployment, J. Am. Coll. Cardiol. 40 (12) (2002) 2072–2081.
[10] E. Schönherr, et al., Effects of platelet-derived growth factor and transforming growth factor-beta 1 on the synthesis of a large versican-like chondroitin sulfate proteoglycan by arterial smooth muscle cells, J. Biol. Chem. 266 (1991) 17640–17647.
[11] S.P. Evanko, et al., Formation of hyaluronan and versican-rich pericellular matrix is required for proliferation and migration of vascular smooth muscle cells, Arterioscler. Thromb. Vasc. Biol. 19 (1999) 1004–1013.
[12] C.A. de La Motte, et al., Mononuclear leukocytes preferentially bind via CD44 to hyaluronan on human intestinal mucosal smooth muscle cells after virus infection or treatment with poly(I.C), J. Biol. Chem. 274 (43) (1999) 30747–30755.
[13] S. Evanko, et al., Proteoglycan distribution in lesions of atherosclerosis depends on lesion severity, structural characteristics and the proximity of PDGF and TGF-β1, Am. J. Pathol. 152 (1998) 533–546.
[14] A. Hinek, et al., Impaired elastin fiber assembly related to reduced 67-kD elastin-binding protein in fetal lamb ductus arteriosus and in cultured aortic smooth muscle cells treated with chondroitin sulfate, J. Clin. Invest. 88 (1991) 2083–2094.
[15] M.J. Merrilees, et al., Retrovirally mediated overexpression of versican v3 by arterial smooth muscle cells induces tropoelastin synthesis and elastic fiber formation in vitro and in neointima after vascular injury, Circ. Res. 90 (4) (2002) 481–487.

International Congress Series 1262 (2004) 407–410

www.ics-elsevier.com

Regulation of extracellular matrix production and degradation of endothelial cells by shear stress

Tetsu Yamane[a], Noriko Yamaguchi[b], Yoji Yoshida[a], Masako Mitsumata[c,*]

[a] *Department of Pathology, School of Medicine, University of Yamanashi, Yamanashi, Japan*

[b] *Department of Molecular Pathogenesis, Medical Research Institute, Tokyo Medical and Dental University, Tokyo, Japan*

[c] *Department of Pathology, School of Medicine, Nihon University, 30-1 Oyaguchikamicho, Itabashi, Tokyo 173-8610, Japan*

Abstract. Extracellular matrix (ECM) including subendothelial basement membranes developed more in the anti-atherosclerotic regions, which were exposed to laminar shear stress, than in the atherosclerotic-prone regions, which were exposed to turbulent low mean shear stress. Here we present evidence that the laminar shear stress influence the subendothelial ECM formation through the regulation of endothelial collagen metabolism. *Methods*: Confluent endothelial cells (EC) obtained from bovine aorta or human umbilical veins were exposed to laminar shear stress using parallel-plate flow chamber. After exposure, collagenase-sensitive products labeled with 3H-proline in both media and cells were measured as collagenous protein, and analyzed by fluorography. Expression of matrix metalloproteinase 2 (MMP2), which degrades type IV collagen in basement membrane, in EC was analyzed by gelatin zymography, Western blotting and Northern blotting. *Results*: (1) Over 90% of collagenous protein produced by EC was collagen type IV. (2) Collagen synthesis of EC was increased by shear stress time-dependently. (3) The MMP2 secretion from EC into medium was interrupted completely by shear stress, although the levels of intracellular protein and mRNA expression of MMP2 were unchanged. (4) Albumin changed MMP2 secretion from EC. *Conclusion*: Our data suggest that laminar shear stress contribute to the formation of anti-atherosclerotic microenvironment in vessel through the regulation of collagen type IV metabolism of EC.

Keywords: Endothelial cell; Shear stress; Type IV collagen; Matrix metalloproteinase 2

1. Introduction

Hemodynamic forces have been implicated in the initiation and localization of atherosclerosis. In the human aorta, atherosclerotic lesions were initially developed at

Abbreviations: EC, endothelial cell; MMP, matrix metalloproteinase; GFP, green fluorescent protein.

* Corresponding author. Tel.: +81-33972-8111x2252; fax: +81-33972-8830.

E-mail address: masakom@med.nihon-u.ac.jp (M. Mitsumata).

0531-5131/ © 2004 Published by Elsevier B.V.
doi:10.1016/j.ics.2003.12.031

the proximal area of bifurcations where the low mean shear stress was exposed. However, the atherogenic lesions hardly occurred at high shear stress regions, such as the leading edge of the flow divider of bifurcations. There were many attractive functions in the vascular endothelial cells which were exposed blood flow derived shear stress. Recently, the character of the shear stress might alter the function of EC. These were responsible for the localization of atherosclerotic lesion.

Collagen type IV is a major component of the basement membrane of blood vessel, which is associated with laminin, entactin and heparan sulfate to form the sheet-like basement membrane, which has the attractive function in EC, as the agent to alter the permeability, tube like formation differentiation and anti-angiogenic activity.

Basement membrane of EC forms a barrier between blood and extravascular tissue components. Remodeling of the basement membrane during embryogenesis, wound repair and metastasis is mediated by the matrix metalloproteinases (MMPs). MMP2 (Gelatinase A), which degrades collagen type IV and V, is secreted as a Mr 72,000 latent proenzyme. MMP2 is proteolytically processed to the Mr 66,000 activating with membrane bound type MMP (MT-MMP). To disclose the influences of mechanical stress on the formation of anti-atherogenic architecture, we examined the effects of laminar shear stress on the metabolism of type IV collagen in EC.

1.1. Materials and methods

Confluent endothelial cells obtained from bovine aorta or human umbilical veins were exposed to laminar shear stress using parallel-plate flow chamber. After exposure to laminar shear stress, collagenase-sensitive products labeled with 3H-proline (50 μCi/ml) in both media and cells were measured as collagenous protein, and analyzed by fluorography. Briefly, radiolabeled proteins were detected by 5% SDS-PAGE using with Amplify (Amersham Pharmacia Biotech) as fluorography enhancer. Expression of matrix metalloproteinase 2 (MMP2), which degrades type IV collagen in basement membrane, was analyzed by gelatin zymography, Western blotting and Northern blotting.

The secretions of MMP2 from EC under various conditions were estimated with gelatin zymography. Briefly, MMP2 activities in the conditioned media, Dulbecco's modified Eagle's medium (DME) without fetal calf serum (FCS), were analyzed. The samples, derived from EC under shear stress 30 dyn/cm^2 for 0.5–72 h, were performed by gelatin-substrate gel electrophoresis with 5% SDS-PAGE.

To analyze the intracellular transportation of MMP2, cDNA of MMP2 (accession No. AX481493) were fused with pEGFP-N1 expression vector (BD Bioscience Clontech Laboratories, New York, USA). The constructed cDNA of MMP2 fused with pEGFP-N1 was transfected into EC and continuously cultured for further experiments. Localization of MMP2 tagged with green fluorescent protein (GFP) was visualized with Laser Scanning Confocal Microscopy (Carl Zeiss, IBAS-2000).

1.2. Results

(1) The synthetic collagen labeled with 3H-proline of EC was analyzed. Over 90% of collagenous protein were collagen type IV which was detected with two main bands, 69

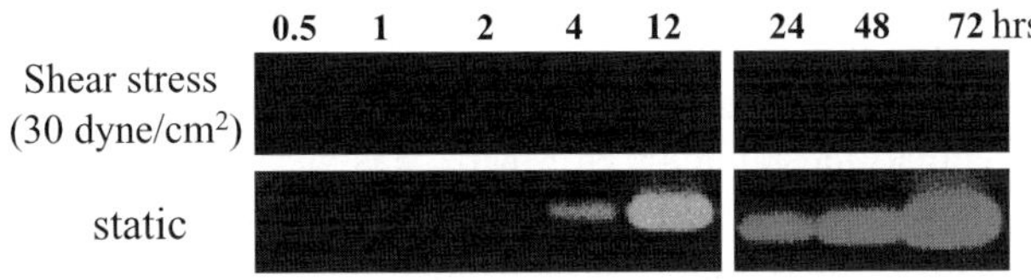

Fig. 1. Gelatin zymography showed the secretion of MMP2 in conditioned medium of EC. The gelatinase activities were clearly visible in the static control media from 30 min to 72 h. However, shear stress completely suppressed these secretions, even in the medium of 30 min exposure to shear stress.

and 98 kDa, in fluorography and Western blotting. Type IV collagen synthesis in BEC was significantly increased by 30 dyn/cm^2 laminar shear stress over 300% compared with static control. These stimulations of shear stress on collagen synthesis occurred duration-dependent within 6 h.

(2) One remarkable finding in this study was that the gelatin zymography revealed the MMP2 secretion of EC into conditioned medium was interrupted completely by shear stress exposure. However, the levels of intracellular protein and mRNA expression of MMP2 were unchanged. Even 30-min exposure of 30 dyn/cm^2 laminar shear stress suppressed the secretion of MMP2 completely (Fig. 1).

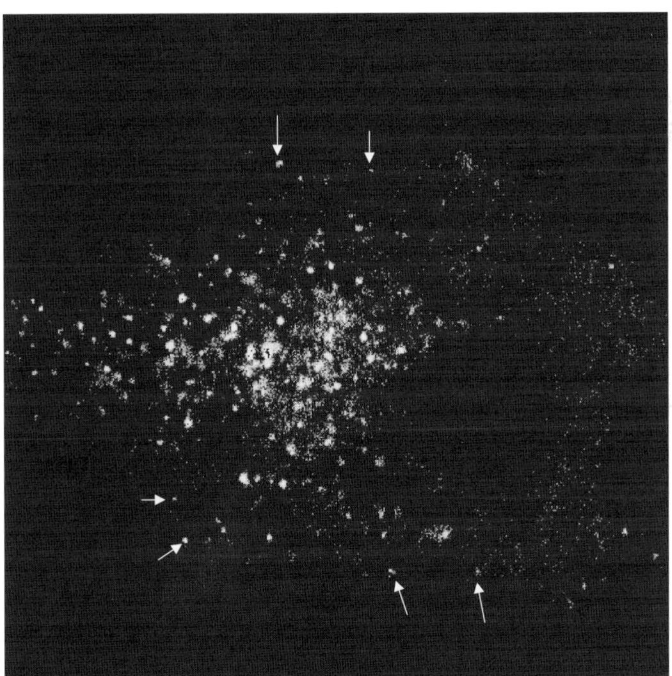

Fig. 2. An expression vector of pEGFPN1 fused with MMP2 were transfected in EC. Many large fluorescent granules were recognized in the cytoplasm and several granules were nearby cell membrane. Observation under Laser Scanning Confocal Microscopy.

(3) On the contrary, mRNA expression of MMP2 and protein level in the cells were unchanged during all exposure periods of shear stress and remained the same level as control. The intracellular transportation of MMP2 was visualized by the method of fused MMP2 tagged with GFP (MMP2/GFP). Under the static condition, many large fluorescent granules were recognized nearby the cell membrane. These were the transported vesicles just in the process of the secretion (Fig. 2).

Under the shear stress, the MMP2/GFP granules were localized under the cell membrane, but the secretion of MMP2 was suppressed from the results of zymography of conditioned medium.

(4) To clarify the mechanisms of suppressive effects of shear stress on the secretion of MMP2, we used albumin. During the search of regulatory proteins of MMP2 secretion, we incidentally found that from 0.01% to 0.1% of albumin in DMEM completely inhibits these suppressive effects of shear stress and induces the secretion of MMP2 into the medium. This albumin effect was confirmed by the confocal microscopy. GFP-fused MMP2 granules were formed under shear stress, because MMP2 exocytosis in the condition without albumin was suppressed by the shear stress exposure. Furthermore, when 0.1% albumin was added into the media, these MMP2 granules were significantly faded away from cells under the shear stress. These results suggested that albumin stimulated the exocytosis of MMP2 even under the suppression by the shear stress.

2. Discussion

The important event in the initiation of the atherosclerosis was the lipid permeation to aortic wall. The lipid deposition is barriered by the function of endothelial cells. The architecture of the endothelial basement membrane affects the differentiation of EC. The results of the present study demonstrate that the synthesis of type IV collagen was enhanced by the laminar shear stress exposure to EC. mRNA expressions of type IV collagen were also enhanced by laminar shear stress exposure. MMP2 has the gelatinase activity to digest the type IV collagen that was the main component of basement membrane. Secretion of MMP2 was strikingly suppressed by the shear stress exposure. These results suggested the hemodynamic force regulated the collagen metabolism of EC and laminar shear stress contributed the formation of resistance to atherosclerotic architecture.

ELSEVIER

International Congress Series 1262 (2004) 411–413

www.ics-elsevier.com

The elastin–laminin receptor-mediated matrix degradation. Effect of glucose concentration. Role in atherosclerosis

Gilles Faury[a], J. Verdetti[a], T. Fülöp[b], L. Robert[c,*]

[a] *Laboratoire de Dévelopement et Vieillissement de l'endothélium, Université Joseph Fourier, Grenoble, France*
[b] *Département de Gérontologie, Université de Sherbrooke, Sherbrooke, Québec, Canada*
[c] *Laboratoire d'Ophtalmologie, Hôtel-Dieu, 1 place du parvis Notre Dame, 75181 Paris cedex 04, France*

Received 7 September 2003; received in revised form 16 October 2003; accepted 20 October 2003

Abstract. *Background*: We further explored the role of the elastin–laminin receptor (ELR)-mediated reactions in matrix remodeling and atherogenesis. The progressive increase of life expectancy and the increasing prevalence of diabetes type II motivated the study of the potential influence of extracellular glucose (glc) concentration on ELR-mediated calcium homeostatic reactions as related to atherogenesis. *Methods*: Most methods using cell cultures were described previously. Glc-variation effects on the vessel wall were studied by tension myography on rat aorta rings and on Ca^{+}-influx using patch clamp technology on endothelial cells. *Results*: Previous results suggested an important role for the ELR-mediated reactions in vascular remodeling and atherogenesis. Upregulation of elastase-type endopeptidases and free-radical release plays a special role in this respect. Coupling of ELR to NO-synthase (NOS) in endothelial cells results in a vasodilation which is age- and NO-dependent. This effect was shown to vanish at low (0 mM) and high (33 mM) [glc] in adult (6-month-old) rat aortas, but is maintained in old (30-month) aortas at the high [glc]. In addition, Ca^{+}-channel activity (Ba^{2+} influx) triggered by elastin peptides was maximal at normal [glc] (11 mM) and decreased at lower and higher [glc] in adult aortas. High [glc] was shown also to increase elastase production and the biosynthesis of several matrix components such as collagen III and fibronectin. *Conclusions*: Our recent results show that high [glc] is a risk factor for ELR-mediated matrix remodeling also. The maintained ELR-NOS coupling in old aortas at high [glc] should further increase ROS-production (free radical release) as shown previously. Superoxide combines with NO yielding the highly toxic peroxinitrite anion with a further increase of degrading protease production. © 2003 Published by Elsevier B.V.

Keywords: Elastin; Elastase; Elastin receptor; Diabetes; Hyperglycemia; NOS; NO

* Corresponding author. Tel.: +33-143860240; fax: +33-143860219.
E-mail address: lrobert5@wanadoo.fr (L. Robert).

0531-5131/ © 2003 Published by Elsevier B.V.
doi:10.1016/S0531-5131(03)01734-5

1. Introduction

Matrix remodeling, degradation and inadequate resynthesis are strongly involved in the age-dependent modifications of the vascular wall. Increasing stiffness and atherosclerotic plaque formation regularly accompany these processes [1,2]. Among the risk factors of emerging importance in the 21st century, diabetes type II appears to take a leading role. An age-dependent increase of fasting blood glucose levels, loss of insulin sensitivity (the «metabolic syndrome»), together with the rapid increase of the «senior» population worldwide, substantiate this claim. Age-dependent remodeling of the vascular extracellular matrix (ECM) plays an important role in this respect. A number of factors were identified as important players in age-dependent vascular remodeling, among them the reaction mediated by the elastin–laminin receptor (ELR) [1,2]. Some of these reactions will be briefly recapitulated. We shall describe some recent experiments which show that extracellular glucose concentration [glc] plays an important role in age-dependent, vascular modifications mainly by acting on the Ca^{2+}-homeostatic mechanisms.

2. Materials and methods

Most experiments on the ELR were carried out on cell cultures and on isolated WBCs, monocytes and lymphocytes, as described [1,2]. The effect of elastin peptides on vascular tension was recorded on noradrenaline precontracted rat aorta rings as described [3]. Cellular Ca^{+}-fluxes were monitored on endothelial cells by the patch clamp technique [4]. Elastase-type, endopeptidase activity was determined on a synthetic substrate (*N*-succinyl-ala3-pNA) and also by zymography [5]. Statistical comparisons were performed by the distribution-free Mann–Whitney *U*-test.

3. Results

Matrix remodeling involves degradation and uncoordinated biosynthesis of the macromolecular components of the vascular ECM. The role of the ELR in the above processes was demonstrated by the following experiments. First, the presence of ELR in freshly excised human atherosclerotic lesions was demonstrated by immunocytochemical methods [6]. It is present on vascular smooth muscle cells (SMC) and lesion-localized mononuclear cells, monocytes, and T-lymphocytes as documented by double labeling of the adequate receptors [6]. Second, its role in the upregulation of matrix-degrading endopeptidase production was shown on cell cultures of fibroblasts, SMCs and lymphocytes [5]. The liberated elastin peptides (EP) acting as agonists on the ELR further stimulate matrix degradation initiating a vicious cycle: EP added to fibroblasts or T-lymphocytes were shown to increase also cell proliferation, an important phase in atherosclerotic modifications. Increasing further EP-concentration produced cell death by necrosis and at higher concentrations by apoptosis [7].

All ELR-mediated reactions were shown to be preceded by an increase of intracellular free Ca (Ca_i^{2+}). Ca^{2+}-transient recordings on human mononuclear cells showed an age-dependent decline of peak values and a progressive slowdown of the extrusion of excess Ca_i^{2+} (see Ref. [8], for review). For cells obtained from older pathological donors, an increase of Ca_i^{2+} was not followed at all by its extrusion, interpreted as a complete loss of Ca_i^{2+}-homeostatic regulation in these cells.

In recent experiments we could show that [glc] also regulates the Ca^{2+}-homeostatic processes [4]. Using the patch-clamp technique on HUVECs, it appeared that Ba^{2+} influx was maximal at normal [glc] (11 mM) and decreased strongly at low (0 mM) or high (33 mM) [glc]. Similar optimal responses to EP were also observed on the EP-triggered vasorelaxation of noradrenaline-precontracted aorta rings. This effect is the result of age-dependent modifications of ELR-NOS coupling in endothelial cells [3,4]. At normal [glc] (11 mM) this effect was obtained by adding 1.10^{-3} mg/ml EPs to the Ringer solution, which is maximal for young adult animals and decreased with age. It is undetectable at 0 mM glc and also for adult (6-month-old) aortas at high [glc] (33 mM). For old (30-month) animals, the ELR–NOS coupling was preserved, as shown by a pressure drop after adding EPs [9].

4. Discussion

ELR-mediated reactions include stimulation of cell proliferation, upregulation of elastase-type endopeptidase production and ROS-release and apoptosis [1,2,5]. It was also shown to produce cell death attributed to the last two processes [7]. Most cells of the atherosclerotic plaque, including SMC and mononuclear cells, express ELR [6]. All these effects were attributed to elastin peptides, agonists of ELR, liberated by elastase action [5]. Now we show that [glc] is also an important determinant in the triggering of these reactions by acting on the first step, Ca-signaling [4]. We previously showed that high [glc] produces an overexpression of collagen and fibronectin [9]. All these data further support the contention concerning the importance of ELR-mediated reactions in atherogenesis.

References

[1] L. Robert, Aging of vascular wall and atherogenesis. Role of the elastin–laminin receptor, Atherosclerosis 123 (1996) 169–179.

[2] L. Robert, Aging of the vascular-wall and atherosclerosis, Exp. Gerontol. 34 (1999) 491–501.

[3] G. Faury, A. Chabaud, M.T. Ristori, L. Robert, J. Verdetti, Effect of age on the vasodilatory action ofelastin peptides, Mech. Ageing Dev. 95 (1997) 31–42.

[4] G. Faury, L. Robert, J. Verdetti, The age-dependent vasodilation and endothelial calcium influx induced by elastin peptides are modulated by extracellular glucose level, Biomed. Pharmacother. 57 (2003) 216–222.

[5] L. Robert, A.M. Robert, B. Jacotot, in: Elastin–Elastase–Atherosclerosis Revisited 140 (1998) 281–295.

[6] G. Peterszegi, C. Mandet, S. Texier, L. Robert, P. Bruneval, Lymphocytes in human atherosclerotic plaque exhibit the elastin–laminin receptor: potential role in atherogenesis, Atherosclerosis 135 (1997) 103–107.

[7] G. Peterszegi, S. Texier, L. Robert, Cell death by overload of the elastin–laminin receptor on human activated lymphocytes: protection by lactose and melibiose, Eur. J. Clin. Invest. 29 (1999) 166–172.

[8] Zs. Varga, M.P. Jacob, L. Robert, J. Csongor, T. Fülöp Jr., Age-dependent changes of k-elastin stimulated effector functions of human phagocytic cells: relevance for atherogenesis, Exp. Gerontol. 32 (1997) 653–662.

[9] Y. Benazzoug, C. Borchiellini, J. Labat-Robert, L. Robert, P. Kern, Effect of high-glucose concentrations on the expression of collagens and fibronectin by fibroblasts in culture, Exp. Gerontol. 33 (1998) 445–455.

International Congress Series 1262 (2004) 414–417

www.ics-elsevier.com

The role of extracellular matrix in restenosis after percutaneous coronary intervention

Ick-Mo Chung*

Division of Cardiology, Ewha Women's University Medical Research Center, 70 Jongro 6Ga, Jongro Gu, Seoul 110-783, South Korea

Abstract. Restenosis after percutaneous coronary intervention (PCI) might be a kind of wound healing reaction, involving at least two important processes, vascular remodeling and neointima formation. There is an accumulating amount of evidence to suggest that the dynamic modulation of the extracellular matrix (ECM) contributes significantly to restenosis by interacting with cells and matrices. In this brief review, the expression pattern of ECM and the possible role of these molecules in the restenosis process are discussed. © 2003 Elsevier B.V. All rights reserved.

Keywords: Extracellular matrix; Restenosis; Hyaluronan; Proteoglycan; Neointima

Although the mechanism of restenosis following percutaneous coronary intervention (PCI) has been intensively studied, restenosis is still a difficult problem to solve based on current medical knowledge. Constrictive vascular remodeling and, to a lesser extent, neointimal formation play a key role in restenosis after balloon angioplasty, whereas neointimal formation is a main cause of lumen loss after stent deployment. [1,2]. The increased cell proliferation rate documented in an animal injury model has not been observed in most human restenotic tissues. On the contrary, very low cell proliferation rate (mostly $<1\%$) was observed in human coronary restenotic arteries after balloon angioplasty and stent deployment [3–6]. These data were found to be the case regardless of the time interval after PCI. However, a few studies reported a high cell replication rate of approximately 25% in in-stent neointima [7] and 15% in restenotic tissue after balloon angioplasty [8]. On the other hand, Strauss et al. [3] reported a trend toward a reduction in cell density of the in-stent neointima over time. We also observed in our analysis of 29 in-stent neointima specimens that the frequency of occurrence of cell-depleted areas with abundant extracellular matrix (ECM) tended to increase over time after stenting [5]. These data are consistent with the low cell replication rate observed in the aforementioned studies.

* Tel.: +82-2-760-5076; fax: +82-2-762-7756.
E-mail address: ickmo@mm.ewha.ac.kr (I.-M. Chung).

doi:10.1016/j.ics.2003.11.008

Restenotic arterial specimens were frequently found to contain a neointima composed of cells, predominantly α-actin positive smooth muscle cells (SMC), in an ECM enriched with proteoglycans, especially versican, and hyaluronan [5,6,9,10]. Myxoid tissue characterized by stellate-shaped SMCs in a disorganized pattern in a proteoglycan/hyaluronan-rich ECM was frequently observed in restenotic tissue after balloon angioplasty [8,9,11] and after stenting [5,7], and the frequency of occurrence of myxoid tissue diminished over time after stenting. Although the exact role of myoxoid tissue is not certain, our recent observation that the molecules implicated in cell migration and ECM synthesis were more frequently expressed in restenotic tissue specimens containing myxoid tissue than those without raises the possibility that myxoid tissue may be a provisional tissue in which active cell migration and the synthesis of ECM occur [12].

Serial ECM changes in restenotic arteries were reported recently. In one study using coronary restenotic arteries, the early transient (< 1 month after PCI) expression of tenascin-C, followed by an abundance of loose ECM enriched with versican was reported [13]. In this study, the versican-rich ECM was subsequently replaced by a more mature ECM enriched with collagen type I and type III at a later period (>6 months after PCI). Similar ECM transition was also observed in in-stent restenotic tissue [5]. Several matrix metalloproteinases are activated following vascular injury to facilitate SMC migration, and type I collagen degradation products are known to stimulate the expression of tenascin-C [14]. Tenascin-C is known as a multifunctional protein, which is implicated in cell proliferation, migration, differentiation and apoptosis, and its expression was correlated with the infiltration of macrophages, suggesting that tenascin-C may be implicated in inflammation [15].

Hyaluronan and versican may significantly contribute to the formation of neointima and vascular remodeling after PCI. In restenotic arteries, an inverse relation between staining intensity for hyaluronan and collagen was noted, and a similar reciprocal pattern in the staining for collagen and versican was also reported [5,9,11]. Hyaluronan and versican were found to be abundant, especially in loose ECM such as myxoid tissue, and scarce in the collagen-rich, cell-depleted areas of human restenotic arteries [5,11]. The accumulation of hyaluronan around PCNA-positive SMCs was observed in human restenotic arteries and in injured rat carotid arteries [11]. In experimental animal studies, an increase in the amount of ECM hyaluronan was found to be responsible for the closing of the ductus arteriosus during fetal development [16]. Migrating and proliferating SMCs organized pericellular matrices enriched with hyaluronan and versican, and interference with the binding of hyaluronan to the cell surface, which was caused by hyaluronan oligosaccharides, was known to inhibit SMC proliferation and migration and to alter the cell morphology [17]. In addition, hyaluronan may be responsible for the process of constrictive remodeling. Hyaluronan added to collagen gels promotes collagen gel contraction by SMCs, and this process was found to be mediated by cellular binding to hyaluronan via CD44 receptors [18]. Therefore, it is speculated that an ECM enriched with hyaluronan/versican provides a large, waterlogged loose matrix, due to their hygroscopic property, into which cells will migrate and proliferate so as to facilitate the healing of the wound.

In conclusion, restenosis following PCI might result from a kind of wound healing process, and the dynamic modulation of ECM and the complicated interaction between cells and matrices mediate this process significantly. Further studies of the role of ECM in this process may lead to the development of therapeutic strategies for the treatment of atherosclerosis and restenosis.

Acknowledgements

The author would like to thank Dr. T.N. Wight, Dr. S.M. Schwartz, Dr. M.A. Reidy (University of Washington), and Dr. H.K. Gold (Harvard University) for their important contribution to the restenosis project. The author would also like to thank Dr. Y. Jang, Dr. W.I. Yang, Dr. D. Choi, Dr. S.Y. Cho, Dr. S.S. Kim (Yonsei University, Korea), Dr. S.J. Park, and Dr. S.W. Park (Asan Medical Center, Korea) for the support they provided to the restenosis project.

References

[1] R. Hoffmann, G.S. Mintz, G.R. Dussaillant, J.J. Popma, A.D. Pichard, L.F. Satler, K.M. Kent, J. Griffin, M.B. Leon, Patterns and mechanism of in-stent restenosis. A serial intravascular ultrasound study, Circulation 94 (1996) 1247–1254.

[2] M.J. Post, B.J.G.L. de Smet, Y. van der Helm, C. Borst, R.E. Kuntz, Arterial remodeling after balloon angioplasty or stenting in an atherosclerotic experimental model, Circulation 96 (1997) 996–1003.

[3] B.H. Strauss, V.A. Umans, R. Suylen, P.J. Feyter, J. Marco, G.C. Robertson, J. Renkin, G. Heyndrickx, V.D. Vuzevski, F.T. Bosman, P.W. Serruys, Directional atherectomy for treatment of restenosis within coronary stents: clinical, angiographic and histologic results, J. Am. Coll. Cardiol. 20 (1992) 1465–1473.

[4] E.R. O'Brien, C.E. Alpers, D.K. Stewart, M. Ferguson, N. Tran, D. Gordon, E.P. Benditt, T. Hinohara, J.B. Simpson, S.M. Schwartz, Proliferation in primary and restenotic coronary atherectomy tissue. Implications for antiproliferative therapy, Circ. Res. 73 (1993) 223–231.

[5] I.M. Chung, H.K. Gold, S.M. Schwartz, Y. Ikari, M.A. Reidy, T.N. Wight, Enhanced extracellular matrix accumulation in restenosis of coronary arteries after stent deployment, J. Am. Coll. Cardiol. 40 (2002) 2072–2081.

[6] C. Glover, X. Ma, Y. Chen, H. Miller, J. Veinot, M. Labinaz, E. O'Brien, Human in-stent restenosis tissue obtained by means of coronary atherectomy consists of an abundant proteoglycan matrix with a paucity of cell proliferation, Am. Heart J. 144 (2002) 702–709.

[7] M. Kearney, A. Pieczek, L. Haley, D.W. Losordo, V. Andres, R. Schainfeld, K. Rosenfield, J.M. Isner, Histopathology of in-stent restenosis in patients with peripheral artery disease, Circulation 95 (1997) 1998–2002.

[8] J.G. Pickering, L. Weir, J. Jekanowski, M.A. Kearney, J.M. Isner, Proliferative activity in peripheral and coronary atherosclerotic plaque among patients undergoing percutaneous revascularization, J. Clin. Invest. 91 (1993) 1469–1480.

[9] T.N. Wight, S. Lara, R. Riessen, R.L. Baron, J. Isner, Selective deposits of versican in the extracellular matrix of restenotic lesions from human peripheral arteries, Am. J. Pathol. 151 (1997) 963–973.

[10] A. Farb, G. Sangiorgi, A.J. Carter, V.M. Wally, W.D. Edwards, R.S. Schwartz, R. Virmani, Pathology of acute and chronic coronary stenting in humans, Circulation 99 (1999) 44–52.

[11] R. Riessen, T.N. Wight, C. Pastore, C. Henley, J.M. Isner, Distribution of hyaluronan during extracellular matrix remodeling in human restenotic arteries and balloon-injured rat carotid arteries, Circulation 93 (1996) 1141–1147.

[12] I.M. Chung, Y. Jang, S.J. Park, S.Y. Cho, S.W. Park, C.W. Lee, S.H. Cho, P. Heldin, H.K. Gold, S.M. Schwartz, Myxoid tissue in stent restenosis may be a provisional tissue in which active cell migration and synthesis of extracellular matrix occur, J. Am. Coll. Cardiol. 35 (Suppl. A) (2000) 48A.

[13] K. Imanaka-Yoshida, R. Matsuura, N. Isaka, T. Nakano, T. Sakakura, T. Yoshida, Serial extracellular matrix changes in neointimal lesions of human coronary artery after percutaneous coronary angioplasty: clinical significance of early tenascin-c expression, Virchows Arch. 439 (2001) 185–190.

[14] M.P. Bendeck, C. Irvin, M.A. Reidy, Inhibition of matrix metalloproteinase activity inhibits smooth muscle cell migration but not neointimal thickening after arterial injury, Circ. Res. 78 (1996) 38–43.
[15] K. Wallner, C. Li, P.K. Shah, M.C. Fishbein, J.S. Forrester, S. Kaul, B.G. Sharifi, Tenascin-c is expressed in macrophage-rich human coronary atherosclerotic plaque, Circulation 99 (1999) 1284–1289.
[16] N. Boudreau, E. Turley, M. Rabinovitch, Fibronectin, hyaluronan, and a hyaluronan binding protein contribute to increased ductus arteriosus smooth muscle cell migration, Dev. Biol. 143 (1991) 235–247.
[17] S.P. Evanko, J.C. Angello, T.N. Wight, Formation of hyaluronan- and versican-rich pericellular matrix is required for proliferation and migration of vascular smooth muscle cells, Arterioscler. Thromb. Vasc. Biol. 19 (1999) 1004–1013.
[18] J.A. Travis, M.G. Hughes, J.M. Wong, W.D. Wagner, R.L. Geary, Hyaluronan enhances contraction of collagen by smooth muscle cells and adventitial fibroblasts, Circ. Res. 88 (2001) 77–83.

International Congress Series 1262 (2004) 418–421

www.ics-elsevier.com

Novel anti-inflammatory properties of the Na^+/H^+ exchange inhibitor ethylisopropylamiloride result in attenuation of atherogenesis in apolipoprotein E-deficient mice

Yong-Xiang Chen, Stewart Whitman, Edward O'Brien*

Medicine (Cardiology), University of Ottawa Heart Institute, Vascular Biology Laboratory, 40 Ruskin Street, Ottawa, Ontario, Canada K1Y4W7

Abstract. Amiloride and related derivatives, such as ethylisopropylamiloride (EIPA), are Na^+/H^+ exchange inhibitors that antagonize urokinase plasminogen activator (uPA) activity; however, their effect on the genesis of complex atherosclerotic lesions is unknown. Therefore, we sought to determine if (and how) EIPA reduces lesion formation in atherosclerosis-prone apoE-deficient ($apoE^{-/-}$) mice. Eight-week-old male $apoE^{-/-}$ mice were fed an atherogenic diet with ($n=10$) or without ($n=9$) a continuous infusion of EIPA via a subcutaneous minipump (3 mg/kg/day) for 4 weeks. No significant differences were observed in the serum cholesterol levels, yet there was a 46% reduction in the en face aortic lesion size with EIPA treatment (control: $29.8 \pm 5.9\%$ vs. EIPA: $16.1 \pm 4.8\%$; $p<0.001$), with a 41% reduction in the percentage of subendothelial area occupied by macrophages (control: $45.8 \pm 5\%$ vs. EIPA: $27.2 \pm 3.2\%$; $p<0.001$). Both the number of VCAM-1-expressing aortic endothelial cells and the abundance of adherent monocytes, detected by scanning electron microscopy, were reduced in the EIPA-treated mice. These data demonstrate novel anti-inflammatory properties of EIPA that result in attenuation of atherogenesis. © 2003 Published by Elsevier B.V.

Keywords: Inflammation; Atherosclerosis; Endothelium; Adhesion molecule; Amiloride

1. Introduction

The initial steps in atherogenesis include the adhesion and trans-endothelial migration of circulating blood leukocytes into the subendothelial space [1,2]. Leukocyte–endothelial adhesion is mediated by endothelial cell adhesion molecules, such as vascular cell adhesion molecule-1 (VCAM-1) and the leukocyte integrin very late-acting antigen-4 (VLA-4) [3]. Enhanced expression of VCAM-1 in endothelial cells plays an important role in atherogenesis [4,5]. The Na^+/H^+ exchanger (NHE) is widely known to participate in a

* Corresponding author. Tel.: +1-613-761-5030; fax: +1-613-761-4237.
E-mail address: eobrien@ottawaheart.ca (E. O'Brien).

0531-5131/ © 2003 Published by Elsevier B.V.
doi:10.1016/j.ics.2003.11.040

variety of cellular functions, including the regulation of intracellular Na^+ levels, the adjustment of intracellular pH, the control of cell volume, as well as the regulation of cell growth and division [6]. This transporter also plays an important role in the regulation of macrophage functions [7,8]. Furthermore, experimental studies demonstrate that NHE inhibitors reduce neointimal lesion formation [9,10]. Recently, we demonstrated that a potent and specific NHE inhibitor, ethylisopropylamiloride (EIPA) not only attenuates vascular smooth muscle cell (SMC) proliferation and migration, but augments SMC apoptosis and antagonizes SMC urokinase plasminogen activator (uPA) activity [11]. As the genesis of complex atherosclerotic lesions involves the interplay of several of these processes, we sought to determine if EIPA can reduce lesion formation in the aorta of atherosclerosis-susceptible apoE-deficient ($apoE^{-/-}$) mice.

2. Material and methods

Male $apoE^{-/-}$ mice (Jackson Labs, Bar Harbour, ME) were weaned at 4 weeks of age and fed a regular chow diet for 4 weeks before beginning a 1.25% (wt/wt) cholesterol and 16% (wt/wt) butter fat diet (TD 88051, Harlan Teklad). A continuous infusion of EIPA (3 mg/kg/day in 70% DMSO saline, $n = 10$) or DMSO (70% in saline, $n = 9$) was delivered via a subcutaneous minipump (total volume = 200 μl; Alzet, Palo Alto, CA) that was implanted 48 h prior to commencing the lipid-enriched diet. Four weeks later, the mice were euthanized, the urine pH was measured to ensure that EIPA causing acidification and blood samples were collected to determine serum cholesterol levels. En face preparations of the aorta distal to the aortic root were analyzed by two observers using Image-Pro software (Media Cybernetics, Silver Spring, MD) to determine the percentage of aortic area occupying the atherosclerotic lesion [12]. Immunohistochemistry was performed on serial paraffin-embedded aortic root sections and the percentage of the lesion occupied by macrophages was calculated by dividing the area immunolabeled with the rabbit anti-mouse macrophage antibody (Boehringer Mannheim Biochemical, Indianapolis, IN) by the total cross-sectional vessel wall area (excluding the adventitia and lumen) and multiplying by 100. All results are presented as the mean ± S.D. unless otherwise stated. An unpaired Student's *t*-test was used to compare differences between the two animal groups, while differences amongst multiple parameters were analyzed using a one-way ANOVA.

3. Results

There was no difference in body weight between the control and drug treatment groups (e.g., 28.4 ± 1.7 vs. 29.4 ± 1.8 g, respectively; $p = 0.25$). Similarly, the total cholesterol levels of the two groups were similar (e.g., 1755.8 ± 195.7 vs. 1683.2 ± 223.9 mg/dl, respectively; $p = 0.55$). Mice receiving the EIPA infusion had a urinary pH of 6.0, while the urinary pH of control mice was 6.5. The ascending aorta, aortic arch, as well as descending aorta of the control mice showed widespread, early atherosclerotic changes, with fatty streaks and the accumulation of macrophages. EIPA-treated mice showed a 46% reduction in the percentage of the en face aortic arch area with atherosclerotic changes (e.g., % atherosclerotic lesion area of control: 29.8 ± 5.9% vs. EIPA: 16.1 ± 4.8%; $p < 0.001$). Macrophages were the predominant cells in these early atherosclerotic lesions

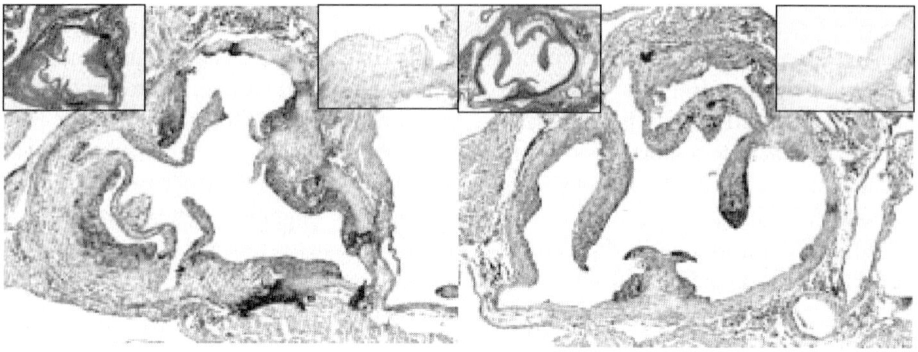

Fig. 1. Photomicrographs of ascending aortic cross-sections immunolabeled with an anti-mouse macrophage antibody (magnification: ×40). For both the control (left) and EIPA-treated (right) tissue specimens, the inset photomicrographs in the top left and right show adjacent tissue sections with Movat pentachrome staining and VCAM-1 immunolabeling (magnification: ×40 and ×400, respectively). Both subendothelial accumulations of macrophages and immunolabeling for VCAM-1 were more abundant in the control mice.

(Fig. 1). The percentage of macrophage area was 41% reduced in EIPA-infused mice compared with control mice (control: $45.8 \pm 5\%$ vs. EIPA: $27.2 \pm 3.2\%$; $p < 0.001$). VCAM-1 immunolabeling was commonly observed in the endothelium lining an atherosclerotic lesion, as well as in some macrophages and medial smooth muscle cells, while more normal segments of the aorta were immunonegative for VCAM-1. In contrast to control mice, EIPA-treated mice showed a marked reduction in VCAM-1 expression in the endothelium lining atherosclerotic lesions (Fig. 1).

4. Discussion

While the amiloride derivative EIPA is known to inhibit smooth muscle growth and migration, these data demonstrate a novel role for this compound as an anti-inflammatory agent capable of reducing early fatty streak lesion formation in mice susceptible to atherosclerosis. The apoE$^{-/-}$ mice in this experiment tolerated the relatively high systemic dosage of this medication without obvious side effects. The mechanisms by which EIPA reduced inflammation appeared to be mediated via the reduced expression of the cell adhesion molecule, VCAM-1, on endothelial cells. VCAM-1 acts to facilitate the transmigration of inflammatory cells into the subendothelium and, therefore, the development of early atherosclerotic lesions. In this acute, primary prevention study, aortic lesion area was reduced with drug treatment. Future studies will determine the potential for this medication to modulate smooth muscle cell growth and extracellular matrix production in chronic lesion formation, as well as the potential role of EIPA in the prevention, or perhaps even regression, of established lesions.

Acknowledgements

This work was supported by grants-in-aid from the Heart and Stroke Foundation of Ontario and the Canadian Institutes for Health Research (CIHR). EOB is a CIHR-UI Investigator and SW is a Research Scholar of the Heart and Stroke Foundation of Ontario.

References

[1] R. Ross, Atherosclerosis—an inflammatory disease, N. Engl. J. Med. 340 (1999) 115–126.

[2] P. Libby, Inflammation in atherosclerosis, Nature 420 (6917) (2002) 868–874.

[3] M.J. Elices, L. Osborn, Y. Takada, C. Crouse, S. Luhowskyj, M.E. Hemler, R.R. Lobb, VCAM-1 on activated endothelium interacts with the leukocyte integrin VLA-4 at a site distinct from the VLA-4/fibronectin binding site, Cell 60 (1990) 577–584.

[4] K.D. O'Brien, M.D. Allen, T.O. McDonald, A. Chait, J.M. Harlan, D. Fishbein, J. McCarty, M. Ferguson, K. Hudkins, C.D. Benjamin, Vascular cell adhesion molecule-1 is expressed in human coronary atherosclerotic plaques. Implications for the mode of progression of advanced coronary atherosclerosis, J. Clin. Invest. 92 (2) (1993) 945–951.

[5] Y. Nakashima, E.W. Raines, A.S. Plump, J.L. Breslow, R. Ross, Upregulation of VCAM-1 and ICAM-1 at atherosclerosis-prone sites on the endothelium in the apoE-deficient mouse, Arterioscler. Thromb. Vasc. Biol. 18 (5) (1998) 842–851.

[6] L. Fliegel, R. Murtazina, P. Dibrov, C. Harris, A. Moor, F.A. Fernandez-Rachubinski, Regulation and characterization of the Na^+/H^+ exchanger, Biochem. Cell. Biol. 76 (1998) 735–741.

[7] M.W. Rolfe, S.L. Kunkel, B. Rowens, T.J. Standiford, E.J. Cragoe, R.M. Strieter, Suppression of human alveolar macrophage-derived cytokines by amiloride, Am. J. Respir. Cell Mol. Biol. 6 (1992) 576–582.

[8] Y. Ohmori, E. Reynolds, T.A. Hamilton, Modulation of Na+/K+ exchange potentiates lipopolysaccharide-induced gene expression in murine peritoneal macrophages, J. Cell. Physiol. 148 (1991) 96–105.

[9] R. Kranzhofer, J. Schirmer, A. Schomig, E. von Hodenberg, E. Pestel, J. Metz, H. Lang, W. Kubler, Suppression of neointimal thickening and smooth muscle cell proliferation after arterial injury in the rat by inhibitors of $Na^+–H^+$ exchange, Circ. Res. 73 (1993) 264–268.

[10] M. Mitsuka, M. Nagae, B.C. Berk, $Na^+–H^+$ exchange inhibitors decrease neointimal formation after rat carotid injury. Effects on smooth muscle cell migration and proliferation, Circ. Res. 73 (1993) 269–275.

[11] Y.-X. Chen, E.R. O'Brien, Ethylisopropyl amiloride inhibits smooth muscle cell proliferation and migration by inducing apoptosis and antagonizing uPA activity, Can. J. Physiol. Pharm. 81 (2003) 730–739.

[12] A. Daugherty, E. Pure, D. Delfel-Butteiger, S. Chen, J. Leferovich, S.E. Roselaar, D.J. Rader, The effects of total lymphocyte deficiency on the extent of atherosclerosis in apolipoprotein $E^{-/-}$ mice, J. Clin. Invest. 100 (1997) 1575–1580.

ELSEVIER

International Congress Series 1262 (2004) 422–425

www.ics-elsevier.com

Infections and atherosclerosis—is serology useful?

Pekka Saikku*

Department of Medical Microbiology, University of Oulu, Oulu, Finland

Abstract. Seroepidemiology has been used to associate infections with atherosclerosis. It does not prove causality, and variability of antibody responses limits its use in risk estimations. © 2004 Published by Elsevier B.V.

Keywords: Seroepidemiology; *Chlamydia pneumoniae*

Seroepidemiology has been used to find out if infectious agents are associated with chemical vapor deposition (CVD). The results have been inconsistent. There are several reasons for this. Antibodies are not well-defined chemical substances, such as C-reactive protein or homocysteine, but a variable group with variable kinds of affinity and avidity. There are individual variations in the immunoreactivity to infections and the persistence of antibodies. Moreover, there may be fluctuations in antibody levels, due to reinfections, reactivations, or healing from chronic infections. Antibodies can also be bound to immunocomplexes [1] or the diseased area [2], thereby affecting their measurement from sera. All this makes the estimation of true risks quite problematic. A further problem is the large variety of methodology used for measurement. Although there are various kits commercially available, international or even national standards are rare, and many laboratories use in-house methods, which makes the comparison of titres difficult. Below, the seroepidemiology of *Chlamydia pneumoniae* in atherosclerosis will be used as an example of the pitfalls in seroepidemiology.

C. pneumoniae is a common respiratory tract pathogen. It is an obligatory intracellular Gram-negative bacterium with a remarkable tendency to cause persistent infections. Antibodies commonly start to appear after 5 years of age, and it is likely that everybody is infected during his or her lifetime, and the majority have several reinfections. Asymptomatic adults often have the agent present in their lungs, and it has been associated with asthma, chronic bronchitis, and chronic obstructive pulmonary disease (COPD). Moreover, DNA of the agent has been found in circulating white blood cells, and monocytes can transmit the pathogen effectively into the vessel wall, where its presence in atherosclerotic lesions has been demonstrated after 14 years of age [3].

* Tel.: +358-8-537-5901; fax: +358-8-335-908.
E-mail address: pekka.saiku@oulu.fi (P. Saikku).

0531-5131/ © 2004 Published by Elsevier B.V.
doi:10.1016/j.ics.2003.12.043

The association of *C. pneumonia* (Cpn) with CVD was found by seroepidemiology [4]. In this study, acute myocardial infarction (AMI) patients showed a seroconversion against an epitope reactive in chlamydial lipopolysaccharide (LPS). After that, both AMI patients and patients with chronic coronary disease were demonstrated to have elevated antibody titers against Cpn. This led to a suggestion that a chronic Cpn infection is associated with atherosclerosis and may exacerbate in AMI.

There are three reasons why this study was successful. Firstly, the enzyme immunoassay (EIA) method used was quite sensitive to IgM antibodies against chlamydial LPS. Secondly, the patients were under 50 years of age and thus without "serological scars." Thirdly, 5 years had elapsed since the *C. pneumonia* epidemic, which led to the discovery of its association with the disease [5]. Antibody levels in the general population had gone down but remained high in those with chronic infection. The next set of material was collected during an ongoing epidemic, and the antibody levels were high in the controls. The problem was avoided by measuring chlamydial LPS immune complexes, which were present in 57% of AMI patients and in 11% of controls [1].

The seroepidemiological association has been repeatedly demonstrated using different methods and varying patient populations [6,7]. Estimated ORs are mostly around 2, but vary markedly, and some large prospective studies have failed to find an association. Some common features are seen in these studies. The risk is higher in younger patients, and it is difficult to demonstrate the risk in a patient population aged 60 years or older. This is natural, since seropositivity usually rises constantly during the lifetime. We noted as early as 1992 that IgG antibodies were not predictive in a prospective study [8], and a recent meta-analysis estimated the risk associated with IgG antibody levels to be minimal (1.15, n.s.) [9]. Moreover, the problem in prospective studies is that a serum sample taken years before the cardiac event does not show how the disease is possibly proceeding due to reactivation or reinfection. Cross-sectional studies usually demonstrate higher risks, and a meta-analysis reported an OR of 2.0 (95% CI 1.5–2.6) [7]. However, the potentially causal exposure variable and the outcome variable are measured at the same time, which makes it impossible to distinguish between them. Meta-analyses also involve the problem of "garbage in, garbage out," and *C. pneumoniae* serology lacks international standards. The micro-immunofluorescence (MIF) test, which is regarded as the gold standard, is technically demanding. This has led to various in-house methods based on EIA. Commercial kits have also been used. They are, however, meant for acute infections, and their performance in chronic infections is unknown. In our hands, the EIA kits tested have so far been disappointing.

One can look for IgA type antibodies, too. These antibodies are short-lived, and their continuous presence points to a chronic infection. Moreover, they tend to form in a Th2-type immune response, which is inefficient in intracellular infections. A meta-analysis of prospective studies using IgA titrations found statistically significant OR (1.25, 95% CI 1.03–1.53) [10]. However, IgA titrations are still less well characterized and may involve unexpected technical difficulties [11]. IgA antibodies are not always present, and even IgG antibodies may be quite low [12], although the pathogen is sitting inside the lesions. We should find better markers. Detection of *C. pneumoniae* DNA in circulating white blood cells is a marker of the agent present [13]. Immune complexes have also been tried, but the techniques remain quite tricky [14].

However, the detection of antibodies in circulation does not indicate directly the activity, or especially the location, of the agent. The possible pulmonary origin of antigens and DNA has not been studied, either. At this moment, hsCRP seems to be a good indicator of the activity of the inflammation, particularly when combined with other titrations. For instance, the combination of elevated IgA antibodies to *C. pneumoniae* and human Hsp 60 with elevated hsCRP, in other words (markers of chronic inflammation, autoimmunity, and active inflammation), predicted a 17-fold risk for cardiac event in the Helsinki Heart Study [15].

C. pneumoniae and herpesviruses are pathogens repeatedly found in atherosclerotic lesions, and electron microscopy seems to exclude bacteria (except L-forms). However, seroepidemiology has yielded the concept of pathogen burden [16,17]. The pathogen need not sit in the lesion, but by inducing an inflammatory reaction, it may aggravate the inflammation going on in atherosclerotic plaques. This type of indirect effect may be present in parodontitis, which allows bacteria and bacterial products easy access into the circulation without a guardian, such as the liver.

Atherosclerosis is a universal phenomenon, especially at old age, and one should think of antibodies against pathogens as markers of this condition. They do not reliably predict cardiac events, which are complications in this process. There are only a few studies where elevated antibody titers have been helpful in identifying the patients who have benefited from antibacterial therapy [18,19]. We need better markers to identify the subjects who could possibly benefit from the eradication of pathogens and to follow up the success of eradication. Seroepidemiology has mostly done its part in studies on infection and atherosclerosis. Some new aspects can, however, be found. Syndrome X has been associated with hsCRP. By studying all young adults born in North Finland in 1966, we could confirm this association, but also found an association of body mass index, systolic and diastolic blood pressure, lowered high-density lipoprotein (HDL), and elevated TG and insulin levels with elevated antibodies against *C. pneumoniae* (to be published).

References

[1] M. Leinonen, et al., Circulating immune complexes containing chlamydial lipopolysaccharide in acute myocardial infarction, Microb. Pathog. 9 (1990) 67–73.

[2] J. Juvonen, et al., Demonstration of *Chlamydia pneumoniae* in the walls of abdominal aortic aneurysms, J. Vasc. Surg. 25 (1997) 499–505.

[3] D. Taylor-Robinson, et al., *Chlamydia pneumoniae* in vascular tissues from heart-transplant donors (research letter), Lancet 351 (1998) 1255.

[4] P. Saikku, et al., Serologic evidence of an association of a novel *Chlamydia*, TWAR, with chronic coronary heart disease and acute myocardial infarction, Lancet ii (1988) 983–985.

[5] P. Saikku, et al., An epidemic of mild pneumonia due to an unusual strain of *Chlamydia psittaci*, J. Infect. Dis. 151 (1985) 832–839.

[6] J. Danesh, et al., Chronic infections and coronary heart disease: is there a link? Lancet 350 (1997) 430–436.

[7] D.G. Bloemenkamp, et al., Meta-analysis of sero-epidemiologic studies of the relation between *Chlamydia pneumoniae* and atherosclerosis: does study design influence results? Am. Heart J. 145 (3) (2003 Mar) 409–417.

[8] P. Saikku, et al., Chronic *Chlamydia pneumoniae* infection as a risk factor for coronary heart disease in the Helsinki Heart Study, Ann. Intern. Med. 116 (1992) 273–278.

[9] J. Danesh, et al., *Chlamydia pneumoniae* IgG titres and coronary heart disease: prospective study and meta-analysis, BMJ 321 (2000) 208–213.

[10] J. Danesh, et al., *Chlamydia pneumoniae* IgA titres and coronary heart disease. Prospective study and meta-analysis, Eur. Heart J. 23 (5) (2002 (March 1)) 371–375.
[11] M. Paldanius, et al., Measurement of *Chlamydia pneumoniae*-specific immunoglobulin A antibodies by the microimmunofluorescence method, Clin. Diagn. Lab. Immunol. 10 (2003) 8–12.
[12] M. Puolakkainen, et al., Serological response to *Chlamydia pneumoniae* in adults with coronary arterial fatty streaks and fibrolipid plaques, J. Clin. Microbiol. 31 (1993) 2212–2214.
[13] J. Boman, C.A. Gaydos, Polymerase chain reaction detection of *Chlamydia pneumoniae* in circulating white blood cells, J. Infect. Dis. 181 (Suppl. 3) (2000 June) S452–S454.
[14] E. Linnanmäki, et al., Presence of *Chlamydia pneumoniae* specific antibodies in circulating immune complexes in coronary heart disease, Circulation 87 (1993) 1130–1134.
[15] T. Huittinen, et al., Synergistic effect of persistent *Chlamydia pneumoniae* infection, autoimmunity, and inflammation on coronary risk, Circulation 107 (2003) 2566–2570.
[16] S.E. Epstein, et al., Infection and atherosclerosis: potential roles of pathogen burden and molecular mimicry, Arterioscler. Thromb. Vasc. Biol. 20 (6) (2000 Jun) 1417–1420.
[17] C. Espinola-Klein, et al., Impact of infectious burden on extent and long-term prognosis of atherosclerosis, Circulation 105 (1) (2002 (January 1)) 15–21.
[18] M. Mosorin, et al., Use of doxycycline to decrease the growth rate of abdominal aortic aneurysms: a randomized, double-blind, placebo-controlled pilot study, J. Vasc. Surg. 34 (4) (2001 October) 606–610.
[19] F. Neumann, et al., Treatment of *Chlamydia pneumoniae* infection with roxithromycin and effect on neointima proliferation after coronary stent placement (ISAR-3): a randomised, double-blind, placebo-controlled trial, Lancet 357 (9274) (2001 (June 30)) 2085–2089.

International Congress Series 1262 (2004) 426–429

www.ics-elsevier.com

Infection and atherosclerosis: mechanisms involving *Chlamydia pneumoniae* in cardiovascular disease

Gerald I. Byrne*, Scot P. Ouellette, Robert J. Belland

Department of Molecular Sciences, University of Tennessee Health Sciences Center, 858 Madison Avenue, Memphis, TN 38163, USA

Abstract. The intracellular bacterium *Chlamydia pneumoniae* is present in atherosclerotic plaques and may contribute to progression and vulnerability of lesions. Results from animal models support a causal role for *C. pneumoniae* in atherosclerosis and virulence attributes ascribed to this organism are consistent with this view. Results from recent antibiotic treatment trials have not proven effective, but additional work is needed to define reasons for these failures. © 2003 Published by Elsevier B.V.

Keywords: *Chlamydia pneumoniae*; Atherosclerosis; Chronic infection; GroEL; Pathogenesis

1. Infection and chronic disease

The hypothesis that infections contribute to a variety of chronic diseases, including cardiovascular disease is not new [1]. The role of infection in chronic disease became clear when *Helicobacter pylori* was found to cause peptic ulcers [2,3], where successful treatment is achieved with antimicrobials that eradicate *H. pylori* [4]. Other chronic diseases, such as atherosclerosis, may not yield easily identified causal factors.

Atherosclerosis and infection is complicated by the possibility that initiation is entirely independent of infections [5], although lesion progression and plaque vulnerability may be influenced by infections. Any number of infections could trigger inflammatory changes locally at the site of lesion development or from a distant site that impacts the status of the plaque [6]. Of the infectious agents suggested to be involved in atherosclerosis, the most compelling evidence implicates the obligate intracellular prokaryotic pathogen, *Chlamydia pneumoniae*.

2. Chlamydiae as infectious agents

The genus *Chlamydia* contains two species that are important human pathogens [7]. *Chlamydia trachomatis* causes ocular infections. In endemic areas the infection can

* Corresponding author. Tel.: +1-901-448-6060; fax: +1-901-448-2044.
E-mail address: gbyrne@utmem.edu (G.I. Byrne).

0531-5131/ © 2003 Published by Elsevier B.V.
doi:10.1016/S0531-5131(03)01862-4

ultimately result in trachoma, a blinding form of the disease that occurs decades after the initial exposure. *C. trachomatis* also causes uncomplicated genital tract infections. Cervical infections in women are particularly troubling because some infected women develop upper genital tract sequelae that can result in tubal scarring and infertility.

The second major human chlamydial pathogen is *C. pneumoniae*. This organism is a respiratory pathogen found worldwide and causes community acquired upper respiratory tract infections. Its role as a chronic pathogen is not firmly established, but it is frequently associated with a significant proportion of cardiovascular disease patients. It is the only pathogen consistently identified and isolated from diseased tissue.

3. *C. pneumoniae* and atherosclerosis

Sero-epidemiologic studies indicate that patients with cardiovascular disease have elevated titers to a chlamydial stress response protein [8,9]. More than half of all atherosclerotic lesions examined contain *C. pneumoniae*, although normal adjacent tissue is free from the presence of the organism [10,11]. Animal models have provided evidence that *C. pneumoniae* respiratory infection can disseminate to developing aortic lesions in atherogenic-prone mice, and infection causes enhanced lesions progression. Infection with other respiratory pathogens or *C. trachomatis* does not contribute to lesion development [12–14].

Direct evidence for *C. pneumoniae* playing a role in heart disease is by demonstrating that patients derive benefit when treated with antibiotics after infarctions or surgical intervention for heart disease. Case-control intervention studies have shown promising results, but a large secondary prevention trial (WIZARD), demonstrated only a 7% reduction in secondary events in the treatment arm versus placebo [15]. The WIZARD study was a well-designed randomized controlled trial that clearly demonstrated no significant long lasting (14 month) benefit in coronary artery disease patients who received an antibiotic against *C. pneumoniae* for 12 weeks. These data suggest that treatment for chlamydiae does not prevent secondary events in heart disease patients. There are other plausible explanations for the WIZARD results [16], and it is noteworthy that use of antibiotics in treatment of heart disease is in early stages of development. Secondary prevention may be difficult to achieve for a variety of reasons [17]. To gain a true understanding of the impact of *C. pneumoniae* eradication on heart disease it will be important to document that the treatment design actually eliminates chlamydiae and reduces critical inflammatory parameters.

4. *C. pneumoniae* biology and atherosclerosis

The organism has been characterized sufficiently to understand how its presence in atherosclerotic lesions can propagate changes as lesions progress from fatty streaks to vulnerable plaques (reviewed in Refs. [18,19]). *C. pneumoniae* can infect and survive in all cell types commonly found associated with atheromatous tissue, including arterial endothelial cells, smooth muscle cells and macrophages. *C. pneumoniae* infection may influence atheroma biology by increasing the levels of oxidized LDL and inducing the production of foam cells. A role for chlamydial GroEL (Hsp60) in this process has been suggested. The presence of GroEL has also been associated with pro-inflammatory activity, and may be an eliciting antigen for autoimmune reactivity. This molecule has thus assumed a central role in the pathogenesis of chronic chlamydial infections.

Monocytes and T lymphocytes are thought to be the principal transporters of *C. pneumoniae* from the lung to the vasculature. The life cycle of this organism depends on invading a susceptible host cell. Productive infections involve the orderly alternation between infectious, metabolically inert elementary bodies and noninfectious metabolically active reticulate bodies. The latter grow and divide within the confines of a cytoplasmic vesicle termed an inclusion. Nonproductive infections can also occur, and these more long-term host cell associations may be more typical of the status of the organism in chronic infections. Genomic studies have provided evidence that clonal variants of *C. pneumoniae* may be selectively adapted to the atheroma [20]. These observations are interesting because respiratory isolates may be inherently heterogeneous with genetic variants that specialize in causing chronic disease in distinct microenvironments.

5. Conclusions

The idea that infections contribute to atherosclerosis is extremely difficult to prove. As with other multifactorial, chronic disease processes, the set of contributing causal factors is complicated and individualized. A large body of correlative evidence exists to implicate *C. pneumoniae* infection in the acceleration of atherosclerosis. The involvement of an infectious agent in the progression rather than the initiation of a disease is a subtle shift in the infectious disease paradigm but is an accurate assessment of the role of *C. pneumoniae* in atherosclerosis.

Acknowledgements

Research activities have been supported by public health service grants AI 19782 (GIB), AI 42790 (GIB), HL 71735 (RJB, GIB), and AI 54875 (GIB).

References

[1] W. Osler, Diseases of the arteries, in: W. Osler (Ed.), Modern Medicine: Its Theory and Practice, Lea & Febiger, Philadelphia, 1908, pp. 426–447.

[2] P.B. Ernst, B.D. Gold, The disease spectrum of *Helicobacter pylori*: the immunopathogenesis of gastroduodenal ulcer and gastric cancer, Annu. Rev. Microbiol. 54 (2000) 615–640.

[3] C. Zimmer, Do chronic diseases have an infectious root? Science 293 (2001) 1974–1977.

[4] E. Rauws, G.N.J. Tytgat, Eradication of *Helicobacter pylori* cures duodenal ulcers, Lancet 337 (1990) 1233–1235.

[5] S.D. Wright, C. Burton, M. Hernandez, H. Hassing, J. Montenegro, S. Mundt, S. Patel, D.J. Card, A. Hermanowski-Vosatka, J.D. Bergstrom, C.P. Sparrow, P.A. Detmers, Y.S. Chao, Infectious agents are not necessary for murine atherogenesis, J. Exp. Med. 191 (2000) 1437–1441.

[6] P. Libby, P.M. Ridker, Novel inflammatory markers of coronary risk. Theory versus practice, Circulation 100 (1999) 1148–1150.

[7] R.S. Stephens (Ed.), *Chlamydia*. Intracellular Biology, Pathogenesis, and Immunity, ASM Press, Washington, DC, 1999, pp. 1–321.

[8] A. Ciervo, P. Visca, A. Petrucca, L.M. Biasucci, A. Maseri, A. Cassone, Antibodies to 60-kilodalton heat shock protein and outer membrane protein 2 of *Chlamydia pneumoniae* in patients with coronary heart disease, Clin. Diagn. Lab. Immunol. 9 (2002) 66–74.

[9] L.M. Biasucci, G. Liuzzo, A. Ciervo, A. Petrucca, M. Piro, D.J. Angiolillo, F. Crea, A. Cassone, A. Maseri,

Antibody response to chlamydial heat shock protein 60 is strongly associated with acute coronary syndromes, Circulation 107 (2003) 3015–3017.

[10] L.A. Jackson, L.A. Campbell, C.C. Kuo, D.I. Rodriquez, A. Lee, J.T. Grayston, Isolation of *Chlamydia pneumoniae* from carotid endarterectomy specimen, J. Infect. Dis. 176 (1997) 292–295.

[11] M. Maass, C. Bartels, P.M. Engel, U. Mamet, H.H. Sievers, Endovascular presence of viable *Chlamydia pneumoniae* is a common phenomenon in coronary artery disease, J. Am. Coll. Cardiol. 31 (1998) 827–832.

[12] T.C. Moazed, L.A. Campbell, M.E. Rosenfeld, J.T. Grayston, C.C. Kuo, *Chlamydia pneumoniae* infection accelerates the progression of atherosclerosis in apolipoprotein E-deficient mice, J. Infect. Dis. 180 (1999) 238–241.

[13] I.W. Fong, B. Chiu, E. Vira, D. Jang, J.B. Mahoney, De Novo induction of atherosclerosis by *Chlamydia pneumoniae* in a rabbit model, Infect. Immun. 67 (1999) 6048–6055.

[14] H. Hu, G.N. Pierce, G. Zhong, The atherogenic effects of chlamydiae are dependent on serum cholesterol and specific to *Chlamydia pneumoniae*, J. Clin. Invest. 103 (1999) 747–753.

[15] C.M. O'Conner, M.W. Dunne, M.A. Pfeffer, J.B. Muhlestein, L. Yao, S. Gupta, R.J. Benner, M.R. Fisher, T.D. Cook, Azithromycin for the secondary prevention of coronary heart disease events. The WIZARD study: a randomized controlled trial, JAMA 290 (2003) 1459–1466.

[16] S.V. Pislaru, F. Van de Werf, Antibiotic therapy for coronary artery disease. Can WIZARD change it all? JAMA 290 (2003) 1515–1516.

[17] J. Gieffers, F. Fullgraf, J. Jahn, M. Klinger, K. Dalhoff, H.A. Katus, W. Solbach, M. Maass, *Chlamydia pneumoniae* infection in circulating human monocytes is refractory to antibiotic treatment, Circulation 103 (2001) 351–356.

[18] J.B. Mahoney, B.K. Coombes, *Chlamydia pneumoniae* and atherosclerosis: does the evidence support a causal or contributory role? FEMS Microbiol. Lett. 197 (2001) 1–9.

[19] M.V. Kalayoglu, P. Libby, G.I. Byrne, *Chlamydia pneumoniae* as an emerging risk factor in cardiovascular disease, JAMA 288 (2002) 2724–2731.

[20] J. Gieffers, L. During, S.P. Ouellette, J. Rupp, M. Maass, G.I. Byrne, H.D. Caldwell, R.J. Belland, Genotypic differences in the *Chlamydia pneumoniae* tyrP locus related to vascular tropism and pathogenicity, J. Infect. Dis. 188 (2003) 1085–1093.

International Congress Series 1262 (2004) 430–433

www.ics-elsevier.com

Interaction of host and microbes in the atherosclerotic plaques

Jan Rupp, Matthias Maass*

Institute of Medical Microbiology and Hygiene, University of Luebeck, Ratzeburger Allee 160, 23538 Luebeck, Germany

Abstract. Atherosclerosis is characterized by chronic inflammation and vascular cell proliferation. The intracellular bacterium *Chlamydia pneumoniae* has been implicated in atherogenesis as it has been recovered from atheromatous plaques. In vitro, *C. pneumoniae* infection initiates activation of the transcriptional factor NF-κB via small GTPases Rac1 and RhoA. This signaling cascade results in the synthesis of numerous proinflammatory and procoagulatory mediators (e.g., IL-6, IL-8, RANTES, MCP-1, PAI-1, TF) that are also characteristically produced in the plaque. In parallel, chlamydiae stimulate vascular cell proliferation via ERK 1/2 MAPkinase and transcription factor Egr-1. Thus, chlamydial infection may have a role in the inflammatory, as well as in the angiogenic, component of atherogenesis. The proinflammatory activity of chlamydial infection is reduced by statins, via suppression of Rho and Rac signalling, indicating a beneficial anti-inflammatory effect of lipid-lowering drugs in vascular infection. *C. pneumoniae* uses blood monocytes as transport vehicles for systemic dissemination. In monocytes the pathogen enters a non-replicative, but viable, state characterized by continuous production of mRNA transcripts. Release of proinflammatory mediators by circulating or transendothelially migrating infected monocytes might promote chronic inflammation and atherogenesis. Interestingly, persistent chlamydiae in monocytes appear to be refractory to conventional antichlamydial treatment, thus posing a challenge to the ongoing experimental treatment studies. The persistent state is likely to have a key role in the pathogenesis of chronic chlamydial infections and requires further examination on a molecular level.

Keywords: *C. pneumoniae*; Atherosclerosis; Inflammation; Statins

1. Introduction

In the last years, the comprehension of the pathogenesis of atherosclerosis has changed fundamentally. Former considerations suggesting atherosclerosis in general as

* Corresponding author. Tel.: +49-0-451/500-2822; fax: +49-0-451/500-2808.
E-mail address: matthias.maass@hygiene.ukl.mu-luebeck.de (M. Maass).

doi:10.1016/S0531-5131(03)01857-0

a static accumulation of lipid-loaded macrophages and adherent thrombocytes were expanded by a more dynamic view of the pathophysiological mechanisms involved. Basic research has established a central role for inflammation and angioproliferation in the pathogenesis of atherosclerotic lesions [1,2], suggesting that other confounders than the known risk factors may initiate and trigger atherosclerosis. Epidemiological studies in patients with coronary artery disease (CAD) indicated that persistent infectious agents like *Chlamydia pneumoniae*, *Helicobacter pylori*, CMV or HSV-1 might be involved in perpetuating the chronic disease.

C. pneumoniae is the only replicative pathogen that has been recovered from atherosclerotic lesions in all clinical stages of CAD [3]. However, it has never been found in healthy arteries. Furthermore, human blood monocytes (PBMC) of CAD patients have been described to be persistently infected with *C. pneumoniae* in up to 26% of cases [4]. Interestingly, the chlamydial infection in PBMC is refractory to current antibiotic treatment due to a non-replicative but viable persistent state of the pathogen [5]. This review summarizes some basic research results of the potential role of *C. pneumoniae* in the pathogenesis of atherosclerosis.

2. *C. pneumoniae* induce vascular inflammation

C. pneumoniae is capable of infecting cell populations present in the atherosclerotic plaques and may implement its characteristic cycle of replication within the cells [6]. Recent studies linked *C. pneumoniae* to the inflammatory component of atherosclerosis by demonstrating a prominent release of proinflammatory and pro-coagulant factors in endothelial cells via the transcription factor NF-κB [7]. *C. pneumoniae* infection of endothelial cells significantly enhanced the release of tissue factor (TF) and interleukin-6 (IL-6) in a time-dependent manner. Thereby, *C. pneumoniae*-induced expression of TF and IL-6 in endothelial cells was centrally mediated via NF-κB p50/65 heterodimer activation [7]. In addition, *C. pneumoniae* infection of endothelial cells was found to increase the chemotactic activity within the vascular wall through enhanced secretion of interleukin-8 (IL-8) and monocyte-chemoattractant protein-1 (MCP-1) [8].

3. *C. pneumoniae* induce pro-atherogenic signal transduction in blood monocytes

The initiation, formation and disruption of atherosclerotic lesions are centrally affected by human PBMC through enhanced vascular recruitment, foam cell formation or secretion of pro-atherosclerotic proteins [2]. Infection of PBMC with *C. pneumoniae* not only initiates the differentiation from blood monocytes into macrophages [9], but also stimulates foam cell formation [10]. It is known that *C. pneumoniae* excites PBMC to an enhanced expression of proinflammatory cytokines and chemotactic factors, and a recent study from Bea et al. described the induction of TF expression in mouse macrophages via activation of the immediate early gene Egr-1 [11]. We could further show that enhanced Egr-1 expression in *C. pneumoniae*-infected human PBMC may be a common step in the regulation of pro-atherosclerotic factors not limited to promoting pro-coagulant activity. *C. pneumoniae*-induced Egr-1 activation was significantly blocked by ERK1/2 MAPkinase inhibition (Fig. 1a), and thus

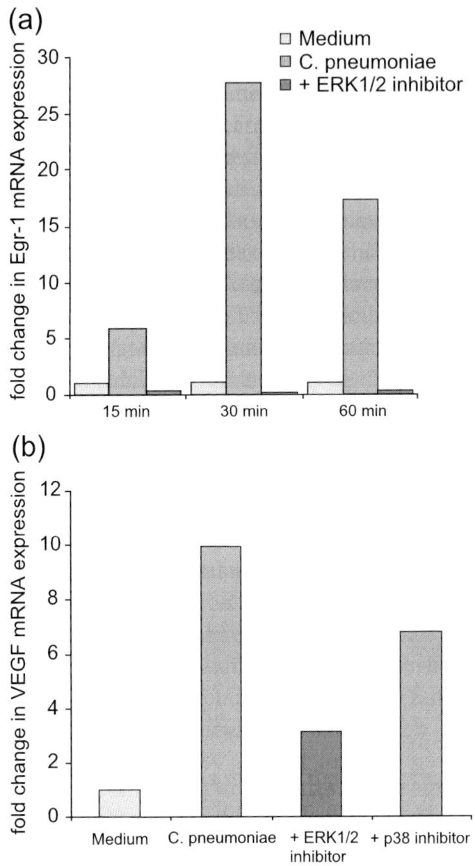

Fig. 1. (a) Shows the mRNA expression of the immediate early gene Egr-1 in *C. pneumoniae*-infected and non-infected human PBMC. Inhibition of the ERK1/2–MAP kinase pathway completely blocked *C. pneumoniae*-induced Egr-1 mRNA (a) and subsequent VEGF mRNA (b) expression in infected blood monocytes (b).

resulted in diminished secretion of the vascular endothelial growth factor (VEGF, Fig. 1b) [12].

4. Statins modify interactions between *C. pneumoniae* and vascular cells

As aforementioned, *C. pneumoniae* might be engaged in the pathogenesis of atherosclerosis through direct stimulatory effects on the secretion of inflammatory and procoagulant factors in the vascular wall but also by induction of an "atherogenic" cross-talk between infected monocytes and vascular cells. Chlamydial infection of PBMC appears refractory to the current antibiotic treatment, and therefore demands a therapeutical approach targeting the pathological signal cascades induced through *C. pneumoniae*. Statins, which are commonly used in CAD patients for cholesterol reduction, have been shown to reduce *C. pneumoniae*-induced secretion of chemotactic IL-8 and MCP-1 in endothelial cells [8], as well as transmission of chlamydial infection from blood monocytes to vascular smooth muscle cells [13]. Furthermore, the *C. pneumoniae*-induced activation profile in VSMC (Rac1 and RhoA prenylation, nuclear transcription factor-κB activation and reactive oxygen species production), which closely reflects the typical profile observed in atherosclerosis, was significantly reduced by statin treatment [13].

5. Conclusions

Atherosclerotic vascular disease is a progressive inflammatory process initiated and maintained by multiple factors. Mechanisms of the innate and adaptive immunity, as well as pathological regulation of vascular cell activity, contribute to its pathogenesis [14].

However, *C. pneumoniae* appears somewhat unique among the potential causal factors as it may simultaneously have a part in several of the most prominent features of atherogenesis; it may initiate a proinflammatory vascular response [7] and promote pro-atherogenic signaling in vascular and mononuclear cells [11,12]. In conclusion, the obtained findings make an infectious component in atherogenesis more plausible but causality remains to be established.

References

[1] P. Libby, P.M. Ridker, A. Maseri, Inflammation and atherosclerosis, Circulation 105 (2002) 1135–1143.

[2] R. Ross, Atherosclerosis: an inflammatory disease, N. Engl. J. Med. 340 (1999) 115–126.

[3] M. Maass, C. Bartels, P.M. Engel, U. Mamat, H.H. Sievers, Endovascular presence of viable *Chlamydia pneumoniae* is a common phenomenon in coronary artery disease, J. Am. Coll. Cardiol. 31 (1998) 823–827.

[4] M. Maass, J. Jahn, J. Gieffers, K. Dalhoff, H.A. Katus, W. Solbach, Detection of *Chlamydia pneumoniae* within peripheral blood monocytes of patients with unstable angina or myocardial infarction, J. Infect. Dis. 181 (2000) 449–451.

[5] J. Gieffers, H. Füllgraf, M. Klinger, K. Dalhoff, H.A. Katus, W. Solbach, M. Maass, *Chlamydia pneumoniae* infection in circulating human monocytes is refractory to antibiotic treatment, Circulation 103 (2001) 351–356.

[6] C.A. Gaydos, J.T. Summersgill, N.N. Sahney, J.A. Ramirez, T.C. Quinn, Replication of *Chlamydia pneumoniae* in vitro in human macrophages, endothelial cells, and aortic artery smooth muscle cells, Infect. Immun. 64 (1996) 1614–1620.

[7] R. Dechend, M. Maass, J. Gieffers, C. Scheidereit, R. Dietz, A. Leutz, D.C. Gulba, *Chlamydia pneumoniae* infection induces NF-κB mediated upregulation of tissue factor and PAI-1 expression in vascular smooth muscle and endothelial cells-A potential link to accelerated arteriosclerotic disease, Circulation 100 (1999) 1369–1373.

[8] H. Kothe, K. Dalhoff, J. Rupp, A. Müller, J. Kreuzer, M. Maass, H.A. Katus, HMG-CoA reductase inhibitors modify the inflammatory response of human alveolar macrophages and endothelial cells infected with *Chlamydia pneumoniae*, Circulation 101 (2000) 1760–1763.

[9] H. Yamaguchi, S. Haranaga, R. Widen, H. Friedman, Y. Yamamoto, *Chlamydia pneumoniae* infection induces differentiation of monocytes into macrophages, Infect. Immun. 70 (2002) 2392–2398.

[10] M.V. Kalayoglu, G.I. Byrne, Induction of macrophage foam cell formation by *Chlamydia pneumoniae*, J. Infect. Dis. 177 (1998) 725–729.

[11] F. Bea, M.H. Puolakkainen, T. McMillen, F.N. Hudson, N. Mackman, C.C. Kuo, L.A. Campbell, M.E. Rosenfeld, *Chlamydia pneumoniae* induces tissue factor expression in mouse macrophages via activation of Egr-1 and the MEK–ERK1/2 pathway, Circ. Res. 92 (2003) 394–401.

[12] J. Rupp, M. Maass, Egr-1, a major link between infection and atherosclerosis? Circ. Res. 92 (9) (2003) e78.

[13] R. Dechend, J. Gieffers, R. Dietz, A. Joerres, J. Rupp, F.C. Luft, M. Maass, HMG-CoA reductase inhibition reduces *Chlamydia pneumoniae*-induced cell interaction and activation, Circulation 108 (2003) 261–265.

[14] G.K. Hansson, P. Libby, U. Schonbeck, Z.Q. Yan, Innate and adaptive immunity in the pathogenesis of atherosclerosis, Circ. Res. 91 (2002) 281–291.

International Congress Series 1262 (2004) 434–437

www.ics-elsevier.com

Detection of infective agents in atherosclerotic tissues

Kazunobu Ouchi*

Department of Pediatrics, Kawasaki Medical School, 577 Matsushima, Kurashiki, 701-0192 Okayama, Japan

Abstract. Many studies demonstrated the presence of *Chlamydia pneumoniae*, cytomegalovirus, and herpes simplex virus in atherosclerotic tissues. The presence of *Helicobactor pylori* and periodontal pathogens in atherosclerotic tissues have been controversial. Among these, only *C. pneumoniae* has been proven to be alive and active in atheromatous tissues and usually associated with histological severity of atherosclerosis. These data indicated *C. pneumoniae* seemed to have the most direct effects to atherogenesis among these microorganisms, followed by cytomegalovirus and herpes simplex virus. © 2004 Published by Elsevier B.V.

Keywords: Atherosclerosis; *Chlamydia pneumoniae*; Cytomegalovirus; Herpes simplex virus; *Helicobactor pylori*

1. Introduction

Recently, many microorganisms and disorders have been listed for the association with atherosclerotic disorders after chronic inflammation has been known to be a key phenomenon in pathogenesis of atherosclerosis [1]. The current interest in atherosclerosis has focused on chronic infections. Many microorganisms such as *Chlamydia pneumoniae*, *Helicobactor pylori*, cytomegalovirus (CMV), herpes simplex virus (HSV), and human immunodeficiency virus have been listed [2]. *C. pneumoniae* had strong association with primary atherosclerosis in seroepidemiological studies. CMV had strong association with atherosclerosis after heart transplantation and restenosis. Several specific disorders, such as periodontal disease, respiratory infection and Kawasaki disease have been researched for association with atherosclerosis [2]. Many seroepidemiologic data indicated these microorganisms were associated with atherosclerosis and ischemic disorders of the cardiovascular system. After these positive findings of seroepidemiologic data, many researchers have tried to demonstrate these infective agents in atherosclerotic tissues. Several microorganisms have been detected in atherosclerotic lesions by various detection methods, such as immuno-histochemical staining (IHC), polymerase chain reaction (PCR), in situ hybridization (ISH), electron microscopy (EM), and isolation. These findings set

* Tel.: +81-86-462-1111; fax: +81-86-462-1199.
E-mail address: kouchi@med.kawasaki-m.ac.jp (K. Ouchi).

doi:10.1016/j.ics.2003.12.096

the investigation sight onto the etiologic role of these infective agents in atherosclerosis. I review the published papers on the detection of these microorganisms in atheromatous tissues and summarize in this report.

2. Detection of infective agents in atherosclerotic tissues

2.1. C. pneumoniae

Among these microorganisms associated with atherosclerosis, *C. pneumoniae* has been most investigated as a research target and substantial data have been accumulated.

To date, *C. pneumoniae* was detected by various detection methods, such as IHC, PCR, ISH, EM, and isolation in atherosclerotic tissues from 32.2% (1415/4395) of the subjects based on the data from 92 published papers. In many data from patients with symptomatic cardiovascular disorders, *C. pnuemoniae* was usually detected from more than 50% of atherosclerotic tissues. Among these detection methods, IHC had highest positive rate, followed by PCR, EM, and culture. There were many discrepant results between PCR and IHC. Identical results were seen only around 40% in many reports [3]. This poor correlation may come from patty distribution of *C. pneumoniae* in atherosclerotic tissues and tissue inhibitor of PCR which was commonly found in atheromatous tissues. Patty distributed nature of *C. pneumoniae* in atherosclerosis tissues was proved by Cochrane et al. [4]. They used consecutive sections of *C. pneumoniae* infected arterial wall and found that PCR of 15 sections lead to 95% chance of getting a positive result, although PCR of one small section lead to only 40% chance. The detection rates of *C. pneumoniae* from atherosclerotic tissues varied from 0% to 100%. This wide variability depended on variable detection methods, samples of variable atherosclerotic tissues, and skill of the researchers. We must follow the recommendation of standardizing *C. pneumoniae* assays for the future study [5].

C. pneumoniae was detected mainly in atheromatous tissues but was rarely found in normal vascular tissues and other organs [3]. Therefore *C. pneumoniae* was site-specifically detected in atherosclerotic tissues.

C. pneumoniae was commonly detected from aorta, iliac artery, and coronary artery, carotid artery, occluded coronary bypass of the saphenous vein, and nonrheumatic aortic stenotic valve [3]. *C. pneumoniae* was rarely found from peripheral artery, such as cerebral artery and radial artery.

The youngest age at which *C. pneumoniae* was detected in the arterial wall was 15 years [6]. A higher detection rate in subjects 25–34 year old (26%) was found than in those 15–24 year old (5%) [7].

Culture of *Chlamydia* from infected tissues has been most difficult among these detection methods. However, *C. pneumoniae* has been isolated from coronary artery, carotid artery, and occluded coronary bypass of the saphenous vein [3]. The other study also found mRNA of *C. pneumonia*e in atherosclerotic tissues [8]. These data clearly indicated *C. pneumoniae* actively infected in atheroma.

Usual serology for *C. pneumoniae* (IgA, IgG), CRP, fibrinogen, and pharyngeal status of the presence of *C. pneumoniae* did not predict the presence of *C. pneumoniae* in atherosclerotic tissues [3]. However, several serology test using specific part of membrane proteins as antigens, such as chlamydial heat shock protein and major outer membrane protein, and PCR of peripheral blood mononuclear cell for *C. pneumoniae* gave promising results, although further studies should be performed to confirm this evidence [9–11].

Substantial data showed the association of *C. pneumoniae* infection with histological severity of atherosclerosis both in younger age group and older age group [3,7]. Several studies using only PCR for detection could not confirm this association.

2.2. Cytomegalovirus

CMV also has been well investigated and substantial data have been accumulated, especially in restenosis and atherosclerosis after heart transplantation rather than primary atherosclerosis [2,12].

To date, CMV was detected by various detection methods, such as PCR, IHC, ISH in atherosclerotic tissues from 38.6% (624/1615) of the subjects based on the data from 27 published papers. In data from patients with symptomatic cardiovascular disorders, CMV was usually detected from more than 50% of atherosclerotic tissues. However, consistent failure to isolate CMV and mRNA in many reports indicated CMV was latent in atherosclerotic tissues [13]. The detection rates of CMV from atherosclerotic arterial wall varied from 0% to 90% in 27 published papers. CMV was detected mainly in atheromatous tissues but was rarely found in normal vascular tissues and other organs as stated in several reports [12]. However, several other reports did not show this trend. Consequently, site-specificity of CMV in atherosclerotic tissues has been controversial. There was no association of CMV infection with histological severity of atherosclerosis.

2.3. Herpes simplex virus

HSV has been rather less investigated than *C. pneumoniae* and CMV [2,12]. To date, HSV was detected by PCR, IHC, ISH in atherosclerotic tissues from 9.2% (38/399) of the subjects based on the data from seven published papers. The detection rate of HSV from atherosclerotic arterial wall varied from 0% to 73% in 7 published papers. HVS mRNA was demonstrated by ISH in aortic specimens from patients with clinically significant atherosclerosis in only one report [14]. HSV was more commonly detected in atheromatous tissues than normal vascular tissues in few reports. We need further study to confirm these data.

2.4. H. pylori

H. pylori has been much less investigated than *C. pneumoniae* and CMV [2,12]. To date, *H. pylori* was detected by only PCR in atherosclerotic tissues from 18.4% (80/434) of the subjects based on the data from nine published papers. However, four papers out of nine did not find any positive sample. There were no data which showed active *H. pylori* infection in atherosclerotic tissues. The detection rate of *H. pylori* from atherosclerotic arterial wall varied from 0% to 53% in nine published papers. *H. pylori* was more commonly detected in atheromatous tissues than normal vascular tissues in few reports.

2.5. Periodontal pathogens

Periodontal pathogens have also been much less investigated than *C. pneumoniae* and CMV [2,12,13]. So far, periodontal pathogens were detected by only PCR in atherosclerotic tissues from 50% (42/82) of the subjects based on the data from two published papers. There were no data which showed active periodontal pathogens in atherosclerotic tissues.

3. Discussion

Numerous studies have demonstrated the presence of *C. pneumoniae*, CMV, and HSV in atherosclerotic lesions. The presence of *H. pylori* and periodontal pathogens in atherosclerotic tissues have been supported by few reports. Among these microorganisms, only *C. pneumoniae* has been proved to infect actively in atheromatous tissues and usually associated with histological severity of atherosclerosis. These data supported that *C. pneumoniae* had the most direct effects to atherogenesis among these microorganisms, followed by cytomegalovirus and herpes simplex virus. *H. pylori* and periodontal pathogens seemed to have rather indirect effect. Although these studies suggested an etiologic role of infective agents, it is not enough to prove a definitive answer about causality by tissue studies. Further observational studies, such as animal model studies, human therapeutic trials, and in vitro studies can only add to the circumstantial evidence.

References

[1] R. Ross, Atherosclerosis—an inflammatory disease, N. Engl. J. Med. 340 (1999) 115–126.

[2] K.J. Mattila, et al., Role of infection as a risk factor for atherosclerosis, myocardial infarction, and stroke, Clin. Infect. Dis. 26 (1998) 719–734.

[3] C.C. Kuo, L.A. Campbell, Detection of *Chlamydia pneumoniae* in arterial tissues, J. Infect. Dis. 181 (2000) S432–S436.

[4] M. Cochrane, et al., Distribution of *Chlamydia pneumoniae* DNA in atherosclerotic carotid arteries: significance for sampling procedures, J. Clin. Microbiol. 41 (2003) 1454–1457.

[5] S.F. Dowell, et al., Standardizing *Chlamydia pneumoniae* assays: recommendations from the centers for disease control and prevention (USA) and the laboratory center for disease control (Canada), Clin. Infect. Dis. 33 (2001) 492–503.

[6] D. Taylor-Robinson, et al., *Chlamydia pneumoniae* in vascular tissues from heart-transplant donors, Lancet 351 (1998) 1255.

[7] C.C. Kuo, et al., *Chlamydia pneumoniae* (TWAR) in coronary arteries of young adults (15–34 years old), Proc. Natl. Acad. Sci. U. S. A. 92 (1995) 6911–6914.

[8] S.C. Johnston, et al., C-reactive protein levels and viable *Chlamydia pneumoniae* in carotid artery atherosclerosis, Stroke 32 (2001) 2748–2752.

[9] I.W. Fong, et al., Chlamydial heat-shock protein-60 antibody and correlation with *Chlamydia pneumoniae* in atherosclerotic plaques, J. Infect. Dis. 186 (2002) 1469–1473.

[10] Y. Kido, et al., Analysis of the serological response to *Chlamydia pneumoniae* in patients with ischemic heart disease by recombinant MOMP-ELISA, J. Infect. Chemother. 7 (2001) 180–185.

[11] F. Blasi, et al., *Chlamydia pneumoniae* DNA detection in peripheral blood mononuclear cells is predictive of vascular infection, J. Infect. Dis. 180 (1999) 2074–2076.

[12] S. O'Connor, et al., Potential infectious etiologies of atherosclerosis: a multifactorial perspective, Emerg. Infect. Dis. 7 (2001) 780–788.

[13] A. Kol, et al., Cytomegalovirus replication is not a cause of instability in unstable angina, Circulation 91 (1995) 1910–1913.

[14] E.P. Benditt, et al., Viruses in the etiology of atherosclerosis, Proc. Natl. Acad. Sci. U.S.A. 42 (80) 6386–6389.

International Congress Series 1262 (2004) 438–441

www.ics-elsevier.com

Trends of cardiovascular diseases among Koreans

Hong Kyu Lee*

Department of Internal Medicine, Seoul National University College of Medicine, 28 Yongon-dong, Chongno-gu, Seoul 110-744, South Korea

Abstract. Mortality, due to cardiovascular diseases in general, declined almost by half from 1984 to 1999, but mortality due to ischaemic heart disease, ischaemic stroke and diabetes increased over the last two decades. Mortality from diabetes increased from 3.4/100,000 in 1983 to 22.3 in 2001; ischaemic heart disease increased from 5.3 in 1987 to 13.8 in 1998; stroke decreased from 62 to about 40 in 2000, with an increase in the proportion of ischaemic stroke, from 2.9% to 14.4%. For risk factors, the prevalence of hypertension declined from 29.3% in 1980 to 27.2% in 1998 (>30 years old), particularly among the younger age group. Diabetes was rare in the 1960s, but 10.2% over the age of 40 are now diabetic. Overweight increased from 15.6% in 1990 to 27.4% in 2001 and obesity tripled in this period. The thrifty phenotype, made by malnutrition during Japanese occupation and Korean War combined with recent rapid economic growth, may explain these trends.

Keywords: Cardiovascular diseases; Korean; Risk factors; Mortality; Prevalence

During the last 20 years, there was a huge increase in the prevalence of obesity, diabetes mellitus and other risk factors of cardiovascular diseases among Koreans, leading to a continuous increase in death due to its complications—coronary heart diseases, stroke, and heart and renal failure. With mortality statistics collected by the National Bureau of Statistics over the last 20 years, the risk factors of cardiovascular diseases collected by several field studies, and a series of National Nutrition surveys conducted in the 1970s through the 1990s, the following summaries are made.

1. Changes in mortality due to cardiovascular diseases among Koreans

The mortality statistics of Koreans are posted on the web pages, http://www.nso.go.kr. With these data and other data sources, Suh [1] made an excellent account on the changes in cardiovascular mortality in Korea.

While total mortality due to cardiovascular diseases declined almost by half from 1984 to 1999 (172.2 to 73.0/100,000 or by 57% in males and 135.5 to 70.2/100,000 or 48% in

* Tel.: +82-2-760-2266; fax: +82-2-762-9662.
E-mail address: hkleemd@plaza.snu.ac.kr (H.K. Lee).

0531-5131/
doi:10.1016/j.ics.2004.01.088

women), the mortality rate due to ischaemic heart disease, ischaemic stroke and diabetes increased over the last two decades. Mortality from diabetes increased relentlessly from 3.4/100,000 in 1983 to 22.3/100,000 in 2001, almost doubling every 3 years. Mortality due to ischaemic heart disease increased from 5.3 in 1987 to 13.8/100,000 in 1998, stabilizing after 1993. Age-adjusted mortality from stroke decreased from 62 to about 40/100,000 in 2000, with a marked increase in the proportion of ischaemic stroke, from 2.9% to 14.4% of all strokes.

Mortality statistics employed by the National Statistics Office were from death certificates, but the validity of the certificates themselves is a little questionable. Many deaths are still diagnosed as "cardiovascular" when there was no clear known cause of death, and 75% of cerebrovascular accidents in 1984 and 53% of those in 1999 are unclassified stroke.

2. Prevalence of cardiovascular disease risk factors

2.1. Hypertension

Suh [1] gave an excellent summary of three nationwide hypertension surveys conducted in Korea, during 1980, 1990, and 1998. For those over the age of 30, the overall prevalence of hypertension was 29.3% in 1980, 26.8% in 1990, and 27.2% in 1998 according to WHO criteria. The decrease of prevalence was more marked among younger ages; in a 1980 survey, 16.4% were hypertensive, while it was 12.4% in 1998. A recent survey in Ansan county, Kyunggi province showed an overall prevalence of hypertension of 33.7%, suggesting the real problem might be bigger [2]. Among these, 64.9% had Grade 1 hypertension, 22.5% Grade 2, and 12.5% Grade 3. The age-specific prevalence of hypertension increased progressively with age, from 14.19% in 18- to 24-year-olds to 71.39% in those 75 years or older. Prevalence was significantly higher in men (41.5%) than in women (24.5%). Isolated systolic hypertension had significantly lower prevalence (4.33%) within the population, although the prevalence was 11.13% in those over 55. Multivariate analysis revealed that age, body mass index and abdomen circumference were significantly associated with hypertension, both in men and women. As much as 78.6% were being treated with antihypertensive medications, and 24.3% of them achieved good control.

2.2. Diabetes mellitus

Diabetes mellitus was a rare disease among Koreans in 1960s, but slowly started to increase in the 1970s (1.5% in those over 30 in 1972) and became rather frequent recently (9.1% in 1993, 10.2% in 2001, ages 40–65) [3,4]. Diabetes frequently appeared as a part of metabolic syndrome in the Yonchon study [4] and National Health and Nutrition Interview survey (NHNIS) [5,6]. Risk factors for diabetes were similar from already known larger studies; ageing, abdominal obesity, insulin deficiency, urbanization and impaired glucose tolerance. Almost half of diabetic subjects did not know they were diabetic.

Diabetes became the most frequent cause (43%) of new dialysis therapy, followed by various types of nephritis (22%) and hypertension (15%).

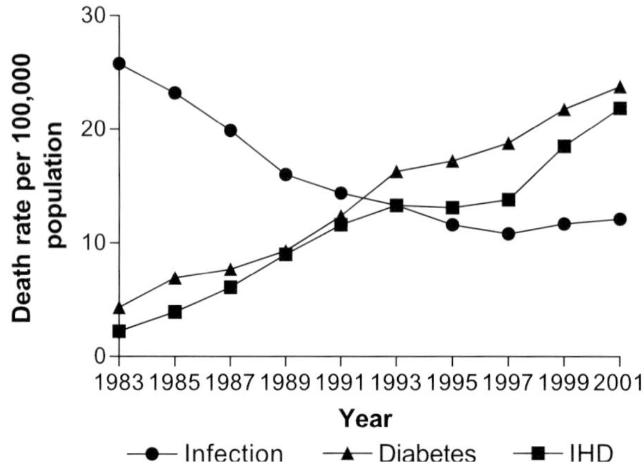

Fig. 1. Death rate from diabetes and ischaemic heart disease compared with infectious disease in Korea (1983–2001). It shows increasing trend of mortalities due to ischaemic heart disease, diabetes mellitus, and decline of death due to infectious disease, over last two decades.

2.3. Obesity

According to Korean National Nutrition surveys and NHNIS, the prevalence of overweight in individuals (defined as BMI > 25 over the age of 20) increased from 15.6% in 1990 to 27.4% in 2001. The prevalence of obesity (BMI>30) tripled in this period from 1.6% to 3.2%. As earlier data might not be representative of all Koreans, caution should be exercised in the interpretation.

Obesity was more prevalent among low-income families and poorly educated people. City dwellers tended to be obese, while people in rural area had more abdominal obesity (unpublished data from Ansan study).

A study on the trend of BMI and obesity in children and adolescents (who attended high school in Seoul over the past 20 years) [7], revealed BMI and the prevalence of obesity increased relentlessly in this period, suggesting an increasing trend of cardiovascular diseases will continue in the foreseeable future.

3. Societal changes associated with the emergence of a cardiovascular disease epidemic

Fig. 1 shows the increasing trend of mortalities due to ischaemic heart disease, diabetes mellitus, and decline of death due to infectious diseases, over the last two decades. The correlation coefficient between ischaemic heart disease mortality and mortality due to diabetes mellitus was 0.95 ($p < 0.001$), suggesting there are common causes behind this trend. An increase in the number of cars, total domestic production and many other social parameters also showed good correlations (Table 1).

I suggested the thrifty phenotype hypothesis of Hales and Barker [8] might explain this trend biologically, based on the mitochondrial hypothesis [9]. Because Korean people lived for a long period of time in a poor nutritional state, it is conceivable that Koreans might have acquired the thrifty genome. Furthermore, Korean people experienced

Table 1
The changes in the number of cars, total domestic production and nutritional status in Korea over last two decades

	GDP (billion dollars)	Number of cars	Total calorie intake (kcal)	Total protein intake (g)	Animal protein intake (g)
1983	82.3	380,993	2 622	86.6	29.1
1985	93.4	556,659	2 687	86.6	28.5
1987	135.2	844,350	2 810	88.4	30.7
1989	220.7	1,558,660	2 825	88.9	30.7
1991	295.1	2,727,852	2 876	88.6	32.4
1993	345.7	4,271,253	2 872	91.7	35.5
1995	489.4	6,006,290	2 959	96.9	39.3
1997	476.6	7,586,474	2 957	97.0	40.2
1999	405.8	7,837,206	2 968	98.2	40.8
2001	427.3	8,889,327	2 994	98.5	45.2

malnutrition during the Japanese occupation (1909 to 1945) and the Korean War (1950–1953), making people thrifty. Combined with rapid economic growth, people became obese, diabetic and many died from cardiovascular complications, while generally people lived longer.

Acknowledgements

This work was supported by a grant of the Korea Health 21 R&D Project, Ministry of Health and Welfare, Republic of Korea (02-PJ1-PG1-CH04-0001).

References

[1] I. Suh, Cardiovascular mortality in Korea: a country experiencing epidemiologic transition, Acta Cardiol. 56 (2) (2001) 75–81.
[2] I. Jo, et al., Prevalence, awareness, treatment, control and risk factors of hypertension in Korea: the Ansan study, J. Hypertens. 19 (9) (2001) 1523–1532.
[3] Y. Park, et al., Prevalence of diabetes and IGT in Yonchon County, South Korea, Diabetes Care 18 (4) (1995) 545–548.
[4] C.S. Shin, et al., Risk factors for the development of NIDDM in Yonchon County, Korea, Diabetes Care 20 (12) (1997) 1842–1846.
[5] Ministry of Health and Welfare, Republic of Korea, Report on 1998 National Health and Nutrition Survey (1998) (in Korean).
[6] Y. Park, et al., Community-based epidemiologic study on atherosclerotic cardiovascular risk factors, Diabetes Res. Clin. Pract. 34 (1996) S65–S72 (Suppl.).
[7] J.H. Park, The current status of maternal and child health in Korea. The Korean Society of Maternal and Child Health Symposium 2003, Seoul, Korea.
[8] C.N. Hales, D.J. Barker, The thrifty phenotype hypothesis, Br. Med. Bull. 60 (2001) 5–20.
[9] H.K. Lee, Method of proof and evidences for the concept that mitochondrial genome is a thrifty genome, Diabetes Res. Clin. Pract. 54 (Suppl. 2) (2001) S57–S63.

International Congress Series 1262 (2004) 442–445

www.ics-elsevier.com

Prevalence of metabolic syndrome among adult Filipinos

Felix Eduardo R. Punzalan[a,1], Rody G. Sy[b,*], Tommy Ty-Willing[c]

[a] National Institutes of Health, University of the Philippines Manila, Taft Avenue, Manila, Philippines
[b] Cardiovascular Section, College of Medicine, University of the Philippines Manila, Taft Avenue, Manila, Philippines
[c] Metropolitan Hospital, Magdalena St., Binondo, Manila, Philippines

Abstract. *Rationale*: Metabolic syndrome is a common condition worldwide. Until recently, there is no universal definition for metabolic syndrome. Its prevalence in the Philippines has never been studied before. *Objectives*: To determine the prevalence of metabolic syndrome among adult Filipino population. *Sample Population*: 4541 individuals aged ≥20 years. *Methods*: Nationwide survey using two-stage stratified sampling design was done in 1998. Measurement of risk factors was done by blood pressure and waist circumference determination; and laboratory testing for lipid profile and fasting blood sugar using Cholestech LDX machine. Metabolic syndrome was defined based on NCEP and International Atherosclerosis Society (IAS) criteria. For IAS criteria, the waist circumference was based on Asia Pacific criterion (>90 and 80 cm, for male and female, respectively). *Results*: Based on NCEP criteria, the prevalence of metabolic syndrome is 14.2% (95% CI: 13.2–15.2). Using the IAS criteria, the prevalence is 19.3% (95% CI: 18.1–20.4). Stratifying the prevalence based on age revealed a prevalence of 6.6%, 17.7%, and 18.3% for ages 20–39, 40–59, 60 years and older, respectively, by NCEP criteria. IAS criteria showed a prevalence of 10.0%, 23.6%, and 24.1% for ages 20–39, 40–59, 60 years and older, respectively. *Conclusion*: Metabolic syndrome is common among Filipino adult population. There is an increasing prevalence with age. Using NCEP criteria instead of the IAS with waist circumference criterion adjusted for Asia Pacific population may underestimate the prevalence of metabolic syndrome. © 2003 Published by Elsevier B.V.

Keywords: Metabolic syndrome; Epidemiology; Asian data

1. Introduction and rationale

In 1998, the World Health Organization [1] proposed clinical diagnosis on metabolic syndrome in patients with type 2 diabetes, impaired glucose tolerance, or

* Corresponding author. Tel./fax: +63-2-726-8579.
E-mail addresses: yobs@pworld.net.ph (F.E.R. Punzalan), rodysymd@info.com.ph (R.G. Sy).
[1] Tel./fax: +63-2-525-9939.

0531-5131/ © 2003 Published by Elsevier B.V.
doi:10.1016/j.ics.2003.12.009

increased insulin resistance if they satisfy two of four criteria, namely: high BP, abnormal lipids, obesity based on BMI or waist–hip ratio, and microalbuminuria. In 2001, the NCEP ATP III [2] based the diagnosis on the presence of at least three of the following criteria: low HDL, increased triglyceride, elevated BP, impaired fasting blood glucose, and increased waist circumference. In 2003, the International Atherosclerosis Society (IAS) [3] came out with Harmonized Clinical Guidelines on Prevention of Atherosclerotic Vascular Disease after a consensus from member societies including the Philippines. IAS adopted the NCEP guideline but adjusted cut-off for the waist circumference according to ethnicity. For Asian countries, the cut-off for waist circumference is reduced to >90 and >80 cm for men and women, respectively. In the Philippines, a nationwide survey was conducted in 1998–1999 by the Food and Nutrition Research Institute with the Department of Health and professional organizations, namely: Philippine Society of Hypertension, Philippine Diabetes Association and Philippine Lipid Society [4]. We used the data from the survey to determine the prevalence of metabolic syndrome among adult Filipinos ≥20 years.

2. Objectives

(1) To determine the prevalence of metabolic syndrome among adult Filipino population. (2) To compare the prevalence of metabolic syndrome using the NCEP and IAS criteria.

3. Methodology

3.1. Study population and sampling strategy

The survey included all the provinces in the country and used a two-stage stratified random sampling design. The barangays (villages) and their members were the first and second stages of selection, respectively; subjects were drawn from the sampled barangays. The final sample size comprised 4541 individuals aged ≥20 years.

3.2. Measurement of risk factors

Determination of blood pressure and waist circumference was done by trained research assistants. Lipid profile and FBS were measured using Cholestech LDX lipid analyzers. Study methodology is described in more detail in separate publication [4].

4. Definition of metabolic syndrome

Metabolic syndrome is considered if three of the following five criteria are present in a subject: (1) elevated triglyceride (>150 mg/dl), (2) reduced HDL (men <40 mg/dl, women <50 mg/dl), (3) elevated BP (Systolic >130 mm Hg or Diastolic >85 mm Hg), (4) impaired fasting glucose (>110 mg/dl), (5) using NCEP criteria, waist circumference of >102 and >88 cm for male and female, respectively. For IAS

Table 1
Prevalence of metabolic syndrome by gender

Criteria	Sex	Prevalence (%)	95% CI
NCEP criteria	All	14.2	13.2–15.2
	Male	14.3	12.8–15.8
	Female	14.1	12.7–15.6
IAS criteria	All	19.3	18.1–20.4
	Male	18.6	17.1–20.3
	Female	19.9	18.3–21.6

criteria, the Asia Pacific cut-off of >90 and >80 cm for male and female, respectively, was used.

5. Analysis

The proportion of subjects with at least any three of the above criteria was determined using both NCEP and IAS criteria. Stratified prevalence based on age was also estimated.

6. Results

Among Filipinos, low HDL level is the most dominant factor with a prevalence of 78.9% in males, 88.9% in females, and 84.0% overall. Next is elevated BP, accounting for 46.4% in males, 36.2% in females, and 41.3% for all. Elevated triglyceride is 22.6% in males, 15.9% in females and 19.2% for all. Impaired fasting blood glucose is similar for both sexes, 7.2% for males, 6.9% for females, and 7.0% for all. Increased waist circumference using NCEP cut-off is 2.0% in males, 8.4% in females, and 5.2% for all. Using the Asian cut-off in IAS, it is present in 12.6% of males, 24.8% of females, and 18.8% of all subjects.

Based on the above findings, the prevalence of metabolic syndrome among adult Filipinos using NCEP criteria is 14.3% for males, 14.1% for females and 14.2% for all. Using the IAS criteria, it goes up to 18.6% for males, 19.9% for females and 19.3% for all (Table 1). For the different age brackets of 20–39 years, 40–59 years, and 60 years or more, the prevalence based on NCEP is 6.6% (95% CI 5.4–7.92), 17.7% (95% CI 15.86–19.7), and 18.3% (95% CI 16.39–20.29), respectively; and based on IAS, is 10.0% (95% CI 8.6–11.65), 23.6% (95% CI 21.49–25.75) and 24.1% (95% CI 22.04–26.35), respectively.

7. Discussion

The most dominant factor among Filipinos is low HDL. This is because our mean HDL based on the national survey in 1998–1999 is only 30.0 mg/dl which is unusually low. Recently Filipino women in California were found to have lower HDL level compared with age-matched Caucasian women [5]. The difference between males and females is magnified for HDL and waist circumference because of higher cut-off for females in both categories.

The prevalence of metabolic syndrome is 14.2% (NCEP) or 19.3% (IAS) in our population. This is comparable with the 14% prevalence in Taiwan [6] using a higher BP cut-off of 140/90 mm Hg and a higher blood glucose value of >126 mg/dl. The prevalence increases with age and our results showed a progressive rise in the three age groupings. In our population, low HDL, elevated triglyceride and BP accounted for the most common combination following NCEP, while with IAS, increased waist circumference displaced elevated triglyceride in the combination.

A lower cut-off for waist circumference for Asians is recommended by the International Obesity Task Force Asian Pacific region [7] because of increased morbidity seen among Asians at lower BMI, waist–hip ratio and waist circumference. Higher prevalence of insulin resistance, diabetes and coronary heart disease among south Asians who migrated to the United Kingdom and the United States has been reported [8,9].

8. Conclusion

This study shows that metabolic syndrome is common among adult Filipinos and maybe one reason why cardiovascular disease ranks as the number one cause of mortality in the country. Intervention can be simple when detected before the appearance of complications. Lifestyle modification, especially on diet, weight loss and exercise, must be emphasized.

References

[1] K.G. Alberti, P.Z. Zimmet, Definition, diagnosis and classification of diabetes mellitus and its complications: Part I. Diagnosis and classification of diabetes mellitus provisional report of a WHO consultation, Diabet. Med. 15 (1998) 539–553.

[2] Executive summary of the third report of the National Cholesterol Education Program (NCEP) expert on detection, evolution and treatment of high blood cholesterol in Adults (Adult Treatment Panel III), JAMA 285 (2001) 2486–2497.

[3] International Atherosclerosis Society (IAS), Harmonized clinical guidelines on prevention of atherosclerotic vascular disease, Exec. Summ. 8 (2003).

[4] R.G. Sy, F.E. Punzalan, The prevalence of dyslipidemia, diabetes, hypertension, stroke and angina pectoris in the Philippines, Philipp. J. Intern. Med. 41 (2003) 1–6.

[5] M.R. Araneta, D.L. Wingard, E. Barrett-Connor, Type 2 diabetes and metabolic syndrome in Filipina–American women: a high-risk nonobese population, Diabetes Care 25 (3) (2002) 494–499.

[6] W.P. Pan, Metabolic syndrome—an important but complex disease entity for Asians, Acta Cardiol. Sin. 18 (2002) 24–26.

[7] Asian Pacific Perspective: Redefining Obesity and its Treatment. Feb 2000. http://www.iotf.org.

[8] T.A. Chowdhury, S.S. Lasker, Complications and cardiovascular risk factors in South Asians and Europeans with early-onset type 2 diabetes, Q. J. Med. 95 (4) (2002) 241–246.

[9] M. Chandalia, N. Abate, A. Garg, J. Stray-Gundersen, S.M. Grundy, Relationship between generalized and upper body obesity to insulin resistance in Asian Indian men, J. Clin. Endocrinol. Metab. 84 (1999) 2329–2335.

International Congress Series 1262 (2004) 446–449

ELSEVIER

www.ics-elsevier.com

Trends in cardiovascular diseases and risk factors in Malaysia

Robaayah Zambahari*

National Heart Institute 145 Jalan Tun Razak, 50400 Kuala Lumpur, Malaysia

Abstract. *Background*: Data from the Information and Documentation System Unit of the Ministry of Health of Malaysia showed that cardiovascular disease had been the principal cause of death in government hospitals over the years, accounting for 23% to 26% of deaths from 1994 to 2001. Heart disease accounted for 14% to 16.6%. Of cardiovascular disease admissions and deaths in government hospitals from 1985 to 2000, ischaemic heart disease accounted for 25% to 33% of admissions and 27% to 35% of deaths. A National Health and Morbidity Survey (NHMS) conducted in 1996 to evaluate health status, health-related behavior and health services utilization in 21,708 individuals aged 30 years or older, of whom 17,390 (80%) agreed to participate, 39% had no risk factors, 34% had one risk factor, 19% had 2 risk factors, 7% had 3 risk factors and 1% had 4 risk factors. *Conclusions*: Cardiovascular disease is the major cause of hospital admissions and death in government hospitals in Malaysia. The National Health and Morbidity survey showed 61% of Malaysians had one risk factor or more.

Keywords: Cardiovascular disease; Survey; Risk factors

1. Introduction

Malaysia, with a population of 23 million, has three major ethnic groups—Malays comprising 55%, Chinese comprising 34% and Indians comprising 10%. Data from the Information and Documentation System Unit of the Ministry of Health of Malaysia showed that cardiovascular disease has been the principal cause of death in government hospitals over the years, accounting for 23% to 26% of deaths from 1994 to 2001. Heart disease accounted for 14% to 16.6%. Of cardiovascular disease admissions and deaths in government hospitals from 1985 to 2000, ischaemic heart disease accounted for 25% to 33% of admissions and 27% to 35% of deaths.

2. Review of publications

In March 1991, a paper on cardiovascular mortality in Peninsular Malaysia: 1950–1989 by Khoo et al. [1] showed that cardiovascular disease, with particular emphasis on

* Tel.: +603-26178435; fax: +603-26928425.
E-mail address: robaayah@ijn.com.my (R. Zambahari).

0531-5131/ © 2003 Published by Elsevier B.V.
doi:10.1016/S0531-5131(03)01818-1

coronary heart disease was an important cause of death. It was observed that among six major disease groups reviewed, cardiovascular diseases which occupied third place as a cause of death in 1950 emerged as the number one killer during the 1970s and has remained so since (with exception in 1980). In contrast, infectious disease which ranked first in 1950 dropped to fourth position in 1980. Between 1960 and 1980, mortality due to cardiovascular diseases was higher in males than in females. This tendency became less apparent during 1985–1989. With reference to race, the incidence of cardiovascular deaths was highest in Indians followed by Chinese and Malays.

A National Health and Morbidity Survey (NHMS) [2] was conducted in 1996 to evaluate health status, health-related behavior and health services utilization for a representative sample of the population of Malaysia. Of 21,708 individuals aged 30 years or older who were eligible, 17,390 (80%) agreed to participate. They were interviewed; blood pressure, capillary blood glucose, blood cholesterol, body weight and height were measured. The following definitions were used.

Hypertension when mean of two blood pressure measurements were ≥ 140 mm Hg systolic (SBP) or ≥ 90 mm Hg diastolic (DBP) or current treatment for hypertension with medication. Abnormal glucose tolerance (diabetes and impaired glucose tolerance) based on the WHO criteria. Hypercholesterolaemia was defined as blood total cholesterol of ≥ 5.2 mmol/l. Overweight was defined as body mass index (BMI) ≥ 25 kg/m^2). Physical activity was graded active if a person engaged in a sporting activity at least three times a week each lasting at least 15 min or a person's daily activity, including occupational activity, is sufficiently rigorous to cause sweating.

Results of the survey showed that 61% had one or two risk factors and 1.2% had all four risk factors.

Distribution of number of risk factors (0–4) among adult Malaysians

Number of risk factor(s)	Prevalence (%)
0	39
1	34
2	19
3	7
4	1

Prevalence of risk factor in isolation and with one or more other risk factors.

	All (%)	Isolated (%)	+1 other (%)	+2 others (%)	+3 others (%)
Hypertension	33.1	12.3	13.3	6.3	1.2
Abnormal glucose tolerance	11.3	2.1	4.1	4.0	1.2
Hypercholesterolaemia	20.1	6.7	7.6	4.6	1.2
Overweight	33.1	6.7	7.6	4.7	1.2

Indian men had a remarkably high prevalence of high blood pressure and abnormal glucose tolerance in association with high blood cholesterol or overweight. Malay women had high prevalence of high blood pressure, high blood cholesterol and overweight. For all four risk factors, the most at risk groups were Indians and Malay women.

In 1996, Malaysia participated in the Asian-Pacific Collaboration on CHD Risk Factor Intervention, coordinated by NHMRC Clinical Trials Centre University of Sydney [3]. This study was to determine and compare rates of measurement and levels of management of traditional coronary risk factors by reviewing the notes of consecutive admissions for myocardial infarction or unstable angina for 6 months up to 30 June 1995. Twenty-three hospitals were selected and the risk factors evaluated were hypertension, obesity, diabetes, hypercholesterolaemia and smoking. Hypercholesterolaemia was defined as history of hypercholesterolaemia or total cholesterol ≥ 5.5 mmol/l and/or cholesterol lowering medication at the time of survey period, diabetes defined as history of diabetes or random blood sugar ≥ 15 mmol/l during first 48 h after admission or ≥ 11 mmol/l at any other time or anti-diabetes medication, hypertension defined as history of hypertension or systolic blood pressure ≥ 140 mm Hg or diastolic blood pressure ≥ 90 mm Hg, obesity/overweight defined as presence of obesity recorded in the notes or body mass index >25 kg/m^2. The results showed that measurements for blood pressure, smoking and blood glucose were generally well established. Measurement rate for cholesterol and overweight were comparably lower. There was a high prevalence rate for hypertension (74%). Treatment rates were high for hypertension (94%) and diabetes (87%), but were much lower for hypercholesterolaemia (27%) and current smokers (19%). Only a few patients were recorded to have received dietary advice for overweight/obesity.

In 1997, Liew et al. [4] reported on the health status of senior citizens of Kuala Lumpur. Senior civil servants (733) with a mean age of 44 years (range 25–56 years) showed that 36% were overweight with 6.5% being obese. 15.2% had systolic hypertension (systolic BP ≥ 140 mm Hg) and 27.6% had diastolic hypertension (diastolic BP ≥ 90 mm Hg). 75.2% had raised cholesterol (total cholesterol ≥ 5.2 mmol/l). 8.4% had elevated blood sugar ≥ 6.7 mmol/l.

In December 2000, Khoo et al. [5] published the results of a health screening program conducted in 10 major centers in Malaysia during the National Heart Week 1995–1997 with 6858 participants aged between 6 and 81 years evaluating body mass index, blood pressure, heart rate and glucose. Results showed that the mean and standard deviation for the body mass index (BMI), systolic blood pressure (SBP), diastolic blood pressure (DBP), heart rate (HR), total cholesterol (TC) and non-fasting (random) blood glucose (GL) of the volunteers studied were 24.3 ± 4.0 kg/m^2, 128.3 ± 21.1 mm Hg, 79.6 ± 1.9 mm Hg, 77.2 ± 12.1 bpm, 5.33 ± 1.37 mmol/l and 5.11 ± 1.97 mm Hg, 77.2 ± 12.1 bpm, 5.33 ± 1.37 mmol/l and 5.11 ± 1.97 mmol/l, respectively. There was a rising trend for BMI, SBP, DBP, TC and GL with age. The Malays, Chinese and Indian seemed to have closely similar mean values for SBP, DBP and HR but the Indians possessed the highest BMI ($25.62 + 3.90$ kg/m^2), TC (5.61 ± 1.48 mmol/l) and GL (5.41 ± 2.43 mmol/l) among the three major ethic groups. While the Ibans had the highest TC ($6.07 + 1.09$ mmol/l), their GL level was the lowest (4.67 ± 1.15 mmol/l). The Kadazans had the lowest TC level (4.94 ± 1.39 mmol/l) among all the ethnic groups.

3. Conclusion

Cardiovascular disease is the principal cause of admission and death in government hospitals in Malaysia. The National Health and Morbidity Survey showed that atherosclerotic risk factors are common among Malaysians with 61% having one or two risk factors. Clustering of risk factors was common.

Indian men had a remarkably high prevalence of high blood pressure and abnormal glucose tolerance in association with high blood cholesterol or overweight. Malay women had high prevalence of high blood pressure, high blood cholesterol and overweight. For all four risk factors, the groups most at risk were Indians and Malay women.

References

[1] K.L. Khoo, et al., Cardiovascular mortality in Peninsular Malaysia: 1950–1989, Med. J. Malays. 46 (1991) 7–20.
[2] T.O. Lim, et al., Clustering of hypertension, abnormal glucose tolerance, hypercholesterolaemia and obesity in Malaysian adult population, Med. J. Malays. 55 (2000) 196–208.
[3] G.M. Ritchie, et al., Asia-Pacific collaboration on coronary heart disease risk factor intervene study design and methods, Heart, Lung and Circulation 10 (2001) 24–29.
[4] Y.M. Liew, et al., Health status of senior civil servants in Kuala Lumpur, Med. J. Malays. 52 (1997) 348–366.
[5] K.L. Khoo, et al., Blood pressure, body mass index, heart rate and levels of blood cholesterol and glucose of volunteers during Nation Heart Weeks, 1995–1997, Med. J. Malays. 55 (2000) 439–450.

ELSEVIER

International Congress Series 1262 (2004) 450–453

www.ics-elsevier.com

The von Hippel-Lindau protein: a key player in oxygen homeostasis and matrix assembly

M.A. Esteban[a], S.J. Mandriota[b], P.H. Maxwell[a,*]

[a] Renal Section, Division of Medicine, Imperial College London, Hammersmith Campus, Du Cane Road, London W12 ONN, UK

[b] Division of Oncology, University Medical Centre, Geneva, Switzerland

Abstract. A key aspect of vascular function is distributing oxygen reliably. Oxygen deficiency is a logical consequence of reducing blood flow, e.g. by an atheromatous plaque. Recently, a transcriptional system centred on the hypoxia-inducible factor-1 (HIF) and the von Hippel-Lindau (VHL) protein has emerged as a major regulator in oxygen homeostasis. HIF regulation in normoxia depends on VHL-mediated destruction. When the oxygen supply is reduced, the HIF pathway is activated. Together with activation of HIF in normoxia, VHL-deficient cells show a striking defect in extracellular matrix assembly, raising the question as to whether HIF underlies this. If so, altered oxygen tension in pathological settings could have major effects on matrix behaviour. © 2003 Elsevier B.V. All rights reserved.

Keywords: Hypoxia; HIF; Prolyl hydroxylases; Extracellular matrix; Fibronectin

1. Regulation of HIF by oxygen

von Hippel-Lindau (VHL) is a tumor suppressor gene underlying hereditary VHL syndrome [1]. VHL is the substrate recognition subunit of a complex with ubiquitin ligase activity. Hypoxia-inducible factor-1 (HIF) is composed of a β subunit, which is constitutively expressed, and an α regulatory subunit. In normoxia, HIFα is recognized by VHL and degraded by the proteasome [2]. Oxygen-dependent regulation of HIFα also occurs at the level of transactivation through preventing the recruitment of coactivators. The basis for the recognition by VHL is the hydroxylation of two proline residues in the central part of the HIFα, and for the control of transactivation the hydroxylation of an asparagine in the carboxy terminal part. The prolyl hydroxylase reaction is carried out by three 2-oxoglutarate-dependent dioxygenases, termed PHD1, PHD2 and PHD3 [1]; the asparagine hydroxylation is mediated by another member of the family, termed FIH. These reactions need molecular oxygen as a cosubstrate and respond exquisitely to oxygen availability. When the oxygen supply is reduced, the hydroxylation steps do not proceed

* Corresponding author. Tel.: +44-208-383-8594; fax: +44-208-383-2062.
E-mail address: p.maxwell@imperial.ac.uk (P.H. Maxwell).

doi:10.1016/j.ics.2003.11.048

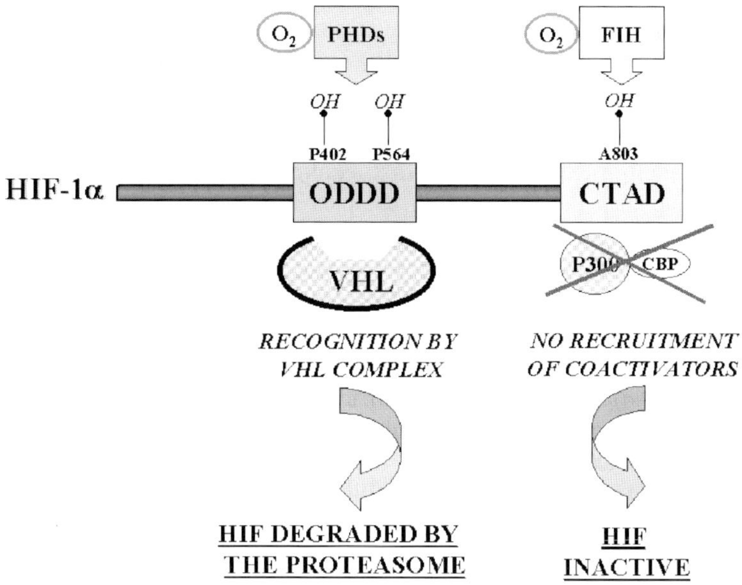

Fig. 1.

and HIF becomes stabilized and recruits transactivators. VHL loss of function not only underlies the VHL syndrome, but also occurs in most sporadic renal cell cancers. Importantly, VHL reexpression suppresses tumor formation by VHL-deficient renal cancer cell lines implanted in nude mice (Fig. 1) [1].

2. VHL(−) renal cancer cells fail to assemble a fibronectin matrix

We observed a striking lack of fibronectin (FN) matrix assembly in VHL-deficient cells as previously documented [3,4]. Stable reexpression of VHL restores effective matrix

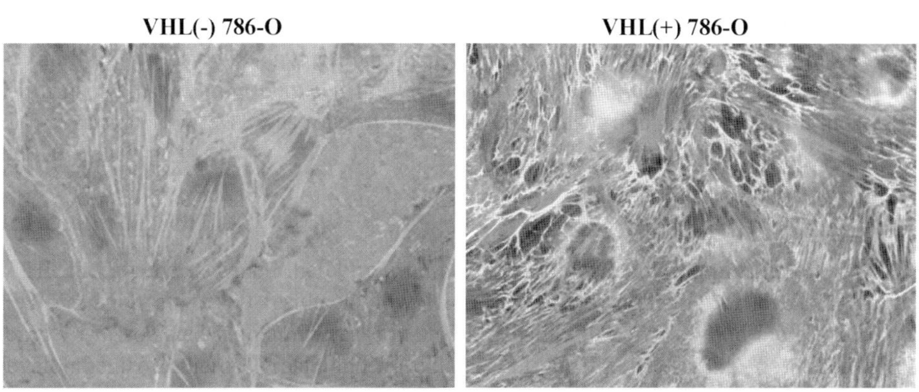

Fig. 2. Immunofluorescence staining of 786-O cells cultured over exogenous FN. FN is presented in green, and actin is presented in red (in colour in the online version).

organization. Importantly, the defect of VHL(−) cells is not reversed by providing exogenous FN (Fig. 2) [4].

2.1. Hypotheses concerning the FN assembly defect

The organization of extracellular FN first requires the binding of soluble FN to α5β1 integrins [4], and then the FN–integrin complex is stretched by the cytoskeleton. FN stretching exposes cryptic internal dimerisation sites and allows fiber growth. Given the role of VHL in proteasomal-mediated degradation, it was proposed that VHL could exert a similar effect on FN [3]. Inactivation of VHL would promote the intracellular accumulation of misprocessed/misfolded FN molecules as a result of the inability to remove them. When secreted, abnormal FN species might interfere with the orderly assembly of normal FN. Support for this came from the fact that FN can be coprecipitated with anti-VHL in VHL(+) cells. We labeled FN in precancerous early lesions of kidneys from VHL patients which represents a very early step after biallelic VHL inactivation [5]. Staining with anti-CAIX (a well-characterised HIF-inducible protein) showed that HIF was activated, but we saw no evidence of intracellular FN accumulation (Fig. 3) which is consistent with a recent study of cultured cells [4].

An alternative mechanism is that extracellular proteases could be degrading FN fibers in VHL(−) cells [1]. Related to this, levels and activity of metalloproteinases 2 and 9 are increased in VHL(−) cells. Abnormalities in the surface organization of integrins could also be important in the phenotype, because VHL(−) cells cannot organize α5β1 integrin fibrillar adhesions, a cell-matrix adhesion structure essential for FN fibrillogenesis [4].

2.2. Is the lack of FN assembly a general feature of VHL(−) cells?

FN matrix defects have been demonstrated in several VHL(−) renal cancer cell lines. Our studies show that VHL reintroduction does not restore a normal matrix phenotype in all of them (data not shown). This suggests that some of these cell lines may carry mutations besides VHL which disturb the matrix formation. Consistent with this, the lack of FN assembly is found in most cancer cell lines of epithelial origin. Importantly, fibroblasts from VHL − / − mice also lack an FN matrix [3]. Therefore, the role of VHL in matrix assembly does not seem to be restricted to the renal epithelium. Elucidating

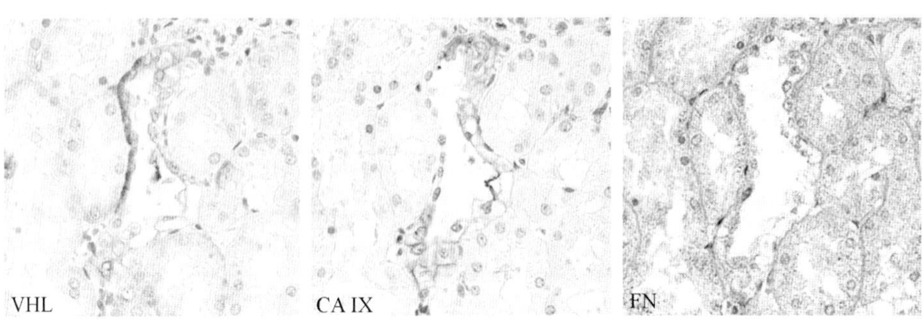

Fig. 3.

whether VHL inactivation influences the organization of other proteins, such as elastin, collagen, laminin or thrombospondin-1, would also be important in understanding the overall effects of VHL on the matrix.

3. Does hypoxia affect the extracellular matrix?

Effects of VHL loss due to HIF should also be seen when HIF is activated by other methods. It is therefore of relevance to assess whether hypoxia influences extracellular FN assembly. In our experiments so far, it appears that lowering oxygen sufficiently to activate HIF in VHL(+) cells does not disturb the matrix assembly. Likewise, stable transfection of specific VHL point mutants (corresponding to type 2C VHL syndromic disease) into VHL(−) renal cancer cells fails to improve their matrix phenotype, despite the fact that they normalize HIF protein levels [1].

4. Conclusions and implications

Abnormal matrix assembly in VHL(−) renal cancers could affect tumor growth by a mechanical effect, facilitating aberrant cell growth outside the tubule. Likewise, reduced interaction between cells and the surrounding environment affects cell behaviour. Notably, VHL loss is unlikely to be the only factor influencing the matrix in cell lines from different tumors. Despite understanding VHL's role in the HIF pathway, it is not yet clear how VHL influences matrix organization. If HIF activation is not involved in the matrix phenotype of VHL-defective cells, understanding how VHL loss promotes this could reveal another molecular action of this tumor suppressor protein.

References

[1] W.G. Kaelin Jr., Molecular basis of the VHL hereditary cancer syndrome, Nat. Rev. Cancer 2 (9) (2002) 673–682.

[2] P.H. Maxwell, M.S. Wiesener, G.W. Chang, S.C. Clifford, E.C. Vaux, M.E. Cockman, C.C. Wykoff, C.W. Pugh, E.R. Maher, P.J. Ratcliffe, The tumour suppressor protein VHL targets hypoxia-inducible factors for oxygen-dependent proteolysis, Nature 399 (6733) (1999) 271–275.

[3] M. Ohh, R.L. Yauch, K.M. Lonergan, J.M. Whaley, A.O. Stemmer-Rachamimov, D.N. Louis, B.J. Gavin, N. Kley, W.G. Kaelin Jr., O. Iliopoulos, The von Hippel-Lindau tumor suppressor protein is required for proper assembly of an extracellular fibronectin matrix, Mol Cell 1 (7) (1998) 959–968.

[4] M.A. Esteban-Barragan, P. Avila, M. Alvarez-Tejado, M.D. Gutierrez, A. Garcia-Pardo, F. Sanchez-Madrid, M.O. Landazuri, Role of the von Hippel-Lindau tumor suppressor gene in the formation of beta1-integrin fibrillar adhesions, Cancer Res 62 (10) (2002) 2929–2936.

[5] S.J. Mandriota, K.J. Turner, D.R. Davies, P.G. Murray, N.V. Morgan, H.M. Sowter, C.C. Wykoff, E.R. Maher, A.L. Harris, P.J. Ratcliffe, et al., HIF activation identifies early lesions in VHL kidneys: evidence for site-specific tumor suppressor function in the nephron, Cancer Cell 1 (5) (2002) 459–468.

International Congress Series 1262 (2004) 454–457

www.ics-elsevier.com

Mechanical stress-related atherosclerosis and functional genomics

Hiromi Rakugi*, Tomohiro Katsuya, Mitsuru Ohishi, Naomichi Matsukawa, Kazuhiko Ishikawa, Toshio Ogihara

Department of Geriatric Medicine, Osaka University Graduate School of Medicine, 2-2 Yamadaoka, #B6, Suita 565-0871, Japan

Abstract. Pulsatile stretch and shear stress in hypertension are reported to participate in atherosclerosis. The relationship between mechanical stress and atherosclerosis has been investigated from the point of biochemical molecules, such as angiotensin, endothelin, cytokines and oxidative stress. In particular, reactive oxygen species are up-regulated by mechanical stretch and participate in advances of atherosclerosis. Furthermore, recent progress in gene analysis has revealed that some specific genes relate to both hypertension and carotid atherosclerosis. It is important to functionally analyze the relations between gene polymorphism and the development of atherosclerosis because atherosclerosis is caused by multiple factors. Plasma homocysteine concentration for the methylenetetrahydrofolate reductase (MTHFR) gene is well reported from the point of functional genomics. C677T polymorphism of this gene is associated with carotid intimal-medial thickness in women smokers in the Japanese general population. The functional genomics that are attempted to intermediate phenotypes of hypertension and atherosclerosis, such as sympathetic activity, oxidative stress, adhesion molecules, endothelial function and arterial stiffness are expected to reveal novel mechanisms of atherosclerosis and to provide more appropriate therapeutic strategies of tailored medicine for hypertension.

Keywords: Mechanical stress; Hypertension; Atherosclerosis; Oxidative stress; Genetics

1. Introduction

Cardiovascular complications due to hypertension are closely related with atherosclerosis. Blood pressure reduction is the most important measure to reduce the mortality and morbidity of cardiovascular complications [1]. Therefore, mechanical stretch to the cardiovascular system is believed to be the leading cause of hypertensive complications. Recently, reactive oxidative species (ROS) are reported to be activated in the cardiovascular systems in hypertensive patients and also participate in atherosclerosis as a key molecule of signal transduction. Furthermore, the functional relations between hyperten-

* Corresponding author. Tel.: +81-6-6879-3852; fax: +81-6-6879-3859.
E-mail address: rakugi@geriat.med.osaka-u.ac.jp (H. Rakugi).

doi:10.1016/j.ics.2003.11.038

sion and atherosclerosis from the perspective of genetic variants have been extensively studied to apply to tailored medicine.

2. Effects of mechanical stress on vascular cells

Fig. 1 presents the previously reported intracellular signals activated by mechanical stretch. Although the molecular mechanisms of these responses are unclear, the evidence has been accumulated that the SA channel acts as a primary sensor for mechanical stimuli [2,3]. Transactivation of the EGF receptor and activation of the Rho/Rho kinase and NADPH/NADH oxidase are very probable molecules activated by mechanical stretch. Increases in intracellular calcium via the SA channel activate production of ROS [3], which participates in most of these pathways. These signals are able to produce an accumulation of extracellular matrix and promote inadequate growth of vascular cells.

ACE inhibitor and angiotensin receptor antagonist are reported to prevent cardiovascular complications beyond the effects of lowering blood pressure [4,5]. Of interest, mechanical stress such as transmural pressure and stretch activates vascular angiotensin generation via interaction between endothelial cells and smooth muscle cells [6]. Many of these substances induce ROS in vascular cells, as well as directly activate ROS by mechanical stress.

3. Genetic analysis of atherosclerosis

Recent progress in gene analysis has revealed that some specific genes relate to both hypertension and atherosclerosis. It is important to functionally analyze the relations between gene polymorphism and the development of atherosclerosis using specific intermediate phenotypes, such as sympathetic activity, metabolites of ROS, expression

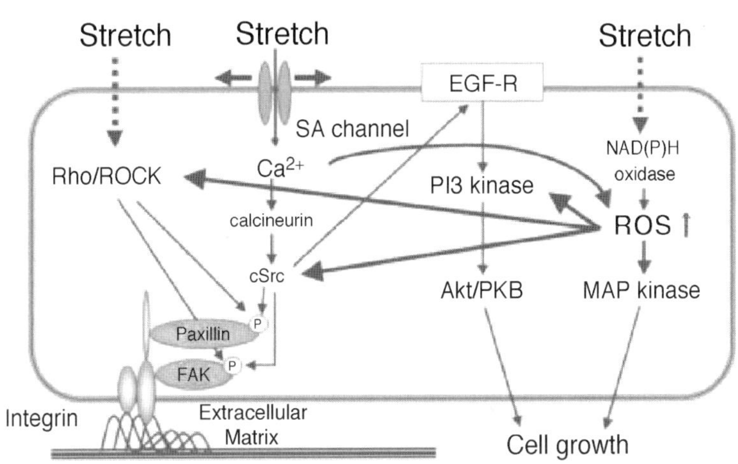

Fig. 1. Signal activation by mechanical stress. It is not clear whether the SA channel-induced cSrc transactivates the EGF receptor as well as angiotensin II-induced cSrc. Interaction between the SA channel and Rho/ROCK system has not been clarified. SA channel, stretch-activated channel; ROS, reactive oxygen species; EGF-R, endothelial growth factor-receptor.

of adhesion molecules, endothelial function and arterial stiffness. These phenotypes are also used as surrogate markers of cardiovascular events. Pharmacogenetic analysis is also important for applying genetic analysis to tailored medicine.

4. Approaches to mechanical, stress-related atherosclerosis

From the point of oxidative stress, hyperhomocysteinemia promotes oxidant injury to the endothelium and is associated with atherosclerotic vascular diseases. Furthermore, homocysteine-lowering therapy with folic acid is only one anti-oxidative intervention that is useful to improve endothelial dysfunction and to decrease the incidence of revascularization after percutaneous coronary intervention [7].

Methylenetetrahydrofolate reductase (MTHFR) is a key molecule of homocysteine metabolism. C677T polymorphism of the MTHFR gene associates with plasma homocysteine levels. Our population study in Japan demonstrated that maximum IMT in the common carotid artery of smokers with the TT genotype was significantly higher than for smokers with the CC genotype and nonsmokers with the TT genotype in women [8]. Significant interactions between the C677T/MTHFR and smoking on the maximum IMT indicate that smoking cessation for subjects with the TT genotype is important in the prevention of cerebrovascular disease.

5. Conclusions

In conclusion, mechanical, stress-related atherosclerosis in hypertension is one of the pathways of atherosclerosis in multi-factorial diseases (Fig. 2). Oxidative stress is well reported as a major risk factor for atherosclerosis in multiple risk factor syndrome, and oxidative stress has been further defined as an important factor also for mechanical, stress-related atherosclerosis. Sufficient blood pressure reduction with antihypertensive drugs is important and clinically useful to reduce mechanical stress. New therapeutic approaches, such as homocysteine-lowering therapy and newly developing anti-oxidative drugs, may additionally reduce the incidence of cardiovascular diseases. Furthermore, genomic analyses for hypertension, oxidative stress and intermediate phenotypes of atherosclerosis provide more appropriate therapeutic strategies for tailored medicine.

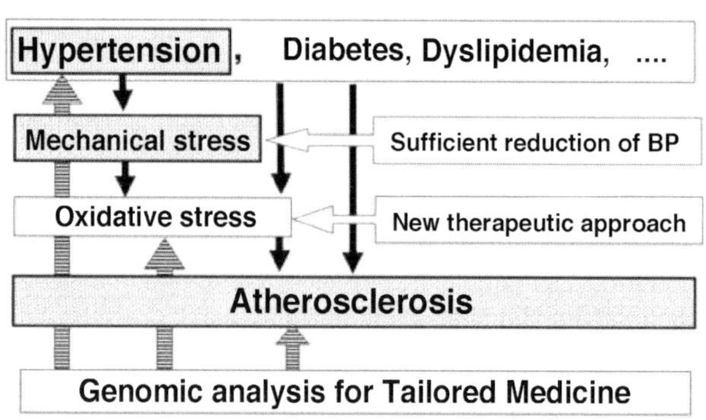

Fig. 2. Therapeutic approaches for hypertension-related mechanical stress and atherosclerosis.

References

[1] J.A. Staessen, J.G. Wang, L. Thijs, Cardiovascular prevention and blood pressure reduction: a quantitative overview updated until 1 March 2003, J. Hypertens. 21 (6) (2003) 1055–1076.
[2] M. Sokabe, K. Naruse, S. Sai, T. Yamada, K. Kawakami, M. Inoue, et al., Mechanotransduction and intracellular signaling mechanisms of stretch-induced remodeling in endothelial cells, Heart Vessels (Suppl. 12) (1997) 191–193.
[3] K. Aikawa, N. Nishikimi, T. Sakurai, Y. Nimura, M. Sokabe, K. Naruse, SA channel mediates superoxide production in HUVECs, Life Sci. 69 (15) (2001) 1717–1724.
[4] S. Yusuf, P. Sleight, J. Pogue, J. Bosch, R. Davies, G. Dagenais, Effects of an angiotensin-converting-enzyme inhibitor, ramipril, on cardiovascular events in high-risk patients. The Heart Outcomes Prevention Evaluation Study Investigators, N. Engl. J. Med. 342 (3) (2000) 145–153.
[5] B. Dahlof, R.B. Devereux, S.E. Kjeldsen, S. Julius, G. Beevers, U. Faire, et al., Cardiovascular morbidity and mortality in the Losartan Intervention for Endpoint Reduction in Hypertension Study (LIFE): a randomised trial against atenolol, Lancet 359 (9311) (2002) 995–1003.
[6] N. Bardy, R. Merval, J. Benessiano, J.L. Samuel, A. Tedgui, Pressure and angiotensin II synergistically induce aortic fibronectin expression in organ culture model of rabbit aorta. Evidence for a pressure-induced tissue renin–angiotensin system, Circ. Res. 79 (1) (1996) 70–78.
[7] G. Schnyder, M. Roffi, Y. Flammer, R. Pin, O.M. Hess, Effect of homocysteine-lowering therapy with folic acid, vitamin B12, and vitamin B6 on clinical outcome after percutaneous coronary intervention: the Swiss Heart Study: a randomized controlled trial, JAMA 288 (8) (2002) 973–979.
[8] N. Inamoto, T. Katsuya, Y. Kokubo, T. Mannami, T. Asai, S. Baba, et al., Association of methylenetetrahydrofolate reductase gene polymorphism with carotid atherosclerosis depending on smoking status in a Japanese general population, Stroke 34 (7) (2003) 1628–1633.

International Congress Series 1262 (2004) 458–461

www.ics-elsevier.com

Hypolipidemic drugs, blood pressure, heart rate, heart rate variability and sympathetic activity

Richard Ceska*, Vojtech Melenovsky, Jan Malik, Eva Kralikova, Tomas Stulc, Michal Vrablik

Department of Internal Med. III., Center Prev. Cardiol, University Hospital Prague, U nemocnice 1 128 08 Prague, Czech Republic

Abstract. Treatment of dyslipidaemia represents a reasonable approach in the prevention and treatment of cardiovascular diseases. Although it is generally accepted that lipid lowering is responsible for the majority of the beneficial effects of treatment, there are also some data demonstrating positive effects of lipid-lowering drugs beyond cholesterol lowering. These pleiotropic effects of statins, but also fibrates and some new hypolipdemic agents (e.g. ezetimibe), are intensively studied. In addition to the influence on CRP and other markers of inflammation, parameters of coagulation, as well as endothelial dysfunction markers, the effects of statins and fibrates on blood pressure, insulin resistance or on the sympathetic activity are under investigation. We discuss the common pathways leading to dyslipidaemia and hypertension and the effects of lipid lowering on blood pressure. Both statins and fibrates have demonstrated a capability to lower blood pressure significantly in some small-scale clinical trials. However, the data from large-scale intervention trials are either absent or ambiguous. Lipid-lowering drugs influence arterial wall structure and, hence, pulse wave velocity. In the Fenofibrate vs. Atorvastatin Trial (FAT), we proved the positive effect of both drugs on heart rate variability (HRV). So far, an explanation of the positive effects of lipid-lowering drugs is not known. But some hypotheses, e.g. modulating of sympathetic activity and/or metabolic syndrome, are available. We can conclude that lipid lowering may serve as an additional method of correcting hypertension in some high-risk patients and that it also has other positive effects on cardiovascular risk.

Keywords: Lipid-lowering drugs; Statins; Fibrates; Blood pressure; Heart rate variability

1. Introduction

Dyslipoproteinaemia and hypertension (along with diabetes and cigarette smoking) represent the most important risk factors for cardiovascular diseases. These disorders are characterised by the high incidence in populations and very often they occur together, e.g.

* Corresponding author. Tel./fax: +42-22-496-2946.
E-mail address: rcesk@lfl.cuni.cz (R. Ceska).

0531-5131/ © 2004 Published by Elsevier B.V.
doi:10.1016/j.ics.2003.11.049

about 40% of patients with hypertension have hyper- or dyslipoproteinaemia. Coincidence of hypertension and dyslipoproteinaemia is a typical feature in patients with the metabolic syndrome [1,2].

Lipid lowering is the almost universally accepted approach in the prevention of cardiovascular diseases. Several large trials have demonstrated that treatment with lipid-lowering drugs is not only safe and well tolerated, but above all, significantly decreases cardiovascular morbidity and mortality [3,4]. These positive effects of treatment have recently been proven across different study populations, and data are available for elderly patients [5], as well as for children and adolescents [6].

2. Lipid-lowering drugs in patients with hypertension

A very important question is whether patients with hypertension will have the same profit from treatment with lipid-lowering drugs as patients irrespective of hypertensive status. Two large trials were published recently answering this question. In the ALLHAT-LLT trial [7], pravastatin did not significantly influence total mortality, and the reduction of cardiovascular risk was also only very limited (9%). An explanation of this result could be due to the small difference in lipids between pravastatin group and "usual care". In the ASCOT-LLA [8], decrease of total and LDL cholesterol by 24% and 35% was accompanied by the reduction in total mortality of 13% and a 29% fall in coronary heart disease. We can conclude that a significant improvement in lipid profile leads to a reduction in cardiovascular morbidity and mortality, even in patients with well-controlled hypertension.

3. Do lipid-lowering drugs reduce blood pressure?

The answer to this question has been summarised recently [9]. This article reviews the common pathways leading to both hypertension and hyperlipoproteinaemia and the effects diet and lipid-lowering drug therapies have had on correcting blood pressure in patients with hypertension. Of the most frequently used lipid-lowering drugs, both statins and fibrates have shown the potential to lower blood pressure by up to 8/5 and 15/10 mm Hg, respectively, in some small-scale clinical trials and affect arterial wall structure and, hence, pulse wave velocity. Therefore, lipid lowering may provide an additional method of correcting essential hypertension in some patients. However, data from the large-scale interventional trials are either missing or ambiguous. Definitive large-scale trials to investigate the anti-hypertensive effects of lipid-lowering drugs are required.

4. Pleiotropic effects of lipid-lowering drugs

In this article, we do not want to discuss the effects of lipid-lowering drugs beyond lipid lowering, as well as whether these effects are clinically relevant. However, it is necessary to mention that both statin and fibrates (and the first data are coming for ezetimibe) have these "pleiotropic effects" [10,11]: 1. endothelial dysfunction improvement 2. anti-inflammatory effects 3. antioxidative effect 4. antiproliferative effect 5. antiaggregatory effect 6. plaque stabilization.

5. Lipid-lowering drugs, heart failure and sympathetic activity

The 4S study has demonstrated, albeit in a post-hoc analysis, a significant reduction in the development of subsequent heart failure in patients with preserved ventricular function at the time of entry into the study [12]. No large-scale clinical trial to date with statins in patients with coronary heart disease has prospectively enrolled patients with chronic heart failure, and no prospective trial of statins has been specifically conducted in patients with chronic heart failure.

Retrospectively, non-randomized subset analyses do, however, suggest a possible benefit of statins in patients with chronic heart failure. In the 4S study, the mortality rate in patients developing chronic heart failure was 25.5% in the simvastatin group compared with 31.9% in the placebo group [12]. In the Heart Protection Study, there were slightly fewer deaths from heart failure in the simvastatin group compared with placebo, but this did not reach significance [3]. The first experimental data were published, providing the pathophysiological explanation of the possible positive effect of statins on experimental heart failure [13]. It is hypothesised, and experimentally proved, that statins exert effects on autonomic function, as assessed by plasma norepinephrine levels, direct recordings of renal sympathetic nerve activity and baroreflex function. Since heart rate variability (HRV) is an important marker of autonomic function and HRV was found depressed in chronic heart failure, several studies have been designed to assess the influence of statin treatment on this parameter. It has been proven that statins improve HRV in patients with previous myocardial infarction [14]. In our clinic, we designed the Fenofibrate vs. Atorvastatin Trial (FAT) study. This randomised, open-label trial investigated whether autonomic cardiovascular control is altered in middle-aged men with combined hyperlipidaemia and whether such alterations are affected by short-term, lipid-lowering therapy with atorvastatin and/or fenofibrate. Compared with normolipidaemic subjects, untreated subjects with familial, combined hyperlipidaemia had several abnormalities of autonomic tone, indicating increased sympathetic tone and decreased baroreflex sensitivity. The alterations in autonomic cardiovascular control were partially reversible by administering both lipid-lowering drugs, fibrate as well as statin [15].

6. Lipid-lowering drugs in prevention of arrhythmia

Interesting data concerning the anti-arrhythmic potential of lipid-lowering drugs came recently from the AVID trial [16]. Lipid-lowering therapy was associated with a reduction in the relative hazard for tachyarrhythmia. It also reduced the relative hazard for all-cause mortality and the hazard for cardiac mortality. These results suggest that part of the benefit from the lipid-lowering treatment may be due to an anti-arrhythmic effect.

7. Conclusions

In patients with known cardiovascular disease, and those at high risk for it, the treatment of atherosclerosis must begin as soon as possible. This treatment should contain a combination of lipid-lowering drugs, anti-platelet treatment, beta-blockers and angiotensin-converting enzyme inhibitors. Some authors suggested recently the use of a "polypill" as a "one size fits all" solution to coronary heart disease prevention. Despite the positive effects of lipid-lowering drugs, including the lipid lowering presented above, they are above all useful for the normalisation of plasma lipids and lipoproteins.

Acknowledgements

This work was supported by the grant NB/7392-3, IGA, Ministry of Health, Czech Republic.

References

[1] H.N. Ginsberg, A.F.H. Stalenhoef, The metabolic syndrome: targeting dyslipidaemia to reduce coronary risk, J. Cardiovasc. Risk 10 (2003) 121–128.
[2] G. Reaven, Metabolic syndrome. Pathophysiology and implications for management of cardiovascular disease, Circulation 106 (2002) 286–288.
[3] MRC/BHF Heart Protection Study of cholesterol lowering with simvastatin in 20 536 high-risk individuals: a randomised placebo-controlled trial, Lancet 360 (2002) 7–22.
[4] S.J. Robins, D. Collins, J.T. Wittes, et al., Relation of gemfibrozil treatment and lipid levels with major coronary events, VA-HIT: a randomized controlled trial, JAMA 285 (2001) 1585–1591.
[5] J. Shepherd, G.J. Blauw, M.B. Murphy, et al., Pravastatin in elderly individuals at risk of vascular disease (PROSPER): a randomised controlled trial, Lancet 360 (9346) (2002 Nov. 23) 1623–1630.
[6] S. deJongh, M.R. Lilien, J. Roodt, et al., Early statin therapy restores endothelial function in children with familial hypercholesterolemia, J. Am. Coll. Cardiol. 40 (2002) 2117–2121.
[7] The ALLHAT Officers and Coordinators for the ALLHAT Collaborative Research Group, Major outcomes in moderately hypercholesterolemic, hypertensive patients randomized to pravastatin vs. usual care, JAMA 288 (2002) 2998–3007.
[8] P.S. Sever, B. Dahlof, N.R. Poulter, et al., Prevention of coronary and stroke events with atorvastatin in hypertensive patients who have average or lower-than-average cholesterol concentrations, in the Anglo-Scandinavian Cardiac Outcomes Trial-Lipid Lowering Arm (ASCOT-LLA): a multicentre randomised controlled trial, Lancet 361 (2003) 1149–1158.
[9] A.S. Wierzbicki, Lipid lowering: another method of reducing blood pressure? J. Hum. Hypertens. 16 (2002) 753–756.
[10] P.O. Bonetti, L.O. Lerman, C. Napoli, A. Lerman, Statin effects beyond lipid lowering–are they clinically relevant? Eur. Heart J. 24 (2003) 225–248.
[11] O. Barbier, I. Pineda Torra, Y. Duguay, Pleiotropic actions of peroxisome proliferator-activated receptors in lipid metabolism and atherosclerosis, Arterioscler. Thromb. Vasc. Biol. 22 (2002) 717–726.
[12] J. Kjekshus, T.R. Pedersen, A.G. Olsson, et al., The effects of simvastatin on the incidence of heart failure in patients with coronary disease, J. Card. Fail. 3 (1997) 249–254.
[13] R.U. Pliquett, K.G. Cornish, J.D. Peuler, I.H. Zucker, Simvastatin normalizes autonomic neural control in experimental heart failure, Circulation 107 (2003) 2493–2498.
[14] S. Riahi, J.H. Christensen, E. Toft, et al., HMG-CoA reductase inhibitors improve heart rate variability in patients with a previous myocardial infarction, Pharm. Res. 45 (2002) 479–483.
[15] V. Melenovsky, D. Wichterle, J. Simek, et al., Effect of atorvastatin and fenofibrate on autonomic tone in subjects with combined hyperlipidemia, Am. J. Cardiol. 92 (2003) 337–341.
[16] L.B. Mitchell, J.L. Powell, A.M. Gillis, et al., Are lipid-lowering drugs also antiarrhytmic drugs? J. Am. Coll. Cardiol. 42 (2003) 81–87.

International Congress Series 1262 (2004) 462–465

www.ics-elsevier.com

Renin–angiotensin system and vasculature—focusing on insulin's action

Kei Kamide[a,*], Michael L. Tuck[b]

[a] *Hypertension and Nephrology, National Cardiovascular Center, 5-7-1 Fujishirodai, Suita, Osaka 565-8565, Japan*

[b] *Sepulveda VA Medical Center, 16111 Plummer St., North Hills, CA 91343, USA*

Abstract. Several recent clinical trials show that blocking agents of the renin–angiotensin system (RAS) reduces cardiovascular events in patients with metabolic syndrome based on insulin resistance. Our laboratory has focused on the relationship between the vascular RAS and the action of insulin on the vasculature. We first revealed that addition of insulin to cultured vascular smooth muscle cells (VSMC) markedly increases angiotensinogen and angiotensin II (Ang II) expression and production. Insulin addition also induces VSMC growth that is inhibited by blockade of the RAS by either an ACEI or an ARB suggesting a role for the RAS in insulin-mediated growth. Insulin has a quite different effect in cultured vascular endothelial cells (EC) as it reduces angiotensinogen and renin expression. However, insulin added to EC induces a marked activation of ACE and the activated ACE promotes the conversion of Ang I to Ang II and cell growth under conditions of high insulin state. Ang II induces the progression of atherosclerosis through the production of oxidative stress that blocks insulin signaling and accelerates atherosclerosis. This paper attempts to clarify the relationship between insulin resistance, the RAS and oxidative stress in vascular tissues to mimic in vivo conditions found in the metabolic syndrome.

Keywords: Renin–angiotensin system; Insulin resistance; Oxidative stress; Atherosclerosis

1. Introduction

The metabolic syndrome is recognized as the relationship of insulin resistance to the clustering of several risk factors for cardiovascular disease. Most guidelines about treatment of hypertension such as the JNC VII [1] and the ESC-ESH2003 [2], recommend the use of angiotensin converting enzyme inhibitor (ACEI) for patients with the metabolic syndrome. The Heart Outcomes Prevention Evaluation (HOPE) study [3] revealed that ACEI treatment with ramapril significantly reduced, by 22%, combined cardiovascular events in patients with multiple cardiovascular risk factors compared with the placebo group. Thus, the clinical indications of ACEI do not just apply to hypertension and congestive heart failure, but have expanded to prevention or regression of atherosclerosis. Furthermore, the angiotensin II type1 receptor blocker (ARB) losartan significantly

* Corresponding author. Tel.: +81-6-6833-5012; fax: +81-6872-7486.
E-mail address: kamide@hsp.ncvc.go.jp (K. Kamide).

0531-5131/
doi:10.1016/j.ics.2003.12.088

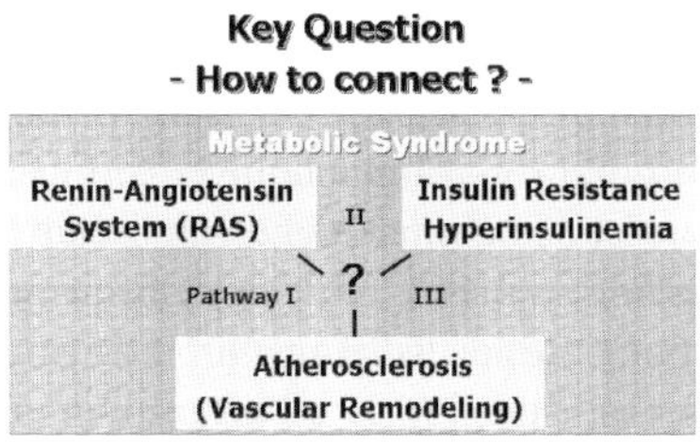

Fig. 1. Key question of this study.

reduces the prevalence of new onset of diabetes mellitus as seen in the LIFE sub-study [4]. These findings mean that blockade of the RAS may lead to improve the insulin sensitivity from the insulin resistant status. In this paper, we try to clarify the interactions between the vascular tissue RAS and the insulin resistance and hyperinsulinemia in the rapid progression of atherosclerosis that is in the metabolic syndrome (Fig. 1).

2. Activation of RAS promotes vascular remodeling and atherosclerosis (pathway I: Fig. 1)

Ang II produced in the vessel walls disrupts the regulatory mechanism of physiologically active substances by impairment of EC function. Ang II affects each stage of atherosclerosis including impairment of EC function, growth of plaque, deposition of lipids, plaque rupture, and obstruction of arteries by thrombus [5].

Recent studies indicated that Ang II-mediated production of reactive oxygen species (ROS) through the NADPH oxidase such as O_2^- and H_2O_2 promotes growth factors, cytokines and chemotactic factors relating to the atherosclerosis [6]. H_2O_2 produced by Ang II mediates regulation of a variety of pro-inflammatory genes including MCP-1, IL-6 and VCAM. Activation of MAPK, PI3/Akt mediates hypertrophic responses. H_2O_2 also activates eNOS and produces NO^-. Thus, ROS activated by Ang II is playing an important role in the progression of atherosclerosis [6]. RAS blocking agents, ACEI and ARB, inhibit these multi-factorial effects of Ang II and reduced cardiovascular events as seen in the HOPE and LIFE studies. However, we still do not know the mechanisms leading to the initial activation of tissue Ang II in high risk conditions such as the metabolic syndrome.

3. Hyperinsulinemia stimulates the vascular RAS (pathway II)

We have proposed that a high level of insulin in insulin resistance states induces the activation of the tissue RAS in blood vessels and heart and leads to the overproduction of Ang II in these tissues. We showed that high level of insulin (≥ 100 μU/ml) directly activates the expression and production of angiotensinogen and cell growth through the AT_1 receptors and the conversion of Ang I to Ang II in VSMC [7]. Insulin can cross-bind to insulin like growth factor-I (IGF-I) receptor because of their similar structural homology. We found that IGF-I also induces the production of vascular angiotensinogen and VSMC growth through the IGF-I receptor since anti-IGF-I receptor antibody could inhibit this response [8]. Administration of insulin increases Ang II level in VSMC as measured by radioimmunoassay and immunocytochemistry [9]. Insulin added to cultured

VSMC upregulates AT_1 receptors by posttranscriptional mechanisms, which are dependent on the stabilization of AT_1 receptor mRNA but not on AT_1 receptor gene transcription [10]. Further investigation in our laboratory examined the effects of insulin on RAS components in cultured EC. Insulin suppressed angiotensinogen and renin production in EC, however, high doses of insulin markedly stimulated ACE activity in these cells [11]. The findings may indicate that low and moderate levels of insulin attenuate RAS activity in the EC to prevent VSMC growth, but that high levels of insulin activate vascular cell growth by increasing ACE activity in EC. These data suggest that high level of insulin, that is, clinically hyperinsulinemic states, induce Ang II production and overexpression of AT_1 receptors in VSMC and upregulation of ACE in EC [11]. This insulin-mediated vascular tissue RAS activation may stimulate the progression of atherosclerosis and hypertension as commonly seen in patients with insulin resistance (Fig. 2).

Insulin resistance and hyperinsulinemia are due to both genetic and environmental (obesity, lack of exercise) influences. It is possible that Ang II itself may promote insulin resistance by inhibiting insulin signal transduction as studied in cultured VSMC. Folli et al. [12] have shown that Ang II addition to VSMC increased serine phosphorylation of the insulin receptor, inhibited insulin-stimulated tyrosine +phosphorylation of IRS-1, increased IRS-1 serine phosphorylation, and inhibited insulin stimulated docking between IRS-1 and PI3 kinase. The mechanism of this Ang II-mediated insulin resistance is postulated to be through the oxidative stress as Ang II is a potent activator of ROS products [13]. Thus, a high insulin state with insulin resistance may induce activation of tissue RAS and production of Ang II, which in turn promotes further progression of insulin resistance and leads to progression of atherosclerosis (Fig. 2).

4. Insulin resistance (hyperinsulinemia) accelerates the progression of atherosclerosis (pathway III)

Both insulin and IGF-I have growth promoting effects on cardiovascular cells [7,8]. In clinical studies, insulin resistance and hyperinsulinemia significantly correlate with the incidence of cardiovascular complications [14]. For example, our laboratory demonstrated

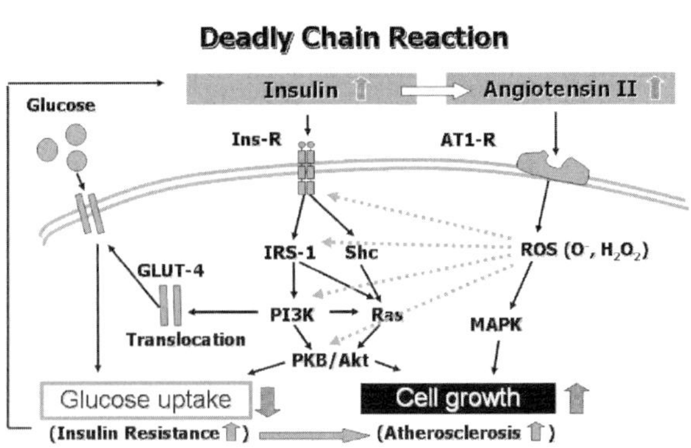

Fig. 2. Our proposed "Deadly Chain Reaction." Ins-R: insulin receptor, AT1-R: angiotensin II type 1 receptor, ROS: reactive oxygen species.

that the severity of left ventricular hypertrophy, thickening of intimal-medial complex, plaque score of the carotid artery, and the number of silent cerebral infarcts correlated with more severe insulin resistance or a lower M-value as determined by the hyperinsulinemic clamp [14,15].

5. Is there a deadly chain reaction in the metabolic syndrome? (Fig. 2)

All pathways for the interaction of the RAS, insulin resistance and hyperinsulinemia and atherosclerosis in vascular tissue are combined in Fig. 2. Initially high levels of insulin due both to genetic factors and obesity that cause insulin resistance induce RAS activation and Ang II production in vascular tissue. This upregulated Ang II produces ROS, which directly promote atherosclerosis, inhibit insulin signal transduction and accelerate insulin resistance. Insulin resistance and hyperinsulinemia further induce vascular hypertrophy and atherosclerosis by insulin's direct growth effect. We propose that this chain reaction plays a very important role in the progression of atherosclerotic cardiovascular disease in the metabolic syndrome. Thus, RAS blockade with ACEI and ARB agents should probably receive more widespread use for the prevention and regression of cardiovascular diseases in patients with the metabolic syndrome.

References

[1] A.V. Chobanian, et al., The seventh report of the joint national committee on prevention, detection, evaluation, and treatment of high blood pressure, J. Am. Med. Assoc. 289 (19) (2003) 2570–2572.

[2] 2003 European Society of Hypertension–European Society of Cardiology guidelines for the management of arterial hypertension, J. Hypertens. 21 (6) (2003) 1011–1053.

[3] S. Yusuf, et al., Effects of an angiotensin-converting-enzyme inhibitor, ramipril, on cardiovascular events in high-risk patients. The Heart Outcomes Prevention Evaluation Study Investigators, N. Engl. J. Med. 342 (3) (2000) 145–153.

[4] B. Dahlof, et al., Cardiovascular morbidity and mortality in the Losartan Intervention For Endpoint reduction in hypertension study (LIFE): a randomized trial against atenolol, Lancet 359 (9311) (2002) 995–1003.

[5] M.R. Weir, V.J. Dzau, The renin–angiotensin–aldosterone system: a specific target for hypertension management, Am. J. Hypertens. 12 (Pt. 3) (1999) 205S–213S.

[6] D.G. Harrison, et al., Interactions of angiotensin II with NAD(P)H oxidase, oxidant stress and cardiovascular disease, J. Renin. Angiotensin Aldosterone Syst. 4 (2) (2003) 51–61.

[7] K. Kamide, et al., Insulin-mediated growth in aortic smooth muscle and the vascular renin–angiotensin system, Hypertension 32 (3) (1998) 482–487.

[8] K. Kamide, et al., Insulin and insulin-like growth factor-I promotes angiotensinogen production and growth in vascular smooth muscle cells, J. Hypertens. 18 (8) (2000) 1051–1056.

[9] F. Villette-Bounoua, et al., Intracrine production of angiotensin II inhibited by insulin, (abstract), Am. J. Hypertens. 14 (Part 2) (2001) 19A.

[10] G. Nickenig, et al., Insulin induces upregulation of vascular AT_1 receptor gene expression by posttranscriptional mechanisms, Circulation 98 (22) (1998) 2453–2460.

[11] K. Kamide, et al., Insulin-mediated modulation of the endothelial renin–angiotensin system and vascular cell growth. J. Hypertens. (in press).

[12] F. Folli, et al., Angiotensin II inhibits insulin signaling in aortic smooth muscle cells at multiple levels. A potential role for serine phosphorylation in insulin/angiotensin II crosstalk, J. Clin. Invest. 100 (9) (1997) 2158–2169.

[13] C.D. Gardner, et al., Hydrogen peroxide inhibits insulin signaling in vascular smooth muscle cells, Exp. Biol. Med. 228 (7) (2003) 836–842.

[14] K. Kamide, et al., Insulin resistance and cardiovascular complications in patients with essential hypertension, Am. J. Hypertens 9 (12 Pt. 1) (1996) 1165–1171.

International Congress Series 1262 (2004) 466–469

www.ics-elsevier.com

Stroke risk factors: recent evidence and new aspects

M. Cubrilo-Turek*

Department of Internal Medicine, Sveti Duh General Hospital, Sveti duh 64, 10 000 Zagreb, Croatia

Abstract. Stroke is an acute medical emergency called "brain attack" representing a disease of the circulatory system, caused by the rupturing or the blockage of an artery. Recent data have shown that about 72–86% of strokes are ischemic, 9–18% are caused by hemorrhage while the rest are undefined. Stroke is one of the leading causes of death worldwide, representing a huge public health concern, because of its high morbidity and long-term disability. It is the third most common cause of death after cardiovascular disease and cancer. Trend of its death rate reduction is observed in many European countries, as well as in North America. This decrease is probably multifactorial. Risk factors for ischemic strokes are multiple and combined (age, hypertension, cigarette smoking, atrial fibrillation, hyperlipidemia, diabetes). Detection and more effective treatment of risk factors as well as improved acute medical care and improvement in diagnostic procedures may play an important role in its prevention. © 2004 Published by Elsevier B.V.

Keywords: Stroke; Risk factors

1. Stroke risk factors

A large number of risk factors for stroke are described, as a reflection of the heterogeneity of the disease. They can be classified as modifiable, potentially modifiable and nonmodifiable (Table 1) [2,3].

Nonmodifiable risk factors for stroke cannot be changed [2]:

- Age is the single most important and most powerful risk factor for stroke. Each 10 years after the age of 55, the stroke rate is more than double both for men and women. Risk of stroke increases with age.
- Gender: stroke is slightly more prevalent in men than in women.
- Race: African-Americans have a higher risk of stroke than Caucasians.
- Positive family history: previous stroke/TIA.

Potentially modifiable risk factors: obesity, physical inactivity, use of cocaine ("crack"), elevated blood cholesterol and lipids, sedentary lifestyle, migraine, use of oral contraceptives (high dose>50 μg).

* Tel.: +385-1-3712-235; fax: +385-1-3712-276.
E-mail address: mcubrilo@mef.hr (M. Cubrilo-Turek).

0531-5131/ © 2004 Published by Elsevier B.V.
doi:10.1016/j.ics.2003.12.036

Table 1
Major nonmodifiable and modifiable risk factors

Nonmodifiable risk factors	Modifiable risk factors
Age	Hypertension
Gender	Cigarette smoking
Ethnicity/race	Cardiac disease (atrial fibrillation, recent myocardial infarction)
Positive family history of stroke/TIA	Diabetes mellitus
	Excessive alcohol consumption
	Asymptomatic carotid stenosis

New tests for risk assessment: elevated homocysteine, high fibrinogen, protein C and S deficiency, C-Reactive Protein (CRP), antiphospholipids antibodies, plasminogen activator inhibitor, lipoprotein Lp(a), IL-6.

2. Hypertension

Hypertension is an important risk factor for stroke which contributes to 70% of all strokes. Hypertension is the strongest modifiable and independent risk factor for both ischemic and hemorrhagic stroke in middle and late age. The risk of stroke rises in proportion to blood pressure, for males as well as for females, and almost doubles for each 7.5 mm Hg increment in diastolic blood pressure (DBP). Isolated systolic hypertension considerably increases stroke risk among the elderly. The relationship between stroke and 'isolated' systolic hypertension in older age may be an even stronger risk factor than diastolic blood pressure. The recommendation and the target goal for general population is $<140/90$. In diabetic hypertensives the target is lower: $<130/85$. Choice of antihypertensive drugs should be individualized according to JNC VII guidelines [4].

3. Smoking

Smoking doubles the risk of stroke and increases both hemorrhagic and ischemic stroke risk. This is particularly important when smoking is combined with hypertension and/or diabetes: doubling a larger number. Smoking is an independent risk factor for ischemic stroke in men and women. The population attributable risk of smoking on stroke is about 15%, six-fold risk compared with nonsmokers. There is a clear-cut dose-response relation between the number of cigarettes smoked, and the risk of stroke. There is 50% risk reduction by quitting smoking.

4. Alcohol

Heavy alcohol consumption is clearly associated with an increased risk in stroke but this association is less clear for moderate and light doses. The relationship between alcohol and hemorrhagic stroke has been clearly demonstrated for heavy drinkers dose-dependently.

5. Asymptomatic carotid stenosis

Asymptomatic carotid stenosis is not really a primary etiologic risk factor, but rather a manifestation of atherosclerosis—"subclinical disease". About 5–10% of people over 65 years of age harbor asymptomatic stenoses >50%-higher with advancing age and in men [3]. While the risk of stroke is doubled with asymptomatic stenosis, the absolute rate of stroke remains relatively low—about 2% per year.

6. Atrial fibrillation

Atrial fibrillation (AF) is responsible for about 10% of ischemic strokes [1]. AF increases stroke risk five-fold. Absolute rate stroke in AF patients varies widely according to the risk stratification. Use of warfarin reduces stroke about 60%, and aspirin reduces stroke about 20%.

The criteria for classifying AF patients as high, low, or intermediate risk are relatively recent and evolving (Table 2).

7. Diabetes mellitus

Diabetes is a strong risk factor for ischemic stroke, probably because of accompanying risk factors, such as obesity, hypertension and lipid abnormalities [5]. About 15% of elderly adults have diabetes which is associated with a two to four-fold increased risk of stroke [1]. The population attributable risk for diabetes causing stroke is 15–20%. Strict control of hypertension (< 130/80 mm Hg, present in at least half of diabetics) is associated with large absolute reductions in stroke. The risk of stroke is increased in patients with diabetes, but there is still no evidence that treatment reduces its risk [1].

8. Hyperlipidemia

The role of hyperlipidemia in stroke risk is uncertain [1]. The lack of a strong relationship between elevation of serum cholesterol and stroke in epidemiologic studies contrasts sharply with its association with myocardial infarction [5]. Cholesterol levels below 180 mg/dl may be at risk for hemorrhagic stroke, particularly in hypertensive individuals. In a large meta-analysis of 45 prospective cohorts including 13,000 strokes, plasma total cholesterol levels were highly significantly associated with the risk of developing stroke, but only in the subset of individuals aged < 45 [6]. In contrast, no association was observed for older groups. Recent meta-analysis showed that statin therapy is associated with a 25% reduction of fatal and nonfatal stroke [7].

Table 2
Risk stratification in atrial fibrillation

High risk	Intermediate risk	Low risk
Age >75 years	Age 65 to 75 years	Age < 65 years
Hypertension	Diabetes	No risk factors
Left ventricular abn	Coronary disease	
>1 moderate risk factor		

9. Obesity

Obesity may increase the risk for both ischemic and hemorrhagic stroke independently of other risk factors because it often coexists with insulin resistance, diabetes, hypertension, and hyperlipidemia [3].

Recommendations for prevention stroke risks [8]:

- Hypertension: prevention (BP < 140/90 mm Hg)
- Smoking: cessation
- Diabetes: keep glucose < 126
- Atrial fibrillation: warfarin
- Cholesterol: statin if LDL < 3.36*, 2.59**
- Carotid stenosis: surgery if 70–99%
- Antiplatelet agents: if atherothrombotic
- Lifestyle changes: diet, exercise, alcohol.

*general population, ** diabetics.

European Stroke Initiative Mission has recommended the following: "To reduce the incidence and impact of stroke by changing the way stroke is viewed and treated" through:

- Public education
- Professional education
- Institutional change.

It is now a clear consensus that stroke is an emergency state which can be prevented by identifying the main risk factors and high-risk individuals. Screening and follow-up programs for more effective education about stroke risk factors, particularly targeting high-risk population remain imperative.

References

[1] Available at: http://www.eusi-stroke.com/recommendations/rc_prevention6.shtml. Accessed October 2003.

[2] R.L. Sacco, American Heart Association Prevention Conference IV: prevention and rehabilitation of stroke: risk factors, Stroke 28 (1997) 1507–1517.

[3] L.B. Goldstein, et al., Primary prevention of ischemic stroke. A statement for healthcare professionals from the stroke council of the American Heart Association, Stroke 32 (2001) 280–299.

[4] A.W. Chobaniann, et al., The seventh report of the joint national committee on prevention, detection, evaluation, and treatment of high blood pressure, JAMA 289 (2003) 2560–2572.

[5] R.T. Benson, R.L. Sacco, Stroke prevention: hypertension, diabetes, tobacco, and lipids, Neurol. Clin. 18 (2000) 309–319.

[6] Prospective Studies Collaboration, Cholesterol, diastolic blood pressure, and stroke: 13.000 strokes in 450.000 people in 45 prospective cohorts, Lancet 346 (1995) 1647–1653.

[7] S. Warshafsky, et al., Efficacy of 3-hydroxy-3-methylglutaryl coenzyme A reductase inhibitors for prevention of stroke, J. Gen. Intern. Med. 14 (1999) 763–774.

[8] AHA scientific statement, primary prevention of ischemic stroke, Circulation 103 (2001) 163–182.

International Congress Series 1262 (2004) 470–473

www.ics-elsevier.com

Stroke–blood pressure and blood pressure-lowering

Andrew Tonkin*

Department of Epidemiology and Preventive Medicine, NHMRC Centre of Research Excellence in Therapeutics, Monash University, Level 3, 553 St Kilda Road, Melbourne, VIC 3004, Australia

Abstract. There is a continuous relationship between blood pressure (BP) and risk of both first and recurrent stroke. Cardiovascular risk approximately doubles with each increment of 20/10 mm Hg, above 115/75 mm Hg. However, most strokes occur in those with "average" BP. In older trials, testing mainly beta-blockers and/or diuretics, lowering BP reduced stroke risk by about one third, within a few years. In more recent trials, ACE inhibitors and calcium antagonists showed similar effects but the more BP is lowered, the greater the stroke reduction. Benefits extend to isolated systolic hypertension in the elderly and the prevention of recurrent stroke. Lifestyle is important. Thiazide diuretics are often recommended as initial treatment, but comorbidities often influence the initial drug choice and most require two or more agents. © 2003 Published by Elsevier B.V.

Keywords: Stroke; Blood pressure; Anti-hypertensive therapy; Burden of disease

1. Burden of disease

1.1 Increased BP (usual SBP> 115 mm Hg) accounts for 4.4% of the global burden, higher than the burden imposed by tobacco, high cholesterol, increased BMI, low fruit/vegetable intake, and inactivity [1].

1.2 BP above 115 mm Hg is associated with 72% of the population attributable fraction related to stroke, the largest of risk factors [1].

2. Epidemiology

2.1 SBP and DBP are related in a continuous, approximate log linear fashion to relative risk of stroke, although the relationship is steeper for haemorrhagic than ischaemic stroke [2]. Increased BP is also related to the risk of recurrent stroke [3]. Because of "regression dilution bias", the strength of the relationship is approximately 60% stronger than in usual population studies [4]. It is estimated that a 5–6 mm Hg decrease in usual diastolic blood pressure is associated with about one third less stroke (and one fifth less coronary heart disease) [5].

* Tel.: +61-3-9903-0044; fax: +61-3-9903-0556.
E-mail address: Andrew.Tonkin@med.monash.edu.au (A. Tonkin).

0531-5131/
doi:10.1016/j.ics.2003.12.010

2.2 The relationship between BP and cardiovascular risk is stronger in males than females. The relative risk associated with increased BP decreases with increasing age but absolute risk increases, such that the BP–stroke relationship is more potent in the elderly [6].
2.3 There is an approximate normal distribution of BP in most populations. Associated with this, most strokes occur in those who have average or only mild increase in BP [7].
2.4 BP interacts with other risk factors such as cholesterol, smoking and increasing age in determining "absolute" cardiovascular risk.

3. Lifestyle and blood pressure levels

3.1 The usual BP increase with aging is not seen in all populations, specifically where lifestyle was characterised by very low salt intake, vegetables were staple and there was a low rate of overweight.
3.2 The DASH diet is rich in fruit, vegetables, whole grains, encourages low fat dairy products rather than saturated fats and poultry and fish rather than red meat. The diet decreased BP over 8 weeks by around 11.4/5.5 mm Hg in hypertensives (>140/90 mm Hg) and by 3.5/2.1 mm Hg in subjects without hypertension [8].
3.3 A more recent study has also examined additional effect of a low (Na) intake. At achieved daily Na intake of 143 mmol/dl (3.3 g), average intake, the DASH diet reduced systolic blood pressure by 5.9 mm Hg; at Na intake of 106 mmol/dl (2.4 g), the upper limit of guidelines, SBP was reduced by 5.0 mm Hg; at Na intake of 65 mmol/dl (1.8 g), possibly "optimal", SBP was reduced by only 2.2 mm Hg [9].
3.4 The PREMIER study [10] showed no additional reduction in BP with the DASH diet (4.3/2.6 mm Hg) above the reduction achieved with lifestyle changes (3.7/1.7 mm Hg). This may have been because fruit and vegetables needed to be purchased, "masking" of effects by BP changes relating to other lifestyle factors, or their "sub-additivity".

4. Anti-hypertensive drug treatment

4.1 Older randomised trials tested diuretics or beta-blockers and showed that a SBP difference of about 10–12 mm Hg and DBP difference of about 5–6 mm Hg was associated with a 39% (SE 4) reduction in the odds of stroke ($p < 0.001$) [5].
4.2 More recent trials have investigated newer anti-hypertensive agents, including ACE inhibitors, calcium antagonists and angiotensin receptor blockers. They showed similar benefits. Trials comparing newer agents have not conclusively shown superiority over older drugs.
4.3 Two recent large-scale trials [11,12] comparing newer agents with diuretic-based regimens yielded apparently conflicting results. The apparent differences in ALLHAT and ANBP-2 are perhaps most explicable by differences in the study cohorts and achieved BP changes. In ALLHAT, the achieved BP difference was 2.4 mm Hg greater for chlorthalidone than lisinopril (and 4 mm Hg greater among the 32% of the cohort who were African-Americans). Thus the greater benefit is probably explicable in terms of the greater BP reduction in ALLHAT in those with treatment based on a diuretic. In ALLHAT there was no difference in BP between treatment limbs based on ACE inhibitor (enalapril in most) and hydrochlorthiazide.

4.4 Recent trials have shown that more aggressive blood pressure lowering decreases stroke and other vascular endpoints. This suggests that BP lowering rather than intrinsic differences in agents is most important.

4.5 A meta-analysis of trials in isolated systolic hypertension in the elderly showed significant reduction in risk of fatal and non-fatal stroke and other major outcomes including all-cause mortality [13]. Diuretics are often recommended as first-line treatment in this context. A meta-analysis in subjects ≥ 80 years has shown a reduction of cardiovascular events but not in cardiovascular or all-cause mortality [14].

4.6 Blood pressure targets.

4.6.1 Most guidelines recommend a BP target of 140/90 mm Hg in the majority. Combination therapy is usually needed.

4.6.2 The target should be lower in those with diabetes and probably also in those with renal parenchymal disease or proteinuria.

4.6.3 Some guidelines recommend a diuretic as first-line therapy, while others give no particular recommendation. In practice, the initial choice is frequently influenced by other co-morbidities.

5. Acute stroke

5.1 Whether to lower BP in acute stroke is unclear. BP is increased in most early after ischaemic stroke but typically settles with bed rest.

5.2 Elevated BP predicts poor outcome but a low normal BP although uncommon, also independently predicts poor outcome. Randomised controlled trials are necessary in this context.

6. Secondary prevention of stroke

6.1 The PROGRESS study established the benefit of BP lowering therapy (based on perindopril but with indapamide also in most) in patients with previous stroke or transient ischaemic attack, both in individuals who were hypertensive and in those without hypertension[15].

7. The challenge of implementation

7.1 Surveys have consistently shown unacceptably low rates of recognition of hypertension and, low rates of treatment, including to target. Future initiatives must concentrate on measures to implement evidence-based and appropriate treatment.

References

[1] M. Ezzati, S.V. Hoorn, A. Rodgers, A.D. Lopez, C.D. Mathers, C.J. Murray, Group CRAC, Estimates of global and regional potential health gains from reducing multiple major risk factors, Lancet 362 (2003) 271–280.

[2] A. Rodgers, S. MacMahon, G. Gamble, J. Slattery, P. Sandercock, C. Warlow, Blood pressure and risk of

stroke in patients with cerebrovascular disease. The United Kingdom Transient Ischaemic Attack Collaborative Group, BMJ 313 (1996) 147.

[3] M. Alter, G. Friday, S. Lai, J. O'Connell, E. Sobel, Hypertension and risk of stroke recurrence, Stroke 25 (1994) 1605–1610.

[4] S. MacMahon, R. Peto, J. Cutler, R. Collins, P. Sorlie, J. Neaton, R. Abbott, J. Godwin, A. Dyer, J. Stamler, Blood pressure, stroke, and coronary heart disease: Part 1. Prolonged differences in blood pressure: prospective observational studies corrected for the regression dilution bias, [comment], Lancet 335 (1990) 765–774.

[5] R. Collins, S. MacMahon, Blood pressure, antihypertensive drug treatment and the risks of stroke and of coronary heart disease, British Medical Bulletin 50 (1994) 272–298.

[6] Collaboration PS, Age-specific relevance of usual blood pressure to vascular mortality: a meta-analysis of individual data for one million adults in 61 prospective studies, Lancet 360 (2002) 1903–1913.

[7] S. MacMahon, A. Rodgers, Blood pressure, antihypertensive treatment and stroke risk, Journal of Hypertension. Supplement 12 (1994) S5–S14.

[8] L.J. Appel, T.J. Moore, E. Obarzanek, W.M. Vollmer, L.P. Svetkey, F.M. Sacks, G.A. Bray, T.M. Vogt, J.A. Cutler, M.M. Windhauser, P.H. Lin, N. Karanja, A clinical trial of the effects of dietary patterns on blood pressure. DASH Collaborative Research Group, [comment], New England Journal of Medicine 336 (1997) 1117–1124.

[9] F. Sacks, L. Svetkey, W. Vollmer, L. Appel, G. Bray, D. Harsha, E. Obarzanek, P. Conlin, Er., P. Miller, D. Simons-Morton, N. Karanja, P. Lin, Effects on blood pressure of reduced dietary sodium and the Dietary Approaches to Stop Hypertension (DSH) diet. DASH-Sodium Collaborative Research Group, New England Journal of Medicine 344 (2001) 3–10.

[10] Writing group of the PREMIER collaborating research group, Effects of comprehensive lifestyle modification on blood pressure control. Main results of the PREMIER clinical trial, JAMA 289 (2003) 2083–2093.

[11] ALLHAT Officers and Coordinators for the ALLHAT Collaborative Research Group, Major outcomes in high-risk hypertensive patients randomized to angiotensin-converting enzyme inhibitor or calcium channel blocker vs diuretic: the antihypertensive and lipid-lowering treatment to prevent heart attack trial (ALLHAT), JAMA 288 (2002) 2981–2997.

[12] L.M. Wing, C.M. Reid, P. Ryan, L.J. Beilin, M.A. Brown, G.L. Jennings, C.I. Johnston, J.J. McNeil, G.J. Macdonald, J.E. Marley, T.O. Morgan, M.J. West, Second Australian National Blood Pressure Study G. A comparison of outcomes with angiotensin-converting-enzyme inhibitors and diuretics for hypertension in the elderly, [comment], New England Journal of Medicine 348 (2003) 583–592.

[13] J.A. Staessen, J. Gasowski, J.G. Wang, L. Thijs, E. Den Hond, J.P. Boissel, J. Coope, T. Ekbom, F. Gueyffier, L. Liu, K. Kerlikowske, S. Pocock, R.H. Fagard, Risks of untreated and treated isolated systolic hypertension in the elderly: meta-analysis of outcome trials, Lancet 355 (2000) 865–872.

[14] F. Gueyffier, C. Bulpitt, J. Boissel, E. Schron, T. Ekbom, R. Fagard, E. Casiglia, K. Kerlikowske, J. Coope, for the INDANA Group, Antihypertensive drugs in very old people: a subgroup meta-analysis of randomised controlled trials, Lancet 353 (1999) 793–796 (INNADA meta-analysis).

[15] PROGRESS Collaborative Group, Randomised trial of a perindopril-based blood pressure lowering regimen among 6,105 individuals with previous stroke or transient ischaemic attack, Lancet 358 (2001) 1033–1041.

International Congress Series 1262 (2004) 474–477

ELSEVIER

www.ics-elsevier.com

Carotid artery disease and risk of ischaemic stroke and coronary events

P.M. Rothwell*

Stroke Prevention Research Unit, Department of Clinical Neurology, University of Oxford, Radcliffe Infirmary, Woodstock Road, Oxford OX2 6HE, UK

Abstract. Carotid artery stiffness, intima-media thickness and early plaque formation are useful predictors of the risk of both ischaemic stroke and coronary heart disease in asymptomatic populations. Early carotid arterial wall disease also predicts coronary artery disease on angiography and subsequent coronary vascular events in populations at risk of coronary heart disease. Carotid stenosis and plaque surface morphology predict both ischaemic stroke and coronary vascular events.

Keywords: Carotid artery stenosis; Intima-media thickness; Ulceration; Atherosclerosis; Stroke

Studies of the prognostic value of carotid artery disease can be divided into studies of early disease (increased carotid wall stiffness, intima-media thickness and early plaque formation) and studies of advanced disease (stenosing or complex plaques).

1. Carotid stiffness, intima-media thickness and early plaque formation

Middle-aged individuals often have evidence of early carotid artery disease, i.e. increased wall stiffness and intima-media thickness (IMT), or early plaque formation [1–3]. The arterial wall undergoes structural changes with increasing age with a decrease in elasticity and an increase in collagen and calcification [4]. This increased wall "stiffness" leads to a rise in pulse pressure and is an independent predictor of stroke [4,5]. Increased carotid IMT and atheromatous plaque may also develop [6–8], both of which are associated with an increased risk of ischaemic stroke [9] and coronary heart disease [1–3]. There is some evidence that increased IMT and early carotid plaque differ in their pathological significance [7], but since the majority of strokes are not caused by carotid disease, the associations with stroke risk are unlikely to be causal.

* Tel.: +44-1865-224237; fax: +44-1865-790493.
E-mail address: peter.rothwell@clneuro.ox.ac.uk (P.M. Rothwell).

0531-5131/ © 2004 Published by Elsevier B.V.
doi:10.1016/j.ics.2003.12.062

2. Carotid stenosis

Although plaque rupture is the main cause of acute vascular events in both the carotid and coronary circulations [10–13], it is mostly associated with severe stenosis in the carotid arteries [10] but often with only mild or moderate stenosis in the coronary arteries [11]. The risk of stroke on medical treatment increases with the severity of the carotid stenosis in symptomatic and asymptomatic individuals [10,14,15], whereas the "background" risk of stroke following successful carotid endarterectomy is unrelated to the degree of carotid stenosis [10,16]. Interestingly, however, the risk of stroke falls very rapidly with time since the last symptomatic ischaemic event and after 2 years is no longer clearly related to the degree of stenosis [16,17], due possibly to "healing" of unstable plaques, the development of collateral circulation, or a censoring artefact in analyses of time to first stroke. Noninvasive measurements of carotid stenosis have also been shown to predict severe coronary artery disease in cohort studies of patients with suspected ischaemic heart disease [18–20] and to predict future coronary vascular events in patients known to have coronary artery disease [21].

3. Carotid plaque surface morphology

The concept derived from coronary artery studies of the stable plaque with a relatively thick fibrous cap versus the unstable plaque with a thin or ruptured cap [11,22] is important in understanding carotid artery disease [23]. Although cerebral infarction may result from the reduction in cerebral perfusion pressure distal to a tight carotid stenosis [24,25], there is evidence that thromboembolism is important [26–29]. Angiographic studies have also shown that patients with irregular or ulcerated carotid plaques have a higher risk of stroke on medical treatment than those with smooth plaques [10,30] and Doppler ultrasound plaque surface morphology may also predict stroke [31]. Carotid plaque surface morphology also predicts the risk of coronary vascular events independently of the degree of carotid stenosis and traditional vascular risk factors, suggesting that other systemic factors determine plaque stability [32].

4. Carotid plaque composition

Lipid rich plaques with a thin cap are associated with instability and rupture [11,12], and are echolucent on carotid ultrasound [33]. Symptomatic plaques are more frequently echolucent than asymptomatic plaques, and echolucent plaques are more frequently associated with surface ulceration [34] and cerebral infarction at baseline [35] than echogenic plaques, but they are not associated with a higher frequency of microemboli [36], and there is only limited evidence that they predict future ischaemic stroke [23]. Intra-plaque haemorrhage, which can be detected on magnetic resonance imaging in vivo [37], is present in a high proportion of carotid plaques but is not clearly associated with plaque instability [23].

5. Other risk factors for ischaemic stroke in patients with carotid stenosis

The predictive value of assessments of carotid artery disease should be studied in the context of other risk factors for ischaemic stroke. Table 1 shows a model for the prediction

Table 1
A Cox's proportional hazards model for the risk of ipsilateral carotid territory major ischaemic stroke (i.e. fatal or lasting longer than 7 days) on medical treatment derived on 1208 patients with 0–99% stenosis in the medical group of the European Carotid Surgery Trial [38]

	Wald statistic[a]	*P*	Hazard ratio	95% CI
Significant terms				
Cerebral events vs. ocular events	7.1	0.008	2.45	1.27–4.75
Residual neurological signs after 7 days	7.4	0.006	1.30	1.08–1.57
Diabetes	7.5	0.007	1.82	1.18–2.80
Any ischaemic event within last 2 months	9.0	0.003	1.71	1.20–2.44
Number of events within last 3 months (per event)	6.6	0.01	1.02	1.01–1.03
Previous myocardial infarction	5.1	0.02	1.31	1.04–1.65
Degree of carotid stenosis (cubic term)[b]	28.9	0.0000	1.34	1.22–1.52
Plaque surface irregularity	6.5	0.01	1.80	1.14–2.83
Post-stenotic collapse of the internal carotid artery	4.5	0.03	0.40	0.17–0.94
Nonsignificant terms				
Age (per year)	0.3	0.62	1.01	0.98–1.03
Male sex	1.0	0.31	1.23	0.83–1.82
Systolic blood pressure (per 10 mm Hg)	0.1	0.82	1.05	0.90–1.15
Diastolic blood pressure (per 10 mm Hg)	0.3	0.61	1.10	0.80–1.30
Peripheral vascular disease	0.0	0.90	1.03	0.65–1.63
Angina without previous myocardial infarction	0.1	0.77	0.96	0.71–1.29
ECG signs of left ventricular hypertrophy	0.0	0.90	1.07	0.40–2.10
Cerebral infarction on symptomatic side on CT brain scan[c]	1.8	0.18	1.32	0.88–1.96
Occlusion of the contralateral internal carotid artery	0.0	0.96	1.00	0.72–1.63

[a] Degrees of freedom for all variables = 1.

[b] Cubic term used in the model shown. For the purpose of illustration, the hazard ratio and confidence interval given in the table refers to the increase in risk for 80% stenosis vs. 70% stenosis.

[c] This term is a significant predictor if residual neurological signs after seven days is omitted from the model: Wald statistic = 5.9, $P = 0.03$, hazard ratio = 1.54, 95% CI = 1.03–2.12.

of ischaemic stroke on medical treatment in patients with carotid stenosis [38]. Both degree of carotid stenosis and plaque surface morphology are independent predictors, but several other factors are equally important. Other assessments, not included in this model, such as transcranial Doppler ultrasound (TCD) detection of microemboli, are also likely to improve prediction [29,39,40]. Microemboli decrease with time after an ischaemic event [29], and are associated with carotid plaque surface thrombus [40], as well as reduced considerably by endarterectomy [39]. Reduction of cerebral perfusion reserve also predicts stroke in patients with carotid occlusion [24,25,41] and may be useful in patients with carotid stenosis. Interestingly, stroke risk only appears to be increased in patients with bilateral severe carotid stenosis who have relatively low systolic blood pressure [42], suggesting that low cerebral perfusion pressure is responsible for some strokes in these patients.

References

[1] L.E. Chambless, et al., Am. J. Epidemiol. 146 (1997) 483–494.
[2] D.H. O'Leary, et al., N. Engl. J. Med. 340 (1999) 14–22.
[3] R. Salonen, et al., Arterioscler. Thromb. 14 (1994) 1631–1640.

[4] M.E. Safar, et al., Stroke 31 (2000) 782–790.
[5] M.J. Domanski, et al., Hypertension 34 (1999) 375–380.
[6] D.H. O'Leary, et al., Stroke 23 (1992) 1752–1760.
[7] S. Ebrahim, et al., Stroke 30 (1999) 841–850.
[8] M.L. Bots, et al., Circulation 96 (1997) 1432–1437.
[9] L.E. Chambless, et al., Am. J. Epidemiol. 151 (2000) 478–487.
[10] P.M. Rothwell, et al., Stroke 31 (2000) 615–621.
[11] V. Fuster, et al., N. Engl. J. Med. 326 (1992) 242–250.
[12] M.J.G. Harrison, et al., Br. Med. J. 1 (1976) 205–207.
[13] B.L. Thiele, et al., Neurology 30 (1980) 1041–1046.
[14] P.M. Rothwell, et al., Lancet 345 (1995) 209–212.
[15] B.R. Chambers, N.W. Norris, N. Engl. J. Med 315 (1986) 860–865.
[16] European Carotid Surgery Trialists' Collaborative Group, Randomised trial of endarterectomy for recently symptomatic carotid stenosis: final results of the MRC European Carotid Surgery Trial (ECST), Lancet 351 (1998) 1379–1387.
[17] North American Symptomatic Carotid Endarterectomy Trialists' Collaborative Group, N. Engl. J. Med. 339 (1998) 1415–1425.
[18] I. Kallikazaros, et al., Stroke 30 (1999) 1002–1007.
[19] P. Giral, et al., Am. J. Cardiol. 84 (1999) 14–17.
[20] J. Nowak, et al., Stroke 29 (1998) 439–446.
[21] H.N. Hodis, et al., Ann. Intern. Med. 128 (1998) 262–269.
[22] R.D. Safian, et al., Circulation 82 (1990) 69–79.
[23] J. Golledge, et al., Stroke 31 (2000) 774–781.
[24] W.J. Powers, Ann. Neurol. 29 (1991) 231–240.
[25] R.L. Grubb, et al., JAMA 280 (1998) 1055–1060.
[26] C.M. Fisher, Neurology 9 (1959) 333–347.
[27] M. Siebler, et al., Neurology 44 (1994) 615–618.
[28] M.J.G. Harrison, et al., Br. J. Surg. 64 (1977) 511–512.
[29] A.M. Forteza, et al., Stroke 27 (1996) 687–690.
[30] M. Eliasziw, et al., Stroke 25 (1994) 304–308.
[31] N. Handa, Stroke 26 (1995) 1781–1786.
[32] P.M. Rothwell, et al., Lancet 355 (2000) 19–24.
[33] M.L.M. Gronholt, Arterioscler. Thromb. Vasc. Biol. 19 (1999) 2–13.
[34] J. Golledge, et al., Br. J. Surg. 84 (1997) 1697–1701.
[35] G.M. Biasi, et al., Eur. J. Vasc. Endovasc. Surg. 17 (1999) 476–479.
[36] D.W. Droste, et al., J. Neurol. Neurosurg. Psychiatry 67 (1999) 525–528.
[37] A.R. Moody, et al., Lancet 353 (1999) 122–123.
[38] P.M. Rothwell, et al., Lancet 353 (1999) 2105–2110.
[39] M. Siebler, et al., Brain 116 (1993) 1005–1015.
[40] M. Sitzer, et al., Stroke 26 (1995) 1231–1233.
[41] R.L. Grubb, et al., JAMA 280 (1998) 1055–1060.
[42] P.M. Rothwell, et al., Stroke 34 (2003) 2583–2590.

ELSEVIER

International Congress Series 1262 (2004) 478–481

www.ics-elsevier.com

Remnant lipoprotein and lipoprotein (a) as risk factors for stroke and carotid disease

Shinichiro Uchiyama*, Masako Yamazaki, Makoto Iwata

Department of Neurology, Neurological Institute, Tokyo Women's Medical University School of Medicine, 8-1 Kawada-cho, Shinjuku, Tokyo 162-8666, Japan

Abstract. Remnant lipoprotein (RLP) and lipoprotein (Lp) (a) are known to promote atherosclerosis and thrombosis. We studied whether these lipoproteins can be risk factors for stroke and carotid disease in 170 consecutive subjects (87 males and 83 females, mean age of 70 years). RLP was significantly higher in patients with ($N=45$) than without ($N=125$) ischemic stroke (Mann–Whitney's U-test, $p=0.01$), while there was no difference in Lp (a) between patients with and without it ($p=0.83$). In contrast, there was a significant difference in Lp (a) ($p=0.003$) but not in RLP ($p=0.26$) between patients with ($N=76$) and without ($N=94$) maximum intima-media thickness (IMT) of 2.0 mm or more at carotid bifurcations. Logistic regression analysis showed that RLP is an independent risk factor for ischemic stroke [7.5 mg/dl or more, relative risk (RR) 2.84, 95% confidence interval (CI) 1.26–6.40]. Multivariate regression analysis showed that Lp (a) ($p=0.032$) but not RLP ($p=0.518$) is significantly correlated with IMT. The results indicate that RLP but not Lp (a) is an independent risk factor for ischemic stroke, while Lp (a) but not RLP is an independent risk factor for carotid disease in our Japanese subjects.

Keywords: Remnant lipoprotein; Lipoprotein (a); Stroke; Carotid disease; Risk factor

1. Introduction

LP (a) and RLP are known to promote atherosclerosis and thrombosis [1]. Molecular structure of Lp (a) is similar to that of plasminogen, which may produce antifibrinolytic effects and effects on vascular smooth muscle proliferation. Many retrospective studies have reported increased Lp (a) in patients with ischemic stroke or carotid disease, although it has not yet been proven by any large prospective study that Lp (a) can be a risk factor for stroke. RLP is known to have a potent atherogenetic effect, and a quantitative assay for chylomicron remnant and VLDL remnant has recently been developed in Japan [2]. We studied whether or not these lipoproteins can be risk factors for stroke and carotid disease in 170 outpatients.

* Corresponding author. Tel.: +81-3-3353-8111; fax: +81-3-5269-7324.
E-mail address: suchiyam@nij.twmu.ac.jp (S. Uchiyama).

0531-5131/
doi:10.1016/j.ics.2003.12.042

2. Subjects and methods

Subjects studied were 170 consecutive patients (87 males and 83 females, mean age of 70 years) suspected of or concerned about stroke or transient ischemic attack (TIA) except those with atrial fibrillation or thrombophilia. We prospectively conducted brain magnetic resonance imaging (MRI) as well as carotid ultrasonography, and determined lipoprotein fractions, triglyceride, RLP, Lp (a), blood glucose, hemoglobin (Hb) A1c, fibrinogen, and hematocrit. We also investigated history and treatment of stroke, hypertension, diabetes mellitus, hyperlipidemia, cigarette smoking, and coronary heart disease. Symptomatic cerebral infarction was diagnosed when stroke or TIA was associated with responsible cerebral infarction confirmed by 1.5 T MRI on both T1 and T2 weighted images. IMT was determined as maximum IMT at both carotid bifurcations including common carotid arteries, carotid bulbs, and internal carotid arteries using duplex ultrasonography with 7.5 MHz probe.

3. Results

RLP was significantly higher in patients with ($N=45$) than without ($N=125$) cerebral infarction with stroke episodes (Mann–Whitney's U test, $p=0.01$), while there was no difference in Lp (a) between patients with and without symptomatic cerebral infarction ($p=0.83$) (Fig. 1). In contrast, there was a significant difference in Lp (a) ($p=0.003$) but not in RLP ($p=0.26$) between patients with ($N=76$) and without ($N=94$) maximum intima-media thickness (IMT) of 2.0 mm or more at carotid bifurcations (Fig. 2). Multiple logistic regression analysis showed that RLP is an independent risk factor for symptomatic cerebral infarction [7.5 mg/dl or more, relative risk (RR) 2.84, 95% confidence interval

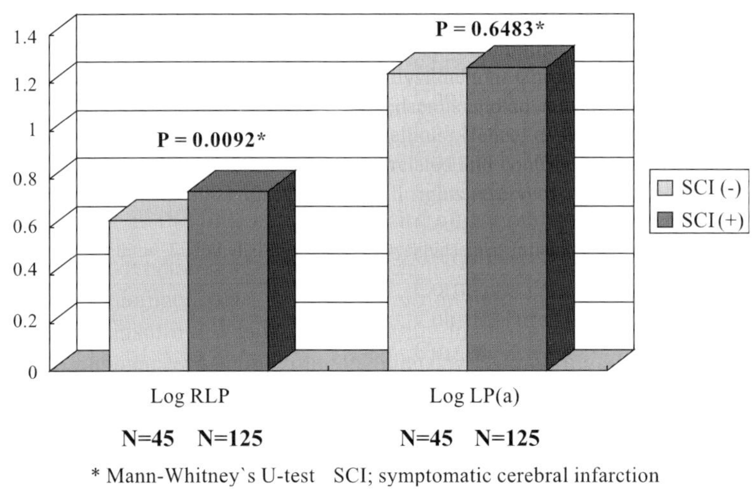

Fig. 1. RLP and Lp(a) in patients with and without symptomatic cerebral infarction. RLP was significantly higher in patients with and without symptomatic cerebral infarction, while there was no significant difference in Lp(a) between patients with than without symptomatic cerebral infarction.

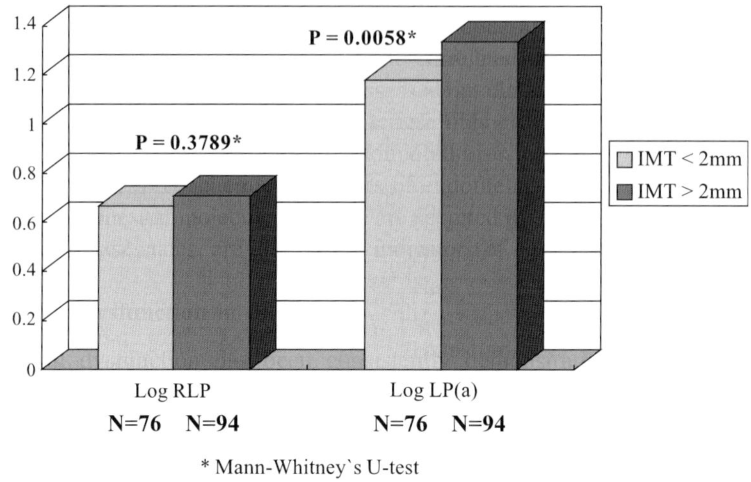

Fig. 2. Remnant lipoprotein (RLP) and lipoprotein (Lp)(a) in patients with maximum thickness (Max-IMT) <2 and ≥2 mm. There was no significant difference in RLP between patients with Max-IMT of 2 mm or more and Max-IMT of less than 2 mm at carotid bifurcation while Lp(a) was significantly higher in patients with Max-IMT of 2 mm or more than those with that of less than 2 mm.

(CI) 1.26–6.40]. Multivariate regression analysis showed that Lp (a) ($p=0.032$) but not RLP ($p=0.518$) is significantly correlated with IMT.

4. Discussion

Though many previous retrospective studies have reported increased Lp (a) in patients with ischemic stroke [1], the result of our study did not show any significant difference in Lp (a) levels between patients with and without symptomatic cerebral infarction. This difference might be due to the difference in included patients with subtypes of ischemic stroke. Majority of our patients with symptomatic cerebral infarction had small subcortical infarction. Cerrato et al. [3] has reported higher lipoprotein (a) levels in atherothrombotic than lacunar stroke. Future prospective studies should investigate correlation of Lp (a) not only with total ischemic stroke but also with specific subtypes of ischemic stroke.

Lp (a) levels were significantly higher in patients with than without carotid plaque with maximum IMT of 2.0 mm or more in our study. Our study also showed a significant correlation of Lp (a) levels with carotid maximum IMTs. When taken together with the results in the previous studies, our result indicates that Lp (a) is a potential risk factor for carotid atherosclerosis. Despite the positive correlation of RLP with symptomatic cerebral infarction, we could not demonstrate any significant correlation of RLP with carotid plaque. Iwamoto et al. [4] have also reported that there was no correlation of RLP with carotid plaque. This discrepancy raises the possibility that RLP can be a risk factor for ischemic stroke separately from carotid atherosclerosis. Our results suggest that RLP can be a risk factor for lacunar stroke but not for atherothrombotic stroke. It remains unclear why RLP can be a risk factor for small artery lacunar stroke. Some possible mechanisms might involve that RLP induces platelet aggregation [5,6] and impairs endothelial function [7,8].

In conclusion, the results of our study indicate that RLP but not Lp (a) is an independent risk factor for symptomatic cerebral infarction (exclusively small subcortical infarction), while Lp (a) but not RLP is an independent risk factor for carotid disease in our series of Japanese patients.

References

[1] S. Uchiyama, Rinsho Shinkeigaku 42 (2002) 1064–1068.
[2] K. Nakajima, et al., Clin. Chim. Acta 223 (1993) 53–71.
[3] P. Cerrato, et al., Neurology 9 (2002) 127–132.
[4] T. Iwamoto, et al., Jpn. J. Stroke 18 (1996) 209–216.
[5] R. Knofler, et al., Thromb. Res. 78 (1995) 161–171.
[6] A.R. Saniabadi, et al., Thromb. Haemost. 77 (1997) 996–1001.
[7] H. Doi, et al., Arterioscler. Thromb. Vasc. Biol., (1999) 1918–1924.
[8] H. Doi, et al., Circulation 102 (2000) 670–676.

International Congress Series 1262 (2004) 482–485

www.ics-elsevier.com

Genetic risk factors for stroke: insights into pathophysiology from candidate gene approaches

Steve E. Humphries*, Laleh Morgan[1]

Cardiovascular Genetics, BHF Laboratories, Department of Medicine, Royal Free and University College London, 5 University Street, London WC1E 6JF, UK

Abstract. Ischaemic stroke and haemorrhagic stroke are believed to result from both shared and different determinants, and thus the genetic variants that influence these clinical endpoints are likely to differ. Studies involving twins, siblings, and families have detected significant evidence for heritability, but to date, the identification of the genes involved is unclear. Study of the genetic determinants of some of the underlying traits known to contribute to risk of stroke may be fruitful. Of these, carotid Intimal–Medial wall Thickness (IMT) is particularly relevant, since it is a surrogate measure of subclinical atherosclerosis and is a strong predictor of future stroke. Some studies have reported that IMT is higher among subjects carrying functional variants in genes related to matrix deposition (stromelysin-1), inflammation (interleukin-6), and lipid metabolism (hepatic lipase, ApoE, CETP, and PON1). The published data will be reviewed to determine the robustness of these associations.

Keywords: Genetics; Stroke

1. Introduction

A stroke is a permanent neurological deficit caused by inadequate perfusion of a region of the brain. Fifteen percent of strokes is caused by haemorrhage. The majority, however, are ischaemic in origin, mainly due to arterial occlusion. There is evidence to suggest important interplays between levels of modifiable risk factors and genetic susceptibility to stroke. Studies involving twins and families have detected significant evidence for heritability [1], indicating that genetic determinants are important, but their identification is unclear. Study of the genetics of some of the underlying traits known to contribute to risk of stroke may be fruitful. Of these, carotid Intimal–Medial wall Thickness (IMT) is particularly relevant, since it is a surrogate measure of subclinical

* Corresponding author. [1]The Victor Horsley Department of Neurosurgery, The National Hospital for Neurology and Neurosurgery, Queen Square, London WC1N 4BG, UK. Tel.: +44-20-7679-6962; fax: +44-20-7679-6912.

E-mail address: rmhaseh@ucl.ac.uk (S.E. Humphries).

doi:10.1016/j.ics.2003.12.024

atherosclerosis and is a strong predictor of future stroke. IMT is measured by ultrasonography and a recent study shows that IMT is a good predictor of stroke in older adults [2]. Studies have identified a number of functional variants in genes coding for proteins likely to be involved in the pathophysiology of intimal medial thickening, and several studies examining their impact on IMT have been published. The results are discussed below.

2. Stromelysin-1

Stromelysin-1 is a matrix metalloproteinase that regulates the extracellular matrix during tissue injury, and thus the growth of the atherosclerotic plaque. There is a common variant in the promoter sequence of its gene, 600 bp upstream from the start of transcription in which one allele has a run of six adenosines (6A) while the other has only five (5A). In vitro studies showed that the 5A allele expressed higher activity than the 6A allele in cells. Thus, individuals homozygous for the 6A allele may have lower stromelysin levels in their arterial walls and this might favour extracellular matrix deposition. The stromelysin genotype was studied in a pilot study of 109 randomly selected middle-aged men without exercise-induced ischaemia [3]. The 6A allele was significantly ($p = 0.033$) associated with higher IMT. The 6A6A genotype was also associated with higher carotid IMT in Finnish men [4]. This suggests that (6A carriers) have increased carotid artery wall thickness and may be at greater risk of stroke.

3. Interleukin-6 (IL-6)

IL-6 is a 28-kDa cytokine derived from diverse tissues including fibroblasts, monocytes, and endothelial cells. It plays a key role in the acute inflammatory response and may thus be pivotal in the pathogenesis of vascular disease including IMT. There are three common variants in the IL-6 gene promoter, of which − 174G>C has been most widely studied. The − 174 G allele at basal levels and after stimulation has the highest IL-6 levels in HeLa cells. In the pilot study described above (Section 2) [3], the IL-6 polymorphism was also significantly associated ($p = 0.036$) with IMT. Men homozygous for the G allele had an IMT that was 11% greater than men homozygous for the C allele [3]. This strongly confirms the association between the GG genotype and higher carotid IMT reported in Finnish men, where IMT was roughly 11% higher in this group compared with those with the CC genotype [4].

4. Hepatic lipase (HL)

HL has a gene in which there are a number of promoter polymorphisms of which the C>T variation at − 480 results in low HL activity and higher HDL levels. High HL activity is associated with an increase in small, dense LDL particles, and increased risk of development of atherosclerosis and vascular events. In the pilot study described above (Section 2) [3], subjects with the HL genotype CC had 13% greater IMT ($p = 0.02$) than the other genotypes combined [3]. To date, these associations have not been confirmed in a second study.

5. Apolipoprotein E (APOE)

APOE gene has a variation that creates the E2, E3, and E4 isoforms. These are important predictors of plasma lipid levels, and have a consistent effect on coronary artery disease (CAD) risk. Several studies have examined this gene with respect to IMT, with some studies showing an association (e.g., Ref. [5]) and others failing to find an effect (e.g., Ref. [6]).

6. Angiotensin-converting enzyme (ACE) gene

ACE gene has an insertion (I)/deletion (D) polymorphism, which has been associated with risk of myocardial infarction (MI). The D allele is associated with higher ACE levels than the I allele. Several studies have examined this gene with respect to IMT, with some studies showing an association (e.g., Ref. [7]) and others failing to find an effect (e.g., Ref. [8]).

7. Paraoxonase (PON1)

PON1 is a 45-kDa glycoprotein that prevents the oxidation of LDL. PON1 knockout mice have higher levels of oxidised LDL and are more susceptible to atherosclerosis. Two common variants within the coding region of the PON1 gene have been reported: L55M (freq 0.37) and Q192R (freq 0.32). Both rare variants are associated with increased risk of CAD. There are inconsistencies in the literature concerning their risk association, which may reflect the small case–control studies that have been used. There have been studies of PON1 with respect to IMT, with some showing an association (e.g., Ref. [9]) and others failing to find an effect (e.g., Ref. [10]).

8. Cholesteryl ester transfer protein (CETP)

CETP is a plasma component important in the metabolism of HDL cholesterol. The protective role of HDL cholesterol against atherosclerosis is well established. Studies have reported an inverse relationship between HDL plasma concentration and CETP activity. A number of polymorphisms in the human CETP gene have been studied, in particular a common variable *Taq*I site (TaqIB), which has been shown to be a silent base change affecting the 277th nucleotide in the first intron of the CETP gene. To date, only one study has examined these CETP polymorphisms with respect to IMT, with a strong association being reported [11].

9. Conclusions

Clearly, we still have a lot of work to do to be able to tease out the genetic factors involved in stroke risk in the population. For the ACE, APOE, and PON genes, where inconsistent associations have been reported, larger studies are required. For HL and CETP, the single reports to date also require further confirmation. For both the stromelysin-1 and IL-6 genotypes, the effects appear consistent in two studies, but further studies are required. It should, however, be possible to include confirmed genetic markers (or specific gene–environment combinations) in risk algorithms. Such has been prepared by Wilson [12] by using essentially nongenetic factors to advise healthy subjects on how best to avoid CAD. If successful, this would give us the ability to give genotype-specific lifestyle advice, or to tailor clinical and therapeutic decisions to an individual's genotype. The use of genetic markers may help identify people at increased stroke risk who require earlier and more aggressive control of other modifiable risk factors (e.g., to diminish the deleterious effects of IL-6 on the cardiovascular system without compromising its beneficial role in innate immune response).

Acknowledgements

The authors were supported by a grant from the British Heart Foundation (RG2000015), and thank colleagues in the CVG group for intellectual input.

References

[1] S. Bak, et al., Genetic liability in stroke: a long-term follow-up study of Danish twins, Stroke 33 (3) (2002) 769–774.
[2] D.H. O'Leary, et al., Carotid-artery intima and media thickness as a risk factor for myocardial infarction and stroke in older adults. Cardiovascular Health Study Collaborative Research Group, N. Engl. J. Med. 340 (1) (1999) 14–22.
[3] T. Rundek, et al., Carotid intima–media thickness is associated with allelic variants of stromelysin-1, interleukin-6, and hepatic lipase genes: the Northern Manhattan Prospective Cohort Study, Stroke 33 (5) (2002) 1420–1423.
[4] R. Rauramaa, et al., Stromelysin-1 and interleukin-6 gene promoter polymorphisms are determinants of asymptomatic carotid artery atherosclerosis, Arterioscler Thromb Vasc. Biol. 20 (12) (2000) 2657–2662.
[5] J.G. Terry, et al., Apolipoprotein E polymorphism is associated with segment-specific extracranial carotid artery intima–media thickening, Stroke 27 (10) (1996) 1755–1759.
[6] C. Sass, et al., Apolipoprotein E4, lipoprotein lipase C447 and angiotensin-I converting enzyme deletion alleles were not associated with increased wall thickness of carotid and femoral arteries in healthy subjects from the Stanislas cohort, Atherosclerosis 140 (1) (1998) 89–95.
[7] M. Hosoi, et al., Angiotensin-converting enzyme gene polymorphism is associated with carotid arterial wall thickness in non-insulin-dependent diabetic patients, Circulation 94 (4) (1996) 704–707.
[8] J. Hung, et al., Angiotensin-converting enzyme gene polymorphism and carotid wall thickening in a community population, Arterioscler Thromb Vasc. Biol. 19 (8) (1999) 1969–1974.
[9] F.R. Leus, et al., Paraoxonase gene polymorphisms are associated with carotid arterial wall thickness in subjects with familial hypercholesterolemia, Atherosclerosis 149 (2) (2000) 371–377.
[10] H. Cao, et al., Lack of association between carotid intima–media thickness and paraoxonase gene polymorphism in non-insulin dependent diabetes mellitus, Atherosclerosis 138 (2) (1998) 361–366.
[11] S. Kakko, et al., Cholesteryl ester transfer protein gene polymorphisms are associated with carotid atherosclerosis in men, Eur. J. Clin. Invest. 30 (1) (2000) 18–25.
[12] P.W. Wilson, et al., Prediction of coronary heart disease using risk factor categories, Circulation 97 (18) (1998) 1837–1847.

International Congress Series 1262 (2004) 486–489

www.ics-elsevier.com

Matrix, matrix metalloproteinases and smooth muscle cell function in atherosclerosis

Michelle P. Bendeck*, Guangpei Hou, Jennifer Chen, Sara Nejat, Eser Adiguzel

Department of Laboratory Medicine and Pathobiology, University of Toronto, Medical Sciences Building, 1 King's College Circle, Rm. 6217, Toronto, ON, Canada M5S 1A8

Abstract. Collagens in the extracellular matrix play important roles modulating the vascular response to injury during the progression of atherosclerosis and restenosis. Collagen can regulate smooth muscle cell (SMC) proliferation, and SMC and macrophage migration and proteinase production. The discoidin domain receptors, DDR1 and DDR2, are novel transmembrane collagen receptors with tyrosine kinase activity, and signal to upregulate matrix metalloproteinase (MMP) expression. Research in our laboratory has been focused on the expression and functions of DDR1 in the cardiovascular system. DDR1 expression is increased following vascular injury. We have shown that DDR1 −/− SMCs have a reduced capacity to proliferate and migrate, and have reduced MMP expression compared with DDR1+/+ cells. We injured the carotid arteries of DDR1 −/− mice and found a dramatic reduction in neointimal thickening. These studies suggest that DDR1 plays a role in arterial wound repair and helps to elucidate the roles of collagen and the DDRs in atherosclerosis and restenosis.

Keywords: Collagen; Matrix metalloproteinase; Atherosclerosis; Smooth muscle cell; Discoidin domain receptor

1. Introduction

Collagens are major matrix constituents in blood vessels. Furthermore, new and exciting research shows that they function as signaling molecules, triggering cellular responses such as migration, proliferation and matrix metalloproteinase (MMP) production in arterial disease [1–4]. Receptors for collagen include integrin receptors and a newly discovered family of receptors the discoidin domain receptors [5]. The DDRs (DDR1 and 2) contain an extracellular discoidin domain, and are the first tyrosine kinase receptors which bind to matrix [6]. Targeted deletion of DDR1 in mice resulted in dwarfism and severe defects in blastocyst implantation and mammary gland development [7], while DDR2-null mice also exhibited dwarfism, skeletal malformation and delayed wound

* Corresponding author. Tel.: +1-416-946-7133; fax: +1-416-978-5959.
E-mail address: michelle.bendeck@utoronto.ca (M.P. Bendeck).

0531-5131/
doi:10.1016/j.ics.2003.12.021

healing [8]. DDR1 upregulates MMP-1 expression in a fibrosarcoma cell line [5], and was required for macrophage invasion of collagen gels, another MMP dependant process [9]. DDR2 positively regulates cell proliferation, migration, MMP-2 expression, and collagen synthesis in fibroblasts and hepatic stellate cells [10–12]. Because the DDRs are important mediators of MMP production and collagen synthesis, we have postulated that they function as collagen sensors, an essential part of the cellular machinery that triggers ECM degradation and renewal in atherosclerosis.

2. Results

We have accumulated substantial evidence supporting a role for DDR1 in arterial wound repair. Using the well-characterized rat carotid balloon catheter injury model, we showed that there was minimal expression of DDR1 in the uninjured carotid, but DDR1 mRNA and protein expression were increased in coincidence with smooth muscle cell (SMC) proliferation and migration into the intima [13]. To test the hypothesis that expression was linked to the process of neointimal formation, we used in vitro assays, which mimic critical steps in intimal thickening, and studied aortic SMCs harvested from DDR1 −/− and wild-type DDR1+/+ mice. Cells must attach to matrix to gain traction for migration, so we measured adhesion to type I and type VIII collagens, and found that DDR1 −/− SMCs showed reduced attachment compared with DDR1+/+ SMCs. Chemotaxis towards collagen types I and VIII was also reduced in DDR1 −/− SMCs. We found that MMP-2 and MMP-9 activity were dramatically downregulated in DDR1 −/− SMCs, suggesting that the DDR1 plays an important role in regulating MMP activity, which is necessary for migration through matrix barriers. Furthermore, DDR1 −/− cells proliferated more slowly than wild-type cells [13]. These studies were the first to demonstrate a functional role for the DDR1 in mediating cell proliferation and migration.

There are no gross abnormalities in cardiac or vascular structure in unstressed DDR1 −/− mice. However, when the carotid arteries of DDR1 −/− and wild-type mice were injured using a copper wire, neointimal area after injury was reduced by 70% in the DDR1 −/− mice, and collagen accumulation in the intimal lesions was also significantly reduced.

To study signaling pathways triggered by the receptor, we transfected DDR1 −/− SMCs with either full-length intact, full-length kinase dead or kinase domain truncated mutants. The intact or kinase dead DDR1 mutants restored cell attachment, bringing adhesion back to levels seen in WT controls; however, cell migration and gelatinase activity were only restored by expression of intact DDR1b [14]. This suggests that kinase activation and downstream signaling is needed for the stimulation of cell migration.

3. Discussion

We conclude that DDR1 plays several important roles in arterial wound repair, illustrated schematically in Fig. 1. DDR1 mediates SMC proliferation and migration via the induction of MMP activity. Furthermore, elimination of DDR1 reduces intimal collagen accumulation, suggesting that DDR1 is also involved in stimulating collagen synthesis. Thus, it seems that inhibiting DDR1 may reduce or prevent lesion formation. However, these observations were made using relatively simple cell culture and mechan-

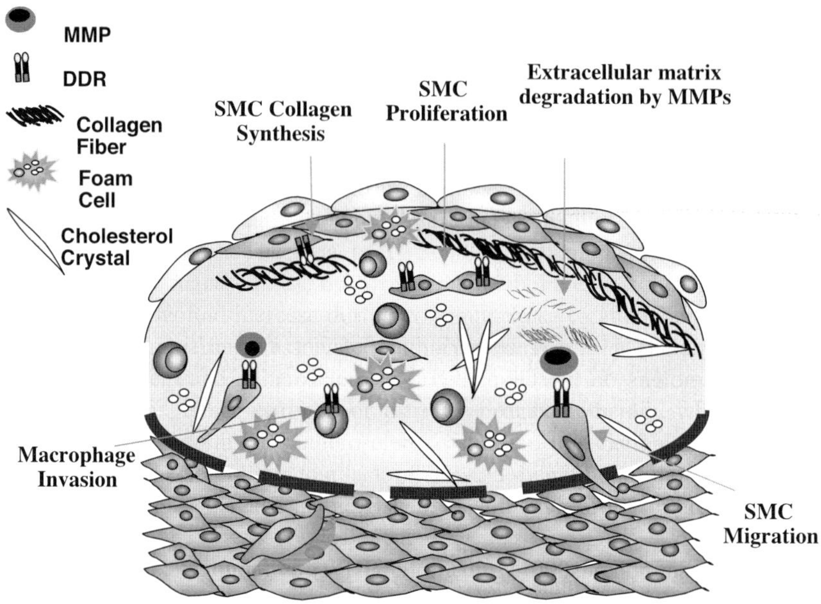

Fig. 1. Schematic diagram of the atherosclerotic plaque. The dotted line indicates the internal elastic lamina. The potential roles of DDR1 in the progression of atherosclerosis include: (a) stimulation of SMC migration from media to intima via increased MMP activity; (b) regulation of SMC proliferation which would increase plaque size; (c) macrophage infiltration into the intima via induction of MMP expression; (d) extracellular matrix degradation mediated by DDR-stimulated MMPs may contribute to plaque destabilization and rupture; (e) stimulation of collagen synthesis by SMCs in the fibrous cap.

ical injury models in vivo. The role of DDR1 in atherosclerosis and models of complex lesion formation remains to be investigated. DDR1 may mediate macrophage infiltration into atherosclerotic plaques, and macrophage-derived MMPs are known to destabilize lesions leading to plaque rupture. On the other hand, DDR1 stimulates an increase in collagen synthesis that may be important to form and maintain the fibrous cap, which would protect against plaque rupture. We are currently investigating the effect of DDR1 gene deletion on plaque progression and fibrous cap formation in the atherosclerotic LDLR −/− mouse model. Results from these studies will be presented.

Acknowledgements

This work was funded by grant # MOP-37847 from the Canadian Institutes of Health Research and a Premier's Research Excellence Award to M. Bendeck. E. Adiguzel was funded by a graduate scholarship from the Heart and Stroke/Richard Lewar Center of Excellence.

References

[1] G. Hou, D. Mulholland, et al., Type VIII collagen stimulates smooth muscle cell migration and matrix metalloproteinase synthesis after arterial injury, Am. J. Pathol. 156 (2000) 467–476.

[2] S. Li, L. Saward, et al., Supermigration of vascular smooth muscle cells on polymerized type I collagen via a matrix autodegradation pathway, Circulation 100 (1999) I-753.

[3] N.O. Carragher, B. Levkau, et al., Degraded collagen fragments promote rapid disassembly of smooth muscle focal adhesions that correlates with cleavage of pp125(FAK), paxillin, and talin, J. Cell Biol. 147 (1999) 619–630.

[4] H. Koyama, E.W. Raines, et al., Fibrillar collagen inhibits arterial smooth muscle cell proliferation through regulation of Cdk2 inhibitors, Cell 87 (1996) 1069–1078.

[5] W. Vogel, G.D. Gish, et al., The discoidin domain receptor tyrosine kinases are activated by collagen, Mol. Cell 1 (1997) 13–23.

[6] W. Vogel, Discoidin domain receptors: structural relations and functional implications, FASEB J. 13 (1999) S77–S82.

[7] W.F. Vogel, A. Aszodi, et al., Discoidin domain receptor 1 tyrosine kinase has an essential role in mammary gland development, Mol. Cell. Biol. 21 (2001) 2906–2917.

[8] J.P. Labrador, V. Azcoitia, et al., The collagen receptor DDR2 regulates proliferation and its elimination leads to dwarfism, EMBO Rep. 2 (2001) 446–452.

[9] H. Kamohara, S. Yamashiro, et al., Discoidin domain receptor 1 isoform-a (DDR1a) promotes migration of leukocytes in three-dimensional collagen lattices, FASEB J. 15 (2001) 2724–2726.

[10] E. Olaso, K. Ikeda, et al., DDR2 receptor promotes MMP-2 mediated proliferation and invasion by hepatic stellate cells, J. Clin. Invest. 108 (2001) 1369–1378.

[11] E. Olaso, P. Labrador, et al., DDR2 receptor regulates fibroblast proliferation and migration through extracellular matrix by transcriptional activation of MMP-2, J. Biol. Chem. 277 (2002) 3606–3613.

[12] K. Ikeda, L.H. Wang, et al., Discoidin domain receptor 2 (DDR2) interacts with Src and Shc following its activation by type I collagen, J. Biol. Chem. 277 (2002) 19206–19212.

[13] G. Hou, W. Vogel, et al., The discoidin domain-receptor tyrosine kinase DDR1 in arterial wound repair, J. Clin. Invest. 107 (2001) 727–735.

[14] G. Hou, W.F. Vogel, et al., Tyrosine kinase activity of discoidin domain receptor 1 is necessary for smooth muscle cell migration and matrix metalloproteinase expression, Circ. Res. 90 (2002) 1147–1149.

International Congress Series 1262 (2004) 490–493

www.ics-elsevier.com

Role of oxidant stress in vascular proteolysis

Zorina S. Galis*

Division of Cardiology, Department of Medicine and Wallace Coulter Department of Biomedical Engineering, Emory University School of Medicine, 1639 Pierce Dr., WMB 319 Cardiology, Atlanta, GA 30322, USA

Abstract. Proteolytic degradation of the matrix scaffold is a necessary component of tissue remodeling. We have proposed that specialized enzymes, called matrix metalloproteinases (MMPs), allow vascular wall remodeling in response to a variety of stimuli, but may ultimately weaken it, bringing about the destabilization and failure responsible for acute cardiovascular events. We are currently briefly reviewing the main evidence we have obtained regarding the key role of oxidative stress in MMP-driven remodeling. An essential finding was that reactive oxygen species (ROS), produced by inflammatory and vascular cells, could trigger activation of latent MMPs, thus leading to vascular matrix degradation. For instance, we showed that lipid-laden macrophages, a major source of both MMPs and ROS, are associated with increased proteolytic activity and drive expansive remodeling, which may explain their association with unstable human atherosclerotic plaques. Of note, vascular cells can also become a source of ROS. We found that active vascular remodeling was characterized by oxidant stress, MMP induction/activation, and matrix degradation. Conversely, we recently demonstrated that introduction of oxidative stress drives arterial lesion progression and angiogenesis. Thus, we propose that the therapeutic decrease of vascular oxidant stress may be used to control vascular remodeling and to increase the stability of atherosclerotic plaques.

Keywords: Matrix metalloproteinases; Oxidant stress; Plaque stability; Vascular remodeling; Inflammation

1. Introduction

Prevention, detection, and treatment of plaque instability have become central for the management of cardiovascular disease. This comes following the new understanding of the common pathway driving atherosclerotic plaques progression toward acute clinical cardiovascular events through destabilization, followed by lumen occlusion due to thrombosis. We have proposed that acute atheroma failure represents a late stage of arterial remodeling initiated by the "good" intention to allow compensatory enlargement of the arterial wall through matrix degradation by enzymes called matrix metalloproteinases (MMPs).

* Tel.: +1-404-727-3754; fax: +1-404-712-8368.
E-mail address: zgalis@emory.edu (Z.S. Galis).

0531-5131/
doi:10.1016/j.ics.2003.12.015

1.1. Vascular sources of MMPs and ROS

The great interest in MMPs, discovered initially for their matrix-degrading capacity assisting tissue invasion by transformed cells, has been sparked by the realization that any cell movement, as well as any structural tissue rearrangement, will require degradation of the matrix scaffold. Such changes, known as "remodeling" in the adult body, occur in response to a variety of stimuli and can have physiological or pathological consequences. We have specifically questioned MMP contributions in relation to main vascular pathological conditions that entail vascular remodeling, including atherosclerosis, development of restenotic lesions, arterial aneurismal dilatation, and failure of vein grafts [1].

MMPs are secreted as latent enzymes with activity controlled by post-translational processing and the presence of natural inhibitors, called TIMPs. Numerous in vitro and in situ observations indicate that vascular and inflammatory cells produce MMPs, but the spectra secreted basally or in response to stimuli is rather distinctive (reviewed in Ref. [1]). Of note, major stimuli of MMP production and activation include mediators of inflammation, growth factors, changes in the hemodynamic environment, and oxidative stress.

Specific stimuli can also increase production of reactive oxygen species (ROS) by vascular and inflammatory cells [2,3]. For instance, investigating the role of hemodynamics in the remodeling of bypass vein grafts, we found that human saphenous vein segments maintained ex vivo under arterial conditions i.e., high shear, pulsatile flow, and high perfusion pressure, experienced oxidative stress [4]. Our results also indicated that superoxide accumulation within the vascular wall, likely due to its deficient scavenging, was related to activation of MMP-2 and MMP-9 and enhanced vein wall remodeling. In relation to atheroma, we demonstrated that the characteristic "foam cell" macrophage is a major source of ROS, including hydrogen peroxide (H_2O_2).

1.2. Reactive oxygen species activate MMPs

We showed that several of the ROS produced by foam cells could trigger in vitro activation of latent MMP-2 and MMP-9 [5], likely explaining MMP activation by isolated foam cells [6]. Mast cell degranulation produces a similar ROS-dependent activation of MMPs in the atheroma shoulder [7]. Thus, ROS provide an important MMP activation pathway. First, this is independent of the availability of other proteases, previously thought to be essential. Second, ROS-dependent MMP activation can occur on a large scale, eliminating the spatial limitation of matrix proteolysis at the pericellular zone, as when due to the action of membrane-associated MT-MMPs. Thus, cells can activate latent MMPs they had secreted, as well as other cells' MMPs, either stored within the matrix or floating around in a soluble phase.

Of note, ROS can easily combine and thus may have different actions depending on the context. For instance, on one hand, we found that production of nitric oxide (NO) by SMC transfected with eNOS gene-reduced expression of MMP-2 and MMP-9, suggesting that NO production may help keep in check MMP expression and matrix degradation in healthy vessels. However, within the diseased arterial wall, NO biological effects are likely modified, for instance through interaction with superoxide. The product, peroxynitrite, interestingly has distinct and completely opposite effects, activating latent MMPs [5] but degrading TIMPs [8], thus likely locally increasing proteolytic activity. Superoxide dismutation through the action of cellular dismutases in fact generates the stable molecule H_2O_2, which also activates MMPs [5].

1.3. MMPs, expansive remodeling, and plaque instability

The arterial expansive remodeling compensates for the development of lesions and thus diminishes lumen loss. However, expansive remodeling was recently associated with human plaque instability [9]. Rich inflammatory infiltrates, previously associated with plaque instability, were more recently associated also with expansive remodeling and MMP activity [10]. We were able to prove the connection by demonstrating experimentally that increasing the macrophage foam cell content of mouse carotid artery lesions enhanced tissue MMP activity and expansive remodeling [11].

1.4. Oxidative stress drives atherosclerotic plaque progression

Numerous lines of evidence suggest that atherosclerotic lesions engender oxidative stress. We recently questioned the potential converse causal relation, i.e., whether oxidative stress drives arterial lesion progression. To test this hypothesis, we studied the effect of inducing vascular ROS production upon formation of mouse carotid artery lesions. We found [12] that carotid artery lesions in the transgenic mouse with smooth muscle cell- (SMC) targeted overexpression of the p22phox subunit of NAD(P)H oxidase, a major vascular source of ROS, had elevated H_2O_2 and MMP activity and caused them to grow larger compared with those of wild type mice (WT). Importantly, lesions presented extensive angiogenesis, clinically associated with culprit lesions [13], likely due to intraplaque hemorrhage, a major mode of failure of human atherosclerotic plaques. Interestingly, a specific polymorphism, increasing vascular p22phox expression, has been associated with the progression of human coronary artery disease [14]. Treatment of SMC with superoxide dismutase (SOD) increased gelatinase levels, further supporting the role of H_2O_2. On the other hand, administration of the antioxidant ebselen inhibited in vitro effects, intra-lesion angiogenesis and carotid artery lesion progression.

2. Discussion

We propose that oxidative stress is a major driver of tissue remodeling, controlling the action of MMPs. Conversely, scavenging ROS will decrease MMP expression, as we demonstrated in experimental atheroma [6]. Lipid lowering has similar effects [15]. In fact, many of the reported beneficial effects of lipid lowering, including improvement of endothelial function, can be obtained directly through decreasing vascular oxidative stress. We propose that decreasing oxidative stress may be a major strategy for the treatment of cardiovascular disease, specifically for increasing plaque stability.

Acknowledgements

Partial funding for these studies was provided through the NIH RO1HL64689, RO1 HL71061, and the American Heart Association Established Investigator Award #0040087N.

References

[1] Z.S. Galis, et al., Matrix metalloproteinases in vascular remodeling and atherogenesis: the good, the bad, and the ugly, Circ. Res. 90 (2002) 251–262.
[2] K. Griendling, et al., Angiotensin II stimulates NADH and NADPH activity in cultured vascular smooth muscle cells, Circ. Res. 74 (1994) 1141–1148.
[3] P.J. Pagano, et al., Localization of a constitutively active, phagocyte-like NADPH oxidase in rabbit aortic adventitia: enhancement by angiotensin II, Proc. Natl. Acad. Sci. U. S. A. 94 (1997) 14438–14488.
[4] K. Mavromatis, et al., Early effects of arterial hemodynamic conditions on human saphenous veins perfused ex vivo, Arterioscler. Thromb. Vasc. Biol. 20 (2000) 1889–1895.
[5] S. Rajagopalan, et al., Reactive oxygen species produced by macrophage-derived foam cells regulate the activity of vascular matrix metalloproteinases in vitro. Implications for atherosclerotic plaque stability, J. Clin. Invest. 98 (1996) 2572–2579.
[6] Z.S. Galis, et al., *N*-acetyl-cysteine decreases the matrix-degrading capacity of macrophage-derived foam cells: new target for antioxidant therapy? (see comments), Circulation 97 (1998) 2445–2453.
[7] J.L. Johnson, et al., Activation of matrix-degrading metalloproteinases by mast cell proteases in atherosclerotic plaques, Arterioscler. Thromb. Vasc. Biol. 18 (1998) 1707–1715.
[8] E.R. Frears, et al., Inactivation of tissue inhibitor of metalloproteinase-1 by peroxynitrite, FEBS Lett. 381 (1996) 21–24.
[9] P. Schoenhagen, et al., Extent and direction of arterial remodeling in stable versus unstable coronary syndromes: an intravascular ultrasound study, Circulation 101 (2000) 598–603.
[10] G. Pasterkamp, et al., Atherosclerotic arterial remodeling and the localization of macrophages and matrix metalloproteases 1, 2 and 9 in the human coronary artery, Atherosclerosis 150 (2000) 245–253.
[11] E. Ivan, et al., Expansive arterial remodeling is associated with increased neointimal macrophage foam cell content: the murine model of macrophage-rich carotid artery lesions, Circulation 105 (2002) 2686–2691.
[12] J. Khatri, et al., Vascular oxidant stress enhances progression and angiogenesis of experimental atheroma. Circulation (in press).
[13] A.N. Tenaglia, et al., Neovascularization in atherectomy specimens from patients with unstable angina: implications for pathogenesis of unstable angina, Am. Heart J. 135 (1998) 10–14.
[14] C. Cahilly, et al., A variant of p22(phox), involved in generation of reactive oxygen species in the vessel wall, is associated with progression of coronary atherosclerosis, Circ. Res. 86 (2000) 391–395.
[15] M. Aikawa, et al., Lipid lowering reduces proteolytic and prothrombotic potential in rabbit atheroma. (Review, 55 refs), Ann. N.Y. Acad. Sci. 902 (2000) 140–152.

ELSEVIER

International Congress Series 1262 (2004) 494–497

www.ics-elsevier.com

The mast cell, a rich source of neutral proteases in atherosclerotic plaques

Petri T. Kovanen*, Miriam Lee, Markus J. Leskinen, Katariina Öörni, Ken A. Lindstedt

Atherosclerosis, Wihuri Research Institute, Kalliolinnantie 4, 00140 Helsinki, Finland

Abstract. Mast cells, an inflammatory cell type highly enriched in intracellular granules containing the neutral proteases, tryptase and chymase, are present in both early and late human coronary atherosclerotic lesions. Our in vitro studies have suggested that activated mast cells promote the conversion of both macrophages and smooth muscle cells (SMCs) into foam cells. In this conversion, the key process is proteolytic modification of low-density lipoproteins (LDL) and high-density lipoproteins (HDL), the former accelerating the cellular influx of cholesterol and the latter preventing the cellular efflux of cholesterol. In addition to effects related to lipid metabolism and foam cell formation, novel functions for mast cells in atherothrombosis are emerging. Experimental studies have shown that chymase and heparin proteoglycans secreted by activated mast cells may destabilize the plaque by inhibiting SMC proliferation and collagen synthesis, and by activating latent interstitial collagenase (MMP-1). Furthermore, by degrading fibronectin with subsequent loss of outside-in survival signaling, chymase induces SMC apoptosis in vitro. Activated mast cells can also induce apoptosis of endothelial cells (ECs) by a mechanism partly involving secretion of tumor necrosis factor-α (TNF-α). These recent findings suggest a role for mast cells both in early and late stages of atherosclerosis. © 2004 Elsevier B.V. All rights reserved.

Keywords: Mast cell; LDL; HDL; Proteases; Apoptosis

1. Mast cells contribute to foam cell formation

Human coronary atherosclerosis is characterized by local accumulations of LDL-derived cholesterol in the arterial intima [1]. Initially, cholesterol accumulates sub-endothelially in the intimal monocyte-derived macrophages, leading to formation of foam cells and fatty streaks. Since cholesterol enters the arterial intima from circulation carried by plasma LDL and is removed by HDL, an imbalance between these two processes results in foam cell formation [2]. Proteolytic modification of LDL and HDL may induce such an imbalance between cholesterol influx and efflux.

* Corresponding author. Tel.: +358-9-681-411; fax: +358-9-637-476.
E-mail address: petri.kovanen@wri.fi (P.T. Kovanen).

0531-5131/
doi:10.1016/j.ics.2003.12.013

In fatty streaks, the increased number of activated mast cells are a significant source of neutral proteases, tryptase and chymase [3,4], which may modify LDL and HDL in a pro-atherogenic fashion. Our in vitro studies, employing rat serosal mast cells and human lipoproteins [4], suggest that activated and degranulated mast cells can accelerate foam cell formation by promoting the uptake of LDL and by inhibiting the release of cellular cholesterol to HDL.

1.1. Mast cells modify low-density lipoproteins (LDL)

Mast cell granule remnants bind LDL via ionic interactions between heparin proteoglycans and apolipoprotein (apo) B-100, and chymase, present in the granule remnants, proteolyze the bound LDL particles, which fuse into larger lipid droplets. Such modified LDL particles bind to proteoglycans more tightly than native LDL particles and are avidly phagocytosed by macrophages, which become foam cells by accumulating LDL-derived cholesterol as cytoplasmic cholesteryl ester droplets. Similarly, cultured rat aortic smooth muscle cells (SMCs) of the synthetic phenotype can phagocytose LDL-coated granule remnants, becoming foam cells. Immunoelectron microscopy has shown that in the human arterial intima, exocytosed mast cell granules bind apoB-100-containing lipoproteins, which are then ingested by the intimal macrophages or smooth muscle cells [4].

Histamine, another well-known mast cell mediator, is capable of enhancing vascular permeability to macromolecules [5], suggesting that activated subendothelial coronary mast cells could facilitate the transport of LDL through the endothelium. Indeed, in a surrogate model of atherogenesis, mast cell activation enhances the transendothelial transport of LDL from plasma to skin during the passive cutaneous anaphylaxis reaction in rats [6].

1.2. Mast cells modify high-density lipoproteins (HDL)

We have shown that chymase, released by activated rat serosal mast cells, induce a minor degradation of HDL apolipoproteins with the lost ability of HDL_3 to induce a high-affinity efflux of cellular cholesterol from mouse or human macrophage foam cells [7]. Further studies with isolated chymase and tryptase revealed rapid depletion of minor HDL subpopulations, i.e. preβ_1-HDL and a fraction of the apoA-IV-containing HDL (LpA-IV), which actively induce cellular cholesterol efflux [8,9].

Both human and rat chymases generate identical proteolytic cleavage sites in apoA-I of reconstituted, preβ-migrating, discoidal HDL, reducing their ability to act as cholesterol acceptors [10]. Furthermore, human chymase is able to effectively deplete the preβ-HDL particles generated by the phospholipid transfer protein (PLTP) of human plasma, thereby impairing this antiatherogenic function of PLTP [11]. Importantly, treatment of HDL_3 with human chymase specifically blocks the ABCA1-dependent pathway of cholesterol efflux from cAMP-stimulated J774 macrophage cells by a mechanism involving depletion of the preβ-migrating, lipid-poor particles present in HDL_3 (unpublished data).

2. Mast cells in plaque remodeling

A possible mechanism causing the rupture or erosion of coronary plaques is apoptotic loss of smooth muscle cells and endothelial cells necessary for plaque stability. We have shown that chymase released from activated rat serosal mast cells is able to induce apoptosis in vascular SMCs in vitro [12]. Chymase degrades the extracellular matrix component, fibronectin, with subsequent disruption of focal adhesions [13]. Interestingly, the mast cell-mediated proapoptotic effect seems to be purely paracrine, since the activated mast cells themselves survive by overexpressing the pro-survival bcl-2 homologue A1 [14]. Similarly, stimulation of rat serosal mast cells with ensuing degranulation down-regulates the expression of bcl-2 in co-cultured, rat cardiac (microvascular) endothelial cells, with subsequent induction of apoptosis [15]. The effect was partially (70%) dependent on the presence of TNF-α and involved the translocation of cytochrome *c* from the mitochondria into the cytoplasm. These results suggest that mast cells may contribute to the erosion and rupture of atherosclerotic plaques by inducing apoptosis in adjacent smooth muscle cells and endothelial cells.

Mast cell-derived chymase may also participate in plaque remodeling by inhibiting SMC growth and collagen expression [16]. In addition, chymase and tryptase are capable of triggering extensive degradation of the surrounding extracellular matrix, by activating locally secreted proMMP-1 [17] and proMMP-3 [18], respectively. Recent studies in carotid endarterectomy specimens indicate that activation of mast cells leads to a significant increase in MMP activity, suggesting that degranulation of mast cells may activate proMMPs in atherosclerotic lesions [19]. Activated mast cells may themselves release MMPs, such as MMP-1 [20] and MMP-9 [21], both of which are present in atherosclerotic lesions [22,23].

3. Conclusions and future challenges

Our present studies suggest a role for activated mast cells in early and late atherosclerotic lesions by: (1) inducing foam cell formation and (2) destabilizing atherosclerotic plaques. In these processes, the neutral proteases, tryptase and chymase, secreted by the activated mast cells play a central role. In contrast to other neutral proteases, chymase and tryptase in their natural form, i.e. bound to heparin proteoglycans, are capable of both degrading LDL and preβ-HDL, and inducing SMC apoptosis, even in the presence of natural protease inhibitors. However, the conceptual framework for the possible functions of mast cell proteases in atherogenesis is based on the data obtained with the aid of immunohistochemical techniques, animal and human cell culture systems, and biochemical experiments. Future challenges should include testing of the actual function of the mast cells in animal models as well as in humans. This could be done by stabilizing the mast cells with drugs or by specifically inhibiting the function of individual components, such as proteases, derived from the activated mast cells present in the arterial wall.

References

[1] R. Ross, Atherosclerosis—an inflammatory disease, N. Engl. J. Med. 340 (1999) 115–126.

[2] P.T. Kovanen, Atheroma formation: defective control in the intimal round-trip of cholesterol, Eur. Heart J. 11 (1990) 238–246.

[3] M. Kaartinen, et al., Accumulation of activated mast cells in the shoulder region of human coronary atheroma, the predilection site of atheromatous rupture, Circulation 90 (1994) 1669–1678.

[4] P.T. Kovanen, Mast cells in human fatty streaks and atheromas: implications for intimal lipid accumulation, Curr. Opin. Lipidol. 7 (1996) 281–286.

[5] N.Z. Wu, et al., Transient venular permeability increase and endothelial gap formation induced by histamine, Am. J. Physiol. 262 (1992) H1238–H1247.

[6] H. Ma, et al., Degranulation of cutaneous mast cells induces transendothelial transport and local accumulation of plasma LDL in rat skin in vivo, J. Lipid Res. 38 (1997) 1877–1887.

[7] L. Lindstedt, et al., Chymase in exocytosed rat mast cell granules effectively proteolyzes apolipoprotein A1-containing lipoproteins, so reducing the cholesterol efflux-inducing ability of serum and aortic intimal fluid, J. Clin. Invest. 97 (1996) 2174–2182.

[8] M. Lee, et al., Mast cell tryptase degrades HDL and blocks its function as an acceptor of cellular cholesterol, Arterioscler. Thromb. Vasc. Biol. 22 (2002) 2086–2091.

[9] M. Lee, et al., Depletion of pre beta 1LpA1 and LpA4 particles by mast cell chymase reduces cholesterol efflux from macrophage foam cells induced by plasma, Arterioscler. Thromb. Vasc. Biol. 19 (1999) 1066–1074.

[10] M. Lee, et al., Apolipoprotein composition and particle size affect HDL degradation by chymase: effect on cellular cholesterol efflux, J. Lipid Res. 44 (2003) 539–546.

[11] M. Lee, et al., Degradation of phospholipid transfer protein (PLTP) and PLTP-generated pre-beta-high density lipoprotein by mast cell chymase impairs high affinity efflux of cholesterol from macrophage foam cells, J. Biol. Chem. 278 (2003) 13539–13545.

[12] M. Leskinen, et al., Mast cell chymase induces apoptosis of vascular smooth muscle cells, Arterioscler. Thromb. Vasc. Biol. 21 (2001) 516–522.

[13] M.J. Leskinen, et al., Mast cell chymase induces smooth muscle cell apoptosis by a mechanism involving fibronectin degradation and disruption of focal adhesions, Arterioscler. Thromb. Vasc. Biol. 23 (2003) 238–243.

[14] A. Karsan, et al., Endothelial cell death induced by tumor necrosis factor-alpha is inhibited by the Bcl-2 family member, A1, J. Biol. Chem. 271 (1996) 27201–27204.

[15] S. Lätti, et al., Mast cell-mediated apoptosis of endothelial cells in vitro: a paracrine mechanism involving TNF-alpha-mediated down-regulation of bcl-2 expression, J. Cell. Physiol. 195 (2003) 130–138.

[16] Y. Wang, et al., Mast cell chymase inhibits smooth muscle cell growth and collagen expression in vitro: transforming growth factor-beta1-dependent and- independent effects, Arterioscler. Thromb. Vasc. Biol. 21 (2001) 1928–1933.

[17] J. Saarinen, et al., Activation of human interstitial procollagenase through direct cleavage of the Leu^{83}-Thr^{84} bond by mast cell chymase, J. Biol. Chem. 269 (1994) 18134–18140.

[18] B.L. Gruber, et al., Synovial procollagenase activation by human mast cell tryptase dependence upon matrix metalloproteinase 3 activation, J. Clin. Invest. 84 (1989) 1657–1662.

[19] J.L. Johnson, et al., Activation of matrix-degrading metalloproteinases by mast cell proteases in atherosclerotic plaques, Arterioscler. Thromb. Vasc. Biol., (1998) 1707–1715.

[20] N. Di Girolamo, et al., In vitro and in vivo expression of interstitial collagenase/MMP-1 by human mast cells, Dev. Immunol. 7 (2000) 131–142.

[21] N. Kanbe, et al., Human mast cells produce matrix metalloproteinase 9, Eur. J. Immunol. 29 (1999) 2645–2649.

[22] S.T. Nikkari, et al., Interstitial collagenase (MMP-1) expression in human carotid atherosclerosis, Circulation 92 (1995) 1393–1398.

[23] M. Kaartinen, et al., Mast cell infiltration in acute coronary syndromes: implications for plaque rupture, J. Am. Coll. Cardiol. 32 (1998) 606–612.

International Congress Series 1262 (2004) 498–501

www.ics-elsevier.com

Role of elastolytic cathepsins in vascular remodeling

Galina K. Sukhova*, Guo-Ping Shi, Peter Libby

Donald W. Reynolds Cardiovascular Clinical Research Center, Cardiovascular Division, Department of Medicine, Brigham and Women's Hospital, 77 Avenue Louis Pasteur, NRB-730J, Boston, MA 02115, USA

Abstract. *Background*: We now appreciate that the pathogenesis of atherosclerosis and abdominal aortic aneurysms (AAA) involves breakdown of extracellular matrix (ECM). We recently implicated certain elastolytic cysteine-dependent cathepsins in these pathological processes. *Results*: We demonstrated over-expression of cathepsins S and K in human atheroma and AAA, and colocalized cathepsin S-positive medial smooth muscle cells (SMC) with sites of internal elastic lamina fragmentation. Moreover, depletion of cystatin C, the most abundant endogenous cysteine protease inhibitor, characterizes both atherosclerotic and aneurysmal lesions. To test directly the role of cathepsin S in atherogenesis, we studied targeted disruption of the cathepsin S gene in atherosclerosis-prone LDLr$^{-/-}$ mice consuming a western diet. Cathepsin S deficiency significantly decreased atherosclerosis. Better-preserved elastin in the tunica media of cathepsin S-deficient mice likely reflected the diminished elastolytic activity in cathepsin S$^{-/-}$ SMC ($p<0.0001$) compared with wild-type SMC. These mice had fewer SMC and less collagen in their intimal lesions, probably because SMC migration requires degradation of elastin. *Conclusions*: Our findings in situ, in vitro and in vivo establish an important role for cathepsins in vascular remodeling.

Keywords: Cysteine proteases; Cathepsin S; Elastolysis; Atherosclerosis; Abdominal aortic aneurysm

1. Introduction

We now appreciate that the structural integrity and function of the vascular wall depends on extracellular matrix (ECM) and that ECM remodeling contributes decisively to the pathogenesis of vascular diseases including atherosclerosis and abdominal aortic aneurysms (AAA) [1].

Our work first implicated cathepsins S and K, members of cysteine proteases family, in atherosclerosis in 1998. These enzymes act inside a highly acidic milieu of lysosomes, and thus did not appear to be involved in extracellular proteolysis [2]. Since then, we

* Corresponding author. Tel.: +1-617-525-4354; fax: +1-617-525-4380.
E-mail address: gsukhova@rics.bwh.harvard.edu (G.K. Sukhova).

doi:10.1016/j.ics.2003.12.087

demonstrated an important role for these enzymes in these diseases in vitro and in vivo, using atherosclerotic mice [3,4].

2. Cathepsins S and K are over-expressed in human atheroma

Several features of cathepsins S and K, including presence in alveolar macrophages, the high elastolytic activity of cathepsin S at neutral pH and their role in emphysema, an inflammatory disease, suggested the potential role of this family in atherosclerosis [2]. Indeed, we detected cathepsins S and K mRNA and protein in human atheroma, although normal arteries expressed very little or no cathepsins. Interestingly, cathepsins S and K localized not only in intimal macrophages, but also in medial smooth muscle cells (SMC) at sites of elastic laminae degradation/fragmentation [3].

These novel and unexpected data provoked further investigation. We demonstrated that cultured human vascular SMC stimulated by pro-inflammatory cytokines express cathepsins S and K. Stimulated SMC produce and, more importantly, release cathepsin S in an active form as demonstrated by active site labeling with [^{125}I]tyr-ala-CHN_2 [3]. Moreover, SMC from cathepsin S-deficient mice showed a 50% reduction ($p < 0.0001$) in elastolytic capacity compared with wild-type cells [4].

3. Reduced levels of cystatin C, the most abundant inhibitor of cysteine proteases, in atherosclerotic and aneurysmal lesions

Cystatin C, the most prominent inhibitor of cysteine proteases that was found in virtually all tissues and body fluids, regulated cathepsin activity [5]. Because inflammatory processes reduce cystatin C [6], and atherosclerosis is an inflammatory disease, we hypothesized that cystatin C levels in human atheromata and AAA might decrease in comparison to the normal vascular wall. Indeed, cystatin C levels decreased dramatically in diseased arteries (Fig. 1) [7]. Consistent with our previously published data [3,7], cathepsin S expression increased in diseased tissue samples (Fig. 1).

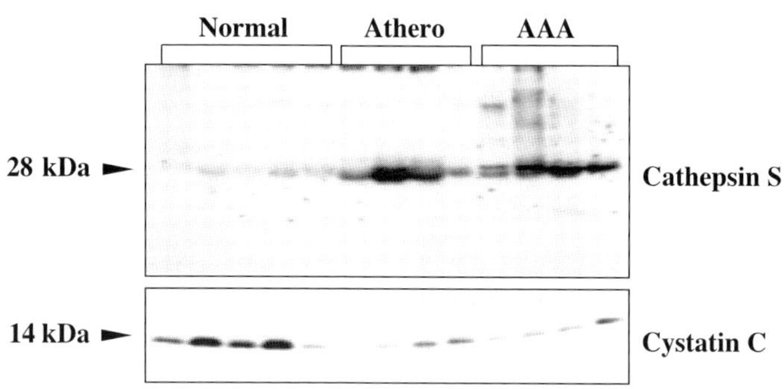

Fig. 1. Reciprocal relationship of cathepsin S and cystatin C in normal and diseased human vascular tissue. Western blot analysis of tissue extracts from normal arteries ($n = 5$), atherosclerotic plaques ($n = 4$) and AAA ($n = 4$) for cathepsin S and cystatin C.

Moreover, cystatin C levels in blood serum decreased significantly (0.52 ± 0.2 μg/ml) in patients with dilated aortas (>2.5 cm) compared with the control group (1.3 ± 1.0, $p<0.003$) [7].

This disturbed enzymes/inhibitor balance in diseased arteries supports a role for cysteine proteases in atherogenesis.

4. Differential regulation of cathepsins and cystatin C expression by vascular SMC

We hypothesized that reciprocal expression of cathepsins and their inhibitor in normal and diseased arteries based on differential regulation of their expression. We demonstrated on cultured human vascular SMC treated by different cytokines that the level of cathepsin S mRNA increased markedly after stimulation by IFN-γ. However, the level of cystatin C mRNA was high and did not change (Fig. 2A). Although the levels of cathepsin S and cystatin C mRNA did not change in SMC stimulated with TGF-β, secretion of cystatin C protein increased (Fig. 2A,B).

5. Cathepsin S deficiency reduces atherosclerosis in LDLr-null mice

To directly test the influence of cathepsin S on atherogenesis, we crossbred Cat $S^{-/-}$ mice with atherosclerosis prone $LDLr^{-/-}$ mice, fed them an atherogenic diet, and evaluated atherosclerotic lesions at 8, 12 and 26 weeks. Cathepsin S deficiency reduced atherosclerosis in the aortas. Lesion area in the abdominal aortas, defined by lipid deposition, was considerably smaller ($p<0.005$) in Cat $S^{-/-}LDLr^{-/-}$ mice. These mice showed substantially reduced intimal thickening ($p<0.02$) and severity of atherosclerosis ($p<0.04$), both evaluated on longitudinal sections of aortic arches. We also colocalized cathepsin S-positive medial SMC with breaks in elastic laminae in these mice, as demonstrated previously in human atheroma [5]. Accordingly, lesions in cathepsin S-deficient mice showed better preservation of elastic laminae ($p<0.004$), and fewer SMC migrated from the tunica media into the intima ($p<0.05$) compared with control. Lack of

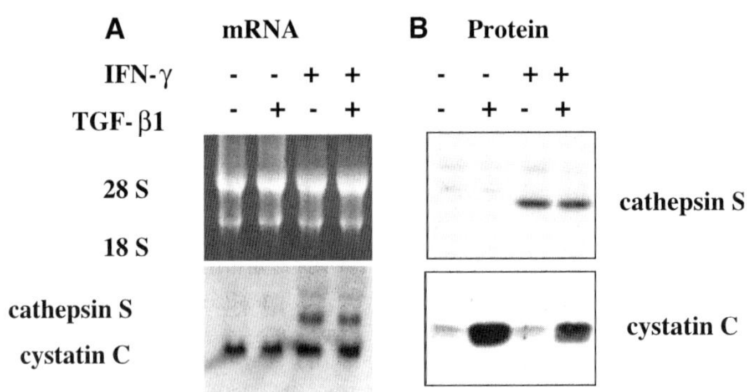

Fig. 2. Differential regulation of cathepsin S and cystatin C expression by human SMC. (A) Northern blot analysis of SMC lysates after stimulation with IFN-γ (500 U/ml), TGF-β (10 ng/ml) or both cytokines. Loading control with ribosomal RNA is shown. (B) Western blot analysis of cultured SMC supernatant for cathepsin S and cystatin C. (From Ref. [7], reproduced with permission).

SMC, the major source of arterial ECM, leads to the substantial decrease in collagen content ($p < 0.01$).

6. Conclusion

We have gained a deeper appreciation of the importance of proteases in vessel remodeling, lesion formation and disruption. In situ, in vitro and in vivo data from animal models of atherosclerosis support our novel view that elastolytic cysteine proteases play an important role in this disease.

References

[1] P. Libby, Vascular biology of atherosclerosis: overview and state of art, Am. J. Cardiol. 91 (2003) 3A–6A.
[2] G.-P. Shi, J.S. Munger, J.P. Meara, D.H. Rich, H.A. Chapman, Molecular cloning and expression of human alveolar macrophage cathepsin S, an elastolytic cysteine protease, J. Biol. Chem. 267 (1992) 7258–7262.
[3] G.K. Sukhova, G.-P. Shi, D.I. Simon, H.A. Chapman, P. Libby, Expression of the elastolytic cathepsins S and K in human atheroma and regulation of their production in smooth muscle cells, J. Clin. Invest. 102 (1998) 576–583.
[4] G.K. Sukhova, Y. Zhang, J.-H. Pan, et al., Deficiency of cathepsin S reduces atherosclerosis in LDL receptor-deficient mice, J. Clin. Invest. 111 (2003) 897–906.
[5] G.S. Merz, Human cystatin C forms an inactive dimmer during intracellular trafficking in transfected CHO cells, J. Cell. Physiol. 173 (1997) 423–432.
[6] A.H. Warfe, D. Zuscer-Franklin, B. Frangione, J. Ghiso, Constitutive secretion of cystatin C (gamma-trace) by monocytes and macrophahes and its downregulation after stimulation, J. Exp. Med. 166 (1987) 1912–1917.
[7] G.-P. Shi, G.K. Sukhova, A. Grubb, et al., Cystatin C deficiency in human atherosclerosis and aortic aneurysms, J. Clin. Invest. 104 (1999) 1191–1197.

ELSEVIER

International Congress Series 1262 (2004) 502

www.ics-elsevier.com

Economic burden of atherosclerosis-related diseases in Korea

Chang-yup Kim*

School of Public Health, Seoul National University, 28 Yongon-dong, Chongno-gu, Seoul 110-799, South Korea

Abstract. *Objective*: To assess the economic burden of atherosclerosis-related diseases in Korea. *Methods and results*: To assess the trend of epidemiologic and economic burdens, mortality statistics and National Health Insurance claims data were analyzed. Atherosclerosis-related diseases include myocardial infarction, angina, TIA, cerebral infarction, peripheral vascular disease, mesenteric ischemia and bowel infarction, renal artery stenosis and renovascular hypertension. About 4.4% of total mortality in 1995 increased to 7.7% in 2001. More recently, cerebral infarct has shown faster increase in mortality and diagnosis of atherosclerosis has decreased, most probably due to more confirmative diagnosis. The insurance data shows rapidly increasing expenditure from atherosclerosis-related diseases. The expenditure had steadily increased in proportion among total expenditure, 2.35% in 1995 to 3.20% in 1999. However, these figures have had fewer shares than epidemiological burden. *Discussion and conlusion*: Economic burden of atherosclerosis-related diseases have rapidly increased recently, but still less than epidemiologic burden. In the near future, more expenditure is expected due to several factors: rapidly aging, changing burden of diseases, and health system factors such as fee-for-services, escalating number of suppliers, and pharmaceuticals.

Keywords: Economic burden; Atherosclerosis; Korea

* Tel.: +82-2-740-8876; fax: +82-2-3673-3955.
E-mail address: cykim@snu.ac.kr (C. Kim).

0531-5131/ © 2003 Published by Elsevier B.V.
doi:10.1016/j.ics.2003.11.039

ELSEVIER

International Congress Series 1262 (2004) 503–506

www.ics-elsevier.com

CETP, a key player in atherogenic dyslipidemia of Type II diabetes

John M. Chapman*, Maryse Guerin

Dyslipoproteinemia and Atherosclerosis Research Unit, INSERM unit 551, Hopital de la Pitié, 83 Boulevard de l'hopital, 75651 Paris, France

Abstract. The WHO has predicted that a worldwide epidemic of Type II diabetes, affecting some 300 million persons, can be envisaged in 2003. The key features of the atherogenic lipid phenotype characteristic of Type II diabetes are low HDL-cholesterol levels, mild to marked hypertriglyceridemia involving VLDL and VLDL remnants, and elevated concentrations of both small dense LDL, and free fatty acids (FFA) in the fasting state; indeed, FFA are implicated in the development of peripheral insulin resistance. Elevated transfer rates of cholesteryl esters (CE) from HDL to atherogenic apoB100 lipoproteins (VLDL, IDL, LDL) mediated by cholesteryl ester transfer protein (CETP) underlie the low HDL-C levels typical of Type II diabetes, identifying CETP as a prime pharmacological target. The future clinical application of CETP inhibitors in Type II diabetic subjects, in association with agents which would act synergistically by reducing concentrations of atherogenic CE acceptor lipoproteins (e.g., statins, fibrates, cholesterol absorption inhibitors), is therefore especially attractive.

Keywords: Dysfunctional HDL; Small dense LDL; Statin; Fibrate; CETP inhibition

Cardiovascular morbi-mortality in Type II diabetes is markedly elevated as a result of a constellation of synergistic risk factors, among which dyslipidemia figures prominently. Diabetic dyslipidemia is characterized by anomalies of the structure, metabolism and biological activities of both atherogenic lipoproteins containing apoB100 (VLDL, IDL and LDL) and of antiatherogenic HDL containing apoAI and/or Apo AII [1]; these anomalies include dysfunctional HDL, a dense LDL phenotype and glycation of apoB and apoAI. Such metabolic and functional anomalies are closely associated with elevated oxidative stress, endothelial dysfunction and premature macrovascular atherosclerotic disease [1,2]. Elevated ratios of atherogenic cholesterol (VLDL, IDL, LDL cholesterol) relative to HDL cholesterol (HDL-C) (>4) are typical of the dyslipidemia of Type II diabetes and are indicative of disequilibrium in proatherogenic versus antiatherogenic plasma lipoprotein

* Corresponding author. Tel.: +33-1-42-17-78-78; fax: +33-1-45-82-81-98.
E-mail address: chapman@chups.jussieu.fr (J.M. Chapman).

0531-5131/ © 2004 Published by Elsevier B.V.
doi:10.1016/j.ics.2003.12.108

levels, frequently due to low HDL-C concentration (≤ 40 mg/dl) [2,3]. Such a disequilibrium favors enhanced deposition of cholesterol in the arterial wall and progression of atherosclerotic disease.

The metabolic anomalies which underlie diabetic dyslipidemia have multiple origins, including (i) defective metabolism of free fatty acid (FFA) by adipose tissue which gives rise to hepatic overproduction of large VLDL (VLDL-1) and results from an elevated FFA flux to the liver, (ii) abnormal intravascular remodelling of apoB-containing lipoproteins (VLDL, VLDL remnants and LDL) which involves CETP-mediated enrichment in cholesteryl esters (CE) transferred from HDL and favors enhanced formation of atherogenic small dense LDL, (iii) formation of small HDL particles of short plasma half-life as a result of initial triglyceride (TG) enrichment via CETP action and subsequent TG hydrolysis by hepatic lipase, and (iv) glycation of apo AI in HDL particles which diminishes their activity in reverse cholesterol transport [4,5]. The mechanisms underlying these metabolic anomalies are summarised in Fig. 1.

In view of the central role of dyslipidemia in the elevated cardiovascular risk typical of Type II diabetes, the therapeutic action of lipid-lowering agents in attenuating such risk is currently attracting worldwide attention. Potent statins correct the atherogenic lipid profile in Type II diabetes by concerted mechanisms which principally result from upregulation of hepatic LDL receptors (LDL-R) via reduction in the intra-hepatic cholesterol pool [4]. Enhanced LDL-R-mediated clearance (up to fourfold) of all atherogenic apoB-containing lipoproteins (VLDL, IDL and LDL), and their major subfractions (including small dense LDL) is a major feature of such action. Importantly, by accelerating catabolism of TG-rich lipoproteins, statins enhance release of surface fragments which sequester to the HDL pool. Elevation in HDL levels is equally favored by diminished CETP-mediated transfer of CE from HDL to atherogenic acceptor lipoproteins (VLDL, LDL), whose particle numbers are markedly reduced (up to − 60%) [6]. Normalisation of the intravascular remodelling of both LDL and HDL particle populations is further enhanced by statin-induced reduction

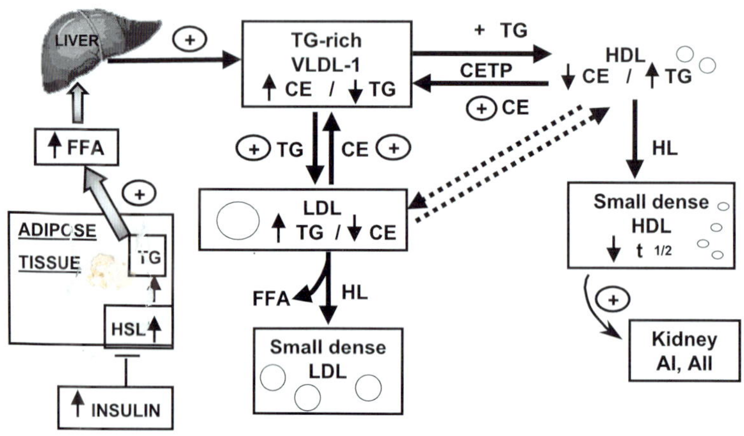

Fig. 1. Metabolic basis of an atherogenic lipoprotein phenotype in Type II diabetes: role of CETP.

in hepatic lipase activity (up to − 25%). Equally, statins upregulate hepatic production of apoAI (+ 15%), thereby contributing further to HDL elevation [6–9]. Finally, the recent data of Guerin et al. [10] suggest that statin treatment may mediate formation of biologically functional HDL particles. Indeed, atorvastatin treatment of subjects displaying combined hyperlipidemia led to significant increase (~ 15%) in the capacity of plasma to facilitate cellular cholesterol efflux via the SR-B1 receptor [10].

Triglyceride levels may vary over a wide range in diabetic patients [3]. We therefore asked the question as to the potential relationship of triglyceride levels to LDL particle phenotype and HDL-C concentrations in Type II diabetics [3]. Our data revealed that progressive elevation in dense LDL levels occurred concomitantly with those of large VLDL (VLDL-1) and apoB across triglyceride tertiles (< 100, 100–200 and >200 mg/dl) and HDL-C [3]. Elevation in triglycerides tertile equally occurred in parallel with increase in BMI and in fasting free fatty acid levels. When physiological CETP-mediated cholesteryl ester (CE) transfer was determined in these patients, a significant elevation was detected in the highest triglyceride tertile, thereby suggesting that elevated CETP activity is a major player whose action underlies the atherogenic particle profile of both LDL and HDL in Type II diabetes [3].

Therapeutically, fibrate treatment has been found to confer significant clinical benefit in mildly hypertriglyceridemic diabetic patients displaying hyperinsulinemia and metabolic syndrome, as exemplified in the VA-HIT trial [11]. Such benefit accrues from reduction in TG-rich lipoprotein levels (VLDL, VLDL remnants), a shift in LDL particle profile from small dense LDL to receptor-active buoyant LDL, and elevation in HDL-C. CETP activity is implicated in the fibrate-mediated normalisation of intravascular LDL modelling, as reduction in circulating levels of triglyceride-rich lipoproteins reduces the number of active CE receptor particles for CETP action [12]. In this way, CETP-mediated CE transfer to LDL from HDL is re-established at the expense of triglyceride transfer from VLDL, restoring a hydrophobic lipid core resistant to hydrolysis by hepatic lipase and resulting in formation of large, buoyant LDL. Finally, fibrate-mediated modulation of lipoprotein profile in Type II diabetes is primarily due to regulation of the expression of key PPARα-responsive genes of lipid metabolism [5,12].

In conclusion, the subnormal levels and dysfunctionality of HDL in diabetic dyslipidemia [5,13] focuses our attention on the clinical relevance of HDL as a major therapeutic target. In this context, it is highly relevant that normalisation of CETP activity—with consequent HDL elevation—via treatment with CETP inhibitors represents an attractive add-on to statin therapy.

References

[1] A.M. Gotto, Lipid management in diabetic patients: lessons from prevention trials, Am. J. Med. 112 (2002) 19S–26S.

[2] R.A. Kreisberg, Diabetic dyslipidemia, Am. J. Cardiol. 82 (1998) 67U–73U.

[3] M. Guerin, W. Le Goff, T.S. Lassel, A. Van Tol, G. Steiner, M.J. Chapman, Atherogenic role of elevated CE transfer from HDL to VLDL(1) and dense LDL in type 2 diabetes: impact of the degree of triglyceridemia, Arterioscler. Thromb. Vasc. Biol. 21 (2001) 282–288.

[4] L.F. Forster, G. Stewart, D. Bedford, J.P. Stewart, E. Rogers, J. Shepherd, C.J. Packard, M.J. Caslake, Influence of atorvastatin and simvastatin on apolipoprotein B metabolism in moderate combined hyperlipidemic subjects with low VLDL and LDL fractional clearance rates, Atherosclerosis 164 (2002) 129–145.

[5] M.R. Taskinen, Diabetic dyslipidemia: from basic research to clinical practice, Diabetologia 46 (2003) 733–749.
[6] M. Guerin, T.S. Lassel, W. Le Goff, M. Farnier, M.J. Chapman, Action of atorvastatin in combined hyperlipidemia: preferential reduction of cholesteryl ester transfer from HDL to VLDL1 particles, Arterioscler. Thromb. Vasc. Biol. 20 (2000) 189–197.
[7] P. Berk II, N. Hoogerbrugge, R.P. Stolk, A.H. Bootsma, H. Jansen, Atorvastatin dose-dependently decreases hepatic lipase activity in type 2 diabetes: effect of sex and the LIPC promoter variant, Diabetes Care 26 (2003) 427–432.
[8] B.F. Asztalos, K.V. Horvath, J.R. McNamara, P.S. Roheim, J.J. Rubinstein, E.J. Schaefer, Comparing the effects of five different statins on the HDL subpopulation profiles of coronary heart disease patients, Atherosclerosis 164 (2002) 361–369.
[9] The DALI Investigators, The effect of aggressive versus standard lipid lowering by atorvastatin on diabetic dyslipidemia: the DALI study: a double-blind, randomized, placebo-controlled trial in patients with type 2 diabetes and diabetic dyslipidemia, Diabetes Care 24 (2001) 1335–1341.
[10] M. Guerin, P. Egger, C. Soudant, W. Le Goff, A. Van Tol, R. Dupuis, M.J. Chapman, Dose-dependent action of atorvastatin in type IIB hyperlipidemia: preferential and progressive reduction of atherogenic apoB-containing lipoprotein subclasses (VLDL-2, IDL, small dense LDL) and stimulation of cellular cholesterol efflux, Atherosclerosis 163 (2002) 287–296.
[11] S.J. Robins, D. Collins, J.T. Wittes, V. Papademetriou, P.C. Deedwania, E.J. Schaefer, J.R. McNamara, M.L. Kashyap, J.M. Hershman, L.F. Wexler, H.B. Rubins, Relation of gemfibrozil treatment and lipid levels with major coronary events: VA-HIT: a randomized controlled trial, JAMA 285 (2001) 1585–1591.
[12] M.J. Chapman, M. Guerin, E. Bruckert, Atherogenic, dense low-density lipoproteins. Pathophysiology and new therapeutic approaches, Eur. Heart J. 19 (Suppl. A) (1998) A24–A30.
[13] G.A. Francis, High density lipoprotein oxidation: in vitro susceptibility and potential in vivo consequences, Biochim. Biophys. Acta 1483 (2000) 217–235.

International Congress Series 1262 (2004) 507–510

www.ics-elsevier.com

Triglycerides rich lipoproteins and atherosclerosis: in vitro and in vivo studies

G.D. Norata[a], S. Raselli[b], L. Grigore[b], F.M. Maggi[a,b], A.L. Catapano[a,b,*]

[a] *Department of Pharmacological Sciences, University of Milan, Milan, Italy*
[b] *Centro per lo Studio e la Prevenzione delle Vasculopatie Periferiche, Ospedale Bassini, Cinisello Balsamo, Italy*

Abstract. The molecular mechanisms underlying the relationship between elevated plasma concentration of triglyceride-rich lipoproteins and coronary artery disease remain uncertain; evidence is accumulating to suggest that endothelial dysfunction is involved. In the present work, we addressed two major questions: First, we investigated the gene expression pattern and intracellular pathways in human endothelial cells incubated with very low density lipoproteins (VLDL) and oxidative modified VLDL (Ox-VLDL). Second, we investigated whether changes in RLP plasma levels during the postprandial phase relate to alterations of the endothelial function. *Results and conclusion:* Among 8411 genes spotted on the array, 1620 (19.2%) were expressed under basal condition. VLDL predominantly activated the ERK1/2 pathway while P38 MAPK was the main target of Ox-VLDL, and CREB and NF-KB were activated by both VLDL and Ox-VLDL. VLDL induced MMP-2 and TGF alpha expression. Ox-VLDL was found to induce IL-15 and MIF expression, promote the generation of reactive oxygen species and exert a cytotoxic effect, thus sustaining inflammation and endothelial damage. These findings confirm the involvement of VLDL and Ox-VLDL in endothelial dysfunction and suggest new genes and molecular mechanisms involved in these actions. Moreover, cholesterol in RLPs contributes significantly to the endothelial dysfunction occurring during the postprandial lipemia.

Keywords: Endothelial cells; Gene expression; Triglycerides; Postprandial phase

1. Introduction

Hypertriglyceridaemia is considered a risk factor for CVD [1]. Although the molecular mechanisms for the relationship between elevated triglyceride-rich lipoproteins and CVD remain uncertain, evidence is accumulating to suggest that endothelial dysfunction is involved [2,3]. Triglyceride-rich lipoproteins can cross the endothelial barrier and enter the arterial wall, placing them in a position where they may promote endothelial damage [4].

* Corresponding author. Department of Pharmacological Sciences, University of Milan, Via Balzaretti, 9, Milan, 20133, Italy. Tel.: +39-2-50318302; fax:. +39-2-50318386.
E-mail address: Alberico.Catapano@unimi.it (A.L. Catapano).

0531-5131/
doi:10.1016/j.ics.2003.12.040

Studies aimed at characterising the endothelial response to triglyceride-rich lipoproteins are required to distinguish how these lipoproteins contribute to the pathophysiology of atherosclerosis. In the present study, we investigated the gene expression pattern in human endothelial cells incubated with very low density lipoproteins (VLDL). Moreover, as VLDL can enter the arterial wall [4] and undergo oxidative modification [5], we compared the VLDL-induced expression pattern with the one of Ox-VLDL.

2. Materials and methods

VLDL was isolated from fresh plasma from normolipidaemic subjects by preparative ultracentrifugation as described [6].

The Eahy 926 line [6], a hybridoma cell line with the characteristics of human endothelial cells, which is widely used as a model of macrovascular endothelium, was cultured and HUVEC were cultured as described [6–8].

Total RNA extraction, retrotranscription, hybridization for the microarray analysis and data analysis was performed as described [6–8].

The immunoblotting was performed as described [9]. ROS was measured as described [6]. Cell viability was evaluated after exposure to VLDL or Ox-VLDL using the MTT test and the LDH release assay [6]. Nuclear morphology was analysed with the fluorescent dye bisbenzimide (Hoechst 33258) as described [9].

For the in vivo studies, 15 patients, all men, with moderate mixed dyslipidemia, were recruited into the study. Fasted patients were given an oral fat load (OFL) and blood samples were collected before the OFL ingestion (T0) and 2, 4, 6, 8 h (T2, T4, T6, T8) thereafter. Cholesterol in RLPs (C-RLPs) was measured after isolation of the fraction by immuno-affinity. Endothelial function, determined as flow-mediated dilatation of the brachial artery (FMD), was assessed at the same time points.

3. Results and discussion

To investigate whether the gene expression in VLDL-treated cells or in Ox-VLDL-treated cells correlate with the expression levels of the individual genes in control cells, the average intensities from four separate experiments in VLDL-treated cells or in Ox-VLDL-treated cells were plotted in a regression analysis against the average intensities of the individual genes from four separate experiments in control cells. The overall gene expressions were highly correlated ($R^2 = 0.85$ for VLDL and $R^2 = 0.87$ for Ox-VLDL) between stimulated and control cells at an interval of approximately three orders of magnitude, however, some genes deviated from the main trend. An agglomerative cluster analysis was used to identify the typical response patterns and establish the relationships between the different gene expression profiles. Seven clusters resulted from the analysis.

The activation of the endothelium is a crucial step in the recruitment of immune cells to the vessel wall. Adhesion molecules play a key role in the early stages of atherosclerosis and the plasma concentrations of soluble adhesion molecules are elevated in individuals with hypertriglyceridaemia. ECs incubated with VLDL showed an increased expression of major histocompatibility complex class II DR beta 5, integrin alpha M, a disintegrin and metalloproteinase domain 15 (ADAM 15) (2.11 ± 1.13) and CD38, all potentially connected with cell–cell adhesion. Of note, toll-like receptor 4, recently identified in atherosclerotic lesions, was increased by VLDL treatment suggesting another mechanism involved in the endothelial cell activation by VLDL. Several growth factors, cytokines, and chemokines and their receptors have been shown to be induced by VLDL and Ox-VLDL as the small inducible cytokine subfamily A member 21, a potent chemoattractant for lymphocytes, the interleukin 12 receptor beta 1 and interleukin 15 (IL-15), a cytokine recently discovered in mouse and human atherosclerotic lesions.

Oxidative stress has been proposed to be a link between the triglyceride-rich lipoproteins and endothelial damage. Ox-VLDL induced the expression of several stress response proteins such as peroxiredoxin 1, glutathione-S-transferase like and the heat shock 27-kDa protein 1. In addition, Ox-VLDL induced the expression of proteins that modulate apoptotic cell death, and upregulated the expression of several DNA damage signaling/repair proteins such as three prime repair exonuclease 2 excision repair cross-complementing rodent repair and RAD23 homolog B. Overall, this suggests a cytotoxic role of Ox-VLDL on endothelial cells. Native VLDL instead induced the expression of small GTP binding protein Rac1, MAPKKK-1, cyclin-dependent kinase 2, myeloid cell nuclear differentiation antigen and serum-inducible kinase, all involved in cell proliferation. This suggests a pro-proliferating role of VLDL in endothelial cells, which is in agreement with recent findings in smooth muscle cells. These findings are also supported by the observation that Ox-VLDL induced a massive ROS generation in ECs while in VLDL-treated cells, the ROS generation was even lower than that observed in control cells. Moreover, the analysis of LDH release and MTT transformation showed that Ox-VLDL induces cell death while VLDL showed an opposite effect. Also, the analysis of cell and nucleus morphology only showed the presence of blebbing and shirking in cells incubated with Ox-VLDL.

In conclusion, we studied the modulation of gene expression in human endothelial cells by VLDL or Ox-VLDL. The expression of several genes implicated in EC activation and damage/proliferation was found to be perturbed confirming ECs as the site of the dysfunction observed in vivo during hypertriglyceridaemia. Different intracellular kinases as well as transcription factors may play a key role in the modulation of the downstream events induced by VLDL, or Ox-VLDL suggesting that these lipoproteins have different targets for the regulation of gene expression.

Under in vivo conditions, the endothelium could face both VLDL and Ox-VLDL, thus, the overall effect could be different from area to area depending on the pro-oxidant microenvironment that promotes conversion of VLDL to Ox-VLDL. We studied the effects of postprandial lipemia on endothelial function, in vivo triglyceridemia peaked between T4 (485 ± 56 mg/dl) and T6 (473 ± 79 mg/dl) and decreased at 8 h (386 ± 77 mg/dl) after the Oral Frat Load (OFL). FMD decreased significantly 6 h after the OFL consumption (from $16.03 \pm 1.32\%$ to $11.53 \pm 1.42\%$, $p<0.01$). Cholesterol in RLPs increased steadily up to 6 h and decreased at 8 h (T0 20.59 ± 3.97, T6 31.11 ± 4.41, T8 28.37 ± 4.95 mg/dl). Fasting levels of TG and C-RLPs correlated significantly with FMD at the baseline. The decrease in endothelial function at 6 h also significantly correlated with the AUC of TG ($R=0.53$, $p=0.04$). Postprandial C-RLPs (AUC), however, showed the best correlation with the decrease of FMD ($R=0.63$, $p=0.012$). The correlation persisted in a multivariate analysis.

We conclude that C-RLPs contribute significantly to the endothelial dysfunction occurring during the postprandial lipemia.

Acknowledgements

We thank Per Eriksson, Karolinska Hospital, Stochkolm for helpful discussions.

References

[1] A.M. Gotto, Triglyceride, The forgotten risk factor, Circulation 97 (1998) 1027–1028.
[2] P. Lundman, M. Eriksson, K. Schenck-Gustafsson, F. Karpe, P. Tornvall, Transient tryglyceridemia decreases vascular reactivity in young, healthy men without risk factors for coronary heart disease, Circulation 96 (1997) 3266–3268.
[3] N. Sattar, J.R. Petrie, A.J. Jaap, The atherogenic lipoprotein phenotype and vascular endothelial dysfunction, Atherosclerosis 138 (1998) 229–235.
[4] B.G. Nordestagaard, R. Wooton, B. Lewis, Selective retention of VLDL, IDL and LDL in the arterial intima of genetically hyperlipidaemic rabbits in vivo, Arterioscler. Thromb. Vasc. Biol. 15 (1995) 534–542.
[5] S. Parthasarathy, M.T. Quinn, D.C. Schewenke, T. Carew, D. Steinberg, Oxidative modification of beta-very low density lipoprotein: potential role in monocyte reruitment and foam cell formation, Arteriosclerosis 9 (1989) 398–404.
[6] G.D. Norata, A. Pirillo, E. Callegari, A. Hamsten, A.L. Catapano, P. Eriksson, Gene expression and intracellular pathways involved in endothelial dysfunction induced by VLDL and oxidised VLDL, Cardiovasc. Res. 59 (2003) 169–180.
[7] G.D. Norata, F. Pellegatta, A. Hamsten, A.L. Catapano, P. Eriksson, Effects of high density lipoprotein subfraction 3 on the expression of matrix-degrading proteases in human endothelial cells, Int. J. Mol. Med. 12 (2003) 73–78.
[8] G.D. Norata, H. Bjork, A. Hamsten, A.L. Catapano, P. Eriksson, High density lipoprotein decrease ADAMTs1 expression induced by LPS and TNFα in human endothelial cells, Matrix Biol. (in press).
[9] G.D. Norata, L. Tonti, P. Roma, A.L. Catapano, Apoptosis and proliferation of endothelial cells in early atherosclerotic lesions: a possible role for oxidized LDL, NMCD, Nutr. Metab. Cardiovasc. Dis. 12 (2002) 297–305.

ELSEVIER

International Congress Series 1262 (2004) 511–514

www.ics-elsevier.com

Dyslipidaemia, inflammation and endothelial dysfunction in diabetes mellitus

Kathryn Tan*

Department of Medicine, University of Hong Kong, Queen Mary Hospital, Pokfulam Road, Hong Kong, Hong Kong

Abstract. Endothelial dysfunction is an early event in atherogenesis and precedes the thickening of the intima and the formation of atherosclerotic plaques. Endothelial dysfunction has also been implicated in the pathogenesis of both micro- and macroangiopathy in diabetes and has been consistently demonstrated in patients with type 1 and type 2 diabetes mellitus. Markers of endothelial dysfunction (e.g. von Willebrand factor, vascular cell adhesion molecules) are elevated in patients with diabetes mellitus, and vasodilation mediated by endothelium-derived nitric oxide is impaired. The aetiology of endothelial dysfunction in diabetes is complex and it has been shown that more than one mechanism is involved. We and others have demonstrated that diabetic dyslipidaemia plays a significant role. The increase in the concentration of small, dense LDL, enhanced susceptibility of LDL to oxidation and exaggerated postprandial lipidaemia found in patients with type 2 diabetes mellitus are associated with impairment of endothelium-dependent vasodilation. We have shown that treatment with atorvastatin improves, but does not completely normalize, endothelial function in patients with type 2 diabetes. In addition to lowering LDL cholesterol, atorvastatin also lowers C-reactive protein (CRP) levels. The magnitude of reduction in CRP correlates with the degree of improvement in endothelium-dependent vasodilation, suggesting that chronic, low-grade inflammation may also be involved in causing endothelial dysfunction. Chronic inflammation is associated with activation of the endothelium and both dyslipidaemia and advanced glycation end products are important triggers for inflammation in diabetes mellitus. Hence, dyslipidaemia, chronic low-grade inflammation and endothelial dysfunction are interrelated and contribute to high cardiovascular risk in subjects with diabetes.

Keywords: Diabetes mellitus; Endothelial dysfunction; Dyslipidaemia; Inflammation

1. Introduction

Endothelial dysfunction is an early marker of cardiovascular disease and has been demonstrated in many states associated with atherosclerosis, such as hypertension,

* Tel.: +852-2855-4769; fax: +852-2816-2187.
E-mail address: kcbtan@hkucc.hku.hk (K. Tan).

doi:10.1016/j.ics.2003.11.028

hypercholesterolaemia, smoking and diabetes [1]. Since abnormalities of vascular reactivity in peripheral circulation are known to be correlated with abnormalities in coronary circulation, endothelial function can be assessed in clinical studies by measuring the vascular reactivity of various peripheral arteries. Changes in the diameter of the blood vessels are determined following stimulation of the endothelium with vasoactive substances or shear stress. Biochemical markers of endothelial activity (e.g. von Willebrand factor, vascular adhesion molecules), which are secreted by the endothelium or shed from its surface in disease states, are also useful indicators of endothelial function.

2. Endothelial dysfunction in diabetes

Endothelial dysfunction has been consistently demonstrated in animal models of diabetes, as well as in patients with type 1 and type 2 diabetes. There was a blunting of the normal vasodilatory response to acetylcholine in isolated arteries from diabetic animals [2]. The defect was at the level of the endothelium rather than reduced sensitivity of the smooth muscle to nitric oxide (NO) because responses of pre-constricted arteries to nitrovasodilators were normal. Clinical studies using venous occlusive forearm plethysmography or high-resolution vascular ultrasound have shown that endothelium-dependent vasodilation is abnormal in both type 1 and type 2 diabetic patients [3,4]. We have measured endothelium-dependent vasodilation in over 200 type 2 diabetic patients using vascular ultrasound. Endothelium-dependent vasodilation was impaired in patients without clinical evidence of diabetic complications (5.4% ± 2.7, $p < 0.01$), in those with microalbuminuria (5.2% ± 2.9, $p < 0.01$), and in those with one or more diabetic complications (4.9% ± 2.4, $p < 0.01$) compared with nondiabetic controls (9.1% ± 3.7). Studies using plasma levels of endothelium-dependent haemostatic factors as an indicator of endothelial dysfunction have also shown similar results [5,6]. Hence, significant abnormalities of endothelial function are present in diabetic patients with or without clinical evidence of vascular complications and it has been suggested that endothelial dysfunction contributes to the pathogenesis of both micro- and macroangiopathy in diabetes [7].

3. Diabetic dyslipidaemia and endothelial dysfunction

A number of factors contribute to the aetiology of endothelial dysfunction in diabetes and diabetic dyslipidaemia has been shown to play an important role. In patients with type 2 diabetes, dyslipidaemia is characterised by hypertriglyceridemia, low HDL and a preponderance of small, dense LDL particles. Watts et al. reported that endothelial dysfunction was independently related to the degree of dyslipidaemia in type 2 diabetes and that small LDL particle size was associated with endothelial dysfunction in these patients [4]. Small, dense LDL particles were more susceptible to oxidation and we have shown that the concentration of small, dense LDL particles and their rate of oxidation ex vivo were independent determinants of endothelium-dependent vasodilation in type 2 diabetic patients [8]. Triglyceride-rich lipoproteins and their remnants can also cause activation of the endothelial cells, and the concentration of remnant lipoproteins inversely correlated with endothelial function [9].

Data from recent randomized, double-blind, placebo-controlled trials suggest that treatment of diabetic dyslipidaemia can lead to an improvement in endothelial function.

Evans et al. reported that ciprofibrate therapy attenuated postprandial lipidaemia and the associated oxidative stress and improved fasting and postprandial endothelial function in type 2 diabetes [10]. We have shown that treatment with atorvastatin also leads to a significant improvement in endothelium-dependent vasodilation in type 2 diabetic patients [11]. Plasma C-reactive protein (CRP) significantly decreased in the atorvastatin-treated group and the percentage change in endothelium-dependent vasodilation correlated with the percentage change in CRP, suggesting that the improvement in endothelium-dependent vasodilation might be partly mediated by the anti-inflammatory effect of atorvastatin.

4. Inflammation and endothelial dysfunction in diabetes

Available evidence suggests that inflammatory processes are involved in the pathogenesis of endothelial dysfunction and atherosclerosis. Levels of CRP, a marker of systemic inflammation, are elevated in patients with impaired glucose tolerance and in those with type 2 diabetes [11,12]. Correlations between CRP and markers of endothelial dysfunction have been reported in both type 1 and type 2 diabetic patients [11,13]. In a recent prospective study of type 2 diabetic patients, inflammatory activity and endothelial dysfunction both increased over time and these increases were strongly interrelated [14]. Factors that may contribute to the state of inflammation in the vasculature in diabetes include oxidative stress, an activated renin angiotensin system, hyperglycaemia, advanced glycation end products and oxidized LDL. Both ongoing intra-arterial inflammation and extravascular stimuli can induce a low level activation of acute phase response, leading to an increase in inflammatory parameters like CRP. In turn, CRP may act not only as a marker of cardiovascular disease but may also have biological properties that cause endothelial dysfunction. In vitro studies have shown that CRP has a direct proinflammatory effect on human endothelial cells and affects endothelial function [15].

5. Conclusion

The aetiology of endothelial dysfunction in diabetes mellitus is complex and involves a number of factors. Whether endothelial function can be used as a surrogate therapeutic target to reduce cardiovascular disease and improve clinical outcomes in patients with diabetes remains to be determined, and prospective studies designed to correlate improvement in endothelial function with improvement in outcome will be required.

Acknowledgements

This work was supported by grants from the Hong Kong Research Grants Council (HKU 483/96M, HKU7350/02M).

References

[1] T.J. Anderson, Nitric oxide, atherosclerosis and the clinical relevance of endothelial dysfunction, Heart Fail. Rev. 8 (1) (2003) 71–86.

[2] L. Rodriguez-Manas, J. Angulo, C. Peiro, et al., Endothelial dysfunction and metabolic control in streptozotocin-induced diabetic rats, Br. J. Pharmacol. 123 (8) (1998) 1495–1502.

[3] P. Clarkson, D.S. Celermajer, A.E. Donald, et al., Impaired vascular reactivity in insulin-dependent diabetes

mellitus is related to disease duration and low density lipoprotein cholesterol levels, J. Am. Coll. Cardiol. 28 (3) (1996) 573–579.

[4] G.F. Watts, S.F. O'Brien, W. Silvester, J.A. Millar, Impaired endothelium-dependent and independent dilatation of forearm resistance arteries in men with diet-treated non-insulin-dependent diabetes: role of dyslipidaemia, Clin. Sci. (Lond.) 91 (5) (1996) 567–573.

[5] M. Greaves, R.G. Malia, K. Goodfellow, et al., Fibrinogen and von Willebrand factor in IDDM: relationships to lipid vascular risk factors, blood pressure, glycaemic control and urinary albumin excretion rate: the EURODIAB IDDM complications study, Diabetologia 40 (6) (1997) 698–705.

[6] M. Koga, M. Otsuki, M. Kubo, J. Hashimoto, S. Kasayama, Relationship between circulating vascular cell adhesion molecule-1 and microvascular complications in type 2 diabetes mellitus, Diabet. Med. 15 (8) (1998) 661–667.

[7] C.D. Stehouwer, J. Lambert, A.J. Donker, V.W. van Hinsbergh, Endothelial dysfunction and pathogenesis of diabetic angiopathy, Cardiovasc. Res. 34 (1) (1997) 55–68.

[8] K.C. Tan, V.H. Ai, W.S. Chow, et al., Influence of low density lipoprotein (LDL) subfraction profile and LDL oxidation on endothelium-dependent and independent vasodilation in patients with type 2 diabetes, J. Clin. Endocrinol. Metab. 84 (9) (1999) 3212–3216.

[9] K. Kugiyama, H. Doi, T. Motoyama, et al., Association of remnant lipoprotein levels with impairment of endothelium-dependent vasomotor function in human coronary arteries, Circulation 97 (25) (1998) 2519–2526.

[10] M. Evans, R.A. Anderson, J. Graham, et al., Ciprofibrate therapy improves endothelial function and reduces postprandial lipemia and oxidative stress in type 2 diabetes mellitus, Circulation 101 (15) (2000) 1773–1779.

[11] K.C. Tan, W.S. Chow, S.C. Tam, et al., Atorvastatin lowers C-reactive protein and improves endothelium-dependent vasodilation in type 2 diabetes mellitus, J. Clin. Endocrinol. Metab. 87 (2) (2002) 563–568.

[12] K.C. Tan, N.M. Wat, S.C. Tam, et al., C-reactive protein predicts the deterioration of glycemia in Chinese subjects with impaired glucose tolerance, Diabetes Care 26 (8) (2003) 2323–2328.

[13] C.G. Schalkwijk, D.C. Poland, W. van Dijk, et al., Plasma concentration of C-reactive protein is increased in type I diabetic patients without clinical macroangiopathy and correlates with markers of endothelial dysfunction: evidence for chronic inflammation, Diabetologia 42 (3) (1999) 351–357.

[14] C.D. Stehouwer, M.A. Gall, J.W. Twisk, et al., Increased urinary albumin excretion, endothelial dysfunction, and chronic low-grade inflammation in type 2 diabetes: progressive, interrelated, and independently associated with risk of death, Diabetes 51 (4) (2002) 1157–1165.

[15] V. Pasceri, J.T. Willerson, E.T. Yeh, Direct proinflammatory effect of C-reactive protein on human endothelial cells, Circulation 102 (18) (2000) 2165–2168.

International Congress Series 1262 (2004) 515–518

ELSEVIER

www.ics-elsevier.com

What are certified scientific findings in HRT? Shall we proceed?

Toshio Hayashi*

Department of Geriatrics, Nagoya University Graduate School of Medicine, 65 Tsuruma-cho, Showaku, Nagoya, Japan

Abstract. During the last 3 years, especially in the last year following the publication of Women's Health Initiative, WHI, many papers reported the ineffectiveness or risk of side effects of hormone replacement therapy (HRT), which is the opposite of previous papers. I have categorized my topic into four parts: (1) megaclinical studies such as PEPI, Nurse's Health Study (NHS), HERS and WHI, (2) the effect of HRT on ischemic cardiovascular disease, (3) the effect of HRT on breast cancer, and (4) the effect of HRT on other disorders such as dementia, quality of life (QOL) and diabetes. Conclusion: Usual HRT using premalin and medroxyprogesterone is not recommended in general (for Asians).

Keywords: Hormone replacement therapy; Estradiol; Megaclinical study

1. Megaclinical study

Below is a brief summary of recent megaclinical studies such as Nurse's Health Study (NHS), HERS and Women's Health Initiative (WHI; Table 1). The Nurse's Health Study may be one of the first megaclinical studies about hormone replacement therapy (HRT) [1]. It is an observational study and the kind of hormone was not considered. However, the number was more than 120,000. The subjects are nurses aged 30 to 55. It reported the risk of coronary heart disease (CHD), especially the mortality decrease which is less than 50% compared with control. However, death from all causes and cancer, including breast cancer, all decreased. These data are subsequently contrasted with other prospective megaclinical studies. That is why the characteristic background of this study, which the subject being nurses, may be relevant. HERS study is a double-blind study against placebo control RCT [2]. There were less than 80 subjects. During the follow-up of 4.1 years, treatment with oral conjugated equine estrogen plus medroxyprogesterone acetate did not reduce the overall rate of CHD events in postmenopausal women with established coronary disease. The treatment did increase the rate of thromboembolic events and gallbladder disease. They do not recommend starting this treatment for the purpose of

* Tel.: +81-52-744-2364; fax: +81-52-744-2371.
E-mail address: hayashi@med.nagoya-u.ac.jp (T. Hayashi).

0531-5131/
doi:10.1016/j.ics.2004.01.017

Table 1
Outline of megaclinical studies of postmenopausal hormone replacement therapy

	Nurse's Health Study	HERS	HERS II	WHI
Literature	N. Engl. J. Med. 336 (1997) 1769–1775	JAMA 280 (1998) 605–613	JAMA 288 (2002) 49–57; JAMA 288 (2002) 58–66	JAMA 288 (2002) 321–333
Research design	Cohort Study	Double-blind against placebo control RCT	Open follow-up after HERS	Double-blind against placebo control RCT
Objectives	Nurse from 30 to 55 years old	50–79 years old, postmenopausal (66.7)	50–79 years old, postmenopausal	50–79 years old, postmenopausal
Number	121,700	2763	2321	16,607
History of CHD	None	+	+	Almost none
Hormone	Any	CEE 0.625 mg+MPA 2.5 mg	CEE 0.625 mg+MPA 2.5 mg (at 6th year, HRT 45%, placebo 8%)	CEE 0.625 mg+MPA 2.5 mg
Results	Less than 50%	No secondary prevention effect, stop at 4.1 years	No secondary prevention effect	No primary prevention effect

secondary prevention of CHD. However, HERS II, although an observational study, showed long-term use of HRT did not show beneficial effect [3]. The impact by Women's Health Initiative study was huge [4]. As you know, overall health risks exceeded benefits from use of combined estrogen plus progestin for an average of 5.2 years follow-up among healthy postmenopausal US women. All-cause mortality was not affected during the trial. The results indicate that this regimen should not be initiated or continued for primary prevention of CHD. However, I would like to point out that the proportion of Asians is only 2.3%. This might mean that the differences between races in the frequency of thrombosis formation are due to gene mutation.

In WHI, hypertensive patients were 36%, for statin, 7% and aspirin was prescribed in 20%. The results indicated that CHD, venous thromboembolic events (VTE) and breast cancer increased. However, colon cancer and femur fracture decreased. I would like to introduce one report (JAMA, 2002; 288:980–987), which reported that CRP and IL-6 independently predict vascular events among apparently healthy postmenopausal women, and that HRT increases CRP. However, use or nonuse of HRT had less importance as a predictor of cardiovascular risk than did baseline levels of either CRP or IL-6.

2. The effect of HRT on ischemic cardiovascular disease

The Nurses' Health Study shows the risk of major coronary heart disease by HRT as a secondary prevention of CHD. The patients receiving HRT for many years show more cardioprotective effect. Relative risk is 1.06 in the less-than-1-year group and 0.38 in longer than 2 years. It also shows the data as a primary prevention. The effect decreases when the HRT is used for longer than 5 years (1–4.9 years, 0.47; 5–9.9 years, 0.51). However, for longer than 10 years, relative risk is 0.69. Stroke did not decrease. Conjugated estrogen (0.3 mg) is also effective in US. In HERS and HERS II, for CHD events, death and nonfatal myocardial infarction, the curves are truncated at year 7 when less than half of the cohort remains in follow-up. Venous thromboembolic events are a major problem in HRT, as with Factor V Leiden mutation for those who were treated with

HRT. The estimated absolute incidence of VTE in women with the mutation who receive HRT was 15.4 per 1000 per year compared with 2.0 of 1000 per year in women without the mutation who were taking placebo. In women with coronary disease, the screening test for V Leiden is necessary to avoid an HRT-associated VTE.

WHI shows that Estrogen plus progestin does not confer cardiac protection and may increase the risk of CHD among generally healthy postmenopausal women, especially during the first year after the initiation of hormone use. Interestingly, in usage longer than 6 years, the ratio decreased less than 1, in other words, 0.7. Further, lipid profile and insulin sensitivity improved with HRT.

The risk of CHD according to biomarker levels was also studied. Age did not have an effect. Shorter term than menopause, hot flush and medication of aspirin and statin use show better for HRT against the CHD disease. Normolipidemia and low fibrinogen are also better for HRT, however CRP was known to increase with HRT and the subjects with high CRP should not become indication for HRT.

3. The effect of HRT on breast cancer

The effect of breast cancer is greater than 1, and endometrial cancer, colorectal cancer and fracture is less than 1. Several meta-analysis data show that benefits of HRT include prevention of osteoporotic fractures and colorectal cancer, while prevention of dementia is uncertain. PEPI study showed the increase in BI–RADS density grade. In other words, there is risk and necessity to check the frequent screening of breast cancer. WHI data conclude that relatively short-term HRT increases the incident of breast cancers, which are diagnosed at a more advanced stage compared with placebo use, and also substantially increases the percentage of women with abnormal mammograms. As what the WHI study shows, progesterone may increase the risk of breast cancer.

4. The other problems such as cognitive function, QOL and diabetes

As an ancillary study of the WHI study, WHI memory study was published. Mean Modified Mini-Mental State Examination (MMSE) Score by treatment assignment showed no significant difference with HRT. Similarly, mean Modified MMSE Score of patients diagnosed as having probable dementia showed no effect with HRT. Quality of life (QOL) was evaluated by HERS and WHI. The trial concluded that HRT has mixed effects on quality of life among older women. The effects of hormone therapy depend on the presence of menopausal symptoms; women without flushing had greater declines in physical measures, while women with flushing had improvements in emotional measures of quality of life. WHI showed data in QOL Scores from Baseline to Year 1. Depression scores, scores for sleep disturbance and scores for satisfaction with sex were rescaled from 0 (worst) to 100 (best). HRT did not show meaningful effect on health-related quality of life. The effects of glucose tolerance in WHI and HERS were shown. In impaired glucose tolerance and diabetics, at the start, HRT showed beneficial effect all over the trial term. In Ontario, Canada, for patients older than 65 years, the number of new users of ERT increased steadily until the publication of the HERS study, after which it began to decrease, and the decline accelerated in the third quarter of 2002, being significantly less than that predicted by the model (p=0.02). Almost all HRT in these data are conjugated ethynyl estrogen, which is mainly estrone, and progesterone. The effect of estrone is quite different from estradiol. Estrogen has pleiotropic effect, e.g., activates endothelial NO synthase. However, it is a biphasic effect on concentration [5]. Estradiol activates eNOS in various sites of cell signaling [6,7], e.g., promoter, stabilization of mRNA, acylation, calmodulin, number of caveolae and decrease of superoxide anion, in NADPH oxidase.

Estiriol improves flow-mediated dilatation (FMD) in octogenarian for 2 years. It also increased NOx and cGMP. This paper summarizes that longer safe treatment is hopeful if HRT should be used for the prevention of atherosclerosis (secondary prevention: longer than 2–4 years; primary prevention: longer than 6 years [WHI] and shorter than 10 years [NHS]). Low dose is also preferable. Factor V Leiden, CRP and IL-6 are also important markers before HRT. Progesterone may increase the risk of breast cancer. Dementia and QOL did not improve.

In conclusion, usual HRT using premalin and medroxyprogesterone is not recommended in general (for Asians).

References

[1] F. Grodstein, M. Stampfer, A. Graham, et al., Postmenopausal hormone therapy and mortality. Nurse' health study, N. Engl. J. Med. 336 (1997) 1769–1776.

[2] S. Hulley, D. Grady, et al., Heart and Estrogen/Progestin Replacement Study Research Group, Randomized trial of estrogen plus progestin for secondary prevention of coronary heart disease in postmenopausal women, JAMA 280 (1998) 605–613.

[3] D. Grady, D. Herrington, et al., HERS Research Group, Cardiovascular disease outcomes during 6.8 years of hormone therapy: heart and estrogen/progestin replacement study follow-up (HERS II), JAMA 288 (2002) 49–57.

[4] Writing Group for the Women's Health Initiative Investigators, Risks and benefits of estrogen plus progestin in healthy postmenopausal women: principal results from the women's health initiative randomized controlled trial, JAMA 288 (2002) 321–333.

[5] T. Hayashi, K. Yamda, T. Esaki, M. Kuzuya, A. Iguchi, Estrogen increases endothelial nitric oxide by a receptor mediated system, Biochem. Biophys. Res. Commun. 214 (1995) 847–855.

[6] D. Sumi, T. Hayashi, A. Iguchi, Estrogen prevents destabilization of endothelial nitric oxide synthase mRNA induced by tumor necrosis factor alpha through estrogen receptor mediated system, Life Sci. 69 (2001) 1651–1660.

[7] T. Hayashi, A. Iguchi, The long-term effect of estriol on endothelial function and bone mineral density in octogenarian women, J. Am. Geriatr. Soc. 50 (2002) 777–778.

International Congress Series 1262 (2004) 519–522

www.ics-elsevier.com

Hormone replacement therapy and atherosclerosis—postmenopausal women and HRT: the fallen myth of the cardiovascular protective effects of hormone replacement therapy

Emilio H. Moriguchi*, José Luiz C. Vieira

WHO/PAHO Collaborating Center for Prevention of Chronic Diseases Associated to Ageing, Pontifical Catholic University of Rio Grande do Sul,Porto Alegre, RS, Brazil

Keywords: Hormone replacement therapy; Atherosclerosis; Coronary heart disease; Cardiovascular prevention

The marked sex difference in risk of coronary heart disease (CHD) has been noted for many decades and was the impetus for early animal experiments of estrogen effects on atherosclerosis [1]. These studies demonstrated that estrogen could prevent atherogenesis in animal models for atherosclerosis. Moreover, in the last 2 decades of the last century, many observational studies have found lower prevalence of CHD both in women taking estrogen or estrogen/progestin than in women not receiving postmenopausal hormone replacement therapy (HRT) [2]. These results, besides the estrogen beneficial changes in intermediate markers such as lipid parameters [3,4], led to a belief that HRT could be an important weapon for preventing CHD.

Regardless of those strong experimental, observational and mechanistic evidences, no large clinical trials had been done to evaluate HRT protection against CHD until 5 years ago. Women taking hormone therapy in observational studies differ from non-users in many aspects like general health status, health awareness (they are "compliant" per definition), profile of coronary risk factors or socioeconomic status. Observational data are not convincing as results from randomized placebo-controlled trials, in which randomization hands out known and unknown biases in an even manner. Guiding therapy by mechanistic evidence is also not safe. The legacy of the CAST study has shown us that treating a patophysiologic processes (suppressing ventricular arrhythmia that is associated with sudden death) is not sufficient to warrant better outcome—patients can die with the surrogate outcome apparently corrected [5].

The results of the first large randomized trial evaluating HRT for prevention of CHD were published in 1998. The Heart and Estrogen/Progestin Replacement Study (HERS)

* Corresponding author. Tel.: +55-51-99012422; fax: +55-51-3315-9323.
E-mail address: emoriguc@pucrs.br (E.H. Moriguchi).

doi:10.1016/S0531-5131(03)01732-1

was a secondary prevention trial that showed no overall cardiovascular benefit and a pattern of early increase in risk of CHD events, with an increase in the rate of thromboembolic events and gallbladder disease for those assigned to 0.625 mg of conjugated equine estrogen (CEE) plus 2.5 mg of medroxyprogesterone acetate (MPA) daily versus those assigned to placebo [6]. Even the apparent time trend of fewer CHD events in years 3–5 did not persist during additional follow-up [7]. Data from earlier observational studies had already shown increase in risk for venous thromboembolism in women taking HRT [8,9]. The data of clinical trials demonstrate a similar increase, indicating a fourfold increase in the risk of thromboembolic events during the first year of use of HRT with a twofold increase during continuous use [6,10]. The selective estrogen receptor modulator raloxifen is associated with a similar risk [11]. The angiographic study Estrogen Replacement and Atherosclerosis (ERA) indicated no angiographic benefit on coronary lesion from either estrogen or estrogen/progestin therapy when compared to placebo [12]. The Papworth HRT atherosclerosis study of transdermal HRT for secondary prevention was stopped early due to a lack of apparent benefit and the possibility of harm (a non-significant 23% increase in the risk of death, myocardial infarction or unstable angina) [13].

The Women's Health Initiative (WHI) enrolled 161,000 predominantly healthy postmenopausal women of 50–79 years old and consists of three different studies: an observational study of 83,000 women to identify predictors of disease; a study of community approaches to developing healthful behaviors; and three randomized, placebo-controlled trials of 68,000 postmenopausal women—a HRT versus placebo trial for the prevention of heart disease; a low-fat dietary pattern trial for the prevention of breast and colorectal cancer; and calcium and vitamin D supplementation trial in the prevention of fractures due to osteoporosis. The HRT trial included two arms: 16,000 women with an intact uterus randomized to receive combined therapy (0.625/day of CEE plus 2.5 mg/day of MPA) versus placebo, and 10,700 women who had had a hysterectomy randomized to receive the same dose of CEE alone or placebo. The same regimen used in HERS was selected for the combined arm as the hormone preparation most commonly used by American women.

During both years of 2000 and 2001, the Data Safety and Monitoring Board recommended reporting to the participants that women taking HRT (in both estrogen and estrogen/progestin arms) had a small increase in cardiovascular events, including myocardial infarction, stroke, deep venous thrombosis and pulmonary embolism, but the increases did not meet statistical criteria for stopping the trial. In July 2002, the estrogen/progestin arm of the WHI hormone trial was discontinued after 5.6 years of the planned 8.5-year trial because women in the hormone treated group were at statistically significant increased risk for myocardial infarction, stroke, pulmonary embolism and breast cancer compared with women receiving placebo, and these risks outweighed the benefits of combined hormone therapy on colon cancer and fractures due to osteoporosis. The results have shown increased risk of CHD (HR, 1.29; 95% CI, 1.02–1.63), stroke (HR, 1.41; 95% CI, 1.07–1.85) and pulmonary embolism (HR, 2.13; 95% CI, 1.39–3.25) [10]. Similar cardiovascular results were found in the final analysis [14]. As the WHI authors have suggested, due to a high rate of discontinuation of therapy, the reported results of the intention-to-treatment analysis may have underestimated the overall harm among women who adhered to treatment. In fact, we could speculate that if an on-treatment criterion was used for interim analysis of harm, maybe the WHI trial would have been stopped 2 years before when a non-significant increase in cardiovascular events associated with active treatment was detected.

Although unopposed estrogen has revealed a non-significant increase in cardiovascular risk on interim analysis, its effect on the prevention of cardiovascular disease is still being evaluated with the ongoing estrogen arm of the WHI. However, if the results of observational studies already had pointed in the past similar effects of "cardioprotection" for both therapies, should we expect that only the results of combined therapy were misleading?

Women are more likely than men to die of stroke, despite of similar stroke rates. In observational studies, HRT has not been consistently linked to stroke prevention. The first clinical trial of HRT in postmenopausal women with previous stroke do not demonstrate reduction in the risk of recurrence of stroke, and even suggested increased risk for fatal stroke [15]. The analysis of the effect of estrogen/progestin effect on stroke rate in generally healthy postmenopausal women of the WHI combined arm have indicated a 31% increase of risk of stroke when compared to placebo. When adjusted for adherence, the increase in risk of stroke raised to 50% [16].

Besides the negative impact of HRT on cardiovascular and cerebrovascular risk, there are recent evidences bringing up more concerns. Recent data showed that estrogen plus progestin therapy increased significantly the risk for probable dementia in postmenopausal women aged 65 years or older [17,18]. Same study data showed also no clinically meaningful effect of HRT on health-related quality of life for postmenopausal women [19]. In conclusion, the set of recent evidences supports the conclusion that the risks of estrogen plus progestin therapy outweigh the benefits for women's health.

Evidence-based medicine has demonstrated that the risk of cardiovascular disease in women can be reduced like in men with the use of beta-blockers, aspirin, statins and ACE inhibitors. The evidence cumulated in the last years is sufficient to warrant recommendation against the use of HRT as a preventive measure for cardiovascular disease both in primary or secondary prevention.

References

[1] E. Barrett-Connor, T. Bush, Estrogen and coronary heart disease in women, JAMA 265 (1991) 1861–1867.

[2] E. Barrett-Connor, D. Grady, Hormone replacement therapy, heart disease, and other considerations, Annu. Rev. Public Health 19 (1998) 55–72.

[3] M.E. Mendelsohn, R.H. Karas, The protective effects of estrogen on the cardiovascular system, N. Engl. J. Med. 343 (1999) 1801–1811.

[4] I.F. Godsland, Effects of postmenopausal hormone replacement therapy on lipid, lipoprotein, and apolipoprotein (a) concentrations: analysis of studies published from 1974–2000, Fertil. Steril. 75 (2001) 898–915.

[5] D.S. Echt, P.R. Liebson, B. Mitchell, et al., Mortality and morbidity in patients receiving encainamide, flecainide, or placebo: the Cardiac Arrythmia Supression Trial, N. Engl. J. Med. 324 (1991) 781–788.

[6] S. Hulley, D. Grady, T. Bush, et al., Randomized trial of estrogen plus progestin for secondary prevention of coronary heart disease in postmenopausal women, JAMA 280 (1998) 605–613.

[7] D. Grady, D. Herrington, V. Bittner, et al., Cardiovascular disease outcomes during 6.8 years of hormone therapy. Heart and Estrogen/progestin Replacement Study Follow-up (HERS II), JAMA 288 (2002) 49–57.

[8] H. Jick, L. Derby, M. Myers, Risk of hospital admission for idiopathic venous thromboembolism among users of postmenopausal oestrogens, Lancet 348 (1996) 981–983.

[9] E. Daly, M.P. Vessey, M.M. Hawkins, J.L. Carson, P. Gough, S. Marsh, Risk of venous thromboembolism in users of hormone replacement therapy, Lancet 348 (1996) 977–980.

[10] Writing Group for the Women's Health Initiative Investigators, Risks and benefits of estrogen plus progestin in healthy postmenopausal women, JAMA 288 (2002) 321–333.

[11] B. Ettinger, D.M. Black, B.H. Mitlak, et al., Reduction of vertebral fracture risk in postmenopausal women with osteoporosis treated with raloxifene: results from a 3-year randomized clinical trial. Multiple Outcomes of Raloxifene Evaluation (MORE) Investigators, JAMA 282 (1999) 637–645.

[12] D.M. Herrington, D.M. Reboussin, B. Brosniham, et al., Effects of estrogen replacement on progression of coronary-artery atherosclerosis, N. Engl. J. Med. 343 (2000) 522–529.

[13] S.C. Clarke, J. Kelleher, H. Lloyd-Jones, M. Slack, P.M. Schofiel, A study of hormone replacement therapy in postmenopausal women with ischaemic heart disease: the Papworth HRT atherosclerosis study, BJOG 109 (2002) 1056–1062.

[14] J.E. Manson, J. Hsia, K.C. Johnson, et al., Estrogen plus progestin and the risk of coronary heart disease, N. Engl. J. Med. 349 (2003) 523–534.

[15] C.M. Viscoli, L.M. Brass, W.N. Kernan, P.M. Sarrel, S. Suissa, R.I. Horwitz, A clinical trial of estrogen-replacement therapy after ischemic stroke, N. Engl. J. Med. 345 (2001) 1243–1249.

[16] S. Wassertheil-Smoller, S. Hendrix, M. Limacher, et al., Effect of estrogen plus progestin on stroke in postmenopausal women: the Women's Health Initiative: a randomized trial, JAMA 289 (2003) 2673–2684.

[17] S.A. Shumaker, C. Legault, L. Thal, et al., Estrogen plus progestin and the incidence of dementia and mild cognitive impairment in postmenopausal women: the Women's Health Initiative Memory Study: a randomized controlled trial, JAMA 289 (2003) 2651–2662.

[18] S.R. Rapp, M.A. Espeland, S.A. Shumaker, et al., Effect of estrogen plus progestin on global cognitive function in postmenopausal women: the Women's Health Initiative Memory Study: a randomized controlled trial, JAMA 289 (2003) 2663–2672.

[19] J. Hays, J.K. Ockene, R.L. Brunner, et al., Effects of estrogen plus progestin on health-related quality of life, N. Engl. J. Med. 348 (2003) 1839–1854.

International Congress Series 1262 (2004) 523–526

www.ics-elsevier.com

Hormone replacement therapy and cardiovascular disease

E. Windler*, B. Eidenmüller, B.-Chr. Zyriax

Universitätsklinikum Hamburg-Eppendorf, Martinistr. 52, 20246 Hamburg, Germany

Abstract. Replacement of estrogen is effective for relief of perimenopausal symptoms. This principle indication appears not to be in conflict with data indicating an increased cardiovascular burden in women of higher age or symptomatic cardiovascular disease. Classical risk factors for cardiovascular disease emerge long before estrogen declines. Thus, the deprivation of estrogen cannot be solely responsible for the increasing risk of atherosclerotic artery disease in postmenopause. Socioeconomic status has a decisive impact on cardiovascular risk and correlates with the use of HRT. This healthy user effect implies no cardiovascular risk provided there is appropriate health care. The increased risk for vascular events in HERS and WHI may only apply to women with clinical or subclinical arteriosclerosis. The unique finding of an overall increased risk for cardiovascular events in the WHI does not apply to the subgroup of women within the first 10 years of postmenopause or those suffering from hot flushes. In essence, HRT can be used for relief of perimenopausal symptoms, but HRT cannot compensate for deficits in the individual lifestyle and health care. Certainly, a healthy lifestyle and good medical care are the basis for preventing cardiovascular disease. © 2004 Published by Elsevier B.V.

Keywords: Hormone replacement therapy (HRT); Cardiovascular disease

Arteriosclerotic, cardio- and cerebrovascular diseases have emerged as the main cause of death in women. Despite an incidence that is now similar to that in men, women still develop arteriosclerotic vascular disease 10–15 years later than men. Inasmuch as the decrease of plasma estrogens in menopause are believed to play a decisive role in this respect, HRT has been expected to be preventive in terms of cardiovascular events. Yet, no causal relationships can be derived from observational trials. Still, undoubtedly women that freely decide to use HRT have a significantly lower risk of cardiovascular events and mortality [8]. Thus, the relationships appear more complex.

As estrogen declines, classical risk factors for cardiovascular disease emerge [13]. Women with coronary artery disease have at least one of the major, classical risk factors, like hypertension, diabetes and insulin resistance, dyslipidemia or smoking (The CORA-

* Corresponding author. Tel.: +49-40-42803-3947, (Mobile) +49-163-557-6082; fax: +49-40-42803-5059.
E-mail address: Prof.Windler@t-online.de (E. Windler).

doi:10.1016/j.ics.2004.01.089

Study, unpublished observation). Indeed, more than 90% of the women are affected by a combination of two, three or even four of these risk factors. Two-thirds meet the criteria of a metabolic syndrome. Even smoking women with coronary artery disease are characterized by additional risk factors. In essence, not only the deprivation of estrogen can be made responsible for the increasing risk for atherosclerotic artery disease in postmenopause.

Still, an influence of decreasing estrogens on the development of these risk factors is not yet excluded. However, LDL-cholesterol and lipoprotein (a) or the incidence of hypertension and diabetes begin to rise clearly before menopause. Women with coronary artery disease typically have gained weight in their early adulthood. From this, it follows that cardiovascular prevention requires correcting the classical risk factors, since estrogens as hormone replacement therapy alone cannot be expected to counteract the entire cardiovascular risk.

Still, it appears not unreasonable to expect certain benefits from HRT on cardiovascular disease. At the same time, it is impossible to predict the overall harm or benefit of HRT on the cardiovascular system, considering the pleiotropic effects of estrogens due to the ubiquitous distribution of estrogen receptors in tissues and the vascular system [3,10]. In addition, the effects of estrogen may vastly differ depending on age and the stage of vascular disease [1]. For example, in the late phase of atherosclerosis, even slight changes in hemostasis may have deleterious consequences as to the size of a thrombus evolving from a ruptured plaque, but may be uncritical as long as the arteries are intact. Thus, only clinical trials can help to decide for which women at which age HRT is beneficial or harmful.

However, this also implies that results of trials cannot be uncritically generalized and transferred to women of different ages and states of vasculature. Generally, women at menopause are still in what may be designated primary prevention for vascular disease. The risk of myocardial infarction increases sharply not before the late fifties followed by cerebrovascular disease a decade later. Considering this, the results of neither HERS, nor the WHI can readily be transferred to the application of HRT in the peri- and early postmenopause [7,11]. WHI may provide some answers from results obtained in that fraction of women at a younger age with perimenopausal symptoms. The results of HERS only apply to women with vascular diseases; however, certain observations and subgroup analyses may still teach a lesson as to problems and risks of HRT.

A particular issue is the increased risk of vascular and thromboembolic events observed in HERS and WHI, predominantly when starting HRT. In HERS, the relative risk for coronary events was increased more than twofold within the first 4 months; however, this normalized within 2 years. In WHI, this time frame is not as clear; however, again the risk increased mostly within the first 2 years of the study. Both reports are based on a very limited, absolute number of additional cardiovascular events. In several secondary prevention studies of similar design, yet smaller size, this phenomenon was not observed. In the Nurses' Health Study, again the cardiovascular risk was increased about twofold within the first year of starting HRT, but normalized within the second year and, from then on, a benefit seemed to appear [5]. This phenomenon may only apply to women with clinical or subclinical arteriosclerosis. This view is in agreement with a recent report on more than 24,000 diabetic patients that showed an increased rate of myocardial infarction within the first year of HRT, only for women who had a previous myocardial infarction

[2]. The assumption that the Nurses' Health Study or WHI comprises only the vasculatures of healthy women is certainly inadequate, since many women at the age of 60 will have silent atherosclerosis.

It is yet noteworthy that the increased risk for cardiovascular events in the WHI is a unique finding. It is neither compatible with the results of one of the large observational trials nor with those of other randomized intervention trials, like HERS, that showed a null-effect. It is noteworthy that the data from the WHI do not show an increased risk of cardiovascular disease for women within the first 10 years postmenopause or for those who suffered from hot flushes [9]. However, this subgroup represents those women that may be eligible for HRT to treat their perimenopausal symptoms. The reported elevated risk is due to older and asymptomatic participants, especially those whose menopause dated 20 or more years back; however, those usually do not have an indication for HRT. Additionally, no prospective study, including HERS and WHI, has reported an elevated cardiovascular mortality. Thus, the results of the WHI should be interpreted with appropriate caution. Some of the uncertainties may be clarified by the results of the estrogen-arm of the WHI, which had so far not been terminated. Some results may turn out to be chance findings, but also the role of progestins may be better understood.

The decisive influence of the dose of estrogens appears to emerge from recent data. Overall, in HERS there was no increase in stroke; however, in the Nurses' Health Study, there appeared to be a gradient towards an elevated risk with the highest dose of 1.25 mg conjugated estrogens [4,12]. In the survey of the Northern California Kaiser Permanente Diabetes Registry, there was an apparent reduction of cardiovascular events with 0.3 mg conjugated estrogens or 2 mg ethinyl estradiol, which vanished with higher doses and even turned into a slightly elevated risk using more than 0.6 or 10 mg, respectively [2]. Thus, the standard dose of 0.6 mg conjugated estrogens in HERS and the WHI is probably the highest acceptable dose, and may be too high to show a positive, long-term effect of HRT on vascular risk.

A recent meta-analysis of the observational trials clearly indicates that socioeconomic status has a decisive impact on cardiovascular risk and correlates with the use of HRT [8]. Thus, the most plausible explanation for much of the observed lower vascular risk of women on HRT is a healthy user effect. This certainly does not exclude a contribution of HRT, however, underscores the importance of lifestyle and medical care. This may explain the differences in outcome of certain subgroups of HERS and WHI [6,9]. For example, those patients in HERS and WHI, likewise who were on a statin, did not show any increased risk. In HERS, women on a statin had a markedly lower rate of myocardial infarction and thromboembolic events, a slightly lower incidence of cerebral events and reduced total mortality as compared with those not on a statin. These effects are not necessarily the consequence of the statin therapy, but rather the result of the overall better health status and medical treatment of those that can afford statins. Thus, medication use is probably a marker of higher socioeconomic status and better health care.

This is also reflected in a recent case-control study (the CORA-Study, unpublished observation). Less women with incident coronary artery disease than healthy controls were on HRT, indicating no principal health hazard due to HRT. It is noteworthy, though, that the women on HRT had less vascular risk factors and a healthier lifestyle on average. However, those few women on HRT who developed a myocardial infarction comprised a subgroup that had the least favorable lifestyle and a markedly adverse risk profile. In essence, HRT can well be part of a healthy lifestyle, including good medical care, but HRT cannot compensate for deficits in individual lifestyle and health care.

References

[1] A. Cano, W.M. van Baal, The mechanisms of thrombotic risk induced by hormone replacement therapy, Maturitas 40 (2001) 17–38.

[2] A. Ferrara, et al., Current use of unopposed estrogen and estrogen plus progestin and the risk of acute myocardial infarction among women with diabetes. The Northern California Kaiser Permanente Diabetes Registry, 1995–1998, Circulation 107 (2003) 43–48.

[3] G. Finking, et al., Die Wirkungen von Östrogen im kardiovaskulären system, Z. Kardiol. 89 (2000) 442–453.

[4] F. Grodstein, et al., A prospective, observational study of postmenopausal hormone therapy and primary prevention of cardiovascular disease, Ann. Intern. Med. 133 (2000) 933–941.

[5] F. Grodstein, J.E. Manson, M.J. Stampfer, Postmenopausal hormone use and secondary prevention of coronary events in the nurses' health study. a prospective, observational study, Ann. Intern. Med. 135 (2001) 1–8.

[6] D.M. Herrington, et al., Statin therapy, cardiovascular events, and total mortality in the Heart and Estrogen/Progestin Replacement Study (HERS), Circulation 105 (2002) 2962–2967.

[7] S. Hulley, et al., Randomized trial of estrogen plus progestin for secondary prevention of coronary heart disease in postmenopausal women. Heart and Estrogen/Progestin Replacement Study (HERS) Research Group, JAMA 280 (1998) 605–613.

[8] L.L. Humphrey, et al., Postmenopausal hormone replacement therapy and the primary prevention of cardiovascular disease, Ann. Intern. Med. 137 (2002) 272–284.

[9] J.E. Manson, et al., Women's Health Initiative Investigators: estrogen plus progestin and the risk of coronary heart disease, N. Engl. J. Med. 349 (2003) 523–534.

[10] M.E. Mendelsohn, R.H. Karas, The protective effects of estrogen on the cardiovascular system, N. Engl. J. Med. 340 (1999) 1801–1811.

[11] J.E. Rossouw, et al., Risks and benefits of estrogen plus progestin in healthy postmenopausal women: principal results from the Women's Health Initiative randomized controlled trial, JAMA 288 (2002) 321–333.

[12] J.A. Simon, et al., Postmenopausal hormone therapy and risk of stroke: the Heart and Estrogen-Progestin Replacement Study (HERS), Circulation 103 (2001) 638–642.

[13] V. Stangl, et al., Coronary atherogenic risk factors in women, Eur. Heart J. 23 (2002) 1738–1752.

International Congress Series 1262 (2004) 527–530

www.ics-elsevier.com

Function and regulation of hepatic scavenger receptor class B type I (SR-BI)

Attilio Rigotti*

Departamento de Gastroenterología, Facultad de Medicina, Pontificia Universidad Católica, Marcoleta 367, Santiago, Chile

Abstract. The scavenger receptor class B type I (SR-BI) was the first functional cell surface high-density lipoprotein (HDL) receptor to be described. SR-BI mediates efficient selective lipid uptake and is highly expressed in the liver. In fact, hepatic SR-BI is critical in regulating plasma HDL cholesterol levels and biliary cholesterol secretion in mice. Recent studies also reveal that various nuclear receptors regulate hepatic SR-BI expression. These findings have implications for understanding the antiatherogenic activity of SR-BI and developing novel HDL-based therapies of atherosclerosis. © 2003 Published by Elsevier B.V.

Keywords: SR-BI; HDL; Liver; Biliary cholesterol; PPARα

High-density lipoproteins (HDL) deliver cholesterol to cells by selective lipid uptake which is mediated by the scavenger receptor class B type I (SR-BI), the first high-affinity cell surface receptor for HDL to be described [1]. Because of its key role in HDL cholesterol metabolism, SR-BI exhibits antiatherogenic activity in murine models of this disease (reviewed in Refs. [2,3]).

SR-BI is highly expressed in the liver [1,4], where it controls the levels of plasma HDL cholesterol and its transport into bile. This article will briefly review the relevance of hepatic SR-BI expression in modulating HDL cholesterol metabolism and its regulation by the peroxisome proliferator-activated receptor α (PPARα).

1. Functional relevance of hepatic SR-BI expression

Numerous studies suggested the importance of SR-BI expressed in the liver for HDL metabolism (reviewed in Refs. [2,3]). Definitive evidence came from studies of mice, in which the levels of SR-BI were genetically manipulated in vivo (reviewed in Refs. [2,3]). Overexpression of SR-BI in the murine liver decreased HDL cholesterol [5–8], accelerated HDL cholesteryl ester clearance and hepatic uptake [6], and increased hepatic and

* Tel.: +56-2-6863832; fax: +56-2-6397780.
E-mail address: arigotti@med.puc.cl (A. Rigotti).

0531-5131/ © 2003 Published by Elsevier B.V.
doi:10.1016/j.ics.2003.12.007

gallbladder bile cholesterol concentrations [5,7]. In contrast, partial or complete SR-BI deficiency in mice increased HDL cholesterol [9,10], impaired selective HDL cholesterol clearance [10], and lowered hepatic and gallbladder bile cholesterol contents [11–13]. Kinetic studies of labeled HDL cholesterol have shown that hepatic SR-BI expression is indeed involved in regulating its transport into bile (Ref. [14] and Rigotti et al., unpublished data). In contrast, hepatic SR-BI expression was not essential for maintaining normal bile acid metabolism [12].

SR-BI might facilitate biliary cholesterol secretion exclusively by increasing cholesterol availability as a consequence of facilitated hepatic uptake of plasma HDL cholesterol. In addition, SR-BI may mediate intrahepatic HDL retroendocytosis leading to HDL cholesterol sorting from the sinusoidal to the canalicular region of hepatocytes [15]. On the other hand, SR-BI, which can facilitate cellular cholesterol efflux (reviewed in Ref. [2]), may also directly participate in biliary cholesterol secretion from the canalicular membrane [5,16]. In fact, SR-BI has been found in the hepatocellular canalicular domain of mice overexpressing SR-BI [5], cultured hepatocyte couplets [15], and canalicular plasma membranes isolated from rodent livers [16,17]; however, differing immunohistochemical findings have been reported on canalicular localization of SR-BI in hepatocytes of wild-type mice [16,18,19]. Thus, a direct role of SR-BI in mediating biliary cholesterol secretion at the canalicular membrane remains to be established.

2. Regulation of hepatic SR-BI expression

Hepatic SR-BI expression is regulated by a variety of dietary, hormonal, metabolic, and pharmacological manipulations (reviewed in Refs. [2,3]). More recently, in vivo and in vitro studies have reported the regulation of SR-BI expression in the liver by nuclear receptors, including FXR (Ref. [20] and Rigotti et al., unpublished data), LXR [21], LRH-1 [22], the PPARγ [23], and HNF4α [23].

The influence of PPAR-α on controlling SR-BI expression in the murine liver has also been studied [19]. Fibrates, which are PPAR-α agonists, reduced SR-BI protein levels in isolated rat hepatocytes and caused a decrease in hepatic SR-BI protein expression in mice [19]. Interestingly, hepatic SR-BI mRNA levels remained unchanged in fibrate-treated mice [19], suggesting a posttranscriptional regulation of SR-BI. This reduced hepatic SR-BI protein expression in fibrate-treated mice was associated with increased HDL particle size which was corrected by restoring normal SR-BI protein levels using recombinant adenoviruses [19]. The posttranscriptional regulation of SR-BI required normal PPAR-α expression because the effect of fibrate treatment on hepatic SR-BI protein levels was abolished in PPAR-α deficient mice [19]. These findings indicate that hepatic SR-BI regulation by fibrates is mediated by PPAR-α activation which is likely leading to transcriptional modulation of a yet unrecognized gene that might be controlling SR-BI mRNA translation and/or SR-BI protein stability.

Interestingly, the expression of CLAMP (a.k.a. PDZK1), a PDZ domain-containing protein apparently involved in stabilizing SR-BI protein in the liver sinusoidal plasma membrane [17], was also down-regulated in livers of fibrate-treated animals [19]. In fact, SR-BI/CLAMP interaction is required for adequate expression of SR-BI in the hepatocellular surface and its functional role in HDL metabolism [24]. These findings suggest that changes in the expression of CLAMP/PDZK1 may cause functionally relevant regulation of SR-BI in the liver.

3. Conclusion

SR-BI expressed in the liver plays a key role in controlling HDL cholesterol metabolism and biliary cholesterol disposal in mice. On the other hand, hepatic SR-BI expression can be modulated by different stimuli including nuclear receptor agonists. These findings have important implications not only for understanding the antiatherogenic activity of SR-BI but also for developing novel HDL-based therapeutic approaches of atherosclerosis.

Acknowledgements

The contributions of many colleagues who have participated in our studies on SR-BI are highly acknowledged. Our work is supported by Fondo Nacional de Desarrollo Científico y Tecnológico (Chile) and NIH Fogarty International Center (USA).

References

[1] S. Acton, et al., Identification of scavenger receptor SR-BI as a high density lipoprotein receptor, Science 271 (1996) 518–520.
[2] A. Rigotti, et al., The role of the high-density lipoprotein receptor SR-BI in the lipid metabolism of endocrine and other tissues, Endocr. Rev. 24 (2003) 357–387.
[3] B.L. Trigatti, et al., Influence of the HDL receptor SR-BI on lipoprotein metabolism and atherosclerosis, Arterioscler. Thromb. Vasc. Biol. 23 (2003) 1732–1738.
[4] K. Landschulz, et al., Regulation of scavenger receptor, class B, type I, a high density lipoprotein receptor, in liver and steroidogenic tissues of the rat, J. Clin. Invest. 98 (1996) 984–995.
[5] K.F. Kozarsky, et al., Overexpression of the HDL receptor SR-BI alters plasma HDL and bile cholesterol levels, Nature 387 (1997) 414–417.
[6] N. Wang, et al., Liver-specific overexpression of scavenger receptor BI decreases levels of very low density lipoprotein ApoB, low density lipoprotein ApoB, and high density lipoprotein in transgenic mice, J. Biol. Chem. 273 (1998) 32920–32926.
[7] E. Sehayek, et al., Biliary cholesterol excretion: a novel mechanism that regulates dietary cholesterol absorption, Proc. Natl. Acad. Sci. U. S. A. 95 (1998) 10194–10199.
[8] Y. Ueda, et al., Lower plasma levels and accelerated clearance of high density lipoprotein (HDL) and non-HDL cholesterol in scavenger receptor class B type I transgenic mice, J. Biol. Chem. 274 (1999) 7165–7171.
[9] A. Rigotti, et al., A targeted mutation in the murine gene encoding the high density lipoprotein (HDL) receptor scavenger receptor class B type I reveals its key role in HDL metabolism, Proc. Natl. Acad. Sci. U. S. A. 94 (1997) 12610–12615.
[10] M.L. Varban, et al., Targeted mutation reveals a central role for SR-BI in hepatic selective uptake of high density lipoprotein cholesterol, Proc. Natl. Acad. Sci. U. S. A. 95 (1998) 4619–4624.
[11] B. Trigatti, et al., Influence of the HDL Receptor SR-BI on reproductive and cardiovascular pathophysiology, Proc. Natl. Acad. Sci. U. S. A. 96 (1999) 9322–9932.
[12] P. Mardones, et al., Hepatic cholesterol and bile acid metabolism and intestinal cholesterol absorption in scavenger receptor class B type I (SR-BI)-deficient mice, J. Lipid Res. 42 (2001) 170–180.
[13] D.Q. Wang, M.C. Carey, Susceptibility to murine cholesterol gallstone formation is not affected by partial disruption of the HDL receptor SR-BI, Biophys. Acta 1583 (2002) 141–150.
[14] Y. Ji, et al., Hepatic scavenger receptor BI promotes rapid clearance of high density lipoprotein free cholesterol and its transport into bile, J. Biol. Chem. 274 (1999) 33398–33402.

[15] D.L. Silver, et al., High density lipoprotein (HDL) particle uptake mediated by scavenger receptor class B type 1 results in selective sorting of HDL cholesterol from protein and polarized cholesterol secretion, J. Biol. Chem. 276 (2001) 25287–25293.
[16] E. Sehayek, et al., Localization of the phosphatidylethanolamine methylation pathway and scavenger receptor class B type I to the canalicular membrane: evidence for apical phosphatidylcholine biosynthesis that may promote biliary excretion of phospholipid and cholesterol, J. Lipid Res. 44 (2003) 1605–1613.
[17] M. Ikemoto, et al., Identification of a PDZ-domain-containing protein that interacts with the scavenger receptor class B type I, Proc. Natl. Acad. Sci. 97 (2000) 6538–6543.
[18] H. Stangl, et al., Effect of estrogen on scavenger receptor BI expression in the rat, J. Endocrinol. 175 (2002) 663–666.
[19] P. Mardones, et al., Fibrates downregulate hepatic scavenger receptor class B type I (SR-BI) protein expression in mice, J. Biol. Chem. 278 (2003) 7884–7890.
[20] G. Lambert, et al., The farnesoid X-receptor is an essential regulator of cholesterol homeostasis, J. Biol. Chem. 278 (2003) 2563–2570.
[21] L. Malerod, et al., Oxysterol-activated LXRalpha/RXR induces hSR-BI-promoter activity in hepatoma cells and preadipocytes, Biochem. Biophys. Res. Commun. 299 (2002) 916–923.
[22] K. Schoonjans, et al., Liver receptor homolog 1 controls the expression of the scavenger receptor class B type I, EMBO Rep. 3 (2002) 1181–1187.
[23] L. Malerod, et al., Hepatic scavenger receptor class B, type I is stimulated by peroxisome proliferator-activated receptor gamma and hepatocyte nuclear factor 4alpha, Biochem. Biophys. Res. Commun. 305 (2003) 557–565.
[24] D.L. Silver, A carboxyl-terminal PDZ-interacting domain of scavenger receptor B, type I is essential for cell surface expression in liver, J. Biol. Chem. 277 (2002) 34042–34047.

International Congress Series 1262 (2004) 531–534

www.ics-elsevier.com

LOX-1, a lectin-like oxidized LDL receptor identified form endothelial cells, in endothelial dysfunction

Tatsuya Sawamura*

Department of Vascular Physiology, National Cardiovascular Center Research Institute, Suita, Osaka 565-8565, Japan

Abstract. Lectin-like oxidized LDL receptor-1 (LOX-1) was initially identified as the major receptor for oxidized LDL in endothelial cells. In vitro, LOX-1 expression is induced by many inflammatory cytokines, oxidative stress, hemodynamic stimuli, and oxidized low-density lipoproteins (OxLDL). In vivo, the expression is enhanced in many proatherogenic settings including, hypertension, hyperlipidemia, and diabetes, and indeed accumulated in the atherosclerotic lesions. LOX-1 activation by OxLDL causes endothelial dysfunction/injury which is characterized by the generation of reactive oxygen species (ROS), subsequently inducing monocytes adhesion to endothelial cells, and endothelial apoptosis. Besides OxLDL, LOX-1 binds multiple classes of ligands including advanced glycation end products (AGE), activated platelets, and leukocytes, which may contribute to the pathogenesis of thrombosis and inflammation related to atherosclerosis. © 2003 Published by Elsevier B.V.

Keywords: Oxidized low-density lipoproteins; LOX-1; Endothelial dysfunction; Inflammation; Atherosclerosis

1. Introduction

Recent studies implicated oxidatively modified low-density lipoproteins (oxidized LDL, OxLDL) in the pathogenesis of atherosclerosis, which is characterized by intimal thickening and lipid accumulation in the arteries [1]. Endothelial dysfunction or activation elicited by OxLDL is assumed to be the key step in the initiation of atherosclerosis. In response to the stimulation of OxLDL, endothelial cells reduced the release of nitric oxide, expressed adhesion molecules, and secreted chemoattractant and growth factors. Subsequently, OxLDL was avidly ingested by macrophages, resulting in foam cell formation. OxLDL was also involved in inducing smooth muscle cells migration, proliferation, and

Abbreviations: LOX-1, lectin-like oxidized LDL receptor-1; LDL, low-density lipoproteins; OxLDL, oxidized low density lipoproteins; BAECs, bovine aortic endothelial cells; NK-cell, natural killer cells; WHHL, Watanabe Heritable Hyperlipidemic rabbit; AGE, advanced glycation end-products; ROS, reactive oxygen species.

* Tel.: +81-6-6833-5012x2518; fax: +81-6-6835-5329.

E-mail address: t-sawamura@umin.ac.jp (T. Sawamura).

doi:10.1016/S0531-5131(03)01816-8

transformation [1]. OxLDL influencing on cellular properties was principally via specific receptors, so-called "scavenger receptors" [2]. Among them, LOX-1, the lectin-like OxLDL receptor-1, is characterized as the major receptor for OxLDL in endothelial cells [3].

2. Molecular cloning of LOX-1

Oxidized LDL is believed to be an essential component of atherogenesis that induces endothelial dysfunction and accumulation of foam cells [1]. Vascular endothelial cells internalize and degrade Ox-LDL through a putative receptor-mediated pathway, which is distinct from macrophage scavenger receptors. I successfully identified a cDNA encoding an endothelial cell-surface receptor for OxLDL, which was designated as lectin-like Ox-LDL receptor-1, LOX-1 [3]. The cDNA for LOX-1 cloned from bovine aortic endothelial cells (BAECs) contained an open-reading frame of 810 base pairs that encodes a protein of 270 amino acid residues. Sequence and structure analysis of LOX-1 revealed that it does not resemble any known scavenger receptors. In contrast, it shares significant identity to NK cell receptors, such as CD94 (KLRD1) and NKR-P1 (KLRB1), which are involved in target-cell recognition and natural killer cell (NK-cell)activation [3,4]. The structure suggested that LOX-1 might induce functional changes and contribute to cell–cell interactions as those exhibited by NK cell receptors [3]. The expression level of LOX-1 is relatively low in basal condition in vitro, but it can be induced by pro-inflammatory and oxidative stimuli [5,6]. In vivo, LOX-1 was overexpressed in several pathological settings including hypertension, hyperlipidemia, diabetes, and even atherosclerosis per se [5,6].

3. Human LOX-1 gene

The human LOX-1 gene is encoded by 6 exons that span approximately 15 kb on the human genome. LOX-1 gene structure indicates a close relationship between exon/intron architecture and protein structure. Exon 1 encoded the mRNA 5′ -untranslated region and the cytoplasmic domain. Exon 2 encoded the remainder of cytoplasmic domain and the transmembrane domain. Exon 3 encoded the neck domain. Exons 4–6 encoded the lectin domain, and the 3′ -untranslated region. LOX-1 gene was mapped to 12p12.3-13.2 region of human chromosomes, where the genes of the natural killer cell receptors cluster. These results showed that the LOX-1 gene is a new member of the lectin-like NK gene complex with a unique expression profile [4]. Recently, an atherosclerosis susceptibility locus called Athsq2 in Ldlr knockout mouse was mapped, and it is residing on a homologous region equivalent to human chromosome 12p13-12. Although the gene encoding Athsq2 has not been identified, it might be LOX-1 [7]. Most recently, association of the polymorphism of human LOX-1 gene with coronary heart diseases has been reported.

4. LOX-1 mediated endothelial responses

OxLDL interacts with endothelial cells, and induced many functional changes, which is characterized as endothelial dysfunction/activation. The highly induced expression of LOX-1 in endothelial cells made it possible to mediate such effects. Cominacini et al. [8]

have shown that OxLDL binding to LOX-1 in endothelial cells generates superoxide anions, decreases NO, and concomitantly activates NF-κB. Li and Mehta [9] reported that OxLDL binding to LOX-1 in human coronary endothelial cells resulted in cellular apoptosis. They also demonstrated that LOX-1 mediates OxLDL-induced upregulation of monocyte chemoattractant protein-1 (MCP-1) and leukocyte adhesion molecules. These data support that oxidized LDL interacts with endothelial cell via LOX-1 could induce multiple functional and phenotype changes relevant to "endothelial dysfunction."

5. Ligands for LOX-1

Advanced glycation end-products (AGEs) are glycooxidatively modified molecules under high glucose conditions in diabetes. Recently, Jono et al. [10] reported that LOX-1 recognizes AGEs besides OxLDL and is a major receptor for AGEs in endothelial cells.

Activated platelets can also be recognized by LOX-1 [11]. The binding of platelets was inhibited by a phosphatidylserine-binding protein, annexin V and enhanced by agonists for platelets. Therefore, the anionic phospholipids exposed on activation on the surface of platelets should be the epitopes for LOX-1. Notably, the binding of platelets to LOX-1 enhanced the release of endothelin-1 from endothelial cells, supporting the induction of endothelial activation. LOX-1-directed platelet–endothelium communication induces the phenotypic changes of endothelial cells that are relevant to atherogenesis. The molecule, which can bind both OxLDL and platelets and affect endothelial function, might provide a clue to solve the endothelial phenomenon observed in hemostasis and atherosclerosis [11].

In a model of endotoxin-induced uveitis, anti-LOX-1 antibody efficiently suppressed leukocyte infiltration and protein exudation. In situ videomicroscopic analyses of leukocyte interactions with retinal veins revealed that anti-LOX-1 antibody reduced the number of rolling leukocytes and increased the velocity of rolling, suggesting that LOX-1 functions as a vascular tethering ligand [12]. The ability of LOX-1 to capture leukocytes under physiologic shear was confirmed in an in vitro flow model. Thus, LOX-1 is a novel adhesion molecule involved in leukocyte recruitment and inflammation.

The property of LOX-1 itself can be understood to directly change endothelial functions, which increase prothrombotic and proinflammatory activity.

6. Role of LOX-1 in atherosclerosis

Histological studies on Watanabe Heritable Hyperlipidemic (WHHL) rabbit atherosclerotic tissues have shown a characteristic pattern of LOX-1 expression. LOX-1 was most prominently stained in the endothelial cells of early atherosclerotic lesions. Importantly, LOX-1 was also observed in the endothelium of non-lesion areas of WHHL rabbit aortas, suggesting the onset of such process seems to be an earliest event in atherogenesis even preceding the lesion formation. The increased expression of LOX-1 is most prominent in the arterial bifurcations in a rat model of diabetes. The anatomical counterparts are generally considered as atherosclerosis-susceptible regions. The endothelium localized in bifurcations is exposed to a combination of complex shear forces and circumferential strain. These findings support that LOX-1 expression is influenced by hemodynamic factors in vivo. Considering the proinflammatory and prooxidative function of LOX-1, it is very likely that LOX-1 works as a proatherogenic factor in vivo, although more detailed analyses in genetic approach are needed.

References

[1] R. Ross, Atherosclerosis—an inflammatory disease, N. Engl. J. Med. 340 (2) (1999) 115–126.

[2] U.P. Steinbrecher, Receptors for oxidized low density lipoprotein, Biochim. Biophys. Acta 1436 (3) (1999) 279–298.

[3] T. Sawamura, N. Kume, T. Aoyama, H. Moriwaki, H. Hoshikawa, Y. Aiba, et al., An endothelial receptor for oxidized low-density lipoprotein, Nature 386 (6620) (1997) 73–77.

[4] T. Aoyama, T. Sawamura, Y. Furutani, R. Matsuoka, M.C. Yoshida, H. Fujiwara, et al., Structure and chromosomal assignment of the human lectin-like oxidized low-density-lipoprotein receptor-1 (LOX-1) gene, Biochem. J. 339 (Pt 1) (1999) 177–184.

[5] M. Chen, T. Masaki, T. Sawamura, LOX-1, the receptor for oxidized low-density lipoprotein identified from endothelial cells: implications in endothelial dysfunction and atherosclerosis, Pharmacol. Ther. 95 (1) (2002) 89–100.

[6] K. Sakurai, T. Sawamura, Stress and vascular responses: endothelial dysfunction via lectin-like oxidized low-density lipoprotein receptor-1: close relationships with oxidative stress, J. Pharmacol. Sci. 91 (3) (2003) 182–186.

[7] C.L. Welch, S. Bretschger, N. Latib, M. Bezouevski, Y. Guo, N. Pleskac, et al., Localization of atherosclerosis susceptibility loci to chromosomes 4 and 6 using the Ldlr knockout mouse model, Proc. Natl. Acad. Sci. U. S. A. 98 (14) (2001) 7946–7951.

[8] L. Cominacini, A. Rigoni, A. Fratta Pasini, U. Garbin, A. Davoli, M. Campagnola, et al., The binding of oxidized low-density lipoprotein (ox-LDL) to ox-LDL receptor-1 in endothelial cells reduces the intracellular concentration of nitric oxide through an increased production of superoxide, J. Biol. Chem. 24 (2001) 24.

[9] D. Li, J.L. Mehta, Upregulation of endothelial receptor for oxidized LDL (LOX-1) by oxidized LDL and implications in apoptosis of human coronary artery endothelial cells: evidence from use of antisense LOX-1 mRNA and chemical inhibitors, Arterioscler. Thromb. Vasc. Biol. 20 (4) (2000) 1116–1122.

[10] T. Jono, A. Miyazaki, R. Nagai, T. Sawamura, T. Kitamura, S. Horiuchi, Lectin-like oxidized low density lipoprotein receptor-1 (LOX-1) serves as an endothelial receptor for advanced glycation end products (AGE), FEBS Lett. 511 (1–3) (2002) 170–174.

[11] M. Kakutani, T. Masaki, T. Sawamura, A platelet–endothelium interaction mediated by lectin-like oxidized low-density lipoprotein receptor-1, Proc. Natl. Acad. Sci. U. S. A. 97 (1) (2000) 360–364.

[12] M. Honjo, K. Nakamura, K. Yamashiro, J. Kiryu, H. Tanihara, L.M. McEvoy, et al., Lectin-like oxidized LDL receptor-1 is a cell-adhesion molecule involved in endotoxin-induced inflammation, Proc. Natl. Acad. Sci. U. S. A. 100 (3) (2003) 1274–1279.

International Congress Series 1262 (2004) 535–537

ELSEVIER

www.ics-elsevier.com

Metabolic syndrome and its relevance to Asia

E.D. Janus*

Wimmera Health Care Group, Baillie Street, Horsham,Vic., 3400, Australia

Abstract. This is a review of metabolic syndrome (MS) and its relevance to Asian countries. MS refers to clustering of metabolic abnormalities with a potential unifying basis, e.g. insulin resistance. There is no uniform agreement defining MS. Most commonly used are the NCEP definition (three or more of abdominal obesity, hypertriglyceridaemia, low HDL, hypertension and hyperglycaemia—criteria specified) and WHO definition (similar but including microalbuminuria, diabetes, impaired glucose tolerance (IGT) and insulin resistance criteria). With increasing overweight MS, which increases risk of cardiovascular disease, may become a major issue in Asia where the prevalence of diabetes is already high. In the Hong Kong 1995–1996 Cardiovascular Risk Factor Prevalence Study, the prevalence of diabetes was 10%, impaired glucose tolerance 14%, MS 17% by NCEP criteria and 21% if WHO recommended Asian waist circumference was used. Prevalences were extremely high in older women: 29%, 26%, 54% and 62%, respectively, at 65–74 years. Agreed definitions for MS in Asia are needed and diet and lifestyle changes including increased physical activity to reduce the epidemic of obesity underlying diabetes and MS are urgent priorities as are novel therapeutic approaches. Published by Elsevier B.V.

Keywords: Asia; Metabolic syndrome; Diabetes; Impaired glucose tolerance

1. Introduction

The best-known major cardiovascular risk factors, apart from smoking, are hypercholesterolaemia, hypertension and diabetes mellitus. These increase with age and with overweight and obesity. The combination of several risk factors is common and conveys a cardiovascular risk comparable to a very high level of a single risk factor such as marked hypercholesterolaemia. The concept of the metabolic syndrome (MS) arises from the coexistence in individuals of clusters of risk factors with a possible common underlying aetiology. Specifically, this includes abdominal obesity, hypertension, high triglycerides, low HDL and hyperglycaemia including impaired glucose tolerance (IGT) and diabetes mellitus (DM) as well as the insulin resistance which is the main candidate for being the underlying aetiology. Patients with MS are at high risk of cardiovascular disease [1].

* Tel.: +61-3-53819167; fax: +61-3-53812537.
E-mail address: januse@netspace.net.au (E.D. Janus).

0531-5131/ Published by Elsevier B.V.
doi:10.1016/S0531-5131(03)01834-X

2. Materials and methods

In 1995–1996, the Hong Kong Cardiovascular Risk Factor Prevalence Study HKRFPS) provided very detailed information on 2900 randomly selected individuals aged 25–74 years who were representative of the Hong Kong Population .The study has been described elsewhere [2]. Measurements included not only the usual cardiovascular risk factors and anthropometric measurements but also glucose tolerance tests and fasting insulin measurements.

3. Results

Insulin resistance means that higher than normal insulin concentrations are required to maintain a given plasma glucose concentration. In insulin-dependent diabetes (IDDM), there is no insulin secretion. Insulin resistance may progress to impaired glucose tolerance (IGT) and non-insulin dependent diabetes (NIDDM), the predominant type of diabetes in Asia. In the HKRFPS, there was a clear, statistically significant decrease in insulin sensitivity, the reciprocal of insulin resistance, as Body Mass Index (BMI) increased. This was apparent even as BMI increased by small increments between 18.5 and 25.0 with further marked reductions as BMI reached 30 and above this. Fasting and 2-h glucoses from oral glucose tolerance tests increased as BMI increased incrementally from below 20 to above 30. Blood pressure also increased incrementally with BMI starting from a BMI as low as 17–20 in Korean studies.

There is no uniformly agreed definition of MS. Most commonly used are the National Cholesterol Education Programme (NCEP) definition and the WHO definition. In the USA in 1988–1994, 23.7% of adults had MS. In Filipinas, the prevalence was a very high 34% compared with 12% in age-matched Caucasian women.

NCEP defines MS as the presence of three or more of the following five criteria: (1) Abdominal obesity-waist circumference >102 cm in males and >88 cm in females, (2) Hypertriglyceridaemia—triglycerides 1.69 mM or greater, (3) HDL cholesterol below 1.04 mM in men and < 1.29 mM in women, (4) Systolic BP 130 mm Hg or greater and/or diastolic BP 85 mm Hg or greater, (5) Fasting glucose 6.1 mM or greater [3]. WHO has the following criteria: (1) Obesity—BMI >30 kg/m^2 and/or waist hip ratio (WHR) >0.90 in men or 0.85 in women, (2) Dyslipidaemia—Plasma triglycerides >1.7 mM and/or HDL Cholesterol < 0.9 in men or < 1.0 in women, (3) Hypertension—On treatment and/or Systolic BP 160 mm Hg and/or diastolic BP >90 mm Hg, (4) Microalbuminuria—urine albumin excretion rate > or = to 20 μg/min. MS is present if two or more of these criteria are present in patients with NIDDM or IGT or if there is impaired fasting glucose (6.0–6.9). MS is also present if two or more of these criteria are present and there is evidence of insulin resistance (highest quartile of fasting insulin or of the HOMA IR index of the population studied). Clearly, prevalences are definition dependent and there is a commonly held view that for Asian populations different definitions of obesity are more appropriate.

In Asian countries, there has been a reduction in physical activity, an increase in energy intake and an increase in overweight and obesity. Along with this has come an increasing prevalence of IGT, NIDDM, hypertension and hyperlipidaemia. In Hong Kong, the prevalence of DM was 10% and IGT 14% in HKRFPS 1995–1996. In China, the prevalence of both IGT and DM has been steadily increasing. By NCEP criteria, the crude prevalence of MS in Hong Kong in this study was 16.7% and 17.1 (15.7–18.5)% age and gender adjusted. It rises from a prevalence of 3.1% at age 25–34 years to 41% in subjects aged over 70 years. In the age group 65–74 years, it is very high, especially in women: 53.7% vs. 27.7% in men. When the NCEP criteria are applied with the WHO recommended modification to the waist circumference criteria for obesity [4], the prevalence rises from 17.1 (1.7–18.5)% to 21.9 (20.4–23.4)%.

In data from Mohan et al. [5] in Chennai in India, formerly Madras, the components of MS were all significantly more prevalent in middle than lower class subjects consistent with their greater caloric intake. This increase in cardiovascular risk in the more affluent is part of economic transition. In more developed societies, the better educated and more affluent usually have the better cardiovascular risk factor profiles.

4. Discussion

The prevalence of the components of the metabolic syndrome is high and rising in Asian countries, and hence, the prevalence of IGT, DM and MS is rising. The criteria used particularly for overweight and obesity (BMI, waist circumference and waist hip ratio) need to be modified for Asians with consequent appropriate Asian criteria for MS. Studies on the prevalence and aetiology of MS in Asia are important and steps to reduce the impending pandemic of overweight, obesity and consequent increases in IGT, DM, MS and cardiovascular disease are urgent. There is also a challenge to provide novel therapeutic approaches.

References

[1] B. Isomaa, P. Almgren, T. Tuomi, et al., Cardiovascular morbidity and mortality associated with the metabolic syndrome, Diabetes Care 24 (2001) 683–689.

[2] T.H. Lam, L.J. Liu, E.D. Janus, C. Bourke, A.J. Hedley, The relationship between fibrinogen and other coronary heart disease risk factors in a Chinese population, Atherosclerosis 143 (1999) 405–413.

[3] Expert Panel on detection and treatment of high blood cholesterol in adults. Executive summary of the third report to the National Cholesterol Education Program (NCEP) Expert Panel on the detection, evaluation and treatment of high blood cholesterol in adults (Adult Treatment Panel III), JAMA 285 (2001) 2486–2497.

[4] World Health Organisation, The Asia Pacific perspective: redefining obesity and its treatment, Health Communications, Australia, (2000) 1–56.

[5] V. Mohan, S. Shanthirani, R. Deepa, G. Premalatha, N.G. Sastry, R. Saroja, Intra-urban differences of the metabolic syndrome in southern India—the Chennai Urban Population Study (CUPS No. 4), Diabetic Medicine 18 (2001) 280–287.

International Congress Series 1262 (2004) 538–541

www.ics-elsevier.com

Dietary habits, obesity status and cardiovascular risk factors in Koreans

Jong Ho Lee[a,*], Yangsoo Jang[b], Ji Young Kim[a]

[a] Department of Food and Nutrition, College of Human Ecology, Yonsei University, 134 Shinchon-Dong, Seodaemun-Gu, Seoul 120-749, South Korea

[b] Division of Cardiology, Cardiovascular Genome Center, Yonsei Medical Institute, Yonsei University, Seoul, South Korea

Abstract. Following the rapid economic development with good food supply, Koreans have changed their lifestyle and food habits. Intake trends illustrate the fall in whole grain intake with the significant rise in animal sources, edible oils and added sugar. Fat-derived energy intake increased rapidly, from about 6% in 1969 to 19% in 1998; however, average calorie intake, approximately 2000 kcal, has changed little over the same period. The 1998 survey showed that the obesity rate among adults was 1.7% for men and 3.0% for women. Although mean values of BMI has only slightly increased from 22.5 kg/m^2 in 1988 to 23.3 kg/m^2 in 1998, the prevalence of the high waist to hip ratio has markedly increased. Similarly, a rapid increase (140%) in mortality rates as a result of CAD was observed. This indicates that obesity is not considered to be of major clinical importance in Korea. Rather, the ability of an individual to cope with an increase in central fat distribution and dietary transition may be important in the development of CAD. Many Koreans appear to be susceptible to the development of excessive abdominal fatness even at low levels of BMI. In addition, the health consequences of visceral fat accumulation including postprandial lipemia, lipid peroxidation and negative antioxidant system appear to occur at much lower levels of BMI and are more intense than in those of European origin. The exact reasons for these ethnic variations in the development of CAD remain unclear. It is likely that genetic differences contribute to this variation in CAD risk, but different dietary and physical activity patterns may also play a role. Therefore, the major goal to prevent CAD should be the reduction of visceral fat through physical exercise and heart-healthy nutrition guidelines, including minimally refined grains and frequent consumption of vegetables and legumes, even for those subjects who are considered at low risk of CAD based on the BMI values.

Keywords: Dietary habits; Obesity status; Cardiovascular risk factors; Visceral fat; Koreans

1. Introduction

The risk factors for coronary artery disease (CAD) at a given BMI are generally higher among Korean people compared with western populations. The risk of obesity-

* Corresponding author. Tel.: +82-2-2123-3122; fax: +82-2-364-9605.
E-mail address: jhleeb@yonsei.ac.kr (J.H. Lee).

doi:10.1016/j.ics.2003.11.034

related diseases among Asians is known to rise from a body mass index (BMI) of 23 kg/ m^2, although there was no clear, single cutoff point for all Asians for high risk [1]. The population of Korea following the rapid economic development with good food supply, similar to other industrialized countries in Asia, is experiencing dramatic and rapid changes in dietary and physical activity habits that are the driving force behind the increase in obesity and obesity-related disease.

2. Changes in dietary intake in Korea

2.1. Consumption pattern of cereal and grain products

Consumption of cereals and grain products, the major contributors to food intake of Koreans, decreased significantly [2]. In 1970, per capita cereal intake accounted for 50% of total grams of food intake. In contrast, cereals accounted for only 27% of total intake in 1998. However, refined rice consumption did not change much throughout the survey period. Legume intake changed little until 1990 but decreased thereafter. Major change in the consumption of cereal and grain products includes a dramatic fall in total intake of whole grains and legume products contrasted with no changes in refined rice intake.

2.2. Carbohydrate and protein intake pattern

Carbohydrate intake decreased gradually after 1970 from 81% of total energy intake to 65% in 1998 [2]. This indicates that carbohydrates still contributed a great proportion of energy but to a much lesser extent. Total protein intake was relatively constant over the past 30 years. The source of intake, however, changed significantly. For example, 15% of protein intake per capita per day came from animal sources in 1970, while 48% came from animal sources in 1998.

2.3. Fat intake pattern

Daily per capita fat intake in Korea more than doubled from 17.2 g in 1970 to 41.5 g in 1998 [3]. Fat intakes derived from plant foods and animal foods are both increasing. However, the animal fat share among total fat intake has increased from 30.6% in 1970 to 48.2% in 1998, while the plant share of fat intake has decreased gradually from 70% in the 1970s to approximately 50% in the 1990s. Fat-derived energy intake increased rapidly, from about 6% in 1969 to 19% in 1998; however, average calorie intake, approximately 2000 kcal, has changed little over the same period. Although fat intake in South Korea is rapidly rising, the proportion of fat-derived energy is still lower than that of many other Asian countries and even much lower than that of most of the Western countries [4].

3. Visceral fat accumulation, postprandial lipemia, lipid peroxidation, DNA damage and endothelial dysfunction in non-obese Korean men

Although mean values of BMI have only slightly increased from 22.5 kg/m^2 in 1988 [4] to 23.3 kg/m^2 in 1998 [2], the prevalence of the high waist to hip ratio has increased markedly with changing food habits and increasingly sedentary lifestyles. Similarly, the mortality rate (per 100,000 of the population) as a result of ischemic heart disease has rapidly increased from 6.8 in 1988 to 13.8 in 1997 [5]. The effects of central obesity on cardiovascular risk factors were determined in a sample of 102 non-obese Korean men [6]. There are significant correlations between abdominal fat distribution, postprandial lipemia and lipid peroxidation. Specifically, data show that visceral fat accumulation at the L4 level is the most significant correlate of impaired postprandial lipid response, lipid peroxidation, DNA damage of lymphocytes and endothelial dysfunction, all of them implicated in cardiovascular morbidity and mortality risk. Visceral adipose tissue accumulation at L4 and L5 has been reported to be a positive association with C-reactive protein levels, suggesting that the expanded abdominal fat depot may induce a low grade inflammatory state, which in turn will stimulate lipid peroxidation. This increased lipid peroxidation could then promote DNA damage, which has been shown to contribute to vascular dysfunction.

4. Body fat distribution and antioxidant status in CAD men with or without diabetes

The differences in visceral fat accumulation and antioxidant status were determined in 64 healthy Korean men and in 56 CAD Korean men with or without diabetes [7]. Findings revealed a significantly greater amount of visceral fat in CAD men with diabetes than in healthy men at both L1 and L4 vertebras. Both groups of CAD men had higher concentrations of plasma homocysteine than did control subjects. Serum beta-carotene and lycopene concentrations were found to be significantly lower in the CAD men with diabetes. This study suggests that further visceral fat accumulation and a relative deficiency of insulin in CAD men may lead to a greater incidence of type 2 diabetes. Also, due to the decreased serum antioxidant levels in patients with CAD when compared with healthy men, it appears that men with CAD should supplement their diet with antioxidant-rich foods.

5. Consumption of whole grains and legumes in CAD men

Increased consumption of whole grains has been recommended to improve insulin sensitivity and to lower serum insulin concentration in CAD men [8]. Jang et al. [9] have recently determined that isocaloric replacement of refined rice with whole grains and other plant products in a powder form reduces CAD risk factors, such as insulin demand and lipid peroxidation in 76 CAD men. After 16 weeks of whole grain consumption, serum concentrations of glucose and insulin decreased by 24% and 14%, respectively. In the whole grain group, plasma MDA and homocysteine and urinary $PGF_{2\alpha}$ concentrations decreased by about 28%. Also, lipid-corrected concentrations of α-carotene, retinol, tocopherols, and lycopene increased by 11–40%, and the percentage composition of n-6 fatty acids of serum phospholipid increased by 14% in the whole grain group. The replacement of refined rice with whole grain and legume powder as a source of carbohydrate in a meal showed significant beneficial effects on glucose, insulin, and homocysteine concentrations and lipid peroxidation in CAD patients. These effects are likely to substantially reduce the risk factors for CAD and diabetes.

6. Conclusion

For the purpose of health promotion, the general public should be advised to be aware of the CAD risk associated with large waist circumference as well as the importance of reducing visceral fat in abdominal obese people. Heart-healthy nutritional guidelines, including minimally refined grains and frequent consumption of vegetables and legumes, and increasing postprandial particle removal with exercise are likely to become part of major goal to reduce the atherogenic risk caused by what we eat.

References

[1] Anonymous, WHO reassesses appropriate body-mass index for Asian populations, Lancet 360 (2002) 235.

[2] South Korean Ministry of Health and Social Affairs, Reports on 1969–1998 National Nutrition Survey; Report on National Health and Nutrition Survey, Ministry of Health and Welfare, Seoul, South Korea, 2000.

[3] Korea Ministry of Health and Social Affairs, National Nutrition Survey Report, Ministry of Health and Welfare, Seoul, South Korea, 1988.

[4] M. Lee, B.M. Popkin, S. Kim, The unique aspects of the nutrition transition in South Korea: the relation of healthful elements in their diet, Public Health Nutr. 5 (2002) 197–203.

[5] South Korea National Statistical Office, Annual Report on the Cause of Death Statistics, National Statistical Office, Seoul, South Korea, 2000.

[6] Y. Jang, O.Y. Kim, H.J. Ryu, J.Y. Kim, S.H. Song, J.M. Ordovas, J.H. Lee, Visceral fat accumulation determines postprandial lipemic response, lipid peroxidation, DNA damage and endothelial dysfunction in non-obese Korean men, J. Lipid Res. 44 (2003) (in press).

[7] Y. Jang, J.H. Lee, E.Y. Cho, N.S. Chung, D. Topham, B. Balderston, Differences in body fat distribution and antioxidant status in Korean men with cardiovascular disease with or without diabetes, Am. J. Clin. Nutr. 73 (2001) 68–74.

[8] Y. Jang, O.Y. Kim, H.Y. Park, J.H. Lee, J.S. Ham, H.J. Ryu, Effect of apolipoprotein E polymorphism on the serum lipid and insulin response to whole grain consumption in coronary artery disease patients, Nutr. Res. 21 (2001) 1463–1473.

[9] Y. Jang, J.H. Lee, O.Y. Kim, H.Y. Park, S.Y. Lee, Consumption of whole grain and legume powder reduces insulin demand, lipid peroxidation, and plasma homocysteine concentrations in patients with coronary artery disease. Randomized controlled clinical trial, Arterioscler. Thromb. Vasc. Biol. 21 (2001) 2065–2071.

ELSEVIER

International Congress Series 1262 (2004) 542–545

www.ics-elsevier.com

Obesity as the key player in the metabolic syndrome

Karen S.L. Lam*, Aimin Xu, Nelson M.S. Wat, Annette W.K. Tso, Mary S.M. Ip

Department of Medicine, University of Hong Kong, Queen Mary Hospital, 102 Pokfulam Road, Rm 419, Block K, Hong Kong, China

Abstract. Metabolic syndrome is a common cardiovascular risk factor in urbanized areas in China. In Hong Kong, it affects 17.1% of the population, increasing to 21.9% if the lower IOTF Asian cut-off values for central obesity were used. This is probably related to the increasing prevalence of excess adiposity. Epidemiological studies, cross-sectional and prospective, suggest that obesity plays a key role in metabolic syndrome in the Chinese, although other factors, such as genetic causes, may also enhance its development. Recent data, including those from Hong Kong and Taiwan, suggest that the adipocytokines, especially adiponectin, provide important links between obesity and various components of metabolic syndrome, through effects on insulin sensitivity, fatty acid synthesis and oxidation, nitric oxide production and inflammatory responses. Raised levels of C-reactive protein, a marker of low-grade chronic inflammation, are independently associated with obesity and predict the development of diabetes in the Chinese. Increased fat in the upper airway also predisposes to obstructive sleep apnea (OSA), sympathetic activation and insulin resistance, accounting for the high prevalence of "Syndrome Z" (metabolic syndrome plus obstructive sleep apnea). Appropriate weight control with regular physical exercise and a healthy diet is, therefore, the best prevention and treatment for metabolic syndrome. © 2003 Published by Elsevier B.V.

Keywords: Metabolic syndrome; Chinese; Obesity; Adiponectin; C-reactive protein

1. Introduction

Metabolic syndrome has been highlighted in the latest guidelines of the National Cholesterol Education Program (NCEP) as an important, modifiable risk factor of cardiovascular diseases [1]. Recent epidemiological data suggest that this condition is highly prevalent among urbanized Chinese, probably attributable to the increasing presence of excess adiposity. Findings from clinical and animal studies have also provided new insight into the mechanisms whereby obesity can lead to various features of metabolic syndrome. In the following sections, selective data of studies performed in Hong Kong, Shanghai and Taiwan will be presented to illustrate how obesity plays a key role in the development of metabolic syndrome.

* Corresponding author. Tel.: +852-2855-4783; fax: +852-2816-2187.
E-mail address: ksllam@hkucc.hku.hk (K.S.L. Lam).

0531-5131/ © 2003 Published by Elsevier B.V.
doi:10.1016/j.ics.2003.11.006

2. High prevalence of metabolic syndrome in urbanized Chinese populations

According to the 1995–1996 Hong Kong Cardiovascular Risk Factors Prevalence Study, the age- and sex-adjusted prevalence of metabolic syndrome, as defined in the NCEP guidelines [1], was 17.1%. Another study conducted in 1998–2001 in Shanghai, a major Chinese city, showed an age-adjusted prevalence of 22% [2], similar to that among US adults, estimated to be 23.7% in the third National Health and Nutrition Examination Survey (NHANES III). These findings are rather surprising, considering the much higher prevalence of obesity (BMI>30 kg/m^2) among US adults: 20.9% compared with only 4% in Shanghai and 5.4% among Hong Kong men (7.4% for women). This may be explained by the observation that Asians, including Chinese, have a higher percentage of body fat for a given BMI, compared with Caucasians [3]. Indeed, the International Obesity Task Force has proposed lower criteria of BMI and waist circumference for diagnosing obesity and central obesity, respectively, in Asians. Thus for Asians, a BMI of ≥ 25 kg/m^2 would be considered as "Obesity I" and, for waist circumference, the upper limits for men and women would be 90 and 80 cm, respectively. Using these criteria, 44% of adults in Shanghai and 40% of Hong Kong men (35% for women) would be considered obese, and the prevalence of metabolic syndrome would reach 21.9% in Hong Kong.

3. Obesity as a major determinant of metabolic syndrome in the Chinese

Cross-sectional studies in Hong Kong and Taiwan have shown that the clustering of variables in metabolic syndrome results from multiple factors linked by adiposity, and that central obesity is an independent determinant of insulin resistance and metabolic risk scores. In a prospective study of 644 non-diabetic subjects, we also found that baseline waist circumference predicted the worsening of glycemia in 2 years [4], while BMI, along with baseline fasting glucose and the Glu298Asp polymorphism of the endothelial nitric oxide synthase (eNOS) gene, predicted the glycemic status of subjects with impaired glucose tolerance in 5 years. BMI was also predictive of blood pressure status in this cohort. These prospective data are supportive of the key role of obesity in the development of diabetes and hypertension, major components of metabolic syndrome, in the Chinese.

4. Adipocytokines as the link between obesity and metabolic syndrome

The fat cell actively secretes various products, which can provide the link between obesity and other components of metabolic syndrome. Free fatty acids, released from lipolysis, promote insulin resistance by increasing intramyocyte fat and induce hyperglycemia through enhanced hepatic gluconeogenesis, competitive reduction in glucose oxidation, reduced glucose transport and decreased glycogen synthesis. They also reduce insulin secretion by increasing uncoupling protein-2 expression, β-cell apoptosis and dysfunction. Another adipocytokine, TNF-α, enhances insulin resistance by reducing insulin receptor kinase activity. Resistin, a fat cell-derived hormone, is another candidate for promoting insulin resistance. However, exciting data on its effects on insulin action and glucose tolerance in rodents [5] remain to be confirmed in humans, even though preliminary data suggest that raised levels are also found in obese and diabetic subjects.

Adiponectin, secreted exclusively from the fat cell, is a more promising link between obesity and metabolic syndrome [6]. In animal and cell studies, this hormone improves insulin sensitivity, reduces atherosclerosis, promotes fatty acid oxidation, decreases fatty acid and fat synthesis [7] and stimulates endothelial nitric oxide production through AMP kinase-mediated phosphorylation of eNOS. Hypoadiponectinemia is found in humans with obesity, diabetes, hypertension, hypertriglyceridemia and low HDL-cholesterol, and predicted cardiovascular events in a study of patients with renal failure. In Taiwanese Chinese, weight loss in obese subjects is accompanied by increases in serum adiponectin. In Hong Kong Chinese, we have found that serum adiponectin is independently associated with insulin resistance and homozygosity for the risk haplotype of two SNPs (45G → T and 276T → G) of the adiponectin gene is associated with increased insulin resistance and hyperinsulinemia. Adiponectin also exhibits anti-inflammatory properties through inhibiting the expression [7] and action of TNF-α, a pro-inflammatory cytokine. The interaction between adiponectin and TNF-α, the expression of which is decreased and increased respectively in obesity, may account for the association between obesity and serum C-reactive protein, a marker of chronic low-grade inflammation. Indeed, C-reactive protein levels vary inversely with those of plasma adiponectin and predict the deterioration of glycemia in Chinese subjects with impaired glucose tolerance [8], supporting the role of chronic low-grade inflammation in linking obesity with other components of metabolic syndrome.

5. Syndrome Z

Obese individuals are more likely to suffer from obstructive sleep apnea (OSA) because of increased fat deposits in the upper airway. On the other hand, OSA is associated with an increased prevalence of metabolic syndrome. Recent findings suggest that this association, also known as "Syndrome Z", is more than the coexistence of two conditions caused by obesity. The US Nurses' Health Study reported that snoring was an independent predictor of type 2 diabetes. We have also demonstrated that indices of OSA, including the apnea–hypnea index and minimum oxygen saturation, are determinants of insulin resistance in OSA subjects, independent of the effect of obesity [9]. Insulin resistance, consequent to sympathetic stimulation induced by hypoxemia, probably contributes to the development of Syndrome Z.

6. Conclusion

These recent data support the key role of obesity in metabolic syndrome although other factors, such as genetic causes, may contribute to its development. Even moderate weight loss has been shown to have beneficial effects on all components of this syndrome. Optimal weight control through regular physical exercise and a healthy diet should be the best way to prevent and treat metabolic syndrome.

Acknowledgements

Clinical studies on adiponectin and the prospective studies were supported by grants from the Hong Kong Research Grant Council 7426/03M and 7290/97M, respectively.

References

[1] Executive summary of the Third Report of the National Cholesterol Education Program (NCEP) expert panel on detection, evaluation and treatment of high blood cholesterol in adults (adult treatment panel III), JAMA 285 (2001) 2486–2497.

[2] K. Xiang, The heavy burden of metabolic syndrome in Shanghai, China, Diabetes Res. Clin. Pract. 56 (Suppl 1) (2002) S2.

[3] M. He, K.C. Tan, E.T. Li, A.W. Kung, Body fat determination by dual energy X-ray absorptiometry and its relation to body mass index and waist circumference in Hong Kong Chinese, Int. J. Obes. 25 (2001) 748–752.

[4] N.M.S. Wat, T.H. Lam, E.D. Janus, K.S.L. Lam, Central obesity predicts the worsening of glycemia in southern Chinese, Int. J. Obes. 25 (2001) 1789–1793.

[5] C.M. Steppan, et al., The hormone resistin links obesity to diabetes, Nature 409 (2001) 307–312.

[6] A.H. Berg, T.P. Coombs, P.E. Scherer, ACRP30/adiponectin: an adipokine regulating glucose and lipid metabolism, Trends Endocrinol. Metab. 13 (2002) 84–89.

[7] A. Xu, Y. Wang, H. Keshaw, L.Y. Xu, K.S.L. Lam, G.J. Cooper, The fat-derived hormone adiponectin alleviate alcoholic and nonalcoholic fatty liver diseases in mice, J. Clin. Invest. 91 (2003) 91–100.

[8] C.B. Tan, N.M.S. Wat, S.C.F. Tam, E.D. Janus, T.H. Lam, K.S.L. Lam, C-reactive protein predicts the deterioration of glycemia in Chinese subjects with impaired glucose tolerance, Diabetes Care 26 (2003) 2323–2328.

[9] M.S.M. Ip, B. Lam, M.M.T. Ng, W.K. Lam, K.W.T. Tsang, K.S.L. Lam, Obstructive sleep apnea is independently associated with insulin resistance, Am. J. Respir. Crit. Care Med. 165 (2002) 670–676.

International Congress Series 1262 (2004) 546–549

www.ics-elsevier.com

The metabolic syndrome: an Asian perspective

Chee-Eng Tan[a,*], Suok-Kai Chew[b], E-Shyong Tai[a]

[a] *Department of Endocrinology, Singapore General Hospital, Block 6 Level 6, Outram Road, Singapore 169608, Republic of Singapore*

[b] *Ministry of Health, College of Medicine Building, Singapore*

Abstract. The phenotypic manifestation of metabolic syndrome (MS) includes central obesity, elevated blood pressure, impaired glucose tolerance, diabetes mellitus (DM), low levels of HDL-C, elevated triglyceride and presence of dense LDL-C. Diagnosis of MS is made when three out of five features are present. We believe that central obesity, as defined by waist circumference above 90 cm in males and 80 cm in females, is more appropriate in an Asian setting. The original ATP III criteria for MS are likely to give a falsely low prevalence of MS in Asia. Using the ATP III criteria, the prevalence of the MS in Singapore was low. When the waist circumference was modified to >90 and >80 cm in males and females, respectively, the prevalence of MS was comparable with those in Western population. Prevalence of MS differed significantly between ethnic groups and was highest in Asian Indians followed by Malays and then Chinese. This pattern was seen in both males and females. It is likely that prevalence of MS will be different across ethnic groups in Asia. Prevalence of MS increases as the population ages but remain significantly higher in Asian Indians compared with the Chinese or Malays across all the age groups. As the population demographic in Asia changes and its population begin to age, the prevalence of MS is also likely to rise. The high prevalence of MS and its associated phenotypic manifestation could play a significant role in the increasing prevalence of CHD as well as burdens of diabetes mellitus in the region. Lifestyle measures and exercises to reduce weight, decrease insulin resistance and increase HDL-C could play a significant role in reducing the impact of MS on cardiovascular diseases (CVD) across Asia.

Keywords: Metabolic syndrome; Chinese; Malays; Asian Indians; Waist circumference

1. The metabolic syndrome: an Asian perspective

The metabolic syndrome (MS) is associated with a number of metabolic derangement including central obesity, glucose intolerance, hyperinsulinemia, low HDL cholesterol (HDL-C), high triglyceride (TG), hypertension [1], obstructive sleep apnea [2] and polycystic ovary disease [3]. Subjects with the MS are also at increased risk of developing diabetes mellitus (DM) [4] and cardiovascular disease (CVD) [5].

* Corresponding author. Tel.: +65-63214654; fax: +65-62273576.
E-mail address: ce_tan@sgh.com.sg (C.-E. Tan).

0531-5131/ © 2004 Published by Elsevier B.V.
doi:10.1016/j.ics.2003.12.089

The third national health and nutrition examination (NHANES III) survey reported that the age-adjusted prevalence of the MS in the United States was 23.7% with the highest prevalence being found among Mexican Americans [6]. The definition of MS was based on the Adult Treatment Panel (ATP III) report [7] where participants having three or more criteria were defined as having the MS. The WHO criteria for MS [8] is more complex because it takes into consideration microalbuminuria, plasma insulin and body mass index (BMI) (in place of waist circumference).

2. Should the ATP III criteria be modified for Asians?

The waist circumference or BMI cut-off used in either definition is inappropriate for the Asian populations. A review of Asian data had concluded that Asians had a higher percentage body fat at a lower BMI compared with Caucasians [9]. Furthermore, subjects of Chinese descent had also been shown to have similar risk of developing glucose intolerance at lower BMI compared with indigenous Europeans [10]. Data from Hong Kong Chinese showed that they are prone to disorders such as DM, hypertension and dyslipidemia at lower levels of BMI than in Caucasian populations [11,12]. For the same reasons, the recommended cut-off for waist circumference in the ATP III is likely to be inappropriate for an Asian population such as ours [11,13]. A more appropriate waist circumference to define central obesity in Asians should be >90 cm in males and >80 cm in females.

Therefore, we believe that modification to the ATP III criteria, and in particular, the waist circumference, is necessary to give a true reflection of the MS in Asians.

3. Definition of metabolic syndrome

The current NCEP ATP III criteria define an individual as having MS when he or she has three or more of the following criteria. 1. Waist circumference >102 cm in men and >88 cm in women. 2. Triglyceride >1.7 mmol/l. 3. HDL cholesterol < 1.0 mmol/l in men and < 1.3 mmol/l in women. 4. Blood pressure >130/85 mm Hg. 5. Fasting glucose of >6.1 mmol/l.

We believe that central obesity in Asians should be defined as waist circumference of greater than 90 cm in males and greater than 80 cm in females. This definition for central obesity has been proposed by Western Pacific WHO in conjunction with the International Association for the Study of Obesity and the International Obesity Task Force [14]. Furthermore, we believe that all subjects on treatment for hypertension should be regarded as having blood pressure >130/85 mm Hg while those being treated for diabetes mellitus should be considered as having fasting glucose >6.1 mmol/l. Therefore, a modification of the ATP III criteria for diagnosing MS should be considered in Asians.

4. Ethnicity and the metabolic syndrome in Asians

The three ethnic groups in Singapore (Chinese, Malay and Asian Indians) represent a large proportion of populations across Asia. We believe that the pattern of MS in the three ethnic groups in Singapore will give us a glimpse of how the MS will pan out in the near future across Asia as the region becomes more urbanized. The prevalence of the MS in

Singapore using a modified waist circumference was comparable with the prevalence reported in the United States (NHANES III) [6].

Prevalence of the MS was highest in the Asian Indians followed by the Malays and then Chinese. Differences in prevalence of the MS between Chinese and the other two ethnic groups were seen in both males and females. Ethnic differences in prevalence of DM or MS are not unique to Singapore as it had been demonstrated in several western populations. The Australian Aborigines [15], American Hispanics [16,17], and migrant Indians [18] have all been shown to have higher prevalence of DM or MS. However, most of these minority ethnic groups have social and lifestyle factors that differ considerably from the European population within their respective countries. In Singapore, all three ethnic groups live in a fairly homogenous, urbanized, city environment. We believe that the difference in prevalence of the MS between ethnic groups cannot be explained solely by environmental factors.

5. Age and the metabolic syndrome

The prevalence of the MS increases as the population ages across all three ethnic groups. In those aged 60–69 years old, about one third exhibited features of the MS. Again, the impact of age on the prevalence of the MS in our population was consistent with data from NHANES III. Since age is an important factor in the phenotypic manifestation of the MS, the young population in Singapore (mean age 34.0 years) implies that as our population ages, the impact of the MS will be significantly greater and may even outstrip those in developed countries such as the United States.

We had previously reported that the increase in prevalence of DM with age appeared to occur approximately 10 years earlier in Asian Indians than in Chinese [19]. If this were also true of the MS, then the earlier age of onset of MS in Asian Indians, coupled with the relatively young age of our population, could explain the higher prevalence of MS in Asian Indians. As the prevalence of the MS was highest in Asian Indians (males and females) across all age groups, we believe that Asian Indians may be particularly prone to develop the MS irrespective of age. We also suggest that genetic factors found in Asian Indians may contribute to the differences in prevalence of the MS between ethnic groups in Singapore through interaction with environmental factors.

6. Implications of the metabolic syndrome

Ethnicity remains a significant predictor of CVD in our population, even after adjustment for DM and other CVD risk factors [20]. We believe that the higher prevalence of the MS in Asian Indians and Malays could be another potential contributory factor to the excess CVD events compared with the Chinese. We had also recently reported that Asian Indians and Malays with DM have almost twice the mortality compared with Chinese with DM [21]. One possible reason for the higher mortality in Asian Indians and Malays with DM could be the longer exposure to DM since the rise in prevalence of DM in Asian Indians occurred at least 10 years earlier than in Chinese. The MS may be present even before the onset of DM. The insulin resistance, low HDL-C, hypertension and central obesity associated with MS means that the atherosclerotic process begins even before IGT or DM is established. Good glycemic control failed to reduce the macrovascular complication in the UKPDS because the atherosclerotic process predates the development of hyperglycemia [22]. The presence of the MS at a younger age in Asian Indians and Malays highlights the need to look beyond DM and IGT if we are to make a significant difference to coronary artery disease events in these two ethnic groups. Lifestyle measures and exercise to reduce weight, decrease insulin resistance and raise HDL-C will be important in reducing coronary risk in Asian Indians and Malays.

In conclusion, we are of the opinion that lowering of the criteria for the diagnosis of central obesity in Asians is necessary. More data are needed to ascertain if lowering the waist circumference to >90 in men and >80 in women is appropriate in identifying individuals with the MS in Asia and whether it could be applied uniformly across different ethnic groups. However, it is likely that ethnic differences in the prevalence of MS exist that could contribute to differences in CVD risk among population groups in Asia.

References

[1] G.M. Reaven, et al., Diabetes 37 (1988) 1595–1607.
[2] S. Coughlin, et al., Obes. Rev. 2 (2001) 267–274.
[3] D.A. Ehrmann, Curr. Diab. Rep. 2 (2002) 71–76.
[4] S.M. Haffner, et al., Diabetes 41 (1992) 715–722.
[5] B. Isomaa, et al., Diabetes Care 24 (2001) 683–689.
[6] E.S. Ford, et al., JAMA 287 (2002) 356–359.
[7] Executive Summary of The Third Report of The National Cholesterol Education Program (NCEP) Expert Panel on Detection, Evaluation, And Treatment of High Blood Cholesterol In Adults (Adult Treatment Panel III), JAMA 285 (2001) 2486–2497.
[8] K.G. Alberti, P.Z. Zimmet, Diabet. Med. 15 (1998) 539–553.
[9] P. Deurenberg, et al., Obes. Rev. 3 (2002) 141–146.
[10] N. Unwin, et al., J. Epidemiol. Community Health 51 (1997) 160–166.
[11] G.T. Ko, et al., Int. J. Obes. Relat. Metab. Disord. 23 (1999) 1136–1142.
[12] G. Li, et al., Obes. Rev. 3 (2002) 167–172.
[13] S.A. Lear, et al., Metabolism 51 (2002) 1427–1432.
[14] WHO/IASO/IOTF: The Asia-Pacific Perspective: Redefining Obesity and its Treatment. Available at: http://www.idi.org.au/home.htm, Access August 21, 2003.
[15] M. Daniel, et al., Diabetes Care 22 (1999) 1993–1998.
[16] J.P. Burke, et al., Arch. Intern. Med. 159 (1999) 1450–1456.
[17] J.B. Meigs, et al., Diabetes 52 (2003) 2160–2167.
[18] H. King, P. Zimmet, World Health Stat. Q. 41 (1988) 190–196.
[19] E.S. Tai, et al., Diabetes Res. Clin. Pract. 49 (2000) 159–168.
[20] J. Lee, et al., Int. J. Epidemiol. 30 (2001 (Oct.) 983–988.
[21] S. Ma, et al., Am. J. Epidemiol. 15 (2003) 2003.
[22] S.M. Haffner, et al., JAMA 263 (1990) 2893–2898.

International Congress Series 1262 (2004) 550–553

www.ics-elsevier.com

Lipoprotein (a) and atherosclerosis: a study from transgenic rabbits

Jianglin Fan[a,*], Teruo Watanabe[b]

[a] *Cardiovascular Disease Laboratory, Department of Pathology, Institute of Basic Medical Sciences, University of Tsukuba, Tenoudai 1-1-1, 305-8575, Tsukuba, Ibaraki, Japan*
[b] *Saga University, Saga, Japan*

Abstract. High levels of lipoprotein (a) [Lp(a)] are an independent risk factor for a number of cardiovascular diseases such coronary heart disease, stroke and restenosis. In addition, numerous clinical and experimental studies indicate that Lp(a), similar to LDL, is an atherogenic lipoprotein, and thus, increased plasma concentrations of Lp(a) may be associated with premature atherosclerosis. Despite the progress in these studies during the past years, the precise physiological functions of Lp(a) is still unknown, and its pathological roles on the pathogenesis of atherosclerosis have not been fully defined. To investigate the functional roles of Lp(a), our laboratory has generated transgenic rabbits expressing human apolipoprotein (a) [apo(a)], and recently, we demonstrated that Lp(a) enhances diet-induced atherosclerosis and vascular calcification in transgenic rabbits. In this article, we summarize the progress in the study of human apo(a) transgenic rabbits. © 2003 Published by Elsevier B.V.

Keywords: Transgenic rabbits; Lp(a); Atherosclerosis; Hypercholesterolemia; Calcification

1. Introduction

The lipoprotein (a) [Lp(a)] particle closely resembles low-density lipoprotein (LDL) in both lipid composition and the presence of apoB. Lp(a) is distinguished from LDL by the presence of an additional unique protein called apolipoprotein (a) [apo(a)]. High levels of Lp(a) have been considered an independent risk factor for a number of cardiovascular diseases such coronary heart disease, stroke and restenosis after PTCA. In addition, numerous clinical and experimental studies indicate that Lp(a), similar to LDL, is an atherogenic lipoprotein, and thus, increased plasma concentrations of Lp(a) may be associated with premature atherosclerosis. Despite the progress in these studies during the past years, the precise physiological functions of Lp(a) is still unknown, and its

Abbreviations: Lp(a), lipoprotein (a); apo(a), apolipoprotein (a); Tg, transgenic; WHHL, Watanabe heritable hyperlipidemic.

* Corresponding author. Tel.: +81-298-53-3165; fax: +81-298-54-9039.
E-mail address: J-LFAN@md.tsukuba.ac.jp (J. Fan).

doi:10.1016/j.ics.2003.12.037

pathological roles on the pathogenesis of atherosclerosis have not been fully understood. This may be due to the complexity of Lp(a) structure, large variations of plasma levels of Lp(a) among the populations, lack of accurate methods to measure Lp(a) concentration in plasma and of appropriate animal models for Lp(a) research [1]. In this respect, our laboratory has developed transgenic (Tg) rabbits that express human apo(a), a unique component of Lp(a), as a novel means to investigate the mechanism of Lp(a) pathogenicity in the process of atherosclerosis. Our recent studies revealed that Lp(a) increases cholesterol-diet-induced atherosclerosis in Tg rabbits. Furthermore, Lp(a) enhances the development of advanced atherosclerosis and vascular calcification in Watanabe heritable hyperlipidemic (WHHL) rabbits. In this article, we summarize the recent findings based on the results from Tg rabbits.

2. Development of transgenic rabbits expressing human apo(a)

Apo(a), a unique component of Lp(a) is only naturally present in primates (monkeys and humans) and hedgehogs; therefore, for a long time, there were no experimental animal models for Lp(a). Tg mice expressing human apo(a) revealed that human apo(a) cannot bind to murine apoB to form Lp(a) [2]. In 1998, our laboratory along with others made the first Tg rabbits expressing human apo(a) as a potential model for the study of Lp(a) [3,4]. Using the full-length of human apo(a) cDNA fragment containing 17 copies of kringle 4 repeats under the control of the mouse transferrin promoter, we generated three lines of Tg rabbits. The plasma levels of Lp(a) in these Tg rabbit were 2–4.5 mg/dl, which are within the average levels of Lp(a) in Japanese population (15 mg/dl). Analysis of the plasma from Tg rabbits showed that human apo(a) can bind to rabbit apoB to form Lp(a)-like particles even though the bondage between human apo(a) and rabbit apoB is not completely covalent, possibly due to the fact that rabbit apoB-100 lacks a compatible Cys-4326 in human [5]. These rabbits did not show any phenotypes and did not develop spontaneous atherosclerosis after 2 years old on a chow diet, suggesting that lower levels of Lp(a) is not atherogenic even in the animals that normally do not have this protein. In the following studies, we fed these Tg and control rabbits a diet containing 0.3% cholesterol and 3% soybean oil for 16 weeks. We found that Tg rabbits developed greater aortic and coronary atherosclerosis than did control rabbits [6]. Immunohistochemical investigation revealed that the enhanced lesion development in Tg rabbits was characterized by increased accumulation of immature smooth muscle cells, suggesting that Lp(a) may mediate smooth muscle cell proliferation and dedifferentiation [7].

3. Lp(a) enhances advanced atherosclerosis and vascular calcification in WHHL rabbits

To further study Lp(a) atherogenicity, we cross-bred Lp(a) Tg rabbits with WHHL rabbits, an animal model for human familial hypercholesterolemia [8]. WHHL rabbits have defective LDL receptor function; therefore, they have high levels of LDL-cholesterol. We envisioned that Tg WHHL rabbits may have high levels of both LDL and Lp(a). Compared with the wild-type Tg rabbits, WHHL Tg rabbits had fourfold increased Lp(a) levels, suggesting that LDL receptors may be involved in the catabolism of Lp(a) in rabbits [8]. In order to elucidate the Lp(a) atherogenicity, we compared the lesions of Tg with non-Tg WHHL rabbits at the age of 7–8 months. Compared with non-Tg WHHL rabbits, the intimal lesion area in WHHL Tg rabbits was significantly increased [9]. Furthermore, the lesions of Tg WHHL rabbits differed markedly from those of non-Tg WHHL rabbits: Tg WHHL rabbits had more complicated lesions such as atheromas and calcification, whereas non-Tg WHHL rabbits had basically fatty streak, an early-stage lesion [9]. We were particularly interested in the vascular calcification seen in Tg WHHL rabbits and made an immunohistochemical study. We found that Lp(a) was frequently associated with vascular calcification in Tg WHHL rabbits. To elucidate the molecular mechanism for Lp(a)-induced calcification, we performed in vitro study using cultured rabbit smooth muscle cells incubated with Lp(a) isolated from normal subjects. These studies showed that incubation with Lp(a), smooth muscle cells showed increased alkaline phosphatase activity and enhanced calcium uptake associated with high expression of matrix Gla protein and Osf2 mRNA [9]. Taken together, these studies suggest that Lp(a) may participate in vascular calcification. Our recent study using human coronary arteries from 40 subjects who had myocardial infarction showed that apo(a) is frequently associated with calcification in the lesion (Sun et al. unpublished data).

In conclusion, our current studies using Tg rabbits provide further evidence that Lp(a) is an atherogenic lipoprotein. Furthermore, we have shown that Lp(a) may be a potential regulator in the vascular calcification. In future study, it will be interesting to determine whether Tg WHHL rabbits have increased incidence of myocardial infarction. We believe that Tg WHHL rabbits may become a useful model for studying the benefits of some drugs in the treatment of atherosclerosis in patients with high levels of Lp(a).

Acknowledgements

This work was supported by the Center for Tsukuba Advanced Research Alliance (TARA) at the University of Tsukuba.

References

[1] S.M. Marcovina, M.L. Koschinsky, J.J. Albers, S. Skarlatos, Report of the national heart, lung, and blood institute workshop on lipoprotein(a) and cardiovascular disease: recent advances and future directions, Clin. Chem. 49 (2003) 1785–1796.

[2] G. Chiesa, H.H. Hobbs, M.L. Koschinsky, R.M. Lawn, S.D. Maika, R.E. Hammer, Reconstitution of lipoprotein(a) by infusion of human low density lipoprotein into transgenic mice expressing human apolipoprotein(a), J. Biol. Chem. 267 (1992) 24369–24374.

[3] J. Fan, M. Araki, L. Wu, M. Challah, H. Shimoyamada, M.R. Lawn, H. Kakuta, H. Shikama, T. Watanabe, Transgenic rabbits expressing human apolipoprotein (a), Circulation 98 (Suppl.) (1998) I–390 (Abstract).

[4] D. Rouy, N. Duverger, S.D. Lin, F. Emmanuel, L.M. Houdebine, P. Denefle, C. Viglietta, E. Gong, E.M. Rubin, S.D. Hughes, Apolipoprotein(a) yeast artificial chromosome transgenic rabbits. Lipoprotein(a) assembly with human and rabbit apolipoprotein B, J. Biol. Chem. 273 (1998) 1247–1251.

[5] J. Fan, M. Araki, L. Wu, M. Challah, H. Shimoyamada, M.R. Lawn, H. Kakuta, H. Shikama, T. Watanabe, Assembly of lipoprotein (a) in transgenic rabbits expressing human apolipoprotein (a), Biochem. Biophys. Res. Commun. 255 (1999) 639–644.

[6] J. Fan, H. Shimoyamada, H. Sun, S. Marcovina, K. Honda, T. Watanabe, Transgenic rabbits expressing human apolipoprotein(a) develop more extensive atherosclerotic lesions in response to a cholesterol-rich diet, Arterioscler Thromb. Vasc. Biol. 21 (2001) 88–94.

[7] T. Ichikawa, H. Unoki, H. Sun, H. Shimoyamada, S. Marcovina, H. Shikama, T. Watanabe, J. Fan, Lipoprotein(a) promotes smooth muscle cell proliferation and dedifferentiation in atherosclerotic lesions of human apo(a) transgenic rabbits, Am. J. Pathol. 160 (2002) 227–236.

[8] J. Fan, M. Challah, H. Shimoyamada, M. Shiomi, S. Marcovina, T. Watanabe, Defects of the LDL receptor in WHHL transgenic rabbits lead to a marked accumulation of plasma lipoprotein[a], J. Lipid Res. 41 (2000) 1004–1012.

[9] H. Sun, H. Unoki, X. Wang, J. Liang, T. Ichikawa, Y. Arai, M. Shiomi, S. Marcovina, T. Watanabe, J. Fan, Lipoprotein(a) enhances advanced atherosclerosis and vascular calcification in WHHL transgenic rabbits expressing human apolipoprotein(a), J. Biol. Chem. 277 (2002) 47486–47492.

International Congress Series 1262 (2004) 554–557

www.ics-elsevier.com

The catabolism of lipoprotein(a)

G.M. Kostner[a,*], A. Hrzenjak[a], S. Frank[a], T. Van Berkel[b], X. Wo[a,1], K.M. Kostner[a]

[a] *Institute of Medical Biochemistry and Medical Molecular Biology, Med-Uni Graz, Harrachgasse 21, A-8010 Graz, Austria*

[b] *Gorlaeus Laboratories, Leiden University, Netherlands*

Abstract. *Background*: Little is known of the catabolism of Lp(a). Although Lp(a) has been found to bind in vitro to numerous receptors, the relevance of these pathways has not been documented in vivo. Here, we investigated the involvement of asialo glycoprotein receptors (ASGPR) in the catabolism of Lp(a). *Methods*: Lp(a) was isolated from donors with various isoforms, radiolabelled and injected in native form or after desialylation into wild-type mice or ASGPR knock out mice ($ASGPR^+$ or $ASGPR^-$ mice). The catabolism from plasma and organ uptake was monitored. In addition, we investigated the metabolic fate of native Lp(a) and Lp(a) incubated for 24 h at 37 °C in human plasma in rats. *Results*: Native Lp(a) was catabolised faster in $ASGPR^+$ mice than in $ASGPR^-$ mice. Desialylation led to a several-fold reduction in the plasma residence time of Lp(a) and most of the asialo-Lp(a) was taken up by the liver. The Lp(a) catabolism in rats could be competitively inhibited by asialo fetoprotein (ASF), yet not by mannan. Preincubation of Lp(a) for 24 h at 37 °C significantly increased the catabolic rate of Lp(a). *Conclusion*: Our data suggest that the Gal-specific asialoglycoprotein receptor might be involved in the Lp(a) catabolism. © 2003 Published by Elsevier B.V.

Keywords: Asialo glycoprotein receptor; Sialidase; Lp(a) metabolism; Transgenic mice

1. Introduction

Little is known of the function and metabolism of Lp(a) [1]. The genetically determined size polymorphism explains approximately 50% of the variation in Lp(a) concentrations, yet there exist numerous additional genetic influences. Also, the efficiency and speed of Lp(a) assembly has an impact on Lp(a) levels [2]. Unfortunately, reliable animal models producing Lp(a) by themselves hardly exist. Work carried out in our laboratory on various animal species revealed that the majority of injected human Lp(a) goes to the liver [3]. It has also been suggested that the kidney plays a role. Many lipoprotein-specific receptors have been suggested to catabolise Lp(a) such as LDL-R, LRP, VLDL-R and GP-330/megalin. Their in vivo relevance for Lp(a) catabolism has not been revealed yet.

* Corresponding author. Tel.: +43-316-3804200; fax: +43-316-3809615.
E-mail address: gerhard.kostner@uni-graz.at (G.M. Kostner).
[1] Present address: Zhejing Traditional Chinese Medical College, China.

doi:10.1016/S0531-5131(03)01891-0

Lp(a), on the other hand, has been found to be proteolytically cleaved in circulating blood and a relatively large amount of high molecular fragments secreted into urine. This pathway, however, accounts for not more than 1% of the removal of Lp(a) from circulation [4,5].

Apo(a), the specific antigen of Lp(a), is a highly glycosylated protein. The most complete characterization of the sugars in apo(a) was recently published by Garner et al. [6] who demonstrated that part of the oligosaccharides are present in a non-sialylated form. This later finding prompted us to elucidate the possibility that Lp(a) may bind to the asialo glycoprotein receptor (ASGPR).

2. Material and methods

Lp(a) was isolated from fasting plasma of healthy individuals with different isoforms in the quickest possible fashion, involving ultracentrifugation (*d* 1.065–1.130 g/ml) and column chromatography over Biogel A-15M in buffers containing 1% proline in the presence of the preservatives EDTA, BHT Thimerosal, PMSF and p-Br-phenacyl bromide [4]. Apo(a) and Lp(a) quantitation was performed by DELFIA [4].

Desialylation of Lp(a) or alpha-fetoprotein was performed by agarose-bound sialidase (51 U/g agarose, incubation for 48 h at room temperature).

2.1. Animals

2.1.1. Mice

We obtained the mice used in this study from Jackson Laboratory. Asialo glycoprotein receptor deficient mice (B6, 129-Asgr2) lacking the lower molecular weight receptor subunit (HL-2) were used. The animals were housed at 22 °C under a constant light–dark cycle and had free access to water and rodent chow.

Anesthetized mice were injected with either native or sialidase-treated Lp(a) in 150 μl of PBS. Blood was collected at different time intervals and the decay of the Lp(a) plasma concentration was followed using DELFIA.

In order to study the uptake of Lp(a) by different tissues, female $ASGPR^-$ and $ASGPR^+$ mice were injected with 0.05 mg of ^{125}I-Lp(a) (180 cpm/ng protein) in 100 μl of PBS. After 15 min, the mice were perfused through the left ventricle with 20 ml PBS. Different organs were harvested and analyzed in the γ-counter.

2.1.2. Rats

Three rats were each injected with 0.5 mg ^{125}I-tyramine-cellobiose-labelled native or neuraminidase-treated Lp(a) in the presence or absence of a 50-fold excess of asialo-alpha fetoprotein (ASF) or of mannan, which specifically block two different types of ASGPR. In addition, freshly drawn plasma was incubated for 24 h at 37 °C prior to the isolation of Lp(a). The decay of the radioactivity from plasma and the uptake into different organs was followed for 60 min.

3. Results and discussion

First, six female $ASGPR^-$ and six $ASGPR^+$ mice were injected with 0.25 mg of freshly prepared Lp(a), each yielding plasma concentration in the physiological rang of 200–250

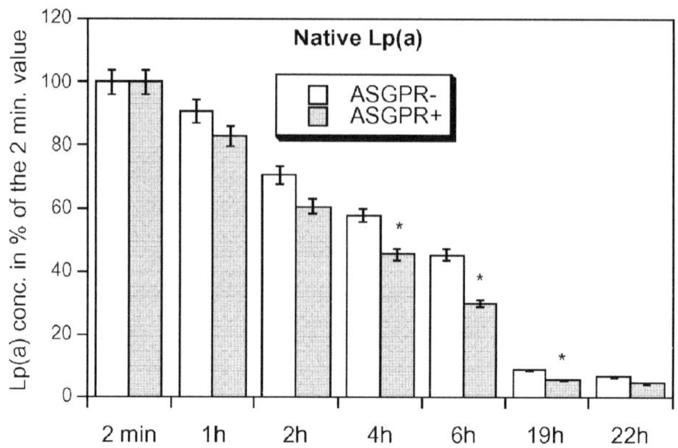

Fig. 1. Catabolism of native Lp(a) in wild-type mice ($n=6$) and in ASGPR$^-$ mice ($n=6$).

mg/l. Plasma Lp(a) decayed with an apparent half-life of 4–6 h (Fig. 1). Lp(a) catabolised faster in ASGPR$^+$ as compared with ASGPR$^-$ mice ($p<0.05$). In order to test whether full desialylation might convert Lp(a) into a more avidly removed substrate by the ASGPR, we injected 0.15 mg of sialidase-treated Lp(a) into control and ASGPR$^-$ mice. As expected, desialylated Lp(a) disappeared from circulation at a very fast rate (data not shown). Interestingly, asialo-Lp(a) was also catabolised significantly faster in the ASGPR$^-$ mice as compared with native Lp(a).

We also studied the uptake of Lp(a) into different organs from ASGPR$^-$ or ASGPR$^+$ mice ($n=5$ for each group). Significantly higher amounts of Lp(a) accumulated in the liver of ASGPR$^+$ mice compared with ASGPR$^-$ mice (2040 ± 146 vs. 508 ± 35 ng/g wet tissue) (data not shown). Much smaller amounts of radioactivity were also found in the spleen and kidney.

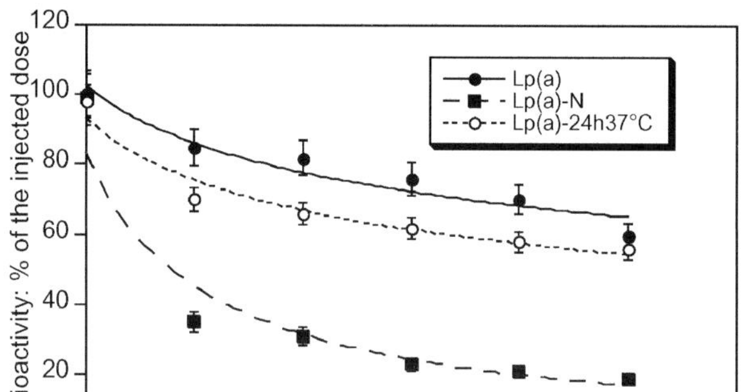

Fig. 2. Catabolism of native Lp(a), asialo-Lp(a) and Lp(a) isolated from plasma, which was preincubated for 24 h at 37 °C in three rats, respectively.

Additional experiments were conducted in rats. First, neuraminidase-treated Lp(a) was injected into rats in the absence or presence of a 50-fold excess of either asialofetoprotein (ASF) or of mannan. Only ASF competitively inhibited the catabolism of neuraminidase-treated Lp(a), whereas mannan had no such effect (data not shown).

Since native, intact glycoproteins are reportedly not catabolised by the ASGPR, we pursued the possibility that Lp(a) might be desialylated in circulating plasma and, in turn, bound and catabolised by the asialo glycoprotein pathway. Freshly drawn plasma containing 810 mg/l of Lp (a) (18 K-IV repeats) was divided into two batches; one was stored at 4 °C, the other incubated for 24 h at 37 °C followed by isolation of Lp(a).

Fig. 2 demonstrates that during incubation of plasma for 24 h Lp(a) is converted into a particle, which is catabolised significantly faster as compared with Lp(a) isolated from fresh plasma.

In summary, we suggest that the ASGPR pathway plays a significant role in the catabolism of Lp(a). Our data from the present study strongly suggest that the galactose-specific asialo glycoprotein receptor is involved in Lp(a) catabolism. It appears that Lp(a) has to be first hydrolysed by sialidases before binding and uptake.

Acknowledgements

This study was made possible by a grant from the Austrian Research foundation, SFB #F702.

References

[1] G.M. Kostner, Lipoprotein(a): still an enigma, Curr. Opinion Lipidol. 13 (2002) 391–396.

[2] L. Becker, B.A. Webb, S. Chitayat, M.E. Nesheim, M.L. Koschinsky, A ligand-induced conformational change in apolipoprotein(a) enhances covalent Lp(a) formation, J. Biol. Chem. 278 (2003) 14074–14081.

[3] K.M. Kostner, S. Frank, G.M. Kostner, Lipoprotein(a), in: Wass, Shalet (Eds.), Oxford Textbook of Endocrinology, 2002, Oxford University Press, pp. 1561–1564.

[4] K.M. Kostner, G. Maurer, K. Huber, T. Stefanelli, H. Dieplinger, E. Steyrer, G.M. Kostner, Urinary excretion of apo(a) fragments: role in apo(a) catabolism, Arterioscler. Thromb. Vasc. Biol. 16 (1996) 905–911.

[5] X. Wo, K.M. Kostner, S. Frank, G.M. Kostner, Assembly and Catabolism of Lipoprotein(a), in: B. Jacotot, D. Mathe, J.-C. Fruchart (Eds.), Proceedings of the 11th International Symposium on Atherosclerosis, Paris, 5–9 Oct., 1997, Raven Press, pp. 163–168.

[6] B. Garner, A.H. Merry, L. Royle, D.J. Harvey, P.M. Rudd, J. Thillet, Structural elucidation of the *N*- and *O*-glycans of human apolipoprotein(a): role of *O*-glycans in conferring protease resistance, J. Biol. Chem. 276 (2001) 22200–22208.

International Congress Series 1262 (2004) 558–561
www.ics-elsevier.com

The effect of methodological differences in the measurement of Lp(a) on the interpretation of clinical data

Santica M. Marcovina*

Northwest Lipid Research Laboratories, University of Washington, 2121 N. 35th Street, Seattle, WA 98103, USA

Abstract. In the majority of clinical studies, Lp(a) levels have been determined by methods affected by apo(a) size heterogeneity. Despite the importance of this topic, no studies have been performed to evaluate the impact of method inaccuracy on the interpretation of clinical data. We have evaluated to what extent method inaccuracy affects the correct classification of subjects for being at risk or not for CAD based on their Lp(a) values. Lp(a) levels were measured in samples from the Framingham study participants by our reference ELISA, by a turbidimetric method and by a commercial ELISA using an Lp(a) value of 75 nmol/l as the clinical decision point. The number of false positive and false negative values obtained by the turbidimetric methods was almost entirely explained by the apo(a) size dependency of this assay. However, the large number of false positive values obtained by the commercial ELISA method was not. To evaluate method differences in the interpretation of clinical data, a study was performed to compare the ability of our ELISA method and a nephelometric method to predict future angina pectoris in men participating in the Physicians' Health Study. Lp(a) values determined by ELISA were associated with increased relative risk for angina while those obtained by the nephelometric method were not. The results of these two studies clearly indicate the importance of using suitable and standardized methods for risk assessment and for the interpretation of clinical outcomes.

Keyword: Lp(a)

1. Introduction

Apo(a), the distinct protein component of Lp(a), is highly heterogeneous in size due to the fact that the kringle 4 (K4) type 2 sequence is present in a variable number of identically repeated copies. This has a marked effect on the immunochemical measurement of Lp(a). In fact, based on the number of apo(a) identical repeats, there will be a variable number of epitopes in plasma samples available to interact with the antibodies used in the immunoassays to measure the concentration of Lp(a). The main

* Tel.: +1-206-685-3331; fax: +1-206-685-3279.
E-mail addresses: smm@u.washington.edu, mcgowan@u.washington.edu (S.M. Marcovina).

doi:10.1016/S0531-5131(03)01856-9

requisite for an immunoassay to provide accurate results are: (1) assay calibrators should have an accuracy-based target value, and (2) the antibodies should possess the same immunoreactivity per particle for the assay calibrator and for the samples being analyzed. This latter requisite is not easily achievable for Lp(a) and it is evident that the size variation of apo(a) affects the development of immunoassays on two fronts: (1) the choice of apo(a) size in the calibrator is arbitrary and, independent of the choice, the calibrator would not be representative of the size of apo(a) in most of the samples; and (2) the immunoreactivity of the antibodies will vary depending on the size of apo(a). As a consequence, the immunoassays will tend to underestimate Lp(a) levels in samples with apo(a) sizes smaller than the apo(a) size of the assay calibrator and conversely overestimate Lp(a) levels in samples with larger apo(a) isoforms.

As the recipients of the National Heart, Lung and Blood Institute (NHLBI) contract for the standardization of Lp(a) measurements, we evaluated a large number of commercially available methods in collaboration with the International Federation of Clinical Chemistry (IFCC) Working Group on Lp(a). Despite the use of a common reference preparation to assign a target value to the assay calibrators, the among-method CV on 30 selected samples ranged from 6% to 31% [1]. A significant apo(a) size-dependent bias was observed for the majority of the assays when the obtained values were compared with those obtained by an assay unaffected by apo(a) size heterogeneity and used as a reference method [2].

The marked difference in Lp(a) values obtained by the different methods, despite the use of a common reference preparation, clearly indicates that the impact of apo(a) isoform size on Lp(a) levels varies among the different methods as a function of the apo(a) size of the assay calibrators. In addition, other factors, such as differences in antibody properties, assay precision and robustness, and sensitivity of the assays to sample handling, storage conditions and length of storage, play a role in and contribute to the lack of comparability of data. Despite the marked among-assay variability, in the majority of clinical studies, Lp(a) levels have been determined by methods affected by apo(a) size heterogeneity. Therefore, for the conclusions of these studies to be valid, we have to rely on the assumption that the distribution of apo(a) isoforms is similar between cases and controls, thus minimizing the potential that method-dependent overestimation or underestimation of Lp(a) values may contribute to the observed difference or lack thereof between cases and controls. Despite the importance of this topic, no studies have been performed to evaluate the impact of method inaccuracy on the interpretation of clinical data.

2. Study design and results

As part of the NHLBI contract on Lp(a) standardization, we evaluated to what extent method inaccuracy affects the correct stratification of subjects for CAD risk, based on their Lp(a) values. In 2940 samples from the participants in the Framingham study collected during the 5th cycle, Lp(a) levels were determined by the reference method and apo(a) isoforms were determined as previously described [3]. During the same cycle, Lp(a) levels were also determined in other laboratories in 2556 of the samples by a turbidimetric method and in 2662 of the samples by a commercially available ELISA. An Lp(a) value of 75 nmol/l was selected as the clinical decision point. Based on the Lp(a) values obtained by the turbidimetric assay, 136 individuals were misclassified as being at increased risk (false positive) and 23 were misclassified as being not at risk (false negative). Based on the Lp(a) values obtained by the commercial ELISA, 329 individuals were misclassified as being at increased risk (false positive) and 25 were false negative. The vast majority of the misclassifications observed by the turbidimetric method were explained by the overestimation or underestimation of Lp(a) values based on the apo(a) size in the samples. The larger number of false positives as compared with the false negatives obtained by this assay is explained by the small apo(a) size in the assay calibrator and by the high frequency of samples in the general population with apo(a) sizes larger than that in the calibrator. This observation is consistent with previously reported data [1]. However, the large number of false positive values generated by the ELISA method was not explained by the apo(a) sizes in these samples. When this method was evaluated in our laboratory, we observed a high degree of intra- and inter-assay imprecision. Additionally, when analyses were performed on fresh samples and on the same samples stored at -70 °C, a significant difference was observed between values obtained on fresh and frozen samples. The values on frozen samples were generally higher than those obtained on fresh samples, but the magnitude of the increase was sample-dependent.

These findings clearly indicate that each assay, in addition to being evaluated for its sensitivity to apo(a) size polymorphism, needs to be optimized in terms of robustness and precision. In addition, assay limitations due to sample preparation and storage need to be evaluated and clearly stated.

To evaluate method differences in the interpretation of clinical data, a study was performed to directly compare the ability of the ELISA reference method [2] and a commercially available latex-based nephelometric method to predict future angina pectoris in men participating in the Physicians' Health Study. Plasma Lp(a) concentration was determined in our laboratory by the ELISA reference method and apo(a) isoform size was also determined as previously published [2,3]. In a different laboratory, Lp(a) levels were determined on the same samples by the nephelometric method. Analyses were performed in samples from 195 study participants who subsequently developed angina and from 195 paired matched controls. As determined by the ELISA method, cases had significantly higher median Lp(a) compared with controls (30.6 vs. 22.5 nmol/l; $p=0.02$). Additionally, Lp(a) was associated with increased relative risk for angina and this association was strengthened after controlling for lipid risk factors. No significant difference in median Lp(a) levels between cases and controls was observed when Lp(a) was measured by the nephelometric method (11.4 vs. 8.8 mg/dl; $p=0.11$). The median Lp(a) level and the association with angina was also not significant.

In conclusion, our data clearly indicate that the impact of apo(a) size heterogeneity and the lack of optimization and standardization of methods used to measure Lp(a) may greatly impact on the correct classification of individual risk status and on the interpretation of clinical data.

Acknowledgements

These studies were performed in collaboration with Ernst Schaefer and Judith McNamara (Framingham Heart Study) and Nader Rifai, Jing Ma, Frank M. Sacks, Paul M.

Ridker, Wendy Jade L. Hernandez and Meir J. Stampfer (Physician's Health Study). The studies were supported by the NHLBI-NIH Contract # N01 HV88175.

References

[1] S.M. Marcovina, J.J. Albers, A.M. Scanu, H. Kennedy, F. Giaculli, K. Berg, et al., Use of a reference material proposed by the International Federation of Clinical Chemistry and Laboratory Medicine to evaluate analytical methods for the determination of plasma lipoprotein(a), Clinical Chemistry 46 (12) (2000) 1956–1967.

[2] S.M. Marcovina, J.J. Albers, B. Gabel, M.L. Koschinsky, V.P. Gaur, Effect of the number of apolipoprotein(a) kringle 4 domains on immunochemical measurements of lipoprotein(a), Clinical Chemistry 41 (2) (1995) 246–255.

[3] S.M. Marcovina, Z.H. Zhang, V.P. Gaur, J.J. Albers, Identification of 34 apolipoprotein(a) isoforms: differential expression of apolipoprotein(a) alleles between American blacks and whites, Biochemical and Biophysical Research Communications 191 (3) (1993) 1192–1196.

International Congress Series 1262 (2004) 562–565

www.ics-elsevier.com

Molecular mechanisms of age-related regulation of genes

Kotoku Kurachi[a,b,*], Sumiko Kurachi[a], Kezhong Zhang[b], Afshin Ameri[b], Jeffrey Huo[b], Mitsuhiro Kuwahara[a], Jean-Marc Fontaine[b], Takahiro Abe[a]

[a] *Age Dimension Research Center, National Institute of Advanced Industrial Science and Technology, Tsukuba, Ibaragi 305-8566, Japan*

[b] *Department of Human Genetics, University of Michigan Medical School, Ann Arbor, MI 48109, USA*

Abstract. Through transgenic mouse analyses of age-related expression of human genes, we recently discovered the first molecular mechanism of age-related regulation of gene expression, a critical finding for understanding the age-dimension homeostasis. In our study, human genes for blood coagulation factor IX (FIX) and anti-coagulant protein C (PC), which show age-dependent increasing and stable expression patterns, respectively, were subjected to systematic in vitro and in vivo analyses. The mechanism found uses two genetic elements, age-related stability elements (ASEs, G/CAGGAAG) and age-related increase element (AIE, a stretch of dinucleotide repeats). ASE is required for age-related stable patterns of gene expression as seen for the human PC (hPC) gene, whereas a combination of ASE and AIE is required for age-related increase patterns of gene expression as seen for the human FIX gene. ASE functions not only for temporal regulation but also for precise spatial regulation of gene expression. Differential and combined usages of ASE and AIE apparently generate specific age-related regulatory patterns of different genes. Transgenic mice persistently over-expressing hFIX at high levels died at much younger ages than expected. These animals developed not only thromboses in tissues such as heart, brain and lung but also generated myocardial fibrosis in the left ventricle, mimicking a type of human myocardial infarction. These findings laid the foundation for developing a new research field, age-dimension technology (ADT), which explores useful applications of the mechanisms of age-dimension homeostasis. © 2004 Published by Elsevier B.V.

Keywords: Molecular; Age-related regulation of genes; Age-dimension technology

Age is a well-known risk factor for many diseases including cardiovascular diseases. Until recently, however, literally nothing was known for the molecular mechanisms of action of age or of age-dimension homeostasis. This deficiency of knowledge was

* Corresponding author. Age Dimension Research Center, National Institute of Advanced Industrial Science and Technology (AIST), AIST Tsukuba Center, Site 6, Higashi 1-1-1, Tsukuba, Ibaragi 305-8566, Japan. Tel.: +81-29-861-2441; fax: +81-29-861-2701.

E-mail address: k.kurachi@aist.go.jp (K. Kurachi).

0531-5131/ © 2004 Published by Elsevier B.V.
doi:10.1016/j.ics.2004.02.166

apparently due to the abstractive nature of age and experimental difficulties. Physiological reactions are maintained stable with small fluctuations over the age, expected characteristics of homeostasis. However, homeostatic states of physiological systems are not constant, but gradually change along with the age dimension, a biological slow dynamic system. Our research efforts were initiated more than a decade ago with an aim towards understanding this phenomenon. Recently, we finally succeeded in discovering the very first molecular mechanism of age-related regulation of gene expression, thus opening a new horizon for understanding the age-dimension homeostasis and its regulation.

In our study, the blood coagulation system was intensively studied as a physiological model system. Human blood coagulation gradually increases its overall activity with age [1–3]. Epidemiological studies suggest that this is presumably due to the increasing imbalance between pro-coagulant activity and anti-coagulant activities with age. Plasma concentration and/or activities of pro-coagulant factors increase with age, whereas those of anti-coagulant as well as fibrinolytic factors do not increase or even decrease slightly with age. Importantly, like most pro-coagulant factors, PAI-1, an inhibitor of tPA, increases its plasma concentration with age. Putting all together, these observations suggested that with advancing age, the balance between the pro-coagulant activity and that of the anti-coagulant activity combined with that of fibrinolysis tips toward a more pro-coagulant state with advancing age. In combination with environmental conditions, this may result in substantial increase in the thrombotic tendency with age [4–7].

As shown by epidemiological studies, the circulatory level of human factor IX (hFIX), a pro-coagulation factor, significantly increases with advancing age in normal populations [3,8,10]. In contrast, the plasma level of human PC (hPC), a key factor in the potent anti-coagulant protein C (PC) pathway, shows only marginal age-associated changes [3,9,11]. Thus, we subjected both hFIX and hPC genes (approximately 40 and 13 kbp in size, respectively) for detailed studies, hoping to obtain critical insights into the molecular mechanisms of age-dimension homeostasis. For analyses of the structure–function–age relationship of these genes, we constructed a series of minigene expression vectors of hFIX and hPC genes [12–17]. All the minigenes were first tested with HepG2 cells to verify their expression activities, and subsequently used to construct transgenic mice. Transgenic animals were then individually, not as age-grouped populations, subjected to ELIA analyses of their circulatory hFIX or hPC protein levels for their entire life spans. Mice have a blood coagulation system similar to that in humans, and furthermore, age-related expression patterns of FIX and PC genes and/or circulatory protein levels are also similar to those of humans [16,17].

Through these studies, we identified two key genetic elements, age-related stability element (ASE) and age-related increase element (AIE) (renamed from our original naming AE5′ and AE3′, respectively; see Refs. [16,17]), essential for age-related stable and increasing patterns of hFIX expression, respectively [16]. ASE was located to the 5′ upstream region, nucleotide (nt)-802 through nt-784, of the hFIX gene by electrophoretic mobility shift assay. ASE has a nucleotide core sequence, GAGGAAG, matching the Ets consensus sequence (G/CAGGAA/TG) [18,19]. AIE, an element necessary for age-related increase in gene expression, was identified in the middle of the hFIX 3′-untranslated region (UTR) [16]. AIE is composed of a 102-bp dinucleotide repeat (AT, GT, CA) and has a potential to form three distinct stem loop structures in its RNA form [12]. Mouse factor IX (mFIX) also shows age-related increase in gene expression [20,21], and its gene contains an ASE sequence identical to the functional ASE in the hFIX gene and an AIE-like stretch of 106-bp dinucleotide repeats in the mFIX 3′-UTR [22]. We showed that the mFIX AIE-like element actually functions as an AIE [17]. These studies demonstrated that the age-related increase in expression of the FIX gene is regulated by a combination of ASE and AIE. In the absence of ASE, minigenes with or without AIE show an age-unstable hFIX gene expression patterns with a rapid decline in expression over puberty and subsequent 3–4 months to low but stable levels or very low basal levels, respectively. In the presence of both ASE and AIE, age-dependent increase patterns of hFIX gene expression, which mimic that of the natural gene, were obtained. Thus, we found the very first molecular mechanism responsible for age-related gene regulation.

hPC and hFIX share significant similarities in protein structures (coding regions), whereas the 5′-flanking regions and 3′-UTRs are grossly dissimilar [12,14,23,24]. The hPC gene has no AIE-like element, whereas at least four ASE consensus elements exist in the hPC minigene under testing. Systematic transgenic mouse testing of these minigenes showed that only CAGGAAG at around the nt-800, but not GAGGAAA at further upstream, functions as age-related regulator. Others in the intron (GAGGATG) and the coding region (CAGGATG) also do not function.

Differential or combined usages of ASE and AIE gives pro- and anti-coagulation factors for their age-related increase or stable pattern of gene expression, respectively. Since clearance rates of circulatory hPC and hFIX proteins from the blood stream were similar to each other in young and old mice, protein clearance from the circulation apparently does not contribute significantly to age-related regulation of hFIX and hPC in the circulation [16,17]. Altogether, these provide a major explanation of how the age-related increasing pattern of the overall blood coagulation activity is generated (Fig. 1).

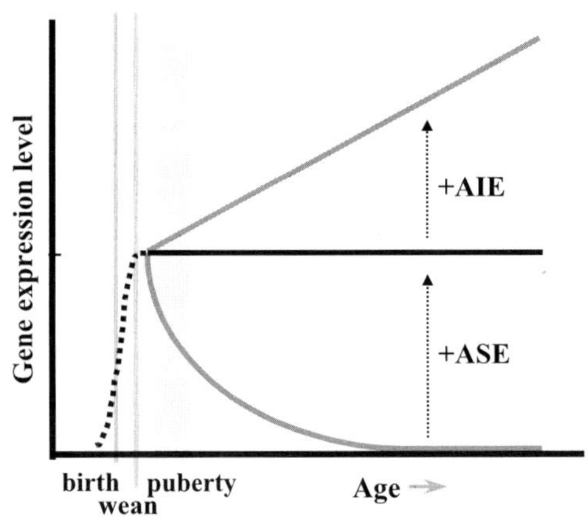

Fig. 1. The molecular mechanism of age-related regulation of genes. Functional roles of ASE and AIE in age-related regulation of gene expression are schematically shown. ASE alone and AIE in combination with ASE were required for age-stable and age-related increase patterns of gene expression, respectively. The mechanisms apparently function with different genes, thus providing the basis for developing a new field, age-dimension technology (ADT).

The mechanisms we found may also function for age-related regulation of many other different genes.

An important observation made in these studies was that animals over-expressing hFIX persistently at high levels die at a much younger age (as early as 3–5 months) than the normal life span (2–3 years) in a FIX level-dependent manner [25]. These animals showed thrombi in tissues including brain, lung and heart, and even myocardial fibrosis in left ventricle, which mimics a type of human myocardial infarction.

In summary, the very first molecular mechanism of age-related gene regulation was found, substantially contributing to understanding of the mechanisms of age-dimension homeostasis. Our studies also laid the foundation for developing age-dimension technology (ADT), a new research field, which aims to develop, for instance, novel preventive and/or therapeutic methods for age-associated diseases, drugs and age-stable gene delivery/expression vectors for gene therapy.

References

[1] M. Andrew, et al., Blood 80 (1992) 998–2005.
[2] D. Marie, et al., Blood 85 (1995) 3144–3149.
[3] G.O.D. Lowe, et al., Br. J. Haematol. 97 (1997) 775–784.
[4] M. Woodward, et al., Br. J. Haematol. 97 (1997) 785–797.
[5] M.G. Conlan, et al., Thromb. Haemost. 70 (1993) 380–385.
[6] M.G. Conlan, et al., Thromb. Haemost. 72 (1994) 551–556.
[7] A.H. Vlieg, et al., Blood 95 (2000) 3678–3682.
[8] C.T. Esmon, Biochim. Biophys. Acta 1477 (2000) 349–360.
[9] B. Dahlback, The Lancet 355 (2000) 1627–1632.
[10] J.D. Sweeney, L.A. Hoernig, Am. J. Clin. Pathol. 99 (1993) 687–688.
[11] K.A. Bauer, et al., J. Clin. Invest. 80 (1987) 1527–1534.
[12] S. Yoshitake, et al., Biochemistry 24 (1985) 3736–3750.
[13] C.H. Miao, et al., J. Biol. Chem. 271 (1996) 9587–9594.
[14] D.C. Foster, S. Yoshitake, E.W. Davie, Proc. Natl. Acad. Sci. U. S. A. 82 (1985) 4673–4677.
[15] S. Kurachi, et al., J. Biol. Chem. 270 (1995) 5276–5281.
[16] S. Kurachi, et al., Science 285 (1999) 739–743.
[17] K. Zhang, S. Kurachi, K. Kurachi, J. Biol. Chem. 277 (2002) 4532–4540.
[18] J.-H. Xin, et al., Genes Dev. 6 (1992) 481–496.
[19] A. Chotteau-Lelievre, et al., Oncogene 15 (1997) 937–952.
[20] S.N. Yao, et al., Thromb. Haemost. 65 (1991) 52–58.
[21] S. Kurachi, E. Hitomi, K. Kurachi, Thromb. Haemost. 76 (1996) 965–969.
[22] S.-M. Wu, D.W. Stafford, J. Ware, Gene 86 (1990) 275–278.
[23] J.-P. Salier, S. Hirosawa, K. Kurachi, J. Biol. Chem. 265 (1990) 7062–7068.
[24] W. Hsu, et al., Thromb. Haemost. 82 (1999) 1782–1783.
[25] A. Ameri, et al., 101 (2003) 1871–1873.

International Congress Series 1262 (2004) 566–569

www.ics-elsevier.com

Vascular cell senescence in human atherosclerosis

Tohru Minamino*, Issei Komuro

Department of Cardiovascular Science and Medicine, Chiba University Graduate School of Medicine, 1-8-1 Inohana, Chuo, Chiba 260-8670, Japan

Abstract. Vascular cells have a finite lifespan when cultured in vitro and eventually enter an irreversible growth arrest called cellular senescence. Many of the changes in senescent vascular cell behavior are consistent with the changes seen in age-related vascular diseases. We have demonstrated the presence of senescent vascular cells in human atherosclerotic lesions, but not non-atherosclerotic lesions. Moreover, these cells express increased levels of proinflammatory molecules and decreased levels of endothelial nitric oxide synthase, suggesting that cellular senescence in vivo contributes to the pathogenesis of human atherosclerosis. One widely discussed hypothesis of senescence is the teleomere hypothesis. An increasing body of evidence has established the critical role of the telomere in vascular cell senescence. Another line of evidence suggests that telomere-independent mechanisms are also involved in vascular cell senescence. Activation of Ras, an important signaling molecule involved in atherogenic stimuli, induces vascular cell senescence and thereby promotes vascular inflammation in vitro and in vivo, while Akt negatively controls the lifespan of human vascular cells, both of which have been known to promote aging in organisms such as yeast and worms. These data suggest that the signaling pathways of longevity are conserved in human vascular cells. Further understanding of the mechanism underlying cellular senescence will provide insights into the potential of antisenescence therapy for vascular aging.

Keywords: Senescence; Aging; Atherosclerosis; Telomere; Ras

1. Introduction

Cellular senescence is the limited ability of primary human cells to divide when cultured in vitro and is accompanied by a specific set of phenotypic changes in morphology, gene expression and function. These changes in phenotype have been implicated in human aging [1]. However, until recently, little attention has been paid to the potential impact of vascular cell senescence in vivo on age-related vascular disorders.

In the past decades, significant progress has been made in our understanding of the mechanisms underlying cellular senescence. One widely discussed hypothesis is the

* Corresponding author. Tel.: +81-43-226-2556; fax: +81-43-226-2096.
E-mail address: t_minamino@yahoo.co.jp (T. Minamino).

0531-5131/
doi:10.1016/j.ics.2003.11.037

telomere hypothesis of senescence [2]. A growing body of evidence has demonstrated the critical role of telomere and telomerase in regulating not only cellular lifespan but also organismal aging. However, recent findings suggest that cellular senescence can also be induced by DNA damage, cellular stress or oncogenic activation, which is independent of replicative age [3]. For example, the constitutive activation of mitogenic stimuli by the expression of oncogenic Ras induces senescent phenotypes. Thus, it is possible that atherogenic stimuli increase cell turnover at the sites of atherosclerosis, thereby promoting telomere shortening, whereas this also results in activation of proliferative signals that potentially induce senescence independent of telomere shortening.

Here we will describe recently accumulating evidence that supports the cell hypothesis of aging in the vasculature.

2. Occurrence of vascular cell senescence in vivo

Human vascular cells have a finite lifespan in vitro and, likely, in vivo as well. The histology of the lesions of human atherosclerosis has been extensively studied, and these studies suggest the occurrence of cellular senescence in vivo. Recently, this notion has been confirmed by cytochemical analysis in vivo using the senescence-associated β-galactosidase (SA β-gal) activity, a biomarker for cellular senescence [4]. We have recently demonstrated SA β-gal positive vascular cells in human atherosclerotic plaque of the coronary arteries obtained from the patients who had ischemic heart disease [5]. SA β-gal positive cells were predominately localized on the luminal surface of atherosclerotic plaque and identified as endothelial cells, but no positive cells were observed in the internal mammary arteries from the same patients where atherosclerotic changes were minimally observed. In advanced plaque, SA β-gal positive VSMCs were detected in the intima, but not in the media [6], which may represent extensive replication in the lesions.

3. Role of cellular senescence in vascular pathophysiology

Aging accelerates vascular dysfunction, such as a decrease in compliance and an increase in inflammatory response, both of which contribute to atherogenesis. This impairment is attributed to age-related functional changes in vascular cells [7,8]. Endothelium-dependent vasodilation is impaired with age due to a decreased production of vasodilators, such as nitric oxide (NO) and prostacyclin in endothelial cells. Moreover, increased expression of pro-inflammatory and pro-thrombogenic molecules was observed in vascular cells of aged arteries. Interestingly, many of the changes in senescent vascular cells in vitro are consistent with known changes seen in age-related vascular diseases. The production of NO and the endothelial NO synthase (eNOS) activity are reduced in senescent human endothelial cells [9]. The levels of prostacyclin production are significantly decreased with in vitro aging of endothelial cells [10], whereas senescent endothelial cells upregulate plasminogen activator inhibitor-1 [11]. More importantly, we have shown that these changes in phenotypes are found in senescent vascular cells of human atherosclerosis as well [6], suggesting a critical role for vascular cell senescence in human atherogenesis.

4. Teleomere-independent vascular cell senescence

We have reported that telomere shortening causes vascular dysfunction associated with senescence [5,12,13]. Recently, signals other than teleomere shortening have been shown to result in cells developing a phenotype indistinguishable from that of senescent cells at the end of their replicative life span. For example, the constitutive activation of mitogenic stimuli induces a senescent phenotype. Cellular senescence triggered by mitogenic stimuli is independent of replicative age, and these signals act before the replicative limits of cells. It is known that various molecules including growth factors, vasoactive peptides and oxidative stresses are induced during the lesion formation and regulate numerous critical cell functions, thereby contributing to atherogenesis [14]. These stimuli function as mitogens for vascular cells through the signaling cascades that activate Ras [14]. In addition to its role in cell proliferation, we have found that constitutive activation of Ras induces vascular cell senescence that is associated with vascular inflammation [6]. Activation of Ras drastically increased expression of proinflammatory cytokines partially through ERK activation in cultured vascular cells. Introduction of Ras into balloon-injured arteries enhanced vascular inflammation as well as senescence compared with control-injured arteries. Moreover, senescent cells express inflammatory molecules in human atherosclerotic plaque, and ERK is activated in these cells, suggesting that teleomere-independent mechanisms may also contribute to vascular cell senescence in human atherosclerosis. It is likely that atherogenic stimuli initially promote cell proliferation, and when overstimulated to proliferate, mitogenic signaling pathways induce teleomere-dependent and teleomere-independent senescence, which results in vascular dysfunction.

5. Conclusion

Accumulating evidence indicates the critical role of cellular senescence in organismal aging and age-related disease, including atherosclerosis. Further understanding of the mechanism underlying cellular senescence will provide new insights into antisenescence therapy for vascular aging.

References

[1] R.G. Faragher, D. Kipling, How might replicative senescence contribute to human ageing? Bioessays 20 (1998) 985–991.

[2] J. Campisi, S.H. Kim, C.S. Lim, M. Rubio, Cellular senescence, cancer and aging: the telomere connection, Exp. Gerontol. 36 (2001) 1619–1637.

[3] M. Serrano, M.A. Blasco, Putting the stress on senescence, Curr. Opin. Cell Biol. 13 (2001) 748–753.

[4] G.P. Dimri, X. Lee, G. Basile, M. Acosta, G. Scott, C. Roskelley, et al, A biomarker that identifies senescent human cells in culture and in aging skin in vivo, Proc. Natl. Acad. Sci. U. S. A. 92 (1995) 9363–9367.

[5] T. Minamino, H. Miyauchi, T. Yoshida, Y. Ishida, H. Yoshida, I. Komuro, Endothelial cell senescence in human atherosclerosis: role of telomere in endothelial dysfunction, Circulation 105 (2002) 1541–1544.

[6] T. Minamino, T. Yoshida, K. Tateno, H. Miyauchi, Y. Zou, H. Toko, I. Komuro, Ras-induced vascular smooth muscle cell senescence in human atherosclerosis. Circulation, (in press)..

[7] L.T. Cooper, J.P. Cooke, V.J. Dzau, The vasculopathy of aging, J. Gerontol. 49 (1994) B191–B196.

[8] J.V. Mombouli, P.M. Vanhoutte, Endothelial dysfunction: from physiology to therapy, J. Mol. Cell. Cardiol. 31 (1999) 61–74.

[9] I. Sato, I. Morita, K. Kaji, M. Ikeda, M. Nagao, S. Murota, Reduction of nitric oxide producing activity

associated with in vitro aging in cultured human umbilical vein endothelial cell, Biochem. Biophys. Res. Commun. 195 (1993) 1070–1076.

[10] M. Nakajima, M. Hashimoto, F. Wang, K. Yamanaga, N. Nakamura, T. Uchida, et al, Aging decreases the production of PGI2 in rat aortic endothelial cells, Exp. Gerontol. 32 (1997) 685–693.

[11] P. Comi, R. Chiaramonte, J.A. Maier, Senescence-dependent regulation of type 1 plasminogen activator inhibitor in human vascular endothelial cells, Exp. Cell Res. 219 (1995) 304–308.

[12] T. Minamino, S. Kourembanas, Mechanisms of telomerase induction during vascular smooth muscle cell proliferation, Circ. Res. 89 (2001) 237–243.

[13] T. Minamino, S.A. Mitsialis, S. Kourembanas, Hypoxia extends the life span of vascular smooth muscle cells through telomerase activation, Mol. Cell. Biol. 21 (2001) 3336–3342.

[14] A.J. Lusis, Atherosclerosis, Nature 407 (2000) 233–241.

International Congress Series 1262 (2004) 570–573

ELSEVIER

www.ics-elsevier.com

Role of inflammation in atherosclerotic calcification, metaplasia and osteoporosis

Linda L. Demer[a,b,*], Yin Tintut[a], Moeen Abedin[a]

[a] *Department of Medicine, The David Geffen School of Medicine at UCLA, USA*
[b] *Department of Physiology, The David Geffen School of Medicine at UCLA, USA*

Abstract. It is not unusual for atherosclerotic lesions to contain ectopic tissue, including bone, cartilage, fat and marrow. It is also common for patients with atherosclerosis to have osteoporosis. Thus, in many elderly patients, bone is forming in their artery walls at the same time as bone is being permanently lost from their skeleton. The stimuli and mechanisms underlying these reciprocal processes are not understood. One clue is that adult tissues, such as bone marrow stroma and adipose tissue, contain mesenchymal stem cells (MSC) with the potential to form bone, cartilage, muscle and fat as well as the potential for self-renewal. We previously found that a subpopulation of cells harvested from normal aortic tunica media have the capacity for differentiation along the osteogenic lineage, which is enhanced by inflammatory factors including cytokines, oxidized lipids, and lipoproteins. But true osteoblasts derived from bone were inhibited by treatment with these same factors, and adipogenesis was favored over osteogenic differentiation in the marrow precursor cells of hyperlipidemic animals. The same inflammatory factors enhanced bone resorptive osteoclastic activity. These findings suggest mechanisms for simultaneous atherosclerotic calcification and osteoporosis. We have now investigated whether the subpopulation of cells with osteogenic potential has the potential to differentiation along other lineages. The findings have important therapeutic implications for use of stem cells in regenerative therapy and tissue bioengineering.

Keywords: Calcification; Atherosclerosis; Mesenchymal stem cell

1. Ectopic tissue in the artery wall

Metaplasia is a well-known phenomenon in atherosclerosis [1–4]. The forms of tissue that occur in atherosclerotic plaque include bone, cartilage, marrow, and fat. These tissues show signs of remodeling and active resorption [5]. While not yet systematically evaluated, the incidence of bone in carotid atherosclerotic lesions is approximately 10–20% [6], with hematopoietic marrow in 1 of 20 cases [3]. Even veins are affected [7], and animal models of atherosclerosis have cartilaginous metaplasia [8–10].

* Corresponding author. Campus Box 951679, UCLA, 10833 LeConte Ave., Los Angeles, CA 90095-1679, USA. Tel.: +1-310-206-2677; fax: +1-310-825-4963.

E-mail address: Ldemer@mednet.ucla.edu (L.L. Demer).

0531-5131/
doi:10.1016/S0531-5131(03)01815-6

2. Bone-like cells in the artery wall

Growing evidence indicates that bone-like metaplasia may be due to osteoblastic differentiation of cells in the artery wall. A cloned subpopulation of cells harvested from bovine aortic medial explants forms aggregates and undergoes osteoblastic differentiation and mineralization in culture [11,12]. Osteoblastic differentiation is evidenced by expression and production of numerous bone-related and bone-specific proteins including the master regulatory transcription factor, core binding factor-a1 [13]. This phenotypic behavior is retained over numerous population triplings. It is also observed in non-cloned bovine and human cells [14–16]. Differentiation and calcification in these cells is highly regulated by a variety of factors including oxidized lipoproteins, parathyroid hormone-related peptide, estradiol, phosphate levels, vitamin D, tumor necrosis factor-α, oncostatin M, and dexamethasone [16–23].

Based on electron microprobe analysis, the mineral produced by these cells is hydroxyapatite, the same mineral as in bone, not merely amorphous calcium phosphate [11,24]. Gene expression during differentiation follows a sequential course [13] closely resembling that of bone-derived osteoblasts [25]. Osteogenesis occurs in cardiac valves as well as artery wall [26]. In vivo, osteoprogenitor cells of the bone marrow are inhibited by hyperlipidemia [27].

3. Reciprocal effects on bone

While inflammatory lipids promote osteoblastic differentiation and mineralization of vascular cells, they have the opposite effect on true bone-derived osteoblasts, inhibiting differentiation and mineralization [23]. This in vitro result would not have in vivo implications unless differentiating bone cells were somehow exposed to lipoprotein particles. Indeed, bone is a vascular tissue; it bleeds significantly when cut, and the marrow space is rich in vascular sinusoids. Lipids may deposit in the subendothelial space of the bone vasculature just as they deposit in the subendothelial space of other vessels. Importantly, the differentiating osteoblasts in bone are located in this subendothelial space. Based on this evidence, we hypothesized that bone is affected by hyperlipidemia. Our studies showed that hyperlipidemic mice had fewer bone progenitors in the marrow precursor cells, as well as reduced bone density [26,28].

4. Mesenchymal stem cells in the vasculature

Mesenchymal stem cells (MSC) are derived from marrow, blood, muscle and fat tissues. The tissues that are sources of MSC also contain vascular tissue, suggesting that vascular cells may contribute, at least in part, to the pluripotentiality. Since the artery wall contains cells with both smooth muscle and osteoblastic potential as well as self-renewal capacity, we hypothesized that these calcifying vascular cells are, in fact, multipotent cells similar to mesenchymal stem cells.

Acknowledgements

This work was funded by NIH Grants HL30568 and HL/AR 69261.

References

[1] C.H. Bunting, The formation of true bone with cellular (red) marrow in a sclerotic aorta, J. Exp. Med. 8 (1906) 365–376.

[2] R. Virchow, Cellular Pathology: As Based Upon Physiological and Pathological Histology (Translated by Frank Chance, 1971), 1863, pp. 404–408, An unabridged and unaltered republication of the English translation, Dover Publications; New York, NY.

[3] T.A. Seemayer, W.L. Thelmo, J. Morin, Cartilaginous transformation of the aortic valve, Am. J. Clin. Pathol. 60 (1973) 616–620.

[4] L. Buerger, A. Oppenheimer, Bone formation in sclerotic arteries, J. Exp. Med. 10 (1908) 354–367.

[5] M. Jeziorska, C. McCollum, D.E. Wooley, Observations on bone formation and remodelling in advanced atherosclerotic lesions of human carotid arteries, Virchows Arch. 433 (6) (1998) 559–565.

[6] J.L. Hunt, R. Fairman, M.E. Mitchell, J.P. Carpenter, M. Golden, T. Khalapyan, M. Wolfe, D. Neschis, R. Milner, B. Scoll, A. Cusack, E.R. Mohler III, Bone formation in carotid plaques: a clinicopathological study, Stroke 33 (5) (2002) 1214–1219.

[7] W.E. Stehbens, Chronic vascular changes in the walls of experimental berry aneurysms of the aortic bifurcation in rabbits, Stroke 12 (5) (1981) 643–647.

[8] J.H. Qiao, M.C. Fishbein, L.L. Demer, A.J. Lusis, Genetic determination of cartilaginous metaplasia in mouse aorta, Arterioscler. Thromb. Vasc. Biol. 15 (12) (1995) 2265–2272.

[9] J. Tse, B. Martin-McNaulty, M. Halks-Miller, K. Kauser, V. DelVecchio, R. Vergona, M.E. Sullivan, G.M. Rubanyi, Accelerated atherosclerosis and premature calcified cartilaginous metaplasia in the aorta of diabetic male Apo E knockout mice can be prevented by chronic treatment with 17 beta-estradiol, Atherosclerosis 144 (2) (1999) 303–313.

[10] M.E. Rosenfeld, P. Polinsky, R. Virmani, K. Kauser, G. Rubanyi, S.M. Schwartz, Advanced atherosclerotic lesions in the innominate artery of the ApoE knockout mouse, Arterioscler. Thromb. Vasc. Biol. 20 (12) (2000) 2587–2592.

[11] K. Bostöm, K.E. Watson, S. Horn, C. Wortham, I. Herman, L.L. Demer, Bone morphogenetic protein expression in human atherosclerotic lesions, J. Clin. Invest. 91 (1993) 1800–1809.

[12] K.E. Watson, K. Boström, B. Norton, T. Lam, L.L. Demer, Transforming growth factor-β1 and 25-hydroxycholesterol stimulate osteoblast-like vascular cells to calcify, J. Clin. Invest. 93 (1994) 2106–2113.

[13] Y. Tintut, F. Parhami, K. Boström, S.M. Jackson, L.L. Demer, cAMP stimulates osteoblast-like differentiation of calcifying vascular cells: potential signaling pathway for vascular calcification, J. Biol. Chem. 273 (1998) 7547–7553.

[14] T. Wada, M.D. McKee, S. Steitz, C.M. Giachelli, Calcification of vascular smooth muscle cell cultures: inhibition by osteopontin, Circ. Res. 84 (2) (1999) 166–178.

[15] D. Proudfoot, J.N. Skepper, C.M. Shanahan, P.L. Weissberg, Calcification of human vascular cells in vitro is correlated with high levels of matrix Gla protein and low levels of osteopontin expression, Arterioscler. Thromb. Vasc. Biol. 18 (3) (1998) 379–388.

[16] A. Shioi, Y. Nishizawa, S. Jono, H. Koyama, M. Hosoi, H. Morii, Beta-glycerophosphate accelerates calcification in cultured bovine vascular smooth muscle cells, Arterioscler. Thromb. Vasc. Biol. 15 (11) (Nov. 1995) 2003–2009.

[17] M. Balica, K. Bostrom, V. Shin, K. Tillisch, L.L. Demer, Calcifying subpopulation of bovine aortic smooth muscle cells is responsive to 17 beta-estradiol, Circulation 95 (7) (1997) 1954–1960.

[18] A. Shioi, M. Katagi, Y. Okuno, K. Mori, S. Jono, H. Koyama, Y. Nishizawa, Induction of bone-type alkaline phosphatase in human vascular smooth muscle cells: roles of tumor necrosis factor-alpha and oncostatin M derived from macrophages, Circ. Res. 91 (1) (2002) 9–16.

[19] K. Mori, A. Shioi, S. Jono, Y. Nishizawa, H. Morii, Dexamethasone enhances in vitro vascular calcification by promoting osteoblastic differentiation of vascular smooth muscle cells, Arterioscler. Thromb. Vasc. Biol. 19 (9) (1999 (Sep.)) 2112–2118.

[20] S. Jono, Y. Nishizawa, A. Shioi, H. Morii, 1,25-Dihydroxyvitamin D3 increases in vitro vascular calcification by modulating secretion of endogenous parathyroid hormone-related peptide, Circulation 98 (13) (1998) 1302–1306.

[21] S. Jono, Y. Nishizawa, A. Shioi, H. Morii, Parathyroid hormone-related peptide as a local regulator of vascular calcification, Arterioscler. Thromb. Vasc. Biol. 17 (6) (1997) 1135–1142.

[22] Y. Tintut, J. Patel, F. Parhami, L.L. Demer, TNF-α promotes in vitro calcification of vascular cells via the cAMP pathway, Circulation 102 (2000) 2636–2642.

[23] F. Parhami, A. Morrow, J. Balucan, N. Leitinger, A.D. Watson, Y. Tintut, J.A. Berliner, L.L. Demer, Lipid oxidation products have opposite effects on calcifying vascular cell and bone cell differentiation: a possible explanation for the paradox of arterial calcification in osteoporotic patients, Arterioscler. Thromb. Vasc. Biol. 17 (4) (1997) 680–687.

[24] L.A. Fitzpatrick, R.T. Turner, E.R. Ritman, Endochondral bone formation in the heart: a possible mechanism of coronary calcification, Endocrinology 144 (6) (2003) 2214–2219.

[25] G.S. Stein, J.B. Lian, T.A. Owen, Relationship of cell growth to the regulation of tissue-specific gene expression during osteoblast differentiation, FASEB J. 4 (13) (1990) 3111–3123.

[26] E.R. Mohler III, M.K. Chawla, A.W. Chang, N. Vyavahare, R.J. Levy, L. Graham, F.H. Gannon, Identification and characterization of calcifying valve cells from human and canine aortic valves, J. Heart Valve Dis. 8 (3) (1999) 254–260.

[27] F. Parhami, S.M. Jackson, Y. Tintut, V. Le, J.P. Balucan, M. Territo, L.L. Demer, Atherogenic diet and minimally oxidized low density lipoprotein inhibit osteogenic and promote adipogenic differentiation of marrow stromal cells, J. Bone Miner. Res. 14 (12) (1999) 2067–2078.

[28] F. Parhami, Y. Tintut, W.G. Beamer, N. Gharavi, W. Goodman, L.L. Demer, Atherogenic high-fat diet reduces bone mineralization in mice, J. Bone Miner. Res. 16 (1) (2001) 182–188.

International Congress Series 1262 (2004) 574–577

www.ics-elsevier.com

Modulation of the ABCA1 transporter activity by protein kinase CK2

Stein Roosbeek[a], Frank Peelman[a], Hans Caster[a], Marc Lensink[a], Joël Vandekerckhove[a], Giovanna Chimini[b], Jan Tavernier[a], Maryvonne Rosseneu[a,*]

[a] *Department of Biochemistry, Ghent University, Hospitaalstr. 13, B-9000 Gent, Belgium*
[b] *Centre d'Immunologie Marseille-Luminy, France*

Abstract. We identified putative protein kinase CK2 phosphorylation sites in the cytoplasmic R1 and R2 domains, downstream of nucleotide binding domains (NBD) of the ABCA1 transporter, and tested their functional significance. In vitro, the recombinant ABCA1 NBD1 + R1 domain, and not the NBD2 + R2 domain, was phosphorylated by CK2. We identified T1242, T1243 and S1255 as the phosphorylated residues in the R1 domain. In HEK-293 cells, ABCA1 flippase activity, apolipoproteins AI and AII binding to the cell, and cellular phospholipid and cholesterol efflux were enhanced by mutations preventing CK2 phosphorylation of the threonine residues. Mutants mimicking threonine phosphorylation had activities close to that of WT ABCA1. Our data therefore suggest that protein kinase CK2 might regulate the transport activity of ABCA1 in vivo. © 2003 Published by Elsevier B.V.

Keywords: ABC transporter; Nucleotide binding domain; Protein kinase CK2

1. Introduction

In ABCA1, a member of the subfamily A of the ATP-binding cassette transporters, the N-terminal transmembrane domain is followed by a cytoplasmic domain, including the nucleotide binding domain (NBD), and a downstream sequence of 80 conserved residues (R-domain), which might have a regulatory function, as proposed for other transporters [1]. These motives are repeated in the C-terminal half of the full-transporter. The 1242-TTLEE and 2211-TTLDQ motives within the R1 and R2 domains are conserved in most members of the human ABCA subfamily [1] and are potential protein kinase CK2 phosphorylation sites. Another potential CK2 phosphor-

Abbreviations: ABC transporter, ATP binding cassette transporter; NBD, nucleotide binding domain.

* Corresponding author. Tel.: +32-9-264-92-74; fax: +32-9-264-94-96.
E-mail address: maryvonne.rosseneu@UGent.be (M. Rosseneu).

0531-5131/ © 2003 Published by Elsevier B.V.
doi:10.1016/j.ics.2003.11.005

ylation site 1255-SGVD is conserved in ABCA4, ABCA6-10, ABCA12, but is absent in R2. Modulation of ABCA1 activity might thus occur through serine or threonine phosphorylation by protein kinase CK2. To test this hypothesis, we studied in vitro phosphorylation of recombinant NBD1 + R1 and NBD2 + R2 by CK2, and the effect of CK2 phosphorylation on ABCA1 activity in transfected cells. ABCA1 activity was enhanced by mutations preventing CK2 phosphorylation of the R1 threonine residues, suggesting that CK2 might play an important role in vivo in regulating ABCA1 activity.

2. Materials and methods

Expression vectors for His-NBD1 + R1 and His-NBD2 + R2 were constructed using the pET28a plasmid, and mutants were made by overlapping PCR. His-NBD + R proteins were expressed in BL21(DE3)pLysS *E. coli*, purified on a Ni-PROBOND™ column by elution at 500 mM imidazole, and desalted on a HiTrap Sepharose column. For in vitro phosphorylation, 2-μg NBD + R was incubated at 22 °C with either [γ-^{32}P] ATP or 10 μM ATP and 10 mM $MgCl_2$ in the presence of 0.3-μg recombinant CK2, and analyzed by SDS gelelectrophoresis and autoradiography.

The construct encoding an ABCA1/GFP fusion protein [2] was used to generate the ABCA1 mutants. After transfection of HEK-293 cells, ABCA1 flippase activity and lipid efflux were measured on a fluorescence plate-reader by labeling the cells with 5 μM fluorescent NBD-lipid at 37 °C, and subsequent incubation either with Na-dithionite at 4 °C for flip-flop or with apo AI or AII for efflux measurements [3]. Cellular apo AI and apo AII binding was measured by flow cytometry after incubation with 20 μg/ml carboxyrhodamine-labeled apolipoprotein AI or AII for 1 h at 4 °C.

3. Results

3.1. Identification of protein kinase CK2 phosphorylation sites in ABCA1

The 39 potential CK2 phosphorylation sites in human ABCA1, 1242TTLE, 1243TLEE and 1255SGVD are located in the R1 domain, while 2211TTLD and 2225SDDD are in R2. In vitro phosphorylation of recombinant NBD + R proteins by CK2 shows that only NBD1 + R1, and not NBD2 + R2, is phosphorylated. MALDI/MS analysis of the native and phosphorylated recombinant proteins identified phosphorylation of T1242, T1243 and S1255. Both threonine residues are better conserved, compared with S1255, which is conserved only in the higher species (Fig. 1). We engineered mutants of the ABCA1 full-transporter, designed at preventing phosphorylation of these threonines: T1242A, T1243A, and T1242A + T1243A. We also mutated the downstream acidic residues (E1245Q + E1246Q) and designed mutants to mimic phosphorylated residues (T1242D, T1243D, T1242D + T1243D).

3.2. Modulation of ABCA1 activity

Transfection with T1242A, T1243A, T1242A + T1243A, and E1245Q + E1246Q mutants increased PE and PS flip-flop to the membrane outer leaflet compared with

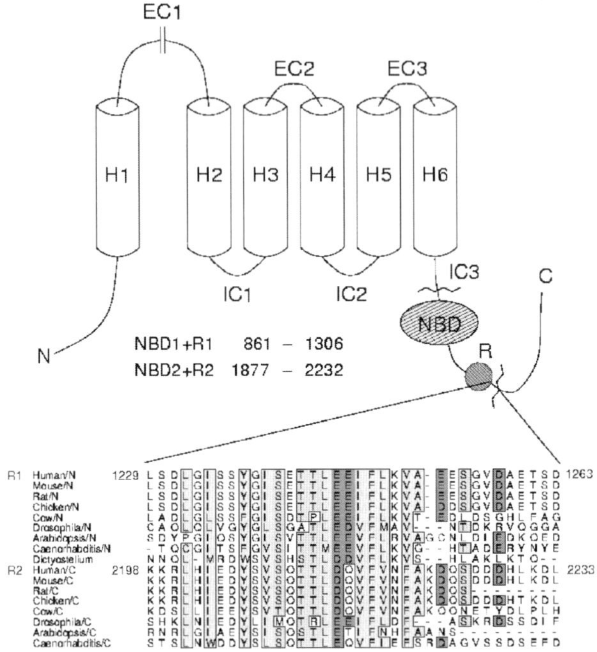

Fig. 1. Topology of the N-terminal domain of an ABCA full-transporter, consisting of two symmetrical halves. The alignment of the R1 and R2 domains shows conservation of CK2 phosphorylation sites at residues T1242, T1243 and S1255 for different ABCA1 species.

WT ABCA1 (Fig. 2). In contrast, when the threonine residues were mutated to aspartic acid, the phospholipid content in the outer leaflet was closer to that of WT. Similar results were obtained for apo AI and apo AII binding to the WT and mutant

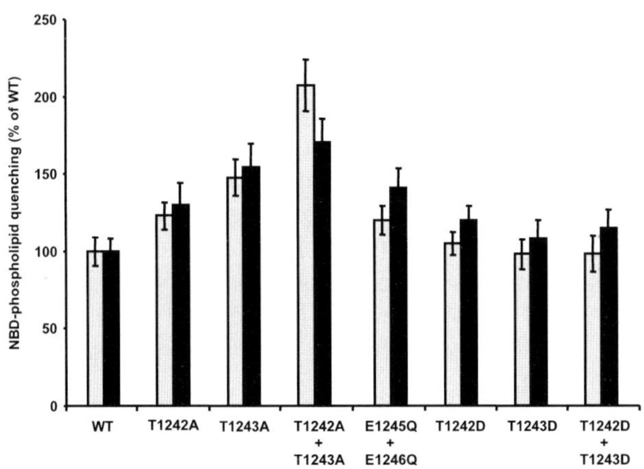

Fig. 2. Na-dithionite quenching of NBD-phospholipid in WT and mutant ABCA1-transfected HEK-293 cells, expressed relative to WT ABCA1. PS (left bar); PE (right bar).

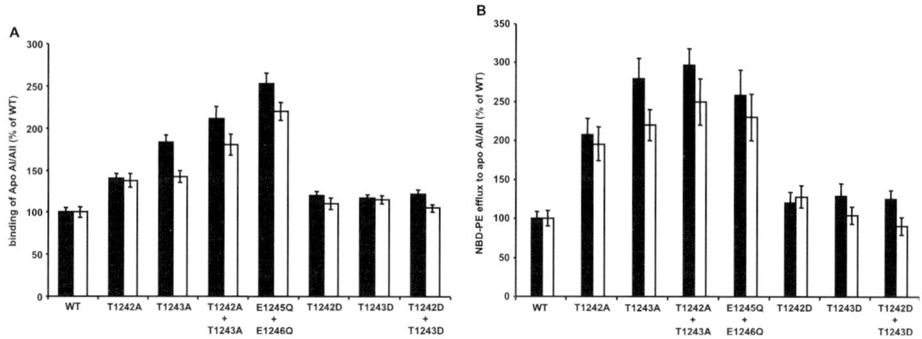

Fig. 3. (A) Binding of carboxyrhodamine-labeled apo AI (left bar) and apo AII (right bar) to HEK-293 cells transfected with WT and mutant ABCA1, expressed relative to WT ABCA1; (B) PE efflux to apo AI (left bar) and apo AII (right bar), expressed relative to WT ABCA1, in HEK-293 cells transfected with WT and mutant ABCA1.

transfected cells (Fig. 3A) for phospholipid efflux (Fig. 3B) and for cholesterol efflux.

4. Discussion

In this paper we showed CK2-specific phosphorylation in the R1 domain affects the major functions of ABCA1, including phospholipid flip-flop, apo AI and apo AII binding and phospholipid and cholesterol efflux, in a coordinated manner. Mutations suppressing the T1242 and T1243 phosphorylation by CK2 increased these activities, whereas mutations mimicking phosphorylation of these residues had activities close to that of WT ABCA1. This suggests that CK2 acts as a down-regulator of ABCA1 function. Besides PKA and PKC [4], CK2 might thus represent a new modulator of ABCA1 activity.

References

[1] F. Peelman, C. Labeur, B. Vanloo, S. Roosbeek, C. Devaud, N. Duverger, P. Denefle, M. Rosier, J. Vandekerckhove, M. Rosseneu, Characterization of the ABCA transporter subfamily: identification of procaryotic and eucaryotic members, phylogeny and topology, J. Mol. Biol. 325 (2003) 259–274.

[2] M. Dean, Y. Hamon, G. Chimini, The human ATP-binding cassette (ABC) transporter superfamily, J. Lipid Res. 42 (2001) 1007–1017.

[3] S. Roosbeek, F. Peelman, A. Verhee, C. Labeur, H. Caster, M. Lensink, C. Cirulli, C. Cochet, J. Vandekerckhove, A. Amoresano, G. Chimini, J. Tavernier, M. Rosseneu, Phosphorylation by protein kinase CK2 modulates the activity of the ATP-binding Cassette A1 (ABCA1) transporter, J. Biol. Chem. (2003) (in press).

[4] R.H. See, R.A. Caday-Malcolm, R.R. Singaraja, S. Zhou, A. Silverston, M.T. Huber, J. Moran, E.R. James, R. Janoo, J.M. Savill, V. Rigot, L.H. Zhang, M. Wang, G. Chimini, C.L. Wellington, S.R. Tafuri, M.R. Hayden, Protein kinase A site-specific phosphorylation regulates ATP-binding cassette A1 (ABCA1)-mediated phospholipid efflux, J. Biol. Chem. 44 (2002) 41835–41842.

ELSEVIER

International Congress Series 1262 (2004) 578–581

www.ics-elsevier.com

Cloning, tissue distribution and function of ABCA transporters

Nobuya Inagaki[a,*], Katsuya Yamada[a], Li-Xia Zhao[a], Gen Yamano[a], Yukiko Tanaka[a], Hisayuki Funahashi[b], Cheng-Ji Zhou[b], Seiji Shioda[b], Nobuhiro Ban[a]

[a] *Department of Physiology, Akita University School of Medicine, 1-1-1 Hondo, Akita 010-8543, Japan*
[b] *Department of Anatomy, Showa University School of Medicine, Tokyo, Japan*

Abstract. We cloned the full-length cDNA of ABCA2. ABCA2 is expressed predominantly in the oligodendrocytes in the brain, and onset of ABCA2 expression in the oligodendrocytes coincides with the appearance of thick myelin basic protein (MBP)-immunolabeled myelin segments. Oligodendrocytes produce the lamellar structure myelin, which is composed of phospholipids and specific myelin proteins. We also cloned ABCA3 from human lung and found that ABCA3 is expressed predominantly at the limiting membrane of the lamellar bodies of alveolar type II cells in human lung. Pulmonary surfactant, composed mainly of phospholipids and specific surfactant proteins, is stored as lamellar bodies before exocytosis into the alveolar space. These data suggest that ABCA2 and ABCA3 are involved in membrane transport of substrates such as the lipids that are closely linked to myelin and surfactant formation processes.

Keywords: ABC transporter; ABCA2; ABCA3; Myelin; Pulmonary surfactant

1. Introduction

The ABC transporter superfamily is one of the largest gene families, encoding highly conserved proteins involved in energy-dependent transport of a variety of substrates across membrane. Among the several subclasses of ABC transporters, the ABCA subclass [1] has received considerable attention because mutation of the ABCA1 or the ABCA4 gene causes Tangier disease accompanying HDL deficiency [2,3] or Stargardt's macular dystrophy [4] in humans, respectively. ABCA1 functions to promote cellular phospholipid and cholesterol efflux to apolipoprotein A-I (apoA-I), initiating the formation of high density lipoprotein [2,3,5], and ABCA4 is proposed to be transmembrane transporters for intracellular *N*-retinylidene-phosphatidylethanolamine [6]. Very recently, ABCA7, whose

* Corresponding author. Tel.: +81-18-884-6069; fax: +81-18-884-6442.
E-mail address: inagaki@med.akita-u.ac.jp (N. Inagaki).

0531-5131/
doi:10.1016/j.ics.2003.12.049

mRNA is upregulated by sustained elevations of cholesterol, has been reported to be involved in ApoA-I-mediated efflux of phospholipids but not of cholesterol [7]. These results suggest that ABCA transporters are involved in transmembrane transport of endogenous lipids.

2. Materials and methods

To isolate the full-length cDNAs of ABCA2 and ABCA3, rat brain and human lung cDNA libraries were screened under standard hybridization conditions [8,9]. RNA blot analysis was performed as previously described [8,9].

The specific antibodies for ABCA2 and ABCA3 were raised in rabbits against the synthetic peptide corresponding to 20 C-terminal amino acid residues of rat ABCA2 and 13 C-terminal amino acid residues of human ABCA3, respectively [8,9].

Culture, transfection and immunoblot analysis were carried out as previously described [8,9]. For double immunofluorescence staining with ABCA2, monoclonal mouse anti-human 2′, 3′-cyclic nucleotide-3′ -phosphodiesterase (CNP), rabbit anti-myelin basic protein (MBP) and rabbit anti-glial fibrillary acidic protein (GFAP) were used; for ABCA3, monoclonal mouse anti-human surfactant protein A (SP-A) IgG antibody was used [9,10].

In situ hybridization, immunohistochemistry and immunoelectron microscopy were performed as previously described [8–10].

3. Results

3.1. ABCA2

We cloned the full-length cDNA of ABCA2 from a rat cDNA library [8]. The predicted 2434 amino acid sequence of ABCA2 shows 44.5%, 40.0% and 40.8% identity with mouse ABCA1, human ABCA3 and human ABCA4, respectively [8].

RNA blotting study revealed that ABCA2 mRNA is expressed at high levels in the brain and at much lower or undetectable levels in other tissues. In in situ hybridization, the signals for ABCA2 mRNA were detected intensely in the white matter such as corpus callosum suggesting that ABCA2 is expressed in oligodendrocytes [8].

In immunohistochemical study using specific anti-ABCA2 antibody, ABCA2-immunostained cells were found to be in the majority in white matter throughout the entire brain. The ABCA2-immunolabeled cell bodies were found to be co-immunostained with an antibody against CNP, a marker protein of oligodendrocytes, suggesting that ABCA2 is expressed mainly in oligodendrocytes. At the ultrastructural level, ABCA2 immunoreactivity was found to be mostly distributed around intracellular vesicles, probably late endosomes and lysosomes, of the oligodendrocytes but not in the myelin sheaths.

Both immunoblot and immunohistochemical results showed a rapid increase in ABCA2 expression, especially during the second and third postnatal week in the developing rat brain [11], when extensive myelination is found in the brain [12,13]. ABCA2-positive cells were detected first in the white matter when short and thick MBP-posotive myelin segments began to appear in the region [11]. These results indicate that the initial

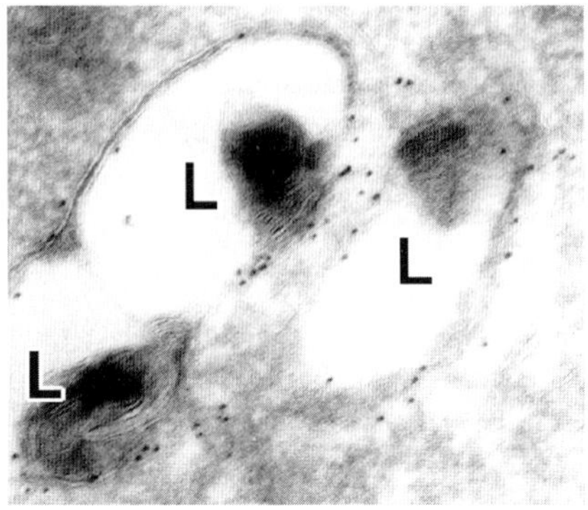

Fig. 1. Immunogold labeling of ABCA3 protein in human alveolar type II cell. ABCA3. Many gold labelings of ABCA3 locate on the limiting membrane of lamellar bodies.

expression of ABCA2 in oligodendrocytes occurs concurrently with the onset of myelin formation, suggesting that ABCA2 may be involved in membrane transport of lipids closely associated with myelination.

3.2. ABCA3

In the present study, we cloned the full-length cDNA of ABCA3 from human lung. ABCA3 protein was analyzed by immunoblotting using the antibody generated against human ABCA3 [9]. A single band at 150 kDa was detected from the crude membrane fraction of human lung tissue.

In immunohistochemical analysis, ABCA3 immunoreactivity appears very intensely in the comparatively large, round or cuboid SP-A-positive cells, scattered in the alveolar epithelium [9]. At the ultrastructural level, immunogold particles were observed mainly in cells with apical microvilli on the plasma membrane, a feature of type II cells. Major labelings are associated with lamellar bodies specific to type II cells, and most are localized exclusively on the limiting membranes and not inside the lamellar bodies (Fig. 1).

4. Discussion

The ABCA2 protein is expressed mainly in oligodendrocytes, and temporal and spatial profiles of ABCA2 expression are in good agreement with those of myelinization. Concurrently with the period of active myelinization, the content of cholesterol, phospholipids and cerebrosides including galactocerebroside and its derivative sulfatide in the brain increases dramatically, indicating active synthesis of these lipids during this period [13] and suggesting that ABCA2 is involved in membrane transport of lipids closely associated with myelination.

Pulmonary surfactant, composed mainly of phospholipids and specific surfactant proteins, reduces the surface tension at the alveolar air/liquid interface, and thereby prevents the lungs from collapsing [14]. Lamellar bodies are dense multilayer structures of surfactant formed in alveolar type II cells and secreted into alveolar space by exocytosis. The mechanism by which phospholipids are packaged into the lamellar body is currently not known, but ABCA3 might well function as a transmembrane transporter of the phospholipid components of pulmonary surfactant. Further studies to clarify the functional roles of ABCA2 and ABCA3 are required.

References

[1] I. Klein, B. Sarkadi, A. Váradi, Biochim. Biophys. Acta 1461 (1999) 237–262.

[2] M.R. Hayden, S.M. Clee, A. Brooks-Wilson, J. Genest Jr., A. Attie, J.J.J. Kastelein, Curr. Opin. Lipidol. 11 (2000) 117–122.

[3] G. Schmitz, T. Langmann, Structure, function, and regulation of the ABC1 gene product, Curr. Opin. Lipidol. 12 (2001) 129–140.

[4] R. Allikmets, Simple and complex *ABCR*: genetic predisposition to retinal disease, Am. J. Hum. Genet., 67 (2000) 793–799.

[5] E. Orsó, C. Broccardo, W.E. Kaminski, A. Böttcher, G. Liebisch, W. Drobnik, A. Götz, O. Chambenoit, W. Diederich, T. Langmann, T. Spruss, M.-F. Luciani, G. Rothe, K.J. Lackner, J. Chimini, G. Schmitz, Transport of lipids from Golgi to plasma membrane is defective in Tangier disease patients and *Abc1*-deficient mice, Nat. Genet. 24 (2000) 192–196.

[6] J. Weng, N.L. Mata, S.M. Azarian, R.T. Tzekov, D.G. Birch, G.H. Travis, Insights into the function of Rim protein in photoreceptors and etiology of Stargardt's disease from the phenotype in *abcr* knockout mice, Cell 98 (1999) 13–23.

[7] N. Wang, D. Lan, M. Gerbod-Giannone, P. Linsel-Nitschke, A.W. Jehle, W. Chen, L.O. Martinez, A.R. Tall, ATP-binding cassette transporter A7 (ABCA7) binds apolipoprotein A-I and mediates cellular phospholipids but not cholesteril efflux. J. Biol. Chem. (in press).

[8] L.X. Zhao, C.J. Zhou, A. Tanaka, M. Nakata, T. Hirabayashi, T. Amachi, S. Shioda, K. Ueda, N. Inagaki, Cloning, characterization and tissue distribution of the rat ATP-binding cassette (ABC) transporter ABC2/ABCA2, Biochem. J. 350 (2000) 865–872.

[9] G. Yamano, H. Funahashi, O. Kawanami, L.X. Zhao, N. Ban, Y. Uchida, T. Morohoshi, J. Ogawa, S. Shioda, N. Inagaki, ABCA3 is a lamellar body membrane protein in human lung alveolar type II cells, FEBS Lett. 508 (2001) 221–225.

[10] C.J. Zhou, L.X. Zhao, N. Inagaki, J.L. Guan, S. Nakajo, T. Hirabayashi, S. Kikuyama, S. Shioda, ATP-binding cassette transporter ABC2/ABCA2 in rat brain: a novel mammalian lysosome-associated membrane protein and a specific marker for oligodendrocytes but not for myelin sheaths, J. Neurosci., 21 (2001) 849–857.

[11] Y. Tanaka, K. Yamada, C.J. Zhou, N. Ban, S. Shioda, N. Inagaki, Temporal and spatial profiles of ABCA2-expressing oligodendrocytes in the developing rat brain, J. Comp. Neurol. 455 (2003) 353–367.

[12] S. Jacobson, Sequence of myelinization in the brain of the albino rat. A. Cerebral cortex, thalamus and related structures, J. Comp. Neurol. 121 (1963) 5–29.

[13] M.L. Cuzner, A.N. Davison, The lipid composition of rat brain myelin and subcellular fractions during development, Biochem. J. 106 (1968) 29–34.

[14] J. Johansson, T. Crustedt, Molecular structures and interactions of pulmonary surfactant components, Eur. J. Biochem. 244 (1997) 675–693.

International Congress Series 1262 (2004) 582–585

www.ics-elsevier.com

Trends in morbidity, mortality, and risk factor levels of coronary heart disease in Japan—Are Japanese living in Japan still protected against coronary heart disease?

Kazunori Kodama*, Fumiyoshi Kasagi

Department of Epidemiology, Radiation Effects Research Foundation, 5-2 Hijiyama-park, Minami-ku, Hiroshima 732-0815, Japan

Abstract. In accordance with the rapid aging of the Japanese population, the number of patients with stroke and heart disease is expected to increase in the 21st century. Continuing rapid westernization of lifestyle, such as dietary habits along with increased hyperlipidemia and diabetes mellitus, presents another concern about a possible future increase in atherosclerotic disease incidence among the male population. A review of mortality from coronary heart disease (CHD) in the mid 1990s revealed that the Japan experienced the lowest mortality among industrialized countries. Japan also belonged to the group of countries with decreased mortality from CHD, with about a 30% reduction observed over the previous 10 years in men. However, recent trends in risk factor levels raise some concerns about the future of CHD in Japan. Compared with the 1990 survey results, the 5th National Survey of Cardiovascular Diseases conducted in 2000 showed an upward trend in the prevalence of hypertension and hyperlipidemia among men in their 30s and 40s. Another report points to an increased DM prevalence in Japan. Therefore, a concern exists about a possible future increase of CHD incidence among young and middle-aged men in Japan. Taking into account the rapid pace of the aging of the population, it is anticipated that, even if the disease's incidence remains unchanged, the number of patients from the ranks of the elderly will rise. Consequently, CHD may become a major issue for Japan's public health care in the 21st Century.

Keywords: Coronary heart disease; Myocardial infarction; Mortality; Incidence; Risk factor

1. Introduction

In accordance with the rapid aging of the Japanese population, the number of patients with atherosclerotic diseases is expected to increase in Japan. In addition, continuing rapid westernization of lifestyle presents another concern about a possible future increase in atherosclerotic disease incidence among young and middle-aged populations in Japan.

* Corresponding author. Tel.: +81-82-261-4723; fax: +81-82-262-9768.
E-mail address: kodama@rerf.or.jp (K. Kodama).

0531-5131/
doi:10.1016/j.ics.2003.12.016

2. Material and methods

Most of the Japanese data mentioned in this article are based on the Vital Statistics, National Survey of Cardiovascular Diseases. Trends of heart disease mortality were obtained from the Vital Statistics of 1950 to 2000 [1]. A series of the National Survey of Cardiovascular Diseases, conducted from 1961 to 2000, was used to describe changes in risk factor levels [2].

3. Results and comments

3.1. Mortality of coronary heart disease

Based on the World Health Statistics Annual, it was revealed that CHD mortality rate in Japan, for both sexes, has been the lowest among industrialized countries, with the rates roughly 1/8 those of East European and Nordic countries and 1/5 those of the United States [3]. In addition, Japan is one of the countries in which CHD mortality has decreased. Over the past 10 years, CHD mortality has decreased by about 30% for males and 40% for females, as is shown in Fig. 1 [1]. However, with further acceleration of the westernization of lifestyle in the metropolitan areas in Japan, CHD mortality may rise in the future.

3.2. Incidence of myocardial infarction (MI)

For making an international comparison of MI incidence, Ueshima [4] reviewed studies conducted in Japan, using diagnostic criteria similar to that used in WHO MONICA Project. He reported that the age-adjusted MI incidence among all Japanese regional groups from Okinawa through Hokkaido is lower than that of other countries, and hence it can be said that Japan belongs to a group with the lowest MI incidence among the world's countries. For example, Japan's MI incidence is 1/10 to 1/5 that of European countries.

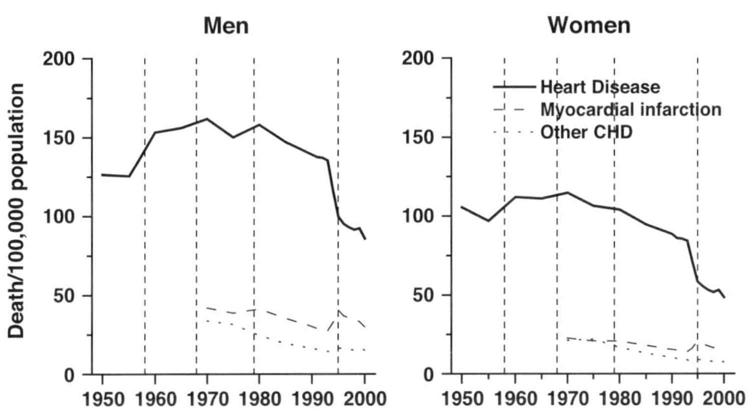

Fig. 1. Trends in age-adjusted death rates for heart disease by sex in Japan, 1950–2000, Vital Statistics.

One possible reason why there is no increase in coronary heart disease in Japan appears to be that the time period during which the Japanese people, as a group, experienced an average total serum cholesterol level of over 200 mg/dl has not been lengthy enough to cause increased incidence.

3.3. Hypertension

According to the National Survey of Cardiovascular Diseases, mean values of systolic blood pressure are liable to decrease for both males and females of each of the over-30 age groups. Such a decreasing trend is becoming more distinct among the higher age groups [2]. However, the survey also showed that the prevalence of hypertension increased among males in their 30s and 40s in the 1990–2000 cycles [2].

3.4. Hyperlipidemia

Based on the National Survey of Cardiovascular Diseases, a rise in cholesterol levels for both males and females in every age group was observed in the 1980–1990 survey cycles. The increased levels were significant, with an annual increase rate of around 1 mg/dl for all age groups. In the 1990–2000 survey cycles, however, such an increasing trend changed, with only a slight rise observed for the majority of male age groups and a decrease observed for the majority of female age groups [2].

Fig. 2 presents the changes in the prevalence of hypercholesterolemia based on the National Survey of Cardiovascular Diseases [2]. The 1980 to 2000 survey cycles show that the rate of those with a serum total cholesterol level of 240 mg/dl or more continued to increase for males in their 30s and 40s, along with a similar upward trend in their mean body mass index (BMI) [2]. For the other male and female age groups, an increase was observed during the period of the 1980 to 1990 survey cycles, with the rates remaining at the same level or decreasing for the 2000 cycle [2].

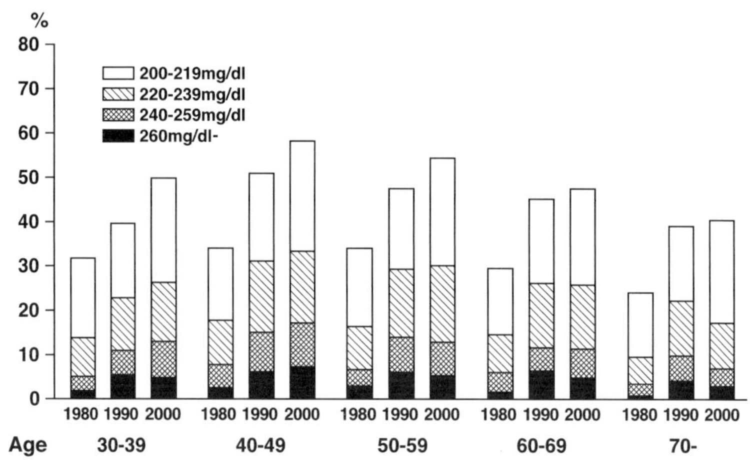

Fig. 2. Trends in prevalence of hypercholesterolemia (Men, 1980–2000, National Survey of Cardiovascular Diseases).

3.5. Smoking

The adult smoking rate in men in Japan has been quite high among industrialized countries. The highest rate was observed in 1966 at 83.7%. The male smoking rate gradually declined thereafter, but it was still above 50% in 2001 [5]. In particular, in 2001, the smoking rate was still 58.9% and 58.1% among men in their 20s and 30s, respectively [2]. The smoking rate among women has been low and showed little change as a whole, but it has been increasing among women in their 20s and 30s.

3.6. Impaired glucose tolerance

In 2002, the MHLW conducted a national survey on the prevalence of diabetes mellitus (DM) as part of the National Nutrition Survey [6]. Based on the survey, it was estimated that there were 7.4 million persons with a strong probability of having DM in Japan. DM, in this case, was defined as either under treatment for DM or having an HbA1c of above 6.1%. The estimated number in the 1997 survey was 6.9 million, indicating a significant increase over a relatively short period [6]. DM will become one of the major health problems in the 21st century in Japan.

Acknowledgements

The authors would like to thank H. Moriwaki, H. Hayashi, and S. Ishii for help with manuscript preparation.

References

[1] Statistics and Information Department, Minister's Secretariat, Ministry of Health, Labor and Welfare, Vital Statistics, 1950–2000, Japan, Tokyo: Statistics and Information Department, Minister's Secretariat, Ministry of Health, Labor and Welfare, 2001 (in Japanese).

[2] Health Service Bureau, Ministry of Health, Labor and Welfare, The 5th National Survey of Cardiovascular Diseases, Ministry of Health, Labor and Welfare, Tokyo, Japan, 2002, in Japanese with English summary.

[3] National Heart, Lung, and Blood Institute (NHLBI), Chart Book on Cardiovascular, Lung and Blood Disease, NHLBI, Bethesda, 2001.

[4] H. Ueshima, General aspects of cardiovascular disease in Japan, in: F. Takaku (Ed.), Textbook of New Clinical Medicine, 8th ed., Igaku Shoin, Tokyo, 2000, pp. 385–391, in Japanese.

[5] Health and Welfare Statistics Association, Trends of National Hygiene, J. Health Welfare Stat. 50 (2003) 81 (in Japanese).

[6] Ministry of Health, Labor and Welfare, National Survey of Diabetes Mellitus in 2002, Available from: http://www.mhlw.go.jp/shingi/2003/08/s0806-4.html.

International Congress Series 1262 (2004) 586–589

www.ics-elsevier.com

Coronary heart disease in Japanese and Japanese Americans: does it provide clues for prevention?

J. David Curb[a,b,*], Hirotsugu Ueshima[c], Beatriz L. Rodriguez[a,b], Robert D. Abbott[a,d], Akira Sekikawa[e], Gina Belleau[a], Katsuhiko Yano[a]

[a] *Pacific Health Research Institute, Honolulu, HI, USA*

[b] *Departments of Medicine and Geriatrics, John A. Burns School of Medicine, University of Hawaii at Manoa, Honolulu, HI, USA*

[c] *Department of Health Science, Shiga University of Medical Science, Otsu, Japan*

[d] *Division of Biostatistics and Epidemiology, University of Virginia School of Medicine, Charlottesville, VA, USA*

[e] *University of Pittsburgh, Pittsburgh, PA, USA*

Abstract. Dramatic lifestyle changes in Japan in recent years have had a major impact on the risk factors for coronary heart disease (CHD). The NI-HON-SAN study was initiated to investigate observed differences in stroke and CHD rates among Japanese in Japan and Japanese emigrants in Hawaii and California. Stroke prevalence was high in Japan, intermediate in Hawaii and lowest in California. CHD prevalence had exactly the opposite trend. Comparisons of risk factors between Japanese in Japan and Hawaii in the INTERLIPID study indicates that, except for smoking, middle-aged Japanese in Hawaii still may have somewhat higher levels of CHD risk factors than those in Japan. It is possible that there are protective factors operating in individuals of Japanese descent associated with the CHD differences between the Japanese and other populations. Further studies to assess differences in coronary calcium scores in the populations are underway.

Keywords: Coronary heart disease; Risk factors; Japan

1. Introduction

In recent years, many Asian countries have shifted toward a Western lifestyle. One result of these lifestyle changes appears to be a significant negative impact on the risk factors for coronary heart disease (CHD) in many countries. While the negative impact appears to be consistent, the corresponding impact of these changes on atherosclerotic disease varies among Asian countries. Some countries appear to have had declines in the

* Corresponding author. CEO, Pacific Health Research Institute, 846 South Hotel Street, Suite 303, Honolulu, HI 96817, USA. Tel.: +1-808-524-4411; fax: +1-808-524-5559.

E-mail addresses: jdcurb@phrihawaii.org (J.D. Curb), gcbelleau@phrihawaii.org (G. Belleau).

0531-5131/
doi:10.1016/j.ics.2003.11.024

rates of both CHD and stroke, while at the same time the population's risk factor levels approached those seen in the US.

2. Comparison of CHD in Japan and the US

2.1. The NI-HON-SAN study

As early as 1950, studies around the world were reporting geographic differences in CHD mortality, pathology, prevalence and incidence [1]. Reported CHD mortality among Japanese was approximately 20% that of US Caucasians, but stroke mortality appeared to be substantially higher among the Japanese.

Differences in mortality and disease patterns could be secondary to differing criteria for hospitalization, diagnosis, death certification or other factors. These facts led to the initiation of the NI-HON-SAN study in 1965 to investigate reported differences in stroke and heart attack rates in Japanese living in the US (Honolulu and San Francisco) and Japan (Hiroshima and Nagasaki) [2,3]. The NI-HON-SAN study confirmed that the prevalence of self-reported stroke in 45–68-year-old men was high in Japan, intermediate in Hawaii and lowest in California, with the opposite pattern present for CHD, as shown in Fig. 1 [4].

The Japanese study population was followed by the Radiation Effects Research Foundation as part of the Adult Health Study of the atomic bomb survivors from Hiroshima and Nagasaki [5,6]. The Honolulu cohort became the basis for the Honolulu Heart Program, a long-term prospective study of cardiovascular disease and its risk factors. It was composed of 8006 first- and second-generation Japanese immigrants who were residents of the island of Oahu. Information on mortality and cardiovascular events occurring after the baseline examination has been obtained through a comprehensive surveillance of hospital discharges, death certificates and autopsy records. Additional data were gathered at repeat examinations at irregular intervals.

2.2. The NI-HON-MAJIC study

Mortality follow-up procedures in both the Japanese and Hawaiian cohorts have differed. The methodology for classification of death from cancer and traumatic death

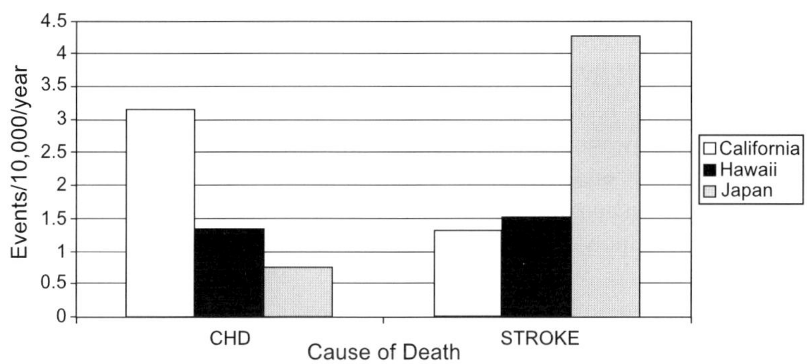

Fig. 1. Prevalence of stroke and CHD in NI-HON-SAN study. Japanese men aged 45–68 years at baseline.

(violent death, accident, etc.) has been verified to be relatively accurate [7], but there were known differences in diagnostic practices for cardiovascular disease. In the NI-HON-MAJIC study, 23-year mortality by age and classification of death was calculated. For comparison purposes, deaths were classified as traumatic, cancer related or non-cancer related. Other factors considered included systolic blood pressure, body mass index (BMI), serum cholesterol, cigarette smoking, alcohol consumption, saturated fat intake, 1-h post-load serum glucose and radiation dose in 1945. The death rates for every age group were significantly higher in Japan for both cancer and non-cancer death. That difference is reduced by risk factor adjustment in the cancer deaths, but not in the non-cancer deaths.

2.3. The INTERLIPID study

Despite recent increases in total cholesterol and higher smoking rates in Japan, CHD incidence continues to be substantially lower at all ages in Japanese than in US Caucasians. To better understand these differences, the CHD risk factors and dietary variables in Japanese living in Japan (Aito, Toyama, Sapporo, Wakayama) and third and fourth generation Japanese emigrants in Hawaii were compared in the INTERLIPID study (an ancillary of the INTERMAP study).

Men and women, aged 40–59 years, were examined by standardized methods. Average systolic and diastolic blood pressures and smoking prevalence were significantly higher in men in Japan than in Hawaii, while treatment rate of hypertension and levels of several—especially lipid—CHD risk factors were lower in Japan. These differences between Japan and Hawaii were smaller for women than men.

2.4. The ERA-JUMP study

Data from national sample surveys in Japan demonstrate risk factor profiles for CHD are similar to those in the US in a post-WWII cohort, except for higher prevalence of cigarette smoking in Japan and higher prevalence of obesity in the US. CHD mortality among men in this age group in Japan is still less than half that in men of the same age in the US [8]. In the ERA-JUMP study (*E*BCT and *R*isk Factor *A*ssessment among *J*apanese and *U*S *M*en in the *P*ost-World-War II birth cohort), risk factors and atherosclerosis are being compared in Japanese in Japan and Hawaii, Caucasians and African Americans in the US, and Koreans in Korea. The measures of subclinical disease in these 40–49-year-old men include calcium scores of coronary artery and aorta measured by electron beam-computed tomography (EBCT), carotid intima thickness measured by ultrasound and pulse wave velocity measured by the Colin's vascular profile (VP-2000). Other measures include dietary intake by food frequency questionnaire, total cholesterol, LDLc, HDLc, blood pressure, cigarette smoking, alcohol consumption, body mass index, intra-abdominal fat and others. Understanding the reasons for the low Japanese CHD rates may lead to new methods for prevention of CHD in all populations.

3. Conclusions

Many factors contribute to international differences in cardiovascular mortality rates. These include body fat, diet, smoking habits, lack of physical activity and the control of high blood pressure. Much of the difference still remains unexplained. A better understanding of the pathophysiology behind these differences may assist in the prevention of cardiovascular disease for all in the 21st century.

Acknowledgements

Supported by the National Heart, Lung and Blood Institute (contract N01-HC-05102, grants U01-HL-56274, 5-R01-HL54868-03, 2-R01-HL50490-06, 1-R01 HL71561-01, R01-HL-46696 and T32-HL-07594), the National Institute on Aging (contract N01-AG-4-2149), the American Heart Association of Hawaii (grant HIGS-16-97), the Robert Perry Fund and the Hawaii Community Foundation.

References

[1] World Trends in Cardiology: I. Cardiovascular Epidemiology, Hoeber-Harper, New York, 1956.

[2] J.L. Belsky, A. Kagan, S.L. Syme, Epidemiologic studies of coronary heart disease and stroke in Japanese men living in Japan, Hawaii and California. Research Plan. Atomic Bomb Casualty Commission Technical Report (1971) 12–71.

[3] T.L. Robertson, H. Kato, T. Gordon, A. Kagan, G.G. Rhoads, C.E. Land, et al., Epidemiologic studies of coronary heart disease and stroke in Japanese men living in Japan, Hawaii and California. Coronary heart disease risk factors in Japan and Hawaii, Am. J. Cardiol. 39 (2) (1977) 244–249.

[4] J.D. Curb, K. Kodama, The NI-HON-SAN study, Ann. Epidemiol. 6 (4) (1996) S197–S201.

[5] K. Kodama, H. Sasaki, Y. Shimizu, Trend of coronary heart disease and its relationship to risk factors in a Japanese population: a 26-year follow-up, Hiroshima/Nagasaki study, Jpn. Circ. J. 54 (4) (1990) 414–421.

[6] K. Kodama, K. Mabuchi, I. Shigematsu, A long-term cohort study of the atomic-bomb survivors, J. Epidemiol. 6 (3 Suppl.) (1996) S95–S105.

[7] E. Ron, R. Carter, S. Jablon, K. Mabuchi, Agreement between death certificate and autopsy diagnoses among atomic bomb survivors, Epidemiology 5 (1) (1994) 48–56.

[8] A. Sekikawa, T. Okamura, T. Kadowaki, K. Mitsunami, K. Murata, A. Kashiwagi, et al., Electron-beam computed tomography for identification of high-risk persons in primary prevention of coronary heart disease in the United States and its implication for Japan, Nippon Koshu Eisei Zasshi 50 (3) (2003) 183–193.

International Congress Series 1262 (2004) 590

ELSEVIER

www.ics-elsevier.com

The pandemic of atherosclerosis in the Mediterranean area

Osama Abdel Aziz*

Department of Cardiology, Tanta University, 98 Mohamed Farid Street, Cairo 00202, Egypt

Keywords: Pandemic; Atherosclerosis; Mediterranean

1. Introduction

The pandemic of atherosclerosis is a threat to humanity all over the world and the people in the Middle East and the Mediterranean area are no exception. Risk factors vary from place to place, town to town and country to country.

The prevalence of such factors and their frequency are also different and necessitate a special search in each country in order to know the real risk factors and how best to combat them.

A specific study has been designed in Egypt—as a model of the Mediterranean countries. All RFs have been determined throughout Egypt, including almost 7000 people from various governorates ranging in age from 25 to 75 years.

The lipid profile was assessed and its relation to other RFs was also determined.

It has been clarified that the RFs definitely vary from country to country and, in our study, even from place to place.

The parameters for women were different from those among men.

This may have an impact on the prognoses and offer an explanation for the different prognostic outcomes and differences in therapeutic approaches.

The total cholesterol levels were higher than the upper limit of normal among almost 40% of the total adult population in Egypt.

The same problem was noticed with LDL-cholesterol, as well as the high prevalence of low HDL.

Genetic factors may play a role, as well as dietary factors and the lack of exercise. Data from other Mediterranean countries will also be discussed and compared.

* Tel.: +20-12-2171436; fax: +20-2-3958000.
E-mail address: osama200@worldnet.com.eg (O.A. Aziz).

doi:10.1016/S0531-5131(03)01861-2

Meet the Professor session

International Congress Series 1262 (2004) 593–596

www.ics-elsevier.com

What is the most important in treating hypertension?

Kikuo Arakawa*

Kawanami Hospital, Fukuoka University School of Medicine, 1-2-36 Noke, Sawara 814-0171, Fukuoka, Japan

Abstract. Essential hypertension is a typical lifestyle disease. Lifestyle factors, especially excess salt intake, "germinate" hypertension; genotype only influences susceptibility to the condition. Hence lifestyle modifications, especially reducing salt intake or performing activities that promote the removal of sodium from the body, are most important in treating hypertension. However, if blood pressure targets cannot be achieved by lifestyle modification, antihypertensive medications that remove excess sodium such as diuretics or calcium antagonists in combination with renin–angiotensin system (RAS)-suppressing drugs may be beneficial. © 2003 Published by Elsevier B.V.

Keywords: Salt; Renin–angiotensin system; Rice diet; Physical exercise; Adenosine–dopamine system

1. Introduction

The latter half of the 20th century was an era of much development in antihypertensive medicine, from the first sympathetic ganglionic blocker in 1950 to angiotensin receptor blockers (ARB) in the 1990s. With the development of ARB, pharmacologic antihypertensive therapy appears to have reached a ceiling of effectiveness [1]. Thanks to these developments, lowering blood pressure has become quite easy.

The effectiveness of antihypertensive drugs in preventing hypertensive vascular diseases has been established by many large-scale clinical trials. However, >50% of patients who receive medical treatment do not fully respond and exhibit hypertensive vascular complications [2,3]. The two major reasons for this seem to be:

(a) blood pressure is not lowered enough [3];
(b) antihypertensives lower blood pressure but do not cure hypertension [4].

Hence, it appears that in the 21st century antihypertensive treatment should focus on preventing onset of the disease. What is the etiology of essential hypertension? Many theories have been postulated but none convincingly points to any single cause. The polygenic theory (Fig. 1) is probably the most widely accepted [5].

* Tel.: +81-92-861-2780; fax: +81-92-861-2111.
E-mail addresses: arakawa@kawanami.com, arakawak@jcom.home.ne.jp (K. Arakawa).

0531-5131/ © 2003 Published by Elsevier B.V.
doi:10.1016/j.ics.2003.12.019

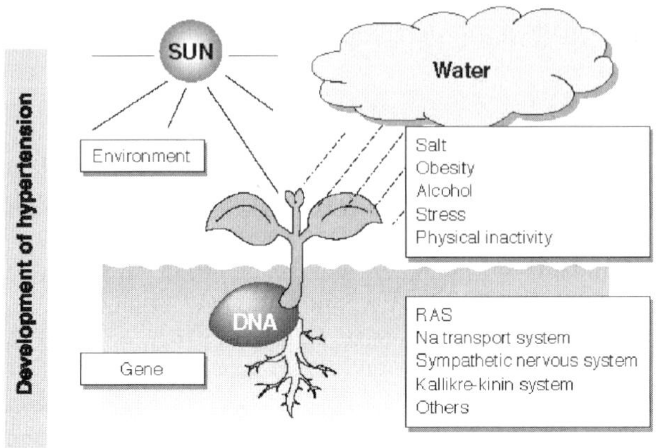

Fig. 1. The polygenic theory: multiple genetic and environmental factors "germinate" hypertension.

More than 20 candidate genes have been investigated as possibly predisposing individuals to hypertension. Among them, angiotensinogen gene polymorphism M235T has gained wide recognition as a determining factor [6]. Angiotensinogen is more readily transcribed in individuals with the mutant gene than in those with the normal M235 variant leading to more active renin–angiotensin systems (RAS).

Excess salt intake is more likely responsible for causing hypertension in the majority of cases. In African Americans, who exhibit a high incidence of hypertension and salt sensitivity, the angiotensinogen M235T gene polymorphism has been detected in 90% of individuals. However, in native Africans, who have the same mutant gene frequency, the incidence of hypertension is much lower [7] Thus, a high-salt diet such as is commonly encountered in the USA appears decisive.

The role of dietary salt in causing hypertension has long been suspected. In 1904, Ambard and Beaujurd [8] demonstrated that salt restriction lowers blood pressure in patients with Bright's disease. Kempner [9] applied this principle to 500 severely hypertensive patients who were advised to adopt a no-salt rice diet with beautiful results in 1948. No-salt rice diet lowered mean blood pressure by ≥ 11 mm Hg in 95% of patients. More recently, the DASH study [10] using modern methodology confirmed the effects of sodium restriction as first suggested by Ambard and Kempner.

Controversy over salt-restriction therapy existed concerning the long time intervals for benefits to appear. For example, Kempner [9] noted that ≥ 3 weeks were required for the no-salt rice diet to take effect. This implied the involvement of some unknown mechanism of salt hypertension other than mere expansion of body fluid. Cailar et al. [11] showed that excess salt intake causes left ventricular hypertrophy and albuminuria independent of blood pressure. These pathologic conditions both suggest a contributing role of angiotensin [12].

Angiotensin has been attributed a chief offender in cardiovascular complications since both angiotensin-converting enzyme (ACE) inhibitors and ARB prevent their acceleration beyond that which may be expected from lowering blood pressure alone [12]. On the other hand, Yanomamo Indians, whose diet contains no salt, have activated RAS [13]. Patients with essential hypotension also have high plasma renin activity [14] although they do not generally exhibit a high incidence of cardiovascular complications. RAS seems primarily to play a role in recycling the body's sodium. Blocking RAS by ACE inhibitor and ARB kills animals on dietary salt restriction; addition of salt reverses the course [15].

Angiotensin is only an assistant of salt in maintaining the balance of body fluid and blood pressure. Thanks to the action of angiotensin, humans can survive without taking excess salt. It is only recently in history that humans discovered a taste for salt, leading to widespread hypertension.

Lifestyle modification, especially reduction of salt intake, is most important in treating hypertension. No-salt rice diet not only lowers blood pressure but also improves left ventricular hypertrophy and funduscopic findings [9]. DASH diet, which is rich in fiber and potassium and promotes natriuresis, is also recommended [16]. DASH diet combined with sodium restriction is even move effective [10,16]. Physical exercise is natriuretic by activating the renal adenosine–dopamine system [4,17,18] and antihypertensive [19].

If lifestyle modification does not achieve blood pressure goals, antihypertensive drugs may be used. Diuretics work in the same way as dietary salt restriction. Many clinical trials including ALLHAT have shown that diuretics not only lower blood pressure but also prevent hypertensive vascular complications more effectively than ACE inhibitor [20]. However, diuretics should always be given together with RAS blockers such as ACE inhibitor or ARB to prevent adverse reactions [20]. Calcium antagonists may be preferred in patients who cannot tolerate diuretics. Calcium antagonists have natriuretic action although they are weaker than diuretics [21].

References

[1] L. Hansson, The future role of losartan, J. Hum. Hypertens. 9 (1995) S55–S58.

[2] R. Collins, R. Peto, S. MacMahon, et al., Blood pressure, stroke, and coronary heart disease. Parts, short-term reductions in blood pressure: overview of randomized drug trials in their epidemiological context, Lancet 335 (1990) 827–838.

[3] A.V. Chobanian, G.L. Bakris, H.R. Black, et al., The seventh report of the Joint National Committee on prevention, detection, evaluation, and treatment of high blood pressure. The JNC 7 report, JAMA 289 (2003) 2560–2572.

[4] K. Arakawa, Let us return to a more natural lifestyle, Curr. Hypertens. Rep. 1 (1999) 363–364.

[5] G. Pickering, High Blood Pressure, J. & A. Churchill, London, 1968.

[6] X. Jeunemaitre, F. Soubreir, Y.V. Kotelevstev, et al., Molecular basis of human hypertension: role of angiotensinogen, Cell 71 (1992) 169–180.

[7] R.S. Cooper, C.N. Rotini, R. Ward, The puzzle of hypertension in African-Americans, Sci. Am. 280 (1999) 56–63.

[8] L. Ambard, E. Beaujurd, Causes de l'hypertension arterielle, Arch. Gén. Med. 1 (1904) 520–533.

[9] W. Kempner, Treatment of hypertensive vascular disease with rice diet, Am. J. Med. 4 (1948) 545–577.

[10] F.M. Sacks, L.P. Svetkey, W.M. Vollmer, et al., Effects on blood pressure of reduced dietary salt and the Dietary Approaches to Stop Hypertension (DASH), NEJM 344 (2001) 3–10.

[11] G. Cailar, J. Ribstein, A. Mimran, Dietary sodium and target organ damage in essential hypertension, Am. J. Hypertens. 15 (2002) 222–229.

[12] V. Dzau, E. Braunwald, Resolved and unresolved issues in the prevention and treatment of coronary artery disease: a workshop consensus statement, Am. Heart J. 121 (1991) 1244–1263.

[13] W.J. Oliver, E.L. Cohen, J.V. Neel, et al., Blood pressure, sodium intake, and sodium related hormones in the Yanomamo Indians, a "no-salt" culture, Circulation 52 (1975) 146–151.

[14] M. Imagawa, H. Kamei, K. Arakawa, High renin low blood pressure and its treatment with calcium glycyrrhetinyl-glycinate, Jpn. Heart J. 23 (1982) 201–209.

[15] C.D. Griffiths, T.O. Morgan, L.M. Delbridge, Effects of combined administration of ACE inhibitor and angiotensin II receptor antagonist are prevented by a high NaCl intake, J. Hypertens. 19 (2001) 2087–2095.

[16] S. Akita, F.M. Sacks, L.P. Svetkey, et al., Effects of the Dietary Approaches to Stop Hypertension (DASH) diet on the pressure–natriuresis relationship, Hypertension 42 (2003) 8–13.

[17] T. Takezako, K. Noda, E. Tsuji, et al., Adenosine activates aromatic L-amino acid decarboxylase activity in the kidney and increases dopamine, J. Am. Soc. Nephrol. 12 (2001) 29–36.

[18] K. Arakawa, Mild physical exercise may activate the adenosine–dopamine system: a new natriuretic mechanism, Curr. Hypertens. Rep. 4 (2002) 1–2.

[19] K. Arakawa, Antihypertensive mechanism of exercise, J. Hypertens. 11 (1993) 223–229.

[20] The ALLHAT Officers and Coordinators for ALLHAT Collaboration Research Group, The Antihypertensive and Lipid-lowering Treatment to Prevent Heart Attack Trial (ALLHAT). Major outcomes in high-risk hypertensive patients randomized to angiotensin-converting enzyme inhibitor or calcium channel blockers vs. diuretic, JAMA 288 (2002) 2981–2997.

[21] G. Licata, R. Scaglione, A. Ganguzza, et al., Effects of amlodipine on renal haemodynamics in mild to moderate hypertensive patients. A randomized controlled study versus placebo, Eur. J. Clin. Pharmacol. 45 (1993) 307–311.

ELSEVIER

International Congress Series 1262 (2004) 597–602

www.ics-elsevier.com

Possible molecular mechanisms regulating endothelial repair in unstable fibroinflammatory atheroma

Joanne S.Y. Lee, Brendan Dickson, Avrum I. Gotlieb*

Department of Pathology, Toronto General Research Institute, University Health Network, Toronto, ON, Canada
Department of Laboratory Medicine and Pathobiology, University of Toronto, Toronto ON, Canada

Abstract. Endothelial repair is essential in preventing or limiting fibroinflammatory atheroma formation and growth as well as limiting the complications of erosion, fissure formation, and rupture from occurring. The integrity of the endothelium depends to a large extent on the integrity of the cytoskeleton in the cell. It is likely that the repair of the integrity of the endothelium will depend, at least in part, on the ability of the endothelial cell (EC) to regulate patterns of interaction between cytoskeletal networks, especially microfilaments (MFs) and microtubules (MTs). A well-integrated cytoskeleton is believed to be required for efficient cell spreading, cell migration, and cell proliferation—the essential processes for endothelial repair. Thus, the endothelial cytoskeleton is indeed a potential treatment target for the prevention and treatment of atherosclerotic disease at the endothelial level. © 2004 Published by Elsevier B.V.

Keywords: Atherosclerosis; Endothelial repair; Actin; Microtubules; Plaque rupture

1. Introduction

The fibroinflammatory atheroma is considered to be a vulnerable atherosclerotic plaque, and thus an important precursor to advanced atherosclerotic lesions [1]. This lesion is characterized by a fibrous cap superimposed on a core of necrotic debris containing lipids and inflammatory cells. As the fibrous cap develops, there is an increase in the amount of smooth muscle cells (SMC) and matrix comprising the lesion. The endothelial cell (EC) layer interfacing with the blood stream is thought to lack normal physiological function and structural integrity. Macrophages, foam cells, T cells, mast cells, and neovascularization are present in the fibrous cap and around the necrotic core [2]. The fibrous cap, the inflammatory infiltrate and the necrotic core may all, either singly or synergistically, influence the

* Corresponding author. Department of Laboratory Medicine and Pathobiology, Banting Institute, University of Toronto, 100 College Street, Room 110, Toronto, ON, Canada M5G 1L5. Tel.: +1-416-978-2557; fax: +1-416-971-2130.

E-mail address: avrum.gotlieb@utoronto.ca (A.I. Gotlieb).

0531-5131/ © 2004 Published by Elsevier B.V.
doi:10.1016/j.ics.2004.01.097

evolution of the fibroinflammatory atheroma into an unstable atherosclerotic lesion characterized by erosion, fissure, or rupture, which in turn may result in an acute coronary syndrome (ACS). The loss of structural integrity of the intact endothelial monolayer and the failure of the endothelium to maintain one or more of its normal physiologic functions are thought to be exacerbated by the inability of the endothelium to restore integrity and function through physiologic repair processes. Thus, injury and failure to repair lead to atheroma initiation and growth. Loss of integrity occurs in both frank denudation of EC and also when cell–cell junctions are disrupted and gaps form between cells. Frank denudation, although unlikely to be the cause of the initial lesions, is seen on the surface of fibroinflammatory atheromas, resulting in ulceration and fissure formation which may promote thrombosis in the vessel lumen and/or rupture of the atheroma through the fibrous cap. Unfortunately, endothelial denudation also occurs following interventional treatments of coronary artery atherosclerosis such as angioplasty, stenting, atherectomy, and saphenous vein by-pass grafting and is thus implicated in the serious complications of acute thrombosis, restenosis, and vein graft atherosclerosis [2]. Thus, once denudation has occurred, understanding how the vascular endothelium repairs itself in a rapid and efficient manner is important in limiting vascular disease and improving responses to treatment.

2. Actin microfilaments and endothelial integrity and repair

Actin microfilaments (MFs) are essential in maintaining the structural integrity of the endothelium [3] through association with cell-substratum and cell–cell adhesion complexes. ECs in confluent monolayers contain both a dense peripheral band of actin MF bundles and central MF or ‘stress fibers’ [3]. Dense peripheral bands are important in cell–cell adhesion while stress fibers are contractile and serve to develop strong substrate anchorage in association with both classical focal adhesion complexes and motile fibrillar adhesions [4]. MFs are also present in the lamellipodia and filopodia at the cell periphery and are required for cell spreading and motility.

F-actin continuously polymerizes and depolymerizes within the cell [5]. Two chains of spherical G-actin monomers wind around each other to form a 7 nm helix of filamentous actin or F-actin. Each actin subunit has defined polarity and one end (plus end) assembles faster than the other (minus end). ATP-dependent formation of these actin filament arrays is regulated by members of the Ras-homologous (Rho) family of small GTPases. Three important regulatory proteins that act on the Rho family are guanine nucleotide dissociation inhibitors (GDIs), guanine nucleotide exchange factors (GEFs) and GTPase activating proteins (GAPs). GDIs slow the rate of GDP dissociation from the GTPase, GEFs activate Rho GTPases by enhancing the exchange of GDP for GTP, and GAPs stimulate GTPase activity. GEF-H1 has been shown to mediate cross-talk between microtubules (MTs) and actin-MFs in HeLa cells [6] and may be responsible for regulating Rho activity in response to MT depolymerization. The classical function of the three isoforms of Rho, RhoA, B, and C is to regulate stress fiber formation whereas lamellipodia and filopodia formation are regulated by Rac and Cdc42, respectively. These three proteins also regulate the assembly of integrin-containing focal adhesion complexes which promotes cell–matrix interactions [7]. Rho proteins also enhance endothelial barrier dysfunction by inhibition of myosin phosphatase, thus disrupting actin myosin interactions at the EC periphery via Ca^{2+}/calmodulin-dependent activation of myosin light chain kinase (MLCK) [8] and by regulation of adherens junctions. RhoA/Rho kinase is also important in vascular SMC migration and intimal thickening [9].

There are numerous actin-binding proteins which regulate the structure and function of F-actin including myosin, vinculin, α-actinin, filamin, cofilin, severin, to name a few. They function as bundling or severing proteins, and in polymerization and depolymerization of MFs. For example, myosins are a large family of molecular motor proteins that are actin-based. An individual myosin converts energy derived from ATP hydrolysis into unidirectional movement towards one specified end of the MF. The action of the myosin motor is important in pushing the leading lamellipodia at the front of the cell. The motor may also promote the flow of actin toward the cell center and away from the leading edge to regulate cell migration. ARP 2/3, another actin-binding protein, is important in actin nucleation. The Arp 2/3 complex consists of seven polypeptides and is associated with regions of actin motility and dynamic assembly [5]. In directed cell migration, p120 Ras–GAP helps in polarizing cells by regulating the reorientation of actin stress fibers and focal adhesion sites [10].

Following wounding, EC in monolayer culture undergo three sequential stages of MF remodeling to become activated migrating cells [11]. Following injury, EC at the wound edge enter stage I (0–2 h) of early repair. This is characterized by the disruption of dense peripheral bands, partial detachment of cells from their neighbors at the wound edge, and spreading by lamellipodia extension into the wound. Lamellipodia protrusion in wound edge cells is driven by a Rac-regulated dendritic array of MFs [12]. The cells then enter stage II (2–4 h), which is characterized by central MF organized in an orientation parallel to the wound edge. The EC spread laterally as well. EC then enter stage III (6–8 h), which is characterized by the redistribution of central MFs to a perpendicular orientation relative to the wound edge and by the initiation of cell migration into the wound. The perpendicular stress fibers are likely important in the transmission of forces generated by actin contractility inside the cell to the matrix outside the cell by means of dissolution and formation of cell substrate adhesion sites. The mechanisms that regulate this reorientation of the MF from parallel to perpendicular are not known.

The monolayer becomes reestablished over time by continued migration and proliferation of EC. There are several factors which have been identified as promoting or inhibiting endothelial repair. The promoters include basic fibroblast growth factor (bFGF) [13], insulinlike growth factor (IGF)-1 [14], glucose [15], nitric oxide (NO) [16], thrombin [17], and vascular endothelial growth factor (VEGF) [18]. Some of the inhibitors of endothelial repair are infection [19], low shear stress [20], NO [21], oxidized LDL [18], smoking [22], transforming growth factor (TGF)-β [23], and thrombin [24]. We have also shown that FGF-2 is an important factor in promoting effective rapid repair. Although different patterns of MF organization appear, the dynamics of MF polymerization and depolymerization, which regulate the reorganization of EC MF spatial structure, have yet to be defined. New methods are available to visualize cytoskeletal dynamics in living cells that may answer some of these questions. Molecular candidates to study include changes in the Rho GTPases, integrins, and associated matrix binding, actin-binding proteins, focal adhesion complexes, and the influence of the other major cytoskeletal system involved in repair, the MT cytoskeleton. Tyrosine phosphorylation of adhesion proteins, such as paxillin, may be important in regulating actin and focal adhesion reorganization during repair [25].

3. Microtubules and endothelial integrity and repair

MTs play a role in maintaining cell shape and directional migration of ECs [3,26]. MTs are formed by self-assembly of alpha–beta ($\alpha\beta$) tubulin heterodimers. They shorten by addition and removal of tubulin subunits from their ends. The faster growing end is the plus end and has a β tubulin exposed while the slower end or the minus end has an α tubulin exposed. The plus ends exhibit dynamic instability, alternating between phases of growing and shrinking [27]. Minus ends are frequently located at a single site in the cell called the MT organizing center [28]. Many proteins bind to tubulin and regulate MT dynamics [29,30].

MTs are essential for regulating EC migration. We showed that ECs at the edge of a wounded monolayer reposition their centrosome to a position between the cell nucleus and the leading edge of the cell [3,26]. Failure to reposition their centrosome leads to impaired EC migration at wound edges and markedly delays repair of the endothelial monolayer [26]. We have shown that FGF-2 released from EC promote centrosome redistribution and enhance EC migration [13]. Cdc 42, dynein, and dynactin regulate MT organizing center reorientation independent of Rho-regulated MT stabilization [31]. Disruption of actin MFs resulted in a long delay in the reorientation of centrosomes in cells at the wound edge [26], suggesting that cooperation between cytoskeletal networks is important. In the presence of normal hemodynamic shear stress, distribution of MTs and centrosomes are similar in vivo and in vitro. Upon reduction in shear forces, there is loss of cell polarity, disruption of interendothelial adhesion, and significant slowing of repair of an in vivo endothelial denuded wound [20]. Thus, low shear disrupts and delays wound repair, allowing the thrombogenic subendothelial matrix to be exposed for longer times to the circulation. This may be one mechanism by which low shear acts as a risk factor for atherosclerotic plaque formation.

4. Microtubule–actin microfilament interaction

MT growth and shortening have been shown to activate Rac1 and RhoA signaling, respectively, which then regulate actin MF structure and function [8]. RhoA activity itself may in turn regulate MT dynamics by inducing the formation of a subset of stabilized MTs [27,32]. Inhibitors of RhoA have recently been shown to block MT-depolymerization-induced formation of stress fibers, focal adhesions, and clustering of integrins by fibronectin [27]. Furthermore, MT breakdown has been shown to stimulate stress fiber formation accompanied by the assembly of focal adhesions and FAK tyrosine phosphorylation [27,32]. Rho regulates centrosome redistribution in addition to central MF remodeling during the early stages of repair. FGF-2 regulates centrosome distribution, at least in part, by a Rho-independent pathway while FGF-2 promotes actin MF remodeling through a downstream Rho-dependent pathway [33]. Wittmann [34] and Waterman-Storer (2001) explore the interplay of MT, actin, and Rho GTPase signalling in cell polarization and motility and suggest that MT may be part of a positive feedback mechanism that regulates the stable polarization of a directionally migrating cell.

5. Microtubule–actin microfilament cross-linking

It is likely that MT–MF structural and/or functional interactions are essential for the effective function of the endothelial cytoskeleton. There are many examples in the literature where coordination and physical interaction between the actin and MT cytoskeleton systems seems to occur either through bifunctional linker proteins or through a series of protein–protein interactions that form a physical bridge between MTs and MFs. These include the MT interacting protein (Mip)-90 [35], coronin1p (Crn1p) [36], D-CLIP-190 [37], CLIP-associated proteins (CLASPs) [38], plakins [39], a receptor for hyaluronic acid-mediated motility/intracellular hyaluronic acid-binding protein (RHAMM/IHABP) [40], p21-activated kinase (PAK) [41], MT-associated protein-2c (MAP2c) [42], and mDia (mDiaphenous) [43,44].

Acknowledgements

JSYLee received a Heart and Stroke Richard Lewar Centre of Excellence/Ontario Graduate Scholarship in Science and Technology and a Heart and Stroke Foundation of Canada Doctoral Research Award. The work was supported by a Medical Research Council of Canada grant.

References

[1] B.C. Dickson, et al., Cardiovasc. Pathol. 12 (2003) 237–248.
[2] A.I. Gotlieb, et al., in: M.D. Silver, A.I. Gotlieb, F.J. Schoen (Eds.), Atherosclerosis: Pathology and Pathogenesis in Cardiovascular Pathology, Churchill Livingstone, New York, 2001, pp. 68–106.
[3] M.K.K. Wong, et al., J. Cell Biol. 107 (1988) 1777–1783.
[4] R. Pankov, et al., J. Cell Biol. 148 (2000) 1075–1090.
[5] J. Condeelis, Trends Cell Biol. 11 (2001) 288–293.
[6] M. Krendel, et al., Nat. Cell Biol. 4 (2002) 294–301.
[7] V.M.M. Braga, et al., Mol. Biol. Cell 10 (1999) 9–22.
[8] V.W.M. Van Hinsbergh, Arterioscler. Thromb. Vasc. Biol. 17 (1997) 1018–1023.
[9] Y. Eto, et al., Am. J. Physiol. 278 (2000) H1744–H1750.
[10] S.V. Kulkarni, et al., J. Cell Biol. 149 (2000) 457–470.
[11] T.-Y.J. Lee, et al., J. Vasc. Res. 33 (1996) 13–24.
[12] C.M. Waterman-Storer, et al., Nat. Cell Biol. 1 (1999) 45–50.
[13] D.S. Ettenson, et al., Arterioscler. Thromb. Vasc. Biol. 15 (1995) 515–521.
[14] W.R. Taylor, et al., Am. J. Physiol. 265 (3 Pt. 1) (1993) C801–C805.
[15] J. Nakao-Hayashi, et al., Atherosclerosis 92 (1992) 141–149.
[16] J.P. Guo, et al., Am. J. Physiol. 269 (1995) H1122–H1131.
[17] S. Bassus, et al., Arterioscler. Thromb. Vasc. Biol. 21 (2001) 1550–1555.
[18] E. Chavakis, et al., Circulation 103 (2001) 2102–2107.
[19] M. Aepfelbacher, et al., Arterioscler. Thromb. Vasc. Biol. 17 (1997) 1623–1629.
[20] S. Vyalov, et al., Am. J. Pathol. 149 (1996) 2107–2118.
[21] P.V. Gade, et al., J. Vasc. Surg. 26 (2) (1997) 319–326.
[22] R.M. Snajdar, et al., J. Surg. Res. 96 (1) (2001) 10–16.
[23] R.L. Heimark, et al., Science 233 (4768) (1986) 1078–1080.
[24] P.J. DiMuzio, et al., J. Vasc. Surg. 20 (4) (1994) 621–628.
[25] T.-Y.J. Lee, et al., Cell Tissue Res. 297 (1999) 435–450.
[26] D.S. Ettenson, et al., Arterioscler. Thromb. 13 (1993) 1270–1281.
[27] C.M. Waterman-Storer, et al., Curr. Opin. Cell Biol. 11 (1999) 61–67.
[28] L. Cassimeris, Curr. Opin. Cell Biol. 11 (1999) 134–141.

[29] C.E. Walczak, Curr. Opin. Cell Biol. 12 (2000) 52–56.
[30] K. Kinoshita, et al., Trends Cell Biol. 12 (2002) 267–273.
[31] A.F. Palazzo, et al., Nat. Cell Biol. 3 (2001) 723–729.
[32] G.G. Gundersen, et al., Curr. Opin. Cell Biol. 11 (1999) 81–94.
[33] T.-Y.J. Lee, et al., J. Vasc. Surg. 35 (2002) 1242–1252.
[34] T. Wittmann, et al., J. Cell Sci., Suppl. 114 (2001) 3795–3803.
[35] M. Gonzalez, et al., Exp. Cell Res. 239 (1998) 243–253.
[36] B.L. Goode, et al., J. Cell Biol. 144 (1999) 83–98.
[37] V.A. Lantz, et al., J. Cell Biol. 140 (1998) 897–910.
[38] A. Akhmanova, et al., Cell 104 (2001) 923–935.
[39] I. Karakesisoglou, et al., J. Cell Biol. 149 (2000) 195–208.
[40] V. Assmann, et al., J. Cell Sci., Suppl. 112 (1999) 3943–3954.
[41] J. Cau, et al., J. Cell Biol. 155 (2001) 1029–1042.
[42] C.C. Cunningham, et al., J. Cell Biol. 136 (1997) 845–857.
[43] T. Ishizaki, et al., Nat. Cell Biol. 3 (2001) 8–14.
[44] A.F. Palazzo, et al., Curr. Biol. 11 (2001) 1536–1541.

International Congress Series 1262 (2004) 603–606
www.ics-elsevier.com

Use of plasma markers as indices of sterol metabolism

Gilbert R. Thompson*

Metabolic Medicine, Division of Investigative Science, Faculty of Medicine, Imperial College, Hammersmith Hospital, Du Cane Road, London W12 0HS, UK

Abstract. Plasma markers of sterol metabolism provide a means of assessing the synthesis of cholesterol and bile acids and the absorption of cholesterol and plant sterols. Synthetic markers are products of the rate-limiting enzymes HMG CoA reductase and cholesterol 7α-hydroxylase, whereas absorptive markers are usually exogenous, exemplified by plant sterols. Markers of cholesterol synthesis include plasma levels of mevalonic acid (MVA) and lathosterol. We have measured both in order to investigate pathophysiological influences on cholesterol synthesis and to monitor the effects of lipid-lowering interventions, such as LDL apheresis and statins. Plasma levels of plant sterols provide a surrogate marker of cholesterol absorption but also reflect other influences including the plant sterol content of the diet and therapeutic interventions, such as plant stanols, statins and ezetimibe. Plasma levels of 7α-hydroxycholestenone, the product once removed of cholesterol 7α-hydroxylase, reflect rates of bile acid synthesis. We have used this marker to monitor the effects of statin therapy on the latter and of feeding plant sterols and stanols. © 2003 Published by Elsevier B.V.

Keywords: Mevalonic acid; Lathosterol; Sitosterol; Campesterol; 7α-Hydroxycholestenone

Although not as quantitative as isotopic turnover studies or faecal excretion of sterols, plasma markers have the advantages of simplicity and convenience and can detect short-term changes in sterol absorption and synthesis. All have been validated against classical methods of measuring cholesterol and bile acid turnover under steady-state conditions. Synthetic markers are endogenous products of the rate-limiting enzymes HMG CoA reductase and cholesterol 7α-hydroxylase, whereas absorptive markers are usually exogenous, in this instance plant sterols.

1. Cholesterol synthesis

Plasma levels of mevalonic acid (MVA) and lathosterol, or better the lathosterol/cholesterol ratio, are both well-validated markers of cholesterol synthesis. We have used

* Tel./fax: +44-20-8383-2322.
E-mail address: g.thompson@imperial.ac.uk (G.R. Thompson).

0531-5131/ © 2003 Published by Elsevier B.V.
doi:10.1016/j.ics.2003.11.018

GC-MS to assay MVA in plasma and urine [1] and capillary column GC to assay lathosterol in plasma. We showed an excellent correlation between changes in MVA concentrations and lathosterol/cholesterol ratios in patients 24 h after LDL apheresis [2]. Acutely reducing the LDL cholesterol level below 1.8 and 2.3 mmol/l resulted in an increase in cholesterol synthesis in control subjects [3], and patients on statins [2], but chronic LDL apheresis synthesis did not increase synthesis in the long term.

Using stable isotopes and the measurement of MVA, a direct correlation was demonstrated between VLDL apoB secretion and cholesterol synthesis in normal subjects [4]. Inhibition of cholesterol synthesis by simvastatin resulted in a corresponding decrease in apoB secretion [5]. Changes in MVA and the lathosterol/cholesterol ratio were shown to precede changes in LDL cholesterol during short-term administration of simvastatin [6].

By monitoring plasma and urinary MVA levels for 24 h after single 40 mg doses, it could be shown that atorvastatin exerted a more prolonged inhibition of HMG CoA reductase than did simvastatin, which accounted for the former's greater LDL-lowering efficacy [7].

In a study of patients with homozygous familial hypercholesterolaemia (FH) undergoing LDL apheresis, treatment with atorvastatin (80 mg daily) resulted in well-correlated decreases in both LDL cholesterol and MVA [8]. Kinetic analysis of the post-apheresis rebound in LDL cholesterol suggested that the decrease in LDL was due to decreased production.

An investigation of the variable response of patients with heterozygous FH to statin therapy showed that poor responders had lower baseline levels of MVA and a smaller decrease in MVA on statins than did good responders [9]. This suggests that HMG CoA reductase is downregulated in poor, compared with good, responders and less susceptible to pharmacological inhibition.

2. Cholesterol absorption

Plasma levels of plant sterols are surrogate markers of cholesterol absorption [10]. However, they are non-specific in that they are influenced by other factors such as the plant sterol content of the diet and therapeutic interventions such as ezetimibe.

Plant sterols can be conveniently measured by GC and, like lathosterol, are best expressed as ratios to cholesterol. As well as correlating positively with cholesterol absorption efficiency, plasma sitosterol and campesterol correlate inversely with the rate of cholesterol synthesis [10]. Hence, subjects who absorb cholesterol efficiently have low rates of cholesterol synthesis.

Using these markers it has been shown that cholesterol absorption is less efficient and cholesterol synthesis is higher in obese than in non-obese subjects [11]. VLDL apoB secretion was inversely correlated with cholesterol absorption, which, in turn, was inversely correlated with cholesterol synthesis. However, it remains to be shown whether decreased absorption of cholesterol upregulates cholesterol synthesis in obese subjects or vice versa.

The influence of dietary and other influences on plasma plant sterol levels is exemplified by the effects of feeding plant sterol or stanol esters to control subjects and patients with FH on statins (O'Neill FH, Brynes A, Mandeno R, Rendell N, Taylor G,

Seed M, Thompson GR, Comparison of the effects of dietary plant sterol and stanol esters on lipid metabolism, submitted for publication). Rises in plasma plant sterols during plant sterol ester feeding were especially marked in FH patients on statin therapy, which itself causes levels to rise [12], whereas plant stanols reduced them.

3. Bile acid synthesis

Plasma levels of 7α-hydroxycholestenone (7α OHC), the product once removed of cholesterol 7α-hydroxylase, is a proven marker of bile acid synthesis.

The original method of assay [13] was recently simplified and improved [14]. Using this approach, it has been shown in FH patients off and on cholestyramine and in those with partial ileal bypass that statin therapy decreased bile acid synthesis only if the latter had been previously upregulated [15]. In the study previously alluded to (O'Neill et al. Comparison of the effects of dietary plant sterol and stanol esters on lipid metabolism, submitted for publication), it was observed that the LDL-lowering effect of plant sterol ester was no longer significant after 2 months. Measurement of plasma 7α-OHC showed a significant decrease in those on plant sterol esters, especially in FH patients on statins. This implies that feeding plant sterols downregulates bile acid synthesis and thereby attenuates their cholesterol-lowering efficacy.

Acknowledgements

This review reflects the work and collaboration of many individuals, especially D. Chan and G. Watts (Australia), M. Pfohl (Germany), A. Sussekov (Russia), D. Marais and F. O'Neill (South Africa) and R. Naoumova, M. Seed and G. Taylor (UK).

References

[1] A. Scoppola, V.M.G. Maher, G.R. Thompson, N.B. Rendell, G.W. Taylor, Quantitation of plasma mevalonic acid using gas chromatography–electron capture mass spectrometry, J. Lipid Res. 32 (1991) 1057–1060.

[2] M. Pfohl, R.P. Naoumova, C. Klass, W. Knisel, B. Jakober, T. Risler, G.R. Thompson, Acute and chronic effects on cholesterol biosynthesis of LDL-apheresis with or without concomitant HMG-CoA reductase inhibitor therapy, J. Lipid Res. 35 (1994) 1946–1955.

[3] M. Pfohl, R.P. Naoumova, C. Neuwirth, A. Sussekov, J. Smykowski, N.B. Rendell, C.W. Taylor, F.J. Seif, G.R. Thompson, Upregulation of cholesterol synthesis after acute reduction of low density lipoprotein by apheresis in normocholesterolaemic subjects: evidence for a threshold effect, Atherosclerosis 135 (1997) 257–262.

[4] G.F. Watts, R. Naoumova, M.H. Cummings, A.M. Umpleby, B.M. Slavin, P.H. Sönksen, G.R. Thompson, Direct correlation between cholesterol synthesis and hepatic secretion of apolipoprotein B-100 in normlipidaemic subjects, Metabolism 44 (1995) 1052–1057.

[5] G.F. Watts, R.P. Naoumova, J.M. Kelly, F.M. Riches, K.D. Croft, G.R. Thompson, Inhibition of cholesterogenesis decreases hepatic secretion of apolipoprotein B-100 in normolipidaemic subjects, Am. J. Physiol. 273 (1997) E462–E470 (Endocrinol. Metab. 36).

[6] M. Pfohl, R.P. Naoumova, K.-D. Kim, G.R. Thompson, Use of cholesterol precursors to assess changes in cholesterol synthesis under non-steady-state conditions, Eur. J. Clin. Investig. 28 (1998) 491–496.

[7] R.P. Naoumova, S. Dunn, L. Rallidis, O. Abu-Muhana, C. Neuwirth, C. Rendell, N.B. Rendell, G.W. Taylor, G.R. Thompson, Prolonged inhibition of cholesterol synthesis explains the efficacy of atorvastatin, J. Lipid Res. 38 (1997) 1496–1500.

[8] A.D. Marais, R.P. Naoumova, J.C. Firth, C. Penny, C.K.Y. Neuwirth, G.R. Thompson, Decreased produc-

tion of low density lipoprotein production by atorvastatin after apheresis in homozygous familial hypercholesterolaemia, J. Lipid Res. 38 (1997) 2071–2078.

[9] F.H. O'Neill, D.D. Patel, B.L. Knight, C.K.Y. Neuwirth, M. Bourbon, A.K. Soutar, G.W. Taylor, G.R. Thompson, R.P. Naoumova, Determinants of variable response to statin treatment in patients with refractory familial hypercholesterolemia, Arterioscler. Thromb. Vasc. Biol. 21 (2001) 832–837.

[10] T.A. Miettinen, R.S. Tilvis, Y.A. Kesaniemi, Serum plant sterols and cholesterol precursors reflect cholesterol absorption and synthesis in volunteers of a randomly selected male population, Am. J. Epidemiol. 131 (1990) 20–31.

[11] D.C. Chan, G.F. Watts, P.H.R. Barrett, F.H. O'Neill, G.R. Thompson, Plasma markers of cholesterol homeostasis and apolipoprotein B-100 kinetics in the metabolic syndrome, Obes. Res. 11 (2003) 591–596.

[12] T.A. Miettinen, T.E. Strandberg, H. Gylling, for the Finnish Investigators of the Scandinavian Simvastatin Survival Study Group, Noncholesterol sterols and cholesterol lowering by long-term simvastatin treatment in coronary patients. Relation to basal serum cholesterol, Arterioscler. Thromb. Vasc. Biol. 20 (2000) 1340–1346.

[13] M. Axelson, A. Aly, J. Sjövall, Levels of 7alpha-hydrox-4-cholesten-3-one in plasma reflect rates of bile acid synthesis in man, FEBS Lett. 239 (1988) 324–328.

[14] C. Galman, I. Arvidsson, B. Angelin, M. Rudling, Monitoring hepatic cholesterol 7alpha-hydroxylase activity by assay of the stable bile acid intermediate 7alpha-hydroxy-4-cholesten-3-one in peripheral blood, J. Lipid Res. 44 (2003) 859–865.

[15] R.P. Naoumova, F.H. O'Neill, S. Dunn, C.K.Y. Neuwirth, G.W. Taylor, M. Axelson, G.R. Thompson, Effect of inhibiting HMG-CoA reductase on 7alpha-hydroxy-4-cholesten-3-one, a marker of bile acid synthesis: contrasting findings in patients with and without prior up-regulation of the latter pathway, Eur. J. Clin. Investig. 29 (1999) 408–412.

In Memoriam

ELSEVIER

International Congress Series 1262 (2004) 609–611

www.ics-elsevier.com

In Memoriam

Donald S. Fredrickson (August 8, 1924–June 7, 2002)

Donald S. Fredrickson, MD, not only discovered the relationship between coronary heart disease and cholesterol, but also headed the National Institutes of Health. Dr. Fredrickson was born in Colorado and received his MD in 1949 from the University of Michigan. He was one of the pioneer scientists investigating the links between lipids and heart disease. Arriving at the National Institutes of Health in Bethesda in 1953 after 2 years of postdoctoral training in lipid chemistry at the Massachusetts General Hospital, he specialized in the study of plasma lipoproteins and their genetic variation in humans.

Abnormal plasma lipid profiles were characterized as one of two conditions, either as too much cholesterol (hypercholesterolemia) or as an excess of another component of lipoproteins, triglycerides (hypertriglyceridemia). Dr. Fredrickson used ultracentrifugation method and other advanced laboratory techniques, as well as clinical and hereditary data, to arrive at a more complex understanding of abnormalities in blood lipoproteins. Ultimately he classified five major types of hyperlipidemia, each of which differed in clinical signs and genetic expression.

He became Clinical Director of the National Heart Institute and Head of its Section on Molecular Diseases in 1961. He concentrated on the study of hereditary abnormalities in plasma lipoproteins, a new discipline he called "Genetic Dyslipoproteinemia". His laboratory also isolated and described several new protein components of the lipoproteins.

He wrote *The Metabolic Basis of Inherited Disease* in 1960, a textbook that became a classic and that continues in print under new editors. His "five phenotypes" became a standard question on medical examinations, and stimulated further research on lipoprotein disorders that continues today. In the 1970s, the World Health Organization adopted the system as a standard of clinical practice in diagnosing conditions linked to hyperlipidemic conditions. The system remains in use throughout the world.

The interest in lipids led Dr. Fredrickson to the discovery of two related diseases linked to the disorders in the metabolism of lipids and lipoproteins. The first of these was "Cholesterol Ester Storage Disease", the result of a deficiency of a fat-splitting enzyme called acid lipase. Another group of patients, the first of whom came from Tangier Island in the Chesapeake Bay in 1960, showed prominent deposits of cholesterol in body tissues, especially in enlarged, orange tonsils, which accumulated due to a lack of HDL. Fredrickson named this condition "Tangier Disease". He concluded that both cholesterol ester storage disease and Tangier disease were hereditary in origin.

Dr. Fredrickson was a driving force behind the establishment of the Lipid Clinics Research Program, which conducted the much-publicized Coronary Primary Prevention

doi:10.1016/j.ics.2004.02.133

Trial. This clinical trial offered conclusive evidence that reduction of cholesterol in the blood alone can prevent heart attack and death due to coronary heart disease. Moreover, the program was the first to measure lipoprotein levels in a large number of Americans of different ages and both sexes.

His research provided a scientific foundation for nutritional guidelines that emphasize the benefits of a low-fat, low-cholesterol diet. His research also established a system for classifying abnormalities in blood lipids. The scientific importance and policy implications of his findings made him the most frequently cited physiologist of the period 1961–1975, according to data from the Institute for Scientific Information. Fredrickson's discoveries about cholesterol have been turned into public policies designed to prevent diseases of the heart and vascular system.

The editors gratefully acknowledge the following websites:
1) http://profiles.nlm.nih.gov/FF/Views/Exhibit/narrative/scientist.html.
2) http://www.nlm.nih.gov/news/press_releases/fredricksonpr02.html.

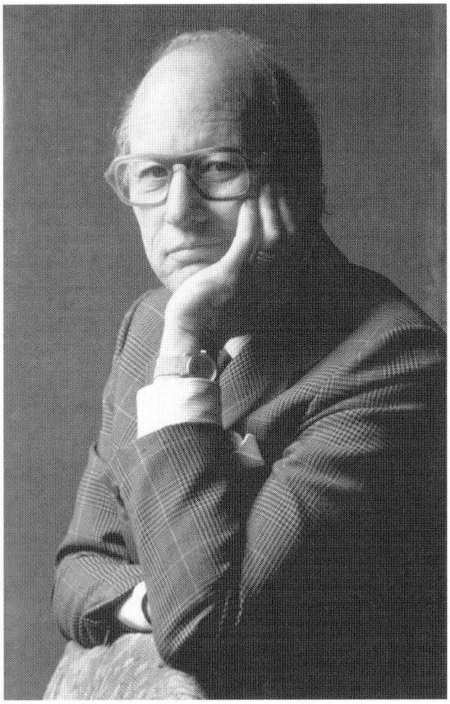

International Congress Series 1262 (2004) 612–614
www.ics-elsevier.com

In Memoriam
Yuichiro Goto (October 6, 1922–May 28, 2003)

Antonio M. Gotto Jr.

I am honored to pay tribute to Professor Yuichiro Goto, a pioneer in the field of atherosclerosis. The most fitting tribute to Professor Goto, however, is the choice of Kyoto as host city for the XIII International Symposium on Atherosclerosis (ISA), signifying Japan's world leadership in the prevention and treatment of cardiovascular disease. This is largely the result of Professor Goto's five decades as a preeminent scientist, educator, author, and public health advocate.

Although westernization of the Japanese diet after World War II led to an increase in ischemic heart disease and diabetes [1], Japan lagged behind the United States and Europe in the study of atherosclerosis. Yuichiro Goto was one of the first in Japan to understand that atherosclerosis, dyslipidemia, and lifestyle are interrelated. In addition to new drug research (most recently pitavastatin, now in development) he emphasized the role of nutrition and the creation of a healthcare system that supports the diagnosis and treatment of presymptomatic disease.

As a Rockefeller Foundation fellow from 1956–1957, Yuichiro Goto trained with Dr. James Alexander at Baylor College of Medicine in Houston, TX. Returning home, he joined the medical school faculties of Keio University and, subsequently, of Tokai University and became one of the first medical educators in Japan to specialize in lipidology.

Although I arrived at Baylor after Professor Goto's departure, our mutual experience there created a bond between us. But it was the similarity of our surnames that first brought us together. While at the 1973 ISA in Berlin, I received an invitation to attend the planning committee meeting for the next triennial symposium in Tokyo—an invitation intended for Professor Goto, the symposium co-chair. Nevertheless, I was urged to join the committee. Thus began our personal and professional relationship. Professor Goto invited me to Japan on several occasions both to lecture on atherosclerosis and to join him in conferences and patient rounds at Keio University Hospital. Everywhere I saw the great respect and admiration that he received from colleagues, students, and patients. My wife and I were honored to meet Professor Goto's lovely wife and daughter and enjoy the hospitality of their home. Subsequently, several of his superb young colleagues came to work with me in Houston. One of the first was Dr. Noriaki Nakaya, whose son, now also a physician, will soon join my colleagues and me at the Weill Cornell Medical College.

Professor Goto was active in numerous medical societies and helped found the International Task Force for Prevention of Coronary Heart Disease and the Japan

0531-5131/
doi:10.1016/j.ics.2003.12.083

Atherosclerosis Society. Also passionate about western classical music, he was the author of books on opera and on the pathographies of 17th and 18th century composers [2].

Yuichiro Goto brought an enlightened and humane perspective to all his endeavors. We had many wonderful times, and I will miss him deeply, as will all his friends and colleagues around the world.

References

[1] Y. Goto, Diseases in the Asia-Pacific region: Japan [abstract], The 5th International Symposium on Clinical Nutrition, Asia Pacific Clinical Nutrition Society Conference, February 4–7, 1996, Asia Pac. J. Clin. Nutr. (1996); 5 (4 sect 2). Available at: http://elecpress.monash.edu.au/APJCN/vol5n4s2p2.htm#v5nr2a11. Accessed August 28, 2003.

[2] Y. Goto, A Promenade to Classical Music, Episodes and Pathographies of Great Composers.

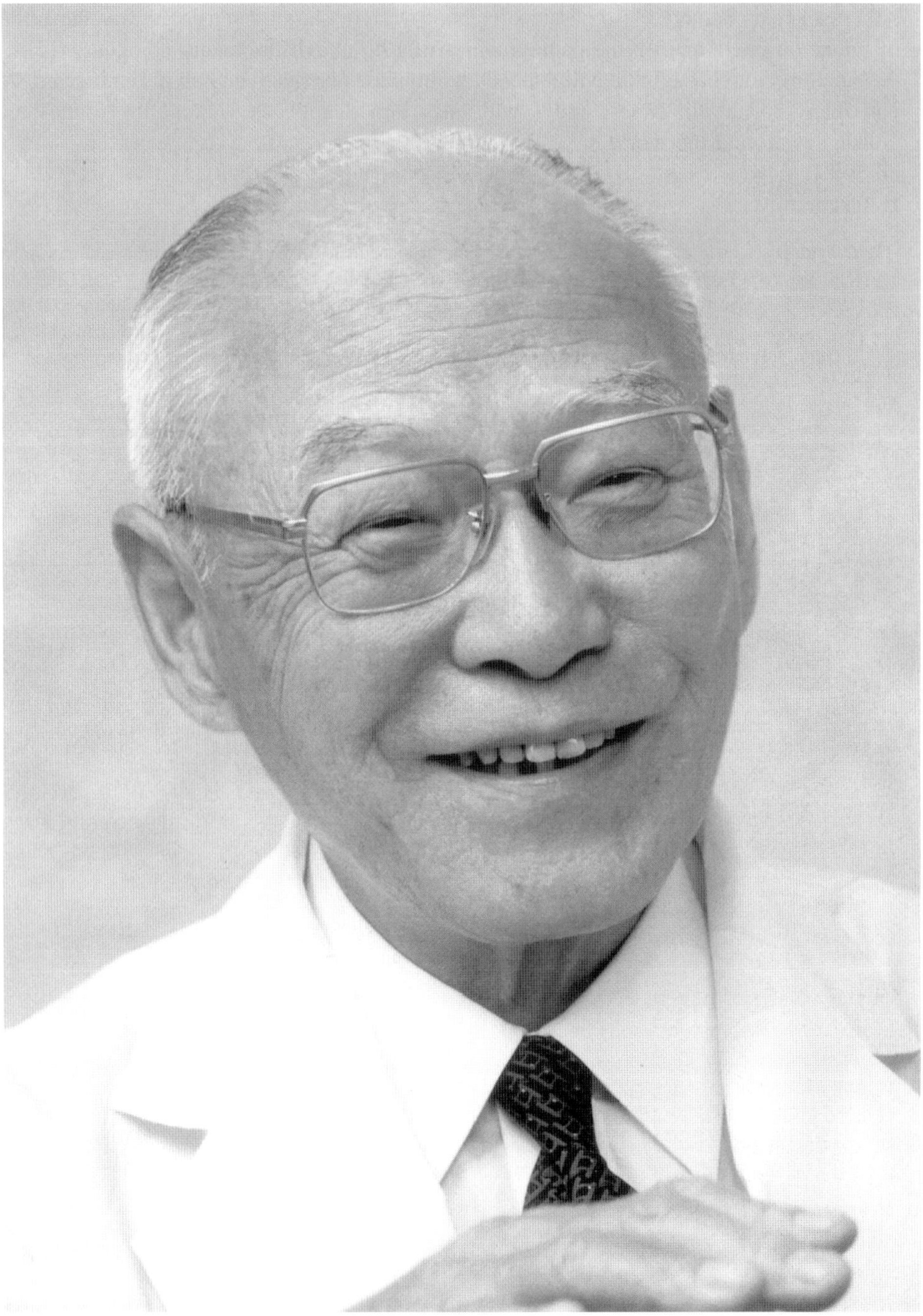

Author index

Keyword index